# Palliative Care in Hematologic Malignancies and Serious Blood Disorders

Christina K. Ullrich • Eric J. Roeland
Editors

# Palliative Care in Hematologic Malignancies and Serious Blood Disorders

## A Clinical Guide

Springer

*Editors*
Christina K. Ullrich
Harvard Medical School
Boston, MA, USA

Eric J. Roeland
Oregon Health and Science University
Portland, OR, USA

ISBN 978-3-031-38057-0 ISBN 978-3-031-38058-7 (eBook)
https://doi.org/10.1007/978-3-031-38058-7



This Springer imprint is published by the registered company Springer Nature Switzerland AG
The registered company address is: Gewerbestrasse 11, 6330 Cham, Switzerland

Paper in this product is recyclable.

# Preface

We are honored to share our colleagues' cumulative work and collective wisdom in caring for patients with hematologic malignancies, including pediatric and adult clinicians. This textbook encapsulates years of relentless effort and dedication to improving the care of patients with hematologic malignancies and their caregivers. Moreover, it demonstrates how clinicians can effectively collaborate to share their expertise to optimize our care for patients with complex medical illness. We are proud of our colleagues who agreed to contribute to this work and demonstrated the fortitude to complete it during COVID.

Emerging evidence—in conjunction with clinical experience—demonstrates that palliative care improves the well-being of seriously ill patients throughout their illness course. Through an interdisciplinary and holistic approach, palliative care improves patients' and their caregivers' physical, psychological, and spiritual distress. Moreover, palliative care promotes care aligned with patients' values and preferences by facilitating effective and compassionate communication and supporting the delineation of treatment goals and informed decision-making. Regardless of prognosis or treatment, such outcomes are relevant throughout the illness trajectory.

Individuals with hematologic malignancies and other serious blood disorders often undergo intensive therapies to find a cure. Others may experience years of chronic and debilitating illness. Both populations often face high uncertainty about the future, intense symptom burden, and impaired function and quality of life. Holistic care of individuals with hematologic malignancies and serious hematologic disorders is challenged by high prognostic uncertainty, wide-ranging ramifications of serious illness, and, at times, a focus on cure and disease-directed care. For example, stem cell and chimeric antigen receptor T cell (CAR-T) therapies now offer the possibility of a cure, even for individuals with advanced blood cancers. In addition, patients with nonmalignant blood disorders experience unmet palliative needs, such as uncontrolled pain among those with sickle cell disease and joint deformity among patients with hemophilia.

Once thought to be the antithesis of hematologic/oncologic care, a palliative care approach, in fact, complements disease-directed therapies by attending to the multidimensional needs of patients and caregivers. While evidence and recognition of the benefit of palliative care in this population are mounting, important clinical and research questions surrounding palliative care integration have emerged. Moreover, there are few resources, and no textbooks, dedicated to the specific needs of individuals with blood cancers and other serious hematologic disorders, highlighting their palliative care needs and best clinical approaches. Likewise, interest in this topic among hematologists is greatly increasing, as evidenced by formal educational symposia at the annual meeting of the American Society of Hematology in 2013 and again in 2015.

This textbook provides a comprehensive yet concise coverage of (1) the unique needs of patients with malignant and nonmalignant blood disorders and outlines specific strategies to optimize hematologist/hematologist-oncologist and palliative care collaboration; (2) issues salient to the provision of palliative care (e.g., communication, decision-making, advance care planning, symptom management, and ethics); (3) special populations (e.g., pediatrics, adolescents and young adults, geriatrics, and caregivers); and (4) issues on the care of patients with blood disorders at the end of life (e.g., care of the imminently dying patient). In keeping with the interdisciplinary nature of palliative care, contributing authors for each chapter represent a range of disciplines, including medicine, nursing, psychology, social work, chaplaincy, pharmacy, and physical and occupational therapists, among others.

We have designed this textbook to serve as a resource for several groups of clinicians. We envision it serving as a reference for hematology-oncology clinicians and trainees seeking to deepen their palliative care knowledge and skills while improving their understanding of the unique needs of patients with blood disorders. This text will also support and guide palliative care clinicians and trainees as they care for this population and their particular needs. Because palliative care is inherently interdisciplinary, covering an array of medical, nursing, and psychosocial topics, clinicians who will utilize this book extend beyond physicians and include advanced practice providers, nurses, social workers, psychologists, chaplains, and allied health professionals caring for this population.

Boston, MA, USA Christiana K. Ullrich
Portland, OR, USA Eric J. Roeland

# Contents

# Contributors

**Yuko Abbott, DSW, LCSW, OSW-C** Moores Cancer Center Radiation Oncology, UC San Diego Health, La Jolla, CA, USA

**Tara A. Albrecht, PhD, ACNP-BC, ACHPN, RN** School of Nursing, Duke University, Durham, NC, USA

**Sharl S. Azar, MD** Department of Medicine, Division of Hematology, Massachusetts General Hospital, Harvard Medical School, Boston, MA, USA

**Holly E. Barron, MSW, LICSW** Division of Social Work, Department of Psychosocial Oncology and Palliative Care, Dana-Farber Cancer Institute, Boston, MA, USA

**Jessica Bordley, MD** Department of Pediatrics, Oregon Health and Science University, Portland, OR, USA

**Julienne Brackett, MD, MS** Department of Pediatrics, Section of Hematology-Oncology, Baylor College of Medicine, Texas Children's Cancer Center, Houston, TX, USA

**Eduardo Bruera, MD** Department of Palliative, Rehabilitation and Integrative Medicine, University of Texas, MD Anderson Cancer Center, Houston, TX, USA

**Darcy E. Burgers, PhD** Division of Pediatric Psychosocial Oncology, Department of Psychosocial Oncology and Palliative Care, Dana-Farber Cancer Institute, Boston, MA, USA

**Heather A. Carlson, MSN, ANP-BC, ACHPN** Department of Palliative Care, Massachusetts General Hospital, Boston, MA, USA

**Melissa K. Cousino, PhD** Department of Pediatrics, C.S. Mott Children's Hospital, Ann Arbor, MI, USA

**Carlos Fernandez Cuartas, MD** Department of Palliative Medicine, Geisinger Medical Center, Danville, PA, USA

**Lysanne Daoust, MSN** Department of Pediatric Palliative Care, Sainte-Justine Hospital, Montreal, QC, Canada

**Mellar Davis, MD, FCCP, FAAHPM** Department of Palliative Care, Geisinger Medical Center, Danville, PA, USA

**Glen Digwood, DO, FACP** Department of Palliative Medicine, Geisinger Community Medical Center, Scranton, PA, USA

**J. Nicholas Dionne-Odom, PhD, RN, ACHPN** School of Nursing, University of Alabama at Birmingham, Birmingham, AL, USA

**Kristin Drouin, MSW, LICSW, APHSW-C** The Wendt Center for Loss and Healing, Washington, DC, USA

**Mallory Fossa, MSN** Department of Pain and Palliative Medicine, Connecticut Children's, Hartford, CT, USA

**George J. Francis, MD, FRCPC, CSCN (EMG)** Department of Clinical Neurosciences, Cumming School of Medicine, University of Calgary, Calgary, AB, Canada

**Emily M. Fredericks, PhD** Department of Pediatrics, C.S. Mott Children's Hospital, University of Michigan Medical School, Ann Arbor, MI, USA

**Jack B. Fu, MD** Department of Palliative, Rehabilitation and Integrative Medicine, University of Texas, MD Anderson Cancer Center, Houston, TX, USA

**Paul Galchutt, MPH, MDiv, BCC** University of Minnesota Medical Center, Minneapolis, MN, USA

**Srila Gopal, MBBS** Department of Medicine, Division of Hematology/Oncology, University of California San Diego, La Jolla, CA, USA

**Dana Guyer, MD** Division of Palliative Medicine, Warren Alpert Medical School of Brown University, Providence, RI, USA

**Elizabeth Hardesty, MSW** Department of Oncology, Children's National Medical Center, Washington, DC, USA

**Steven J. Hardy, PhD** Divisions of Hematology and Oncology, Department of Psychiatry and Behavioral Sciences, Children's National Hospital, George Washington University School of Medicine and Health Sciences, Washington, DC, USA

**Portia Howard, MDIV** Volunteer and Spiritual Care Services, University of California, San Diego Health, San Diego, CA, USA

**David Hui, MD** Department of Palliative Care, Rehabilitation and Integrative Medicine, University of Texas, MD Anderson Cancer Center, Houston, TX, USA

**Shana S. Jacobs, MD** Department of Oncology, Children's National Hospital, Washington, DC, USA

**Natalie Jewitt, MD** Paediatric Advanced Care Team (PACT), Department of Paediatrics, The Hospital for Sick Children, Toronto, Canada

**Courtney W. Johnson, MD, MS** Department of Hospitalist Medicine, Children's National Health System, Washington, DC, USA

**Joshua A. Johnson, M. Div.** Department of Spiritual Care, Carondelet St. Joseph's Hospital, Tucson, AZ, USA

**Danielle Faye Jonas, MSW** Silver School of Social Work, New York University, New York, NY, USA

**Alisha Kassam, MD, MPH** Department of Pediatric Oncology and Palliative Medicine, Southlake Regional Health Centre, Newmarket, ON, Canada

**Daniel J. Kats, MD** Department of Pediatrics, Massachusetts General Hospital, Boston, MA, USA

**Erica Carmen Kaye, MD, MPH** Hospice and Palliative Medicine Fellowship Program, Department of Oncology, St. Jude Children's Research Hospital, Memphis, TN, USA

**Allison Kestenbaum, MA, MPA, BCC, ACPE** Spiritual Care Services/Howell Palliative Care, UC San Diego Health, La Jolla, CA, USA

**Deborah A. Lafond, DNP** PANDA Education Consultants, PLLC, Lakeland, FL, USA

**Shelby Langer, PhD** Edson College of Nursing and Health Innovation, Phoenix, AZ, USA

**Kathleen A. Lee, MD** Section of Palliative Care, Division of General Medicine, Beth Israel Deaconess Medical Center, Boston, MA, USA

**Deena R. Levine, MD, FAAHPM** Department of Oncology, Division of Quality of Life and Palliative Care, St. Jude Children's Research Hospital, Memphis, TN, USA

**Nadine Linendoll, PhD, MDiv, GNP** Division of Hematology/Oncology, Department of Medicine, Institute for Clinical Research and Health Policy Studies, Tufts Medical Center, Tufts University School of Medicine, Boston, MA, USA

**Robert Macauley, MD** Department of Pediatrics, Oregon Health and Science University, Portland, OR, USA

**Kevin Madden, MD** Department of Palliative, Rehabilitation and Integrative Medicine, University of Texas, MD Anderson Cancer Center, Houston, TX, USA

**Marc-Antoine Marquis, MD, MSc, MA** Department of Pediatrics, Sainte-Justine Hospital, Montreal, QC, Canada

Department of Pediatric Palliative Care, Sainte-Justine Hospital, Montreal, QC, Canada

**Jonathan M. Marron, MD, MPH** Department of Pediatric Oncology, Dana-Farber Cancer Institute and the Harvard Medical School Center for Bioethics, Boston, MA, USA

**Samantha D. Martin, MD** Department of Pediatrics, Boston, MA, USA

**Monia Marzouki, MD** Department of Pediatrics, Sainte-Justine Hospital, Montreal, QC, Canada

**Maura A. Miglioretti, PhD** Department of Pediatrics, C.S. Mott Children's Hospital, Ann Arbor, MI, USA

**Pietro Miozzo, BS, MD** Department of Pediatrics, Massachusetts General Hospital, Mass General for Children, Boston, MA, USA

**Li Mo, MD** The Center of Gerontology and Geriatrics, National Clinical Research Center of Geriatrics, West China Hospital, Sichuan University, Chengdu, Sichuan, China

**Gopi S. Mohan, MD, PhD** Department of Pediatrics, Pediatric Critical Care, Massachusetts General Hospital, Boston, MA, USA

Division of Hematology-Oncology, Boston Children's Hospital, Boston, MA, USA

Harvard Medical School, Boston, MA, USA

Department of Pediatrics, Pediatric Critical Care, The University of Texas MD Anderson Cancer Center, Houston, TX, USA

**Jonathan Moreira, MD** Department of Medicine, Division of Hematology/Oncology, Northwestern University Feinberg School of Medicine, Chicago, IL, USA

**Shinichiro Morishita, PhD** Department of Physical Therapy, School of Health Sciences, Fukushima Medical University, Fukushima, Japan

**Sue E. Morris, PsyD** Division of Adult Psychosocial Oncology, Department of Psychosocial Oncology and Palliative Care, Dana-Farber Cancer Institute, Boston, MA, USA

**Carolyn Mulroney** Department of Medicine, University of California San Diego, La Jolla, CA, USA

**Lauren Elizabeth Nicholls, MD** Department of Palliative Care, Geisinger Community Medical Center, Scranton, PA, USA

**Oreofe O. Odejide, MD, MPH** Department of Medical Oncology, Dana-Farber Cancer Institute, Boston, MA, USA

**Judith A. Paice, PhD, RN** Division of Hematology-Oncology, Feinberg School of Medicine, Northwestern University, Chicago, IL, USA

**Susan Parsons, MD, MRP** Department of Medicine, Tufts University School of Medicine, Boston, MA, USA

Division of Hematology/Oncology, Department of Medicine, Institute for Clinical Research and Health Policy Studies, Tufts Medical Center, Boston, MA, USA

**Effie Wang Petersdorf, MD** Division of Hematology and Oncology, University of Washington, Seattle, WA, USA

Division of Translational Science and Therapeutics, Fred Hutchinson Cancer Center, Seattle, WA, USA

**Laura S. Porter, PhD** Department of Psychiatry and Behavioral Sciences, Duke University Hospital, Durham, NC, USA

**Nicholas Purol, MSW** Department of Psychosocial Oncology and Palliative Care, Boston Children's Hospital and Dana-Farber Cancer Institute, Boston, MA, USA

**Vinay Rao, DO** Division of Palliative Medicine, Yale University School of Medicine, New Haven, CT, USA

**Daniel R. Richardson, MD, MA** Department of Medicine, Division of Hematology, University of North Carolina at Chapel Hill, Chapel Hill, NC, USA

**Eric J. Roeland, MD, FAAHPM** Division of Medical Oncology, Section Palliative Care, Department of Medicine,, Knight Cancer Institute, Oregon Health and Science University,, Portland, OR, USA

**Courtney Schroeder, MD** Division of Hematology/Oncology, Department of Medicine, Tufts Medical Center, Boston, MA, USA

**Julie K. Silver, MD** Department of Physical Medicine and Rehabilitation, Harvard Medical School, Massachusetts General Hospital, Boston, MA, USA

**Jennifer M. Snaman, MD, MS** Pediatric Advanced Care Team, Department of Pediatric Oncology, Department of Psychosocial Oncology and Palliative Care, Dana-Farber Cancer Institute, Boston, MA, USA

**Angela Sousa, MSN, ANP-BC, ACHPN** Department of Palliative Care, Newton-Wellesley Hospital, Newton, MA, USA

**Angela Steineck, MD, MS** Department of Pediatrics, Seattle Children's Hospital, Seattle, WA, USA

**Sarah J. Tarquini, PhD** Department of Psychosocial Oncology and Palliative Care, Dana-Farber Cancer Institute, Boston, MA, USA

Division of Pediatric Psychosocial Oncology, Department of Psychosocial Oncology and Palliative Care, Dana-Farber Cancer Institute, Boston, MA, USA

**Kristen Uhl, PhD** Department of Psychosocial Oncology and Palliative Care, Dana-Farber Cancer Institute, Boston, MA, USA

**Christina K. Ullrich, MD, MPH, FAAHPM** Department of Psychosocial Oncology and Palliative Care, Department of Pediatric Oncology, Dana-Farber Cancer Institute, Boston, MA, USA

Division of Hematology/Oncology, Boston Children's Hospital, Boston, MA, USA

Harvard Medical School, Boston, MA, USA

**Melissa K. Uveges, PhD, MA, RN** Boston College Connell School of Nursing, Chestnut Hill, MA, USA

**Nicki Vithalani, MD** Department of Palliative Medicine, Geisinger Lewistown Hospital, Lewistown, PA, USA

**Marcia A. Winter, PhD** Department of Psychology, Virginia Commonwealth University, Richmond, VA, USA

**Lindsay Wooster-Halberg, LCSW, APHSW-C** Department of Pediatrics, Oregon Health and Science University, Portland, OR, USA

# 1 Introduction

Christina K. Ullrich and Eric J. Roeland

Hematologists/oncologists and palliative care specialists have more in common than most think. Both medical fields are intensely focused on the exceptional care of patients with advanced illness. Clinicians gravitate toward these fields driven by "a calling" to engage in medically, emotionally, and psychosocially complex care. It is challenging but rewarding work. Clinicians in both fields provide a highly individualized approach to care, one based on disease risk factors and molecular markers and the other on specific symptoms and psychosocial factors. Neither field can treat a patient in isolation without assessing the whole patient *as a person* and considering the patient's goals, resources, support, and coping. Both also rely on a multi -or interdisciplinary care model drawing on the strengths of other clinician colleagues, including nurses, social workers, pharmacists, spiritual counselors, case managers, psychologists, nutritionists, and physical therapists.

As dual-trained oncologists and palliative care specialists, we have observed a shift in the interactions between hematologists/oncologists and palliative care specialists. Hematologists/oncologists increasingly welcome palliative care clinicians as active clinical team members. The outdated view that cancer-directed therapy and palliative care are mutually exclusive and opposing approaches to care has been replaced by strong evidence supporting the early integration of palliative care, including in the curative setting [1, 2]. Moreover, as trainees continue to gain access to palliative care education and clinical training, we see a generational shift toward increasing cooperation and collaboration.

C. K. Ullrich (✉)
Department of Psychosocial Oncology and Palliative Care, Department of Pediatric Oncology, Dana-Farber Cancer Institute, Boston, MA, USA
e-mail: Christina_Ullrich@dfci.harvard.edu

E. J. Roeland
Division of Medical Oncology, Department of Medicine, Section Palliative Care, Knight Cancer Institute, Portland, OR, USA
e-mail: roeland@ohsu.edu

As we look toward the future, we foresee ongoing uncertainty. As novel therapies become increasingly more effective and their use expands, we will require innovative approaches to predict and manage toxicity while supporting patients, caregivers, and one another. In addition, with patients living longer without a cure and instead with chronic illness, we must meet their needs to live as well as possible and as long as possible. With continued treatment success, we also anticipate that prognostic uncertainty [3] will become increasingly common, and we will have to shift away from historic prognostic trajectories to managing the unknown. *In short, it will be as important as ever that palliative care be based on need, not prognosis*. More specifically, it must not be reserved for the last moments of a patient's life.

Simultaneously, our world has become increasingly more complex. The challenges of delivering cutting-edge, high-quality, individualized care to patients with hematologic malignancies and nonmalignant hematologic conditions have also become increasingly complicated. The post-COVID era has further highlighted inequities in access to medical care in patients experiencing unemployment, housing insecurity, safety concerns, mental health challenges, and substance abuse, all impacting serious illness outcomes and experiences. Similarly, hematology/oncology and palliative care clinicians also share increasingly high rates of moral distress and burnout in caring for these patients in an increasingly fragmented medical system [4–6]. Consequently, we believe there is much we can continue to learn from each other and even more we can do to support one another as we strive to deliver high-quality, comprehensive care in the context of such inequities and challenges.

The path forward is recognizing and supporting patients, caregivers, and clinicians in this uncertainty. This textbook has been structured as a resource for clinicians caring for individuals with a hematologic malignancy or nonmalignant hematologic condition, with both hematology/oncology and palliative care content. We hope this structure makes for a valuable reference for clinicians caring for patients with



C. K. Ullrich, E. J. Roeland (eds.), *Palliative Care in Hematologic Malignancies and Serious Blood Disorders*,
https://doi.org/10.1007/978-3-031-38058-7_1

hematologic malignancies and serious nonmalignant hematologic disorders while also serving as a call for continued inspiration, research, and collaboration in this critical space.

## References


1. El-Jawahri A, LeBlanc T, VanDusen H, et al. Effect of inpatient palliative care on quality of life 2 weeks after hematopoietic stem cell transplantation: a randomized clinical trial. JAMA. 2016;316(20):2094–103. https://doi.org/10.1001/jama.2016.16786.
2. El-Jawahri A, LeBlanc TW, Kavanaugh A, et al. Effectiveness of integrated palliative and oncology care for patients with acute myeloid leukemia: a randomized clinical trial. JAMA Oncol. 2020;7(2):238–45. https://doi.org/10.1001/jamaoncol.2020.6343.
3. Temel JS, Shaw AT, Greer JA. Challenge of prognostic uncertainty in the modern era of cancer therapeutics. J Clin Oncol. 2016;34(30):3605–8. https://doi.org/10.1200/JCO.2016.67.8573.
4. Neumann JL, Mau L-W, Denzen EM, et al. Hematopoietic cell transplantation multidisciplinary care teams: national survey of transplant provider burnout, moral distress and career satisfaction. Biol Blood Marrow Transplant. 2016;22(3):S29–30.
5. Neumann JL, Mau L-W, Virani S, et al. Burnout, moral distress, work–life balance, and career satisfaction among hematopoietic cell transplantation professionals. Biol Blood Marrow Transplant. 2018;24(4):849–60.
6. Dijxhoorn A-FQ, Brom L, van der Linden YM, Leget C, Raijmakers NJ. Prevalence of burnout in healthcare professionals providing palliative care and the effect of interventions to reduce symptoms: a systematic literature review. Palliat Med. 2021;35(1):6–26.

# Part I

# Hematologic Malignancies and Serious Blood Disorders

# Hematologic Malignancies

# 2

Daniel R. Richardson and Carolyn Mulroney

## Introduction

Integrated palliative care within oncology has demonstrated improved outcomes for patients with advanced solid malignancies and, more recently, for those undergoing hematopoietic cell transplantation (HCT) and induction chemotherapy for hematologic malignancies. Historically, palliative care physicians were infrequently asked to see patients with hematologic malignancies; however, it is our hope and expectation that palliative care engagement will continue to improve in the upcoming years. As oncologic hematologists caring for patients with hematologic malignancies, we desire to highlight several unique aspects of caring for patients with hematologic malignancies that may differ from those patients with solid tumors.

First, many hematologic malignancies are highly curable even when "metastatic" at diagnosis. Therefore, risk stratification and treatment intensity for these patients vary significantly from those patients with solid malignancies. There are three major categories of hematologic malignancies—leukemia, lymphoma, and myeloma. The prognosis of each varies widely by the maturity of the cell of origin. Diseases with immature cells of origin often lead to aggressive malignancies (e.g., acute myeloid leukemia [AML]) that can be treated and even cured with chemotherapy. Conversely, diseases with mature cells of origin often lead to more indolent diseases (e.g., multiple myeloma or chronic lymphocytic leukemia [CLL]) that are less aggressive and not generally curable. High-intensity chemotherapy for aggressive hematologic malignancies often results in disease response and functional improvement in many patients. This response can complicate treatment decision-making for patients as high-risk, high-reward scenarios exist, leading to very poor outcomes for patients who experience complications. HCT is perhaps the quintessential high-risk, high-reward treatment offering a chance of cure for some patients while also carrying the risk of high morbidity and mortality. High-risk, high-reward treatment paradigms require a clear understanding of patient preferences and goals. Patients may fear that expressing their preferences, including worries about treatment and its toxicity, may impact the intensity of their treatment. Therefore, having a clinical team outside the HCT team can provide a space for patients and caregivers to express these concerns. Palliative care specialists working alongside the HCT team may substantially improve the patient-centeredness of care in these instances.

Second, staging is different for hematologic malignancies than for patients with solid tumors. Diagnosis commonly involves a bone marrow biopsy where the morphology (i.e., what the cells look like under the microscope), immunophenotype (typically captured through various immunohistochemical stains or flow cytometry), and sometimes cytogenetic (i.e., karyotype abnormalities determined grossly or with fluorescent in situ hybridization [FISH]) or molecular features (i.e., specific mutations within individual genes) inform the final diagnosis. Imaging is uncommonly required for leukemia staging though lymphoma staging and treatment response rely on positron emission tomography (PET) scans. For example, imaging in multiple myeloma helps determine the extent of bony involvement, though prognosis depends mainly on treatment response.

The cell of origin, along with genetic and cytogenetic features, predicts prognosis in most cases. Mutations in specific genes (particularly within *TP53*) may carry heavy prognostic value and may allow for a targeted-treatment approach (e.g., FLT3 targeted therapy in AML). While there are well-developed risk prediction models for some hematologic malignancies involving many of the above criteria, treatment response is the most important dynamic prognostic indicator.

D. R. Richardson (✉)
Department of Medicine, Division of Hematology, University of North Carolina at Chapel Hill, Chapel Hill, NC, USA
e-mail: daniel_richardson@med.unc.edu

C. Mulroney
University of California San Diego, La Jolla, CA, USA
e-mail: camulroney@health.ucsd.edu



C. K. Ullrich, E. J. Roeland (eds.), *Palliative Care in Hematologic Malignancies and Serious Blood Disorders*,
https://doi.org/10.1007/978-3-031-38058-7_2

Primary refractory disease (i.e., a disease that does not respond to initial treatment) portends a poor prognosis. Increasingly, the depth of response to treatment, including the presence or absence of minimal residual disease (MRD), is used to determine prognosis. Older patients generally fare substantially worse than younger patients as they often harbor more high-risk molecular and cytogenetic features and often are unable to tolerate high-intensity therapies.

The most common toxicity of traditional cytotoxic chemotherapies is acute cytopenia, as would be expected. Many patients require infectious prophylaxis, hematopoietic stimulating factors (e.g., granulocyte-colony stimulating factor [GCSF]), and transfusions to complete therapy. Additionally, novel targeted agents have unique toxicities such as "differentiation syndrome," where cells rapidly differentiate and infiltrate organs outside the bone marrow, and "tumor lysis syndrome," where the rapid death of malignant cells can lead to renal and metabolic failure. The recent expansion of available therapies across hematologic malignancies (including some high-risk, high-reward therapies such as chimeric antigen receptor [CAR T]-cell therapy) has substantially increased the available options to patients. Yet, these therapies will likely complicate treatment decision-making and may expose patients to more toxicity.

Because of the potential for good outcomes, even with advanced disease, many patients are treated aggressively near the end of life. Predicting who will respond to therapy and when they will respond is challenging. Even for patients with incurable diseases, prolonged survival and treatment response is possible despite multiple relapses. Unfortunately, these factors often lead to high healthcare utilization at the end of life. Integrated palliative care may improve these outcomes, though fundamental challenges in balancing potential benefits with known risks will likely remain. As palliative care teams are increasingly involved in patient care with hematologic malignancies, these specialists must be aware of their unique clinical aspects. To facilitate an improved understanding of established clinical and prognostic factors, we have summarized critical points regarding lymphoma, leukemia, myeloma, and HCT. We hope this chapter serves as a key reference for palliative care specialists to effectively engage and support patients with hematologic malignancies along with their caregivers and the clinical team.

## Lymphoma

The World Health Organization (WHO) bases the classification of lymphomas on morphology, immunophenotype, genetics, clinical features, postulated normal cell counterpart of the cell of origin, anatomic site, and age. Treatment and prognosis for patients with lymphoma depend on an accurate diagnosis. In 2016, the WHO updated the prior classification from 2008 based on additional genetic data and clinical behavior aspects [1]. In general, on presentation with suspected lymphoma, patients should undergo an excisional biopsy of lymph nodes because fine needle aspirate and core needle biopsies are limited in providing the tissue morphology required for an accurate diagnosis. Staging studies for lymphoma include computed tomography (CT) scans and PET/CT scans. Most cases will require bone marrow aspirate and biopsy. Additional biopsies and evaluation of the central nervous system (CNS) may be necessary depending on the clinical scenario. These same studies, including repeat biopsy, are frequently necessary at the time of relapse. Molecular testing has increasing relevance in the management of lymphoma with the identification of effective targeted therapies.

### Low-Grade B-Cell Lymphoma

Low-grade mature B-cell lymphomas are generally characterized by an indolent clinical course. These entities may not require immediate treatment, and treatment decisions are based on clinical characteristics and disease burden. Treatment for these diseases is non-curative; yet, treatment can lead to extended remissions. Patients with stage I and stage II may obtain long-term cures with radiation therapy alone. The most common form of low-grade lymphoma is follicular lymphoma. The overall survival for patients with follicular lymphoma is about two decades, and the median progression-free survival after front-line therapy is approximately 7 years. Relapse of follicular lymphoma within 2 years of first-line therapy is associated with a decreased overall survival (OS) [2–4].

The International Prognostic Index in first-line follicular lymphoma (FLIPI) is the most common clinical prognostic index used for follicular lymphoma and has been correlated with overall survival, time to treatment failure from diagnosis, risk of transformation to higher grade lymphoma, and 5-year survival from first progression [5]. Identified risk parameters in this scoring include age >60 years, stage III/IV, hemoglobin <12 g/dL, lactate dehydrogenase greater than the upper limit of normal, and more than four nodal areas of involvement. Additional parameters may further improve prognostic scoring systems, including beta-2 microglobulin, bone marrow involvement, lymph node diameter, Eastern Cooperative Oncology Group (ECOG) performance score, and molecular abnormalities.

The decision to initiate therapy for follicular lymphoma and similar low-grade B-cell lymphomas is based on tumor bulk and clinical symptoms. Upfront therapy options commonly use a "watch-and-wait strategy" in low-bulk disease, single-agent rituximab, or rituximab-chemotherapy followed by rituximab maintenance therapy for 2 years. Recently, a "non-chemotherapy" option of rituximab combined with lenalidomide is an option for treatment-naïve patients [6].

Other less common indolent B-cell lymphomas include splenic marginal zone lymphoma, hairy cell leukemia, hairy cell leukemia variant, splenic B-cell lymphoma/leukemia, splenic diffuse red pulp small B-cell lymphoma, lymphoplasmacytic lymphoma, Waldenstrom macroglobulinemia, extranodal marginal zone lymphoma of mucosa-associated lymphoid tissue (MALT), and nodal marginal zone lymphoma. Each follows a similar decision-making paradigm for treatment as follicular lymphoma; however, with increasing treatment alternatives based on each patient's unique features. Newer agents identified, including BTK inhibitors, PI3K inhibitors, and antibody-drug conjugates, are increasingly incorporated into the disease's front line and later relapses. Most low-grade B-cell lymphomas will relapse in the patient's lifetime, and disease transformation and resistant disease are considerations at the time of relapse. Relapsed low-grade lymphomas may respond well to standard chemotherapy and autologous and allogeneic HCT.

Aggressive B-cell lymphomas, described below, include an extensive number of distinct entities with substantially different treatment outcomes with most requiring multiagent chemotherapy. Except for mantle cell lymphoma, treatment in these diseases is with curative intent unless the patient is frail or otherwise unable to receive chemotherapy.

### Mantle Cell Lymphoma

Mantle cell lymphoma (MCL) is an aggressive, incurable small B-cell lymphoma. Despite its aggressiveness, not all patients require initiation of treatment at first diagnosis. The decision to initiate therapy is based on the bulk and clinical characteristics. Classical MCL involves immunoglobulin heavy chain gene (IGHV)-unmutated or minimally mutated B cells that express SOX11 and typically involve nodal and extranodal sites. Acquisition of additional molecular abnormalities is associated with more aggressive forms of the disease, including the blastoid and pleomorphic MCL variants. MCL can also develop from IGHV-mutated SOX 11-negative B cells, and this frequently presents with a clinically indolent course involving the peripheral blood, bone marrow, and spleen. Sox 11-negative MCL tends to be more genetically stable for a longer period than classical MCL, but the acquisition of additional cytogenetic abnormalities and, in particular abnormalities involving TP53, leads to a much more aggressive disease. In situ mantle cell neoplasm (ISMCN), characterized by cyclin D1-positive cells in the inner mantle zones of lymphoid follicles, is frequently discovered incidentally and has a very low proliferative fraction, may be disseminated, and typically have a low rate of progression.

### Large B-Cell Lymphoma

Large B-cell lymphoma is by and large treated with curative intent at diagnosis. The most common large B-cell lymphoma is diffuse large B-cell lymphoma (DLBCL) which can be subclassified based on gene expression profiling into the germinal center (GC) versus activated B-cell (ABC) subgroups. Chromosomal alterations and clinical outcomes differ based on these subtypes. Gene expression profiling is not uniformly available, and commonly used subclassifications in clinical practice are GC and non-GC based on immunohistochemistry. The most common immunohistochemistry algorithm for subclassification is the Hans algorithm based on the expression of CD10, BCL6, and IRF4/MUM1 [7]. While the clinical outcome of ABC/non-GCB DLBCL is worse than GCB DLBCL, clinical treatment decisions cannot be uniformly based on this information.

Molecular/cytogenetic features that are important for determining treatment and outcome in DLBCL/ABC lymphoma include MYC rearrangements seen in 5–15% of DLBCL and when associated with BCL2 or BCL6 rearrangements falls into a distinct category of "double-hit" or "triple-hit" lymphoma. In addition to MYC rearrangements, protein expression in the absence of gene rearrangements may have prognostic significance. MYC protein expression >40% in association with BCL2 or BCL6 protein expression is associated with a more aggressive clinical course than standard DLBCL without molecular rearrangements or protein expression.

High-grade B-cell lymphoma (HGBL) under the current WHO classification includes all large B-cell lymphomas with MYC and BCL2 and/or BCL6 rearrangements unless they otherwise meet the criteria for follicular lymphoma or lymphoblastic lymphoma. HGBL-NOS are morphologically similar to HGBL but lack rearrangements in MYC and BCL2/BCL6 rearrangements.

Anthracycline-based chemotherapy is standard of care for the front-line treatment of large B-cell lymphomas and is curative unless a patient cannot tolerate multiagent chemotherapy. The most commonly used treatment for DLBCL and other aggressive B-cell lymphoma is R-CHOP (rituximab combined with cyclophosphamide, doxorubicin, vincristine, and prednisone). HGBL will frequently be treated with escalated regimens such as dose-adjusted R-EPOCH (rituximab, etoposide, prednisone, vincristine [Oncovin], cyclophosphamide, and doxorubicin [hydroxydaunorubicin]), R-CODOX--M/R-IVAC (rituximab, cyclophosphamide, doxorubicin, vincristine, cytarabine, methotrexate/rituximab, ifosfamide, etoposide, cytarabine), and HyperCVAD/MTX-Cytarabine (cyclophosphamide, vincristine, doxorubicin, [Adriamycin], and dexamethasone). The International prognostic score (IPI) based on PET/CT response at diagnosis and longitudinally is useful in counseling patients regarding expectations [5]. For example, the R-IPI in DLBCL is associated with treatment outcomes and reflects the disease's biological aggressiveness using available clinical markers.

### Primary DLBCL of the Central Nervous System

Primary DLBCL of the central nervous system (PCNSL) is the most common form of lymphoma involving the CNS but represents only 4% of intracranial neoplasms and 4–6% of extranodal lymphomas [8]. The vast majority (>80%) of PCNSL are of the activated B-cell subtype of DLBCL. A definitive diagnosis requires pathologic confirmation. The diagnostic procedure of choice is a stereotactic biopsy of the brain lesion, vitrectomy in the case of vitreoretinal disease, or cerebrospinal fluid (CSF) sampling. A patient may present with a wide variety of symptoms depending on the area of involvement of the CNS, including nonspecific neurocognitive abnormalities, signs of increased intracranial pressure, or neurocognitive deficits.

Hematologic oncologists use two prognostic scoring systems when evaluating patients with PCNSL: (i) the International Extranodal Lymphoma Study Group (IELSG) score [9] and (ii) the Memorial Sloan Kettering Cancer Center (MSKCC) score [10]. The IELSG score includes ECOG performance score, age, CSF protein concentration, lactate dehydrogenase serum level, and deep brain involvement to determine prognosis. Two-year survival rates correlate with the presence of 0–1, 2–3, or 4–5 adverse-risk factors and are 80%, 48%, or 15%, respectively. The MSKCC scoring system identifies three prognostic groups based on the Karnofsky performance status (KPS) and age. Age $\leq$ 50 and KPS $\geq$ 70 correlate with and median overall survival of 5.2–8.5 years. A combination of age >50 and KPS $\geq$70 correlates with median overall survival of 2.1–3.2 years. Patients with age >50 and KPS <70 demonstrate a substantially inferior median survival of 0.9–1.1 years. The median OS of patients with PCNSL in the United States doubled from 1970 to 2010 based on the Surveillance, Epidemiology, and End Results database; however, this was only seen for patients under the age of 70 [11].

Treatment for PCNSL in the modern era relies on multiagent chemotherapy regimens with agents that can achieve effective chemotherapy levels in the CNS [12]. High-dose methotrexate, high-dose cytarabine, 6-mercaptopurine, rituximab, and thiotepa are utilized in various regimens. High-dose chemotherapy followed by HCT with thiotepa may be used in first or second remission or after partial responses to treatment. Whole-brain radiation therapy (WBRT) is most commonly used in the setting of relapsed refractory disease and for patients who cannot tolerate combination chemotherapy regimens. WBRT leads to excellent initial response rates but is associated with a low overall survival of 12–18 months, limited by relapse in the CNS [13, 14]. Combinations of chemotherapy and WBRT improve survival over WBRT alone; however, this is complicated by significant neurologic toxicity [13].

The current standard for treating naïve PCNSL is multiple cycles of induction therapy with rituximab and methotrexate-based polychemotherapy, including rituximab followed by consolidation therapy. The choice of therapy is based on the patients' age, performance status, and comorbidities. In older patients who are not eligible for high-dose chemotherapy consolidation or consolidative WBRT, maintenance therapy may be considered.

The prognosis for primary refractory or relapsed PCNSL remains poor, with a median survival of 2 months without further treatment [15]. Recurrent disease occurs at a median of 10–18 months after the initial treatment, and most relapses develop within the first 2 years of diagnosis. Very late relapsed can also be seen. Patients with PCNSL frequently experience short- or long-term effects of the lymphoma and its treatment, including persistent neurologic deficits, psychomotor slowing, neurocognitive impairments, memory dysfunction, gait ataxia, behavioral changes, and incontinence associated with significant functional decline.

### EBV-Positive Diffuse Large B-Cell Lymphoma

EBV+ DLBCL is an aggressive B-cell lymphoma associated with chronic Epstein–Barr virus (EBV) infection and has a poor prognosis with standard chemotherapeutic approaches. Risk stratification is based on IPI and the Oyama score [5, 16]. The Oyama score includes age >70 years and the presence of B symptoms. CD30 by IHC is an adverse and targetable prognostic factor. Treatment is similar to DLBCL with RCHOP used widely with a low complete response and decreased OS [16].

### Primary Mediastinal (Thymic) Large B-Cell Lymphoma

Primary mediastinal (Thymic) large B-cell lymphoma (PMBL) represents about 2–3% of all NHL and 6–8%of LBCL. The median age is 36 years, and women are affected more frequently (ratio 2:1). This aggressive lymphoma presents with bulky anterior/superior mediastinal mass with 80% having stage I/II disease. Systemic symptoms occur in 20%. Patients may present with symptoms related to bulk and disease location including superior vena cava syndrome. Overall survival at 5 years is 70–85%. CD30 is expressed in approximately 80% of cases, PD-L1 and PD-L2 are positive in approximately 50–75%, and both CD30 and PD-L1/PD-L2 are targetable from a therapeutic perspective [17, 18]. It can be challenging to distinguish PMBL from DLBCL unless an adequate tissue sample is obtained. Initial therapy for curative intent includes dose-adjusted R-EPOCH with or without radiation therapy and RCHOP/radiation therapy.

### Plasmablastic Lymphoma

Plasmablastic lymphoma is a rare B-cell lymphoma representing less than 1% of DLBCL. This lymphoma is composed of immunoblastic or plasmablastic cells and is CD20-negative. EBV positivity is present in 50% to 80% of cases. This lymphoma occurs most commonly in the setting of immunodeficiency, especially human immunodeficiency virus (HIV) infection, and represents approximately 3% of HIV-related lymphoma. The median OS is 15 months.

### Human Herpesvirus-8-Positive Diffuse Large B-Cell Lymphoma

HHV8+ DLBCL is a rare disease and is one of the Human herpesvirus-8 (HHV8)/Kaposi sarcoma herpes virus-positive lymphoproliferative disorders, which also include germinotrophic lymphoproliferative disorder, multicentric Castleman disease (MCD), and primary effusion lymphoma (PEL). Approximately 50% of patients are HIV positive. This lymphoma commonly arises in a background of HHV8+ MCD in patients who are also HIV positive however can present de novo without evidence for MCD. Pathology shows sheets and confluent clusters of plasmablasts and destruction of normal lymph node architecture, and in some cases, a leukemic component may be present. Neoplastic cells are negative for EBV. Patients have an aggressive course and poor prognosis [19, 20].

### Primary Effusion Lymphoma

Primary effusion lymphoma (PEL) is a rare, aggressive B-cell lymphoma typically presenting with effusions without tumor mass, although it can present with solid variants. Reported to have near-universally associated with human herpesvirus-8 (HHV8) and can have concurrent EBV infection. Underlying immunodeficiency including HIV, increased age, and post-organ transplant immunodeficiency predispose to this lymphoma. These patients are most commonly present with symptoms related to effusions. Treatment is anthracycline based as for other high-grade lymphomas, but the prognosis is poor. Treatment of the underlying immunodeficiency is essential, if possible. The involvement of more than one body cavity is associated with OS of 4 months in comparison to 18 months in patients with only one cavity involved [21].

### Burkitt Lymphoma

Burkitt lymphoma is a rare, very aggressive lymphoma with endemic and sporadic variants. The sporadic variant occurs globally and has an increased incidence in HIV. The sporadic variant and HIV-associated form are associated with EBV in 25–40% of cases. The proliferative rate for this lymphoma is near 100%. MYC translocation is pathognomonic of the disease and is typically at 8q24. CNS disease with leptomeningeal involvement occasionally occurs at presentation. Treatment for this disease involves intensive multiagent chemotherapy with curative intent and is frequently complicated by tumor lysis syndrome due to the high-proliferative rate and bulk of disease. There is no validated prognostic score for Burkitt lymphoma. The outcome for relapsed and refractory disease is poor. Common regimens used at diagnosis are intensive multiagent regimens such as modified R-CODOX-M IVAC, reported to have 75% EFS at 3 years [22].

### T-Cell Lymphoma

T-cell lymphomas are a heterogeneous group of lymphomas that can develop within lymphoid tissues such as the spleen and lymph nodes or beyond lymphoid tissues (i.e., gastrointestinal tract, liver, nasal cavity, skin, and others). Natural killer (NK) cell shares many features with T cells and when they become cancerous, the cancer is called NK or NK/T-cell lymphoma. Overall, T-cell lymphomas account for approximately 7% of all lymphomas in the United States [23]. Peripheral T-cell lymphomas (PTCLs) are a group of clinically aggressive diseases associated with poor outcomes. Evaluating effective therapies in PTCL is challenging given its rarity. Types of PTCL include:

- T-cell prolymphocytic leukemia
- T-cell large granular lymphocytic leukemia
- Aggressive NK-cell leukemia
- Indolent large granular NK-cell lymphoproliferative disorder
- Adult T-cell leukemia
- Extranodal NK-/T-cell lymphoma, nasal type
- Enteropathy-type T-cell lymphoma
- Hepatosplenic T-cell lymphoma

Unfortunately, treatment advances in PTCLs have been slow compared to other lymphomas. Therefore, PTCL patients frequently are treated with similar therapies used in B-cell lymphomas with generally poor outcomes. Relapse is common with currently available agents with few effective options available for salvage therapy [24]. Therefore, patients with PTCLs represent a patient population with high risk of relapse and death.

In contrast to PTCLs, primary cutaneous T-cell lymphomas have a 5-year disease-specific survival of over 85–90% [25]. Primary cutaneous T-cell lymphomas included in the 2018 updates for the WHO-EORTC classification include the following:

- Mycoses fungoides
- Mycoses fungoides variants
- Sezary syndrome
- Adult T-cell leukemia lymphoma

Primary cutaneous CD30+ lymphoproliferative disorders include:

- Cutaneous anaplastic large-cell lymphoma and lymphomatoid papulosis (LyP)
- Subcutaneous panniculitis-like T-cell lymphoma
- Extranodal NK/T-cell lymphoma, nasal type

- Chronic active Epstein–Barr Virus (EBV) infection
- Primary cutaneous peripheral T-cell lymphoma, rare subtypes
  - Primary cutaneous gamma/delta T-cell lymphoma
  - CD8+ aggressive epidermotropic cytotoxic T-cell Lymphoma
  - Primary cutaneous CD4+ small/medium T-cell lymphoproliferative disorder
  - Primary cutaneous acral CD8+ T-cell lymphoma
- Primary cutaneous peripheral T-cell lymphoma, NOS

The 5-year disease-specific survival for folliculotropic mycosis fungoides and Sezary syndrome is 75% and 36%, respectively [25]. Extranodal NK/T-cell lymphoma nasal type involving the skin has a 5-year disease-specific survival of 16%. Primary cutaneous gamma delta T-cell lymphoma and CD8+ aggressive epidermotropic T-cell lymphoma have inferior disease-specific survival at 11% and 31%, respectively [25]. Primary cutaneous peripheral T-cell lymphoma 5-year disease-specific survival is only 15% [25]. Cutaneous T-cell lymphoma patients are frequently followed by a multidisciplinary team, including medical oncologists and dermatologists, and may receive topical therapy, single-agent oral or intravenous chemotherapy, novel targeted therapy, radiation therapy, and more rarely combination chemotherapy and HCT.

## Plasma Cell Disorders

Plasma cell disorders refer to a spectrum of disorders characterized by the monoclonal proliferation of lymphoplasmacytic cells in the bone marrow sometimes with tissue deposition of monoclonal immunoglobulins [26]. These disorders include multiple myeloma, Waldenström macroglobulinemia, and light chain deposition disease (e.g., amyloidosis).

### Multiple Myeloma

Multiple myeloma is the most common plasma cell disorder representing approximately 15% of hematologic malignancies with increased incidence in patients of African American descent [27]. It is characterized by immunodeficiency, lytic bone disease, anemia, and renal failure attributed to the underlying plasma cell disorder. Hypercalcemia is also common due to bone demineralization in approximately one-third of patients [28]. Multiple myeloma is largely a cancer of older adults with a median onset of 60 years. Although multiple myeloma can be treated with effective new therapies and advancing treatment approaches, multiple myeloma is by definition incurable. Patients with multiple myeloma have a monoclonal protein >3 g/dL produced and secreted by malignant plasma cells that can be measured by serum-free light chain analysis and protein electrophoresis of the serum (SPEP) and/or urine (UPEP) as well as immunofixation. The most common monoclonal subtype is immunoglobulin G (IgG), followed by IgA, kappa or lambda light chain only (i.e., Bence Jones), IgD, and then IgM [28]. In patients with light chain multiple myeloma, the incidence of kidney failure is much higher. A diagnosis of multiple myeloma requires a bone marrow biopsy with ≥10% clonal plasma cells or a biopsy-proven plasmacytoma, solitary tumors consisting of plasma cells occurring outside the bone, and is associated with a worse prognosis. End-organ involvement (i.e., immunodeficiency, lytic bone disease, anemia, and renal failure) differentiates multiple myeloma from monoclonal gammopathy of undetermined significance (MGUS) and smoldering multiple myeloma.

MGUS has less than 10% plasma cells in the bone marrow, serum M protein <3 g/dL; whereas smoldering multiple myeloma describes patients with a serum monoclonal protein ≥3 g/dL and/or 10–60% plasma cells in the bone marrow without end-organ damage [29].

Multiple myeloma is then categorized into two risk groups: high risk versus standard risk. Laboratory analysis and fluorescence in situ hybridization (FISH) results for specific molecular changes can help determine prognosis and treatment. Patients with high-risk disease are defined by an elevated lactate dehydrogenase level (≥2 times the upper limit of normal), high-risk molecular changes by FISH [t(4;14), t(14;16), t(14;20), del17p13, or gain 1q], and plasma cell leukemia (either ≥2000 plasma cells/microL of peripheral blood or ≥20% on a manual differential count) [30, 31].

After a diagnosis and risk stratification, the hematologic oncologist must determine the patient's eligibility for autologous HCT, which can prolong progression-free and overall survival over chemotherapy alone. Patients who receive an autologous HCT are typically younger (<65 years) with better physical function and lack decompensated heart or liver function. Interestingly, autologous HCT may be safely completed for all patients with kidney disease (even patients receiving dialysis) as no evidence demonstrates an impact on stem cell collection or engraftment [32]. Overall, there are three strategies for patients eligible for autologous HCT: (1) early transplant directly after recovery from stem cell collection; (2) delayed transplant strategy with continued therapy, usually with the same regimen used for induction, reserving autologous HCT until the first relapse; and (3) allogeneic HCT. Of note, the role of allogeneic HCT remains investigational and controversial [33]. The clinical decision between an early versus late autologous HCT depends on multiple factors: patient preference, risk stratification, patient age, response and tolerability to induction chemotherapy, insurance approval, and the medical center's resources for long-term storage of stem cells. If a patient is a candidate for an autologous HCT, the initial chemotherapy should avoid agents that impair stem cell collection or damage stem cells (e.g., melphalan).

Patients with multiple myeloma eligible for HCT receive induction therapy for 3–4 months before stem cell collection to reduce the tumor cell volume in the bone marrow and peripheral blood and improve symptoms. There is no consensus regarding the preferred induction regimen. Patients ineligible for HCT usually receive 8–12 cycles of initial therapy with a triplet regimen followed by maintenance therapy until progression. Common triplet regimens include: VRd (bortezomib [Velcade], lenalidomide [Revlimid], dexamethasone), DRd (daratumumab, lenalidomide, dexamethasone), or VCd (also called CyBorD, bortezomib, cyclophosphamide, dexamethasone) [34]. Frail patients with multiple comorbidities and/or advanced age who cannot safely receive a triple regimen will receive doublet therapy (e.g., lenalidomide and dexamethasone, or bortezomib and dexamethasone). Patients require antimicrobial and thromboembolic prophylaxis for these chemotherapy combinations and are at risk of neuropathy. Patients with multiple myeloma require maintenance therapy after autologous HCT, given that virtually all patients will relapse. Maintenance regimens include lenalidomide (low-risk patients) or bortezomib (high-risk patients).

## Waldenström Macroglobulinemia

Waldenström macroglobulinemia is a rare plasma cell dyscrasia characterized by ≥10% lymphoplasmacytic lymphoma (small lymphocytes that have plasma cell features) in the bone marrow with an excess IgM monoclonal gammopathy in the blood (i.e., "macroglobulinemia"). It is named after a Swedish internal medicine doctor who first described it. Over 90% of patients with Waldenström macroglobulinemia have a mutation of the MYD88 gene [35]. Patients experience symptoms related to the infiltration of the hematopoietic tissues (e.g., hepatosplenomegaly, lymphadenopathy, anemia) and the IgM monoclonal gammopathy (e.g., peripheral neuropathy, hyperviscosity) as well as increased infections, fatigue, weight loss, and bleeding. A minority of patients with Waldenström macroglobulinemia have kidney or gastrointestinal tract involvement and/or cryoglobulinemia. Overall, Waldenström macroglobulinemia is an indolent disease for most patients with modern therapy with a median prognosis of a decade [36].

Typically, treatment is reserved for symptomatic patients. Like multiple myeloma, Waldenström macroglobulinemia is incurable; consequently, treatment focuses on controlling symptoms and minimizing end-organ damage. The initial treatment depends on the patient's age, symptom severity, comorbidities, and patient preference. Symptomatic hyperviscosity requires emergent plasmapheresis. Disease-directed therapy usually includes a combination of rituximab and bendamustine (BR) given up to 6 months in fit patients; alternatively, elderly frail patients may receive a Bruton tyrosine kinase (BTK) inhibitor (e.g., ibrutinib, acalabrutinib). Patients may or may not receive maintenance therapy with rituximab as the most commonly used therapy. At relapse, treatment approaches include re-initiating the original therapy, an alternative first-line agent, and rarely, high-dose chemotherapy followed by autologous HCT maintenance therapy.

## Immunoglobulin Light Chain Amyloidosis

Immunoglobulin light chain (AL) amyloidosis (also called primary amyloidosis) is another plasma cell disorder associated with the overproduction of monoclonal light chains. AL amyloidosis occurs primarily in older adults and is characterized by tissue deposits of amyloid fibrils that can occur in any organ and produce damage, including nephrotic syndrome, restrictive cardiomyopathy, hepatomegaly, peripheral neuropathy, macroglossia, purpura, and bleeding. Patients with amyloidosis can occur in association with other plasma cell disorders mentioned above. A biopsy of the affected tissue establishes the diagnosis of AL amyloidosis.

AL amyloidosis treatment starts with optimizing the function of the symptomatic end-organ, and an evaluation for autologous HCT based on low-quality evidence. In select patients fit for HCT, patients typically receive 2–4 cycles of bortezomib-based induction prior to stem cell mobilization and autologous HCT [37]. However, most patients with newly diagnosed AL amyloidosis are ineligible for transplant due to advanced age, advanced heart failure, renal insufficiency, and/or multiorgan involvement [38]. For patients ineligible for HCT, treatment consists of 4–6 cycles of a bortezomib-based treatment regimen with response assessment at each cycle.

## Acute Myeloid Leukemia

Acute myeloid leukemia (AML) is a heterogeneous hematologic malignancy of myeloid progenitor cells, which results in a proliferation of abnormal, immature cells leading to impaired hematopoiesis and eventually bone marrow failure [1]. The traditional treatment paradigm gives patients intensive cytotoxic chemotherapy to induce remission, followed by further cytotoxic agents to consolidate the response.

AML risk stratification was historically based on immature cells' morphology, cytogenetic abnormalities, and clinical features [2]. However, over the last few decades, molecular profiling has allowed for the further classification of AML into prognostically distinct subtypes. The 2017 European Leukemia Net (ELN) guidelines, widely used clinically and in research, stratify patients into favorable, intermediate, or adverse-risk groups [3]. There are substantial differences in overall survival between these groups. About 60% of younger patients (those less than 60 years) with the favorable-risk disease were alive at 5 years compared to only 10% of younger patients with adverse-risk disease [4]. Older patients fare substantially worse than younger patients owing to an increased risk of treatment-related mortality and more chemotherapy-resistant disease biology. The 2-year overall survival for older patients with AML is 40% for favorable risk and <10% for adverse risk [4].

Currently, there are four genetic abnormalities associated with favorable-risk disease: t(8;21), inversion 16, mutated *NPM1* without *FLT3*-ITD or with a low allelic ratio (<0.5), and biallelic mutated CEBPA. NPM1 is mutated in roughly 20–30% of patients and is the most common mutation seen in AML [5]. Most patients will have either intermediate-risk or adverse-risk disease. Common genetic abnormalities in adverse-risk AML include complex karyotype, monosomal karyotype, mutated *RUNX1*, mutated *ASXL1*, and mutated *TP53*. Mutations in TP53 are present in 6% of patients and confer inferior outcomes (median for patients <60 years: 10.7 months; >60 years: 6.0 months) [6].

The treatment of AML patients, while ultimately resting on patient preference, traditionally relies on the fitness of patients, segregating patients who are fit to receive intense induction versus those who are not. Nearly all young patients receive intensive induction. Alternatively, many older patients and those with considerable comorbidities are at substantial risk of treatment-related mortality with intensive induction strategies and therefore often receive "less-intense" treatments [7]. Intensive induction therapy usually involves a combination of an anthracycline (often daunorubicin) and cytarabine, with the most common dosing consisting of 7 days of continuous infusion cytarabine and 3 days of the anthracycline, respectively (i.e., "7 + 3"). Intensive strategies offer increased remission rates (ranging from 60 to 80%) with the risk of increased acute side effects, such as prolonged neutropenia, mucositis, and gastrointestinal issues [8]. For patients with favorable-risk disease, intense induction followed by intense consolidation can cure many patients. Rates of cure are substantially less in intermediate-risk and adverse-risk patients. HCT is frequently considered for these patients with higher-risk AML if they can achieve remission, as it often is the only curative option. Less-intense therapy usually involves using "hypomethylating agents" (either azacitidine or decitabine) given outpatient for 5–10 days per 28-day cycle [8]. These agents are better tolerated, though remission rates are substantially lower (20–50%) than with intensive induction. Less-intense treatment regimens rarely result in sustained remissions beyond a few years, and patients who receive less-intense treatment strategies seldom receive HCT.

The goals of therapy are vastly different between intensive and less-intense strategies. Less-intense strategies focus on maintaining quality of life and reducing transfusion burden without inducing substantial side effects, while intensive strategies focus predominantly on a cure. Therefore, clarification of patient values, goals, and preferences is critical at the time of treatment decision-making, especially for patients who may be eligible for intensive strategies. Notably, patients who can receive less-intense chemotherapy, such as hypomethylating agents, spend less time in the hospital and experience improved overall survival than patients who did not receive any chemotherapy [9, 10]. These improved outcomes have led most leukemia physicians to offer less-intensive therapy rather than no therapy if patients can tolerate it. Best supportive care alone should therefore only be considered for patients who cannot tolerate less-intense treatment or have strong preferences against chemotherapy.

Clinical prognostication for patients with AML is largely informed by the response to therapy and the development of relapse. Relapse remains the predominant cause of mortality in patients with AML. The development of highly specific testing for MRD using multi-parameter flow cytometry, polymerase chain reaction (PCR), or other techniques has allowed hematologic oncologists to more clearly understand the depth of response to therapy [11, 12]. Multiple studies have illustrated that residual disease confers significantly higher relapse risk and inferior overall survival, though further work remains to standardize clinical interpretation [4].

The development of several novel agents requires mentioning as their availability is changing practice patterns. Eight new therapies were approved for AML between 2017 and 2019. Venetoclax, an oral agent targeting BCL-2, was approved in 2018. When combined with hypomethylating agents or low-dose cytarabine, venetoclax increases remission rates that, in some settings, are similar to those achieved by intensive strategies [13]. Notably, on the trial that led to its approval, which was restricted to patients deemed unfit to receive intensive induction by their oncologist, many patients received HCT. Achieving HCT demonstrated that using venetoclax may be part of a curative intent strategy even for older patients or those with substantial comorbidities [13]. Larger, randomized trials are ongoing to determine the long-term benefit of using venetoclax, but it is now widely adopted due to these remission rates. Single agents targeting mutations in IDH1, IDH2, and FLT3 are now available to patients with relapsed AML. These agents alone can induce remission in a substantial proportion of patients (20–40%), though single-agent therapy responses are often not durable [14–16]. These agents' availability has provided hope to many patients with relapsed disease who may have considered clinical trials as the only therapeutic option.

## Acute Promyelocytic Leukemia

Acute promyelocytic leukemia (APL) is a subtype of AML. Although APL represents only a small fraction of all acute myeloid leukemias, it is important to briefly mention it because newly diagnosed patients with APL are treated in the inpatient setting. Moreover, APL outcomes are vastly different from other subtypes of AML. APL results from a characteristic translocation in the *PML* gene on chromosome 15 with the *RARA* gene on chromosome 17 (i.e., t[15;17]). Patients commonly present with coagulopathies and disseminated intravascular coagulation. The introduction of all-*trans*-retinoic acid (ATRA) and arsenic (ATO) combinations transformed APL treatment from the deadliest of AML subtypes to the most curable. ATRA-ATO therapy results in remission rates over 90% and cures in 80% of patients [17, 18]. Patients with APL can develop "differentiation syndrome" from treatment, which can cause hyperleukocytosis and systemic inflammatory response, potentially leading to respiratory failure. Differentiation syndrome can be fatal though prophylactic treatments have substantially limited its prevalence and severity. In contrast to older non-APL-AML patients, most older individuals with APL will be cured of their disease. Therefore, the benefit-risk ratio of pursuing aggressive supportive care interventions, including mechanical ventilation, vasopressor support, and temporary dialysis, is very different for APL than non-APL-AML.

## Myelodysplastic Syndrome

Myelodysplastic syndrome (MDS) includes a varied group of acquired bone marrow failure syndromes resulting from clonal expansion of malignant cells and leading to ineffective hematopoiesis and cytopenias. Anemia (commonly macrocytic) is the typical presenting cytopenia. MDS shares many clinical, morphologic, mutational, and cytogenetic features with AML and has a 25–30% overall risk of progression to AML. MDS prognosis after progression to AML is limited, with most (60–70%) of disease being refractory to treatment.

Overall prognosis in MDS is highly variable based on certain prognostic features. The revised version of the International Prognostic Scoring System (R-IPSS) accurately predicts the risk of progression to acute leukemia and death based on cytogenetics, bone marrow blast percentage, and cytopenias [19]. Other important prognostic features include individual genetic mutations (e.g., TP53, ETV6, RUNX1, ASXL1, and EZH2), which, when present, increase the risk of progression to AML. Age is also a critical prognostic factor with a median age of diagnosis of 70 years. The median overall survival of patients classified by the R-IPSS with very low or low-risk disease is between 5 and 8 years; 3 years for patients with intermediate-risk disease; 1.5 years for high risk; and 0.8 years for very high-risk disease [19]. These short median survival times demonstrate the severity of higher-risk MDS. Although progression to AML represents a proportion of mortality in these patients, most patients with MDS succumb to complications of ineffective hematopoiesis, leading to infections or less-frequently bleeding or cardiovascular compromise.

Although allogeneic HCT is the only curative option for patients with MDS, it is only offered to patients with high-risk disease due to the associated morbidity. Patients with lower-risk disease benefit from supportive care, including transfusions, infectious prophylaxis, and potentially hematopoietic growth factors (such as erythropoiesis-stimulating agents to reduce transfusion burden). However, no clear survival benefit has been observed with these agents. Azacitidine (a hypomethylating agent) can modestly improve survival (24 months vs. 15 months) in patients with intermediate-2 or high-risk disease, though adequate response requires at least 4–6 months and complete remission rates are low (17%) [10]. Lenalidomide has particular efficacy in patients with low- or intermediate-risk disease with deletion of 5q (del[5q]), leading to transfusion independence in most patients [20].

## Acute Lymphoblastic Leukemia

Acute Lymphoblastic Leukemia (ALL) is a malignant proliferation of lymphoid progenitors in the bone marrow, blood, and often extramedullary sites. Although ALL is most often diagnosed in children (80% of cases), a bimodal distribution of diagnosis is apparent, with a second peak occurring around age 50. The general treatment paradigm is similar to that of AML, where cytotoxic chemotherapy is used to induce remission, and subsequent therapies are used in consolidation to deepen the response to treatment. Relapse is the primary cause of morbidity and mortality in patients, with CNS relapse occurring more frequently than in AML. This CNS involvement has prompted the increased use of maintenance therapy post-consolidation and HCT in many patients.

Appropriate ALL management relies on accurate risk assessment to guide initial treatment and consideration of HCT. Younger and more-fit older patients are typically treated with "pediatric-inspired" multiagent chemotherapy. In contrast, older and more frail patients are treated with less-intense treatments involving high corticosteroid doses [21]. HCT is used for patients with particularly high-risk features or for patients who achieve remission following relapse.

While most children with ALL are cured, patients over 60 years old experience poor outcomes, with only a 10–15% chance of long-term survival [22]. This vast difference in outcomes is likely attributable to unfavorable biology in older patients and acquired comorbidities. Age and white blood count were historically used in risk stratification; now, cytogenetic features play a much more prominent role, with evidence showing that cytogenetic features are more important to predict outcomes than age or white blood count. In particular, the presence of a translocation in the Philadelphia chromosome, t(9;22), has prognostic and therapeutic implications. Historically patients with Ph-positive ALL had dismal outcomes, with overall survival at 1-year of only about 10%. However, the development of tyrosine kinase inhibitors (TKIs) (e.g., imatinib, dasatinib, ponatinib, and nilotinib) has improved the survival of these patients substantially. For Ph-negative patients, the presence of t(4;11), *KMT2A* translocation, t(8;14), a complex karyotype (≥5 abnormalities), and changes in the number of chromosomes (low hypodiploidy [30–39 chromosomes] and near triploidy [60–78 chromosomes]) portend poor outcomes. Additionally, genetic features which are similar to Ph-positive ALL without t(9;22) ("Ph-like ALL") have been associated with inadequate response to induction therapy and reduced overall survival [22].

Clinically, oncologists caring for patients with ALL rely on treatment response to predict overall outcomes. The morphology of bone marrow aspirates historically evaluated treatment response; however, more recently, the development of highly sensitive testing for MRD using molecular techniques such as flow cytometry, immunoglobulin/T-cell receptor gene rearrangements, and PCR is standard practice to evaluate disease response [23]. In fact, MRD is accepted as the strongest independent predictor of outcomes. Patients who have achieved MRD-negativity, especially early within their treatment course, are less likely to relapse and have substantially longer disease-free and overall survival [24].

Although 85–90% of patients with ALL achieve morphologic remission after induction therapy, a substantial proportion will relapse. Recurrence of disease, either by the development of MRD-positivity or morphologic relapse, signifies poor future outcomes. Traditionally, patients with either relapsed or refractory ALL experienced overall survival of less than 6 months. Cytotoxic salvage chemotherapy also known as rescue therapy is often given in this setting, though remission rates are historically low for standard salvage regimens.

However, recent advances in targeted-therapy have significantly improved outcomes for these patients. For example, blinatumomab(a bi-specific t-cell engager), inotuzumab (a CD-22 targeted agent), and CAR T-cell therapies are now frequently utilized for patients in relapse, even among older patients [25–27]. These treatments represent a welcomed therapeutic expansion as they are often more tolerable than traditional cytotoxic salvage regimens. Yet, their availability now adds further uncertainty in decision-making and prognostication in relapsed patients.

## Mixed Phenotype/Ambiguous Lineage Leukemia

Acute leukemia that cannot be clearly delineated into either AML or ALL is classified as mixed-phenotype or ambiguous lineage leukemia. Outcomes for these patients are traditionally worse than for either AML or ALL. Using either AML-like induction chemotherapy regimens or ALL-like chemotherapy regimens are reasonable approaches, though data is emerging that ALL regimens may be better. HCT is considered in the first remission due to the poor overall outcomes [28].

## Chronic Myeloid Leukemia

Chronic myeloid leukemia (CML) is a hematopoietic cell neoplasm characterized by the BCR-ABL fusion gene, which derives from a translocation between chromosomes 9 and 22, t(9;22)(q34;q11) [29]. This translocation results in "the Philadelphia chromosome," named after its discovery in Philadelphia. CML is divided into three phases: chronic phase, accelerated phase, and blast phase. Most patients (85%) present in the chronic phase [30]. Patients classically present with the insidious onset of fatigue, night sweats, splenomegaly, and weight loss. Additionally, workup reveals abnormal blood counts characterized by leukocytosis, neutrophilia, basophilia, eosinophilia, and circulating immature myeloid cells. Elevated lactate dehydrogenase and uric acid levels are also common, leading to gout flares. The acquisition of additional oncogenic mutations over time is associated with progression to accelerated or blast phases and resistance to TKIs [30]. The identification of oncogenic mutations in addition to the characteristic 9;22 translocation at diagnosis (e.g., trisomy 8 or isochromosome 17q) may be associated with a worse overall prognosis [30, 31]. Progressive symptoms or abrupt changes in blood counts represent progression into accelerated phase or blast phase CML, as discussed below.

The introduction of highly effective TKIs has revolutionized CML therapy. Before TKI therapy, many patients underwent HCT. Without HCT, median overall survival was 5–7 years. However, patients now on TKIs who achieve deep cytogenetic or molecular responses have life expectancies similar to the general population [32]. Roughly 80–85% of patients will fall in this category. Patients continue taking TKIs indefinitely, though treatment discontinuation can be considered for some patients with prolonged, deep responses [33].

Prior to developing TKIs, multiple prognostic scoring systems were utilized to predict the chance of response to therapy but are increasingly becoming less valuable to predict outcomes. Currently, the speed and depth of response to TKI therapy and the phase of disease at diagnosis are the most important prognostic features [30, 34, 35]. Patients presenting in accelerated phase, defined by the WHO as 10–19% blasts in the bone marrow, had a substantially worse response to therapy and overall survival than patients who present with chronic phase CML. Patients with blast phase CML, defined by the WHO as ≥20% blasts in the bone marrow, have poor outcomes with a median OS of only 7–11 months, even in the current era of TKIs [36]. Well-defined disease response criteria based on cytogenetic and molecular features at 3, 6, and 12 months predict patients' outcomes [34].

Resistance to TKIs is typically acquired through mutations in the kinase domain of BCR-ABL1. Mutation identification in the tyrosine kinase domain may alter treatment choice [29]. Multiple TKIs exist and patients are transitioned from one TKI to another due to loss of response. HCT is only reserved for patients who present in the accelerated phase or blast phase or who fail available TKIs. HCT outcomes are best in patients with chronic phase CML as compared to accelerated- or blast phase. The 3-year survival probability for patients undergoing HCT in accelerated phase and blast phase is only 51% and 29%, respectively [37].

## Chronic Lymphocytic Leukemia

Chronic lymphocytic leukemia (CLL) is the most common lymphoid malignancy in patients of European descent, representing 25–30% of leukemia cases in the United States (US) or about 22,000 new diagnoses each year [38]. CLL is an indolent, clonal proliferation of mature B cells that often presents with leukocytosis/lymphocytosis, lymphadenopathy, and splenomegaly, although most (80%) of patients are asymptomatic at diagnosis. CLL can also lead to constitutional symptoms, weaken the immune system, and contribute to hemolytic anemia. Diagnosis is typically made by flow cytometry of peripheral blood lymphocytes demonstrating monoclonal lymphocytes with a characteristic immunophenotype.

Patients' outcomes with CLL vary widely and novel, highly effective, and well-tolerated therapies continue to improve outcomes. Median overall survival continues to improve and is well over 10 years. Individual prognostication at the time of diagnosis is challenging given the wide variation in outcomes and the changing therapeutic landscape [39]. The CLL-International Prognostic Index identifies multiple independent markers for overall survival, including age, molecular mutations, lab markers, and clinical staging [40]. In particular, patients with mutations in the *TP53* gene have a substantially inferior prognosis than those without such mutations. Conversely, patients with *IGHV* somatic hypermutation have superior outcomes compared to patients without hypermutation.

Most patients do not require treatment at diagnosis, and the median time from diagnosis to treatment is 5–7 years. Treatment indications include progressive cytopenias, symptom development, and autoimmune complications such as hemolytic anemia or immune-related thrombocytopenia [38]. Various treatments are reasonable at diagnosis, including single agents (e.g., ibrutinib) or combination therapy, including a monoclonal antibody such as rituximab or obinutuzumab. Oral targeted agents (e.g., venetoclax, ibrutinib, acalabrutinib) are preferred over traditional chemotherapy agents due to the high response rates and reduced acute treatment-related side effects. Novel agents can achieve more profound responses, including MRD-negativity, which predicts a longer progression-free survival though the effect on overall survival remains unclear.

Most patients (>90%) will respond to initial therapy though nearly all will eventually relapse. Time to relapse is a useful surrogate for disease aggressiveness, although this information's utility is uncertain in the modern era of multiple effective therapies. Typically, the duration of response to second-line therapy is less than that achieved initially.

CLL can transform into more aggressive diseases such as diffuse large b-cell lymphoma (DLBCL) or Hodgkin lymphoma. The transformation to DLBCL, termed "Richter transformation," occurs in about 1% of patients per year and has a particularly poor prognosis with a median OS of 1 year [41]. Patients are treated with intense chemotherapy regimens initially developed for de novo DLBCL. Most patients who achieve remission with initial therapy will be considered for allogeneic HCT due to the high relapse rates and poor overall survival. Among patients who can undergo HCT, median post-HCT survival is around 4–5 years [41].

## Hematopoietic Cell Transplantation

HCT and cellular therapy are used extensively for the treatment of malignant and non-malignant diseases. In the setting of hematologic malignancies, these therapies are used predominantly for curative intent except for autologous HCT in myeloma and mantle cell, where it is used to increase remission depth and duration. Despite advances in targeted therapy, the number of patients who benefit from HCT continues to increase. Advances in transplant procedures, access to effective alternative hematopoietic cell sources, and improvements in supportive measures have expanded HCT to older patients and patients who do not have fully matched-related sibling donors. The number of transplants performed in the US exceeds 20,000 annually [39]. Indications for allogeneic HCT are shown in Table 2.1. There is little evidence so far that this number will not continue to grow even with the expansion in cellular and immunotherapies.

For many patients with hematologic malignancies, the time course from diagnosis through treatment initiation and subsequent transplant procedure can be relatively short. To maximize the probability of cure, these patients frequently make decisions to undergo high-risk transplant procedures quickly, sometimes without a good understanding of associated early- and late-morbidity and mortality risks. Palliative care supports these settings and has been underutilized despite the known morbidity and mortality associated with HCT. As healthcare delivery evolves to emphasize value-based and patient-centered care, the role of supportive services, including palliative care, in the short- and long-term must grow.

Since 2007 all allogeneic HCT have been reported to the Stem Cell transplant Outcomes Data Base and registered with the Center for International Blood and Marrow Transplant Research (CIBMTR). At present, all allogeneic HCTs are reported to CIBMTR, and it is estimated that over 85% of autologous HCT are reported as well. As a result of this registration process, there exist easily accessible statistics regarding survival and other outcome measures.

The most common indications for transplant in the US have been multiple myeloma and lymphoma, which account

**Table 2.1** Indication for allogeneic stem cell transplant by disease state (based on 2015 Guidelines from American Society for Blood and Marrow Transplantation [ASBMT])

| | |
|---|---|
| **Plasma cell disorders** | |
| Multiple myeloma | Initial response (CR, VGPR, or PR), relapsed/refractory disease, relapse following prior autologous stem cell transplant |
| Plasma cell leukemia | Initial response (CR, VGPR, or PR), relapsed/refractory disease |
| Primary amyloidosis | Initial response (CR, VGPR, or PR), relapsed/refractory disease |
| **Lymphoma** | |
| Hodgkin lymphoma | Chemosensitive relapsed/refractory disease |
| Diffuse large B-cell lymphoma | Chemosensitive relapsed/refractory disease |
| Mantle cell lymphoma | First remission (complete, partial) |
| Peripheral T-cell lymphoma | First remission, chemosensitive relapse/ refractory disease |
| Burkitt lymphoma | First remission |
| Cutaneous T-cell lymphoma | Chemosensitive relapse/refractory disease |
| **Leukemia/MDS** | |
| Acute myeloid leukemia | Good risk t(8;21), t(16;16)/inv(16)—CR2 |
| | Intermediate risk, high risk, and secondary AML–CR1 |
| Chronic myeloid leukemia | Chronic phase—TKI resistant or intolerant |
| | Accelerated phase/blast phase |
| Myelodysplastic syndrome | Intermediate—2/high risk by IPSS |
| | (Can consider in low-/intermediate-risk refractory to therapy) |
| **Lymphoid malignancies** | |
| Acute lymphoblastic leukemia | Adults—CR1 (standard, high risk) |
| DLBCL, mantle cell lymphoma, T-cell lymphomas | Relapse following auto-HCT; primary refractory, CR2 or greater |
| Chronic lymphocytic leukemia | High risk del(17p)—CR1 or beyond; Richter transformation in first chemosensitive response |
| Follicular lymphoma | Primary refractory, CR2 or beyond, relapse following auto-HCT, transformation to high-grade lymphoma |
| **Myeloproliferative neoplasms** | |
| Myelofibrosis and MDS-MPN overlap syndromes | Primary—(intermediate, high risk); secondary |
| **Bone marrow failure syndrome** | |
| Severe aplastic anemia | Newly diagnosed, relapse/refractory |

*CR* complete response; *DLBCL* diffuse large B-cell lymphoma; *inv* inversion; *IPSS* International Prognostic Scoring System; *MDS* myelodysplastic syndrome; *MPN* myeloproliferative neoplasm; *t* translocation; *TKI* tyrosine kinase inhibitor

for 60% of all HCT and are most commonly performed using autologous hematopoietic cells collected from the peripheral blood. In contrast, acute myelogenous leukemia, acute lymphoblastic leukemia, myelodysplastic syndrome, and myeloproliferative neoplasms account for over 75% of allogeneic HCT.

To undergo HCT, all patients must undergo testing to confirm that they can tolerate the transplant procedure. These tests include determining ECOG or Karnofsky performance status, cardiac function, pulmonary function, creatinine clearance, liver function, and evaluation for other comorbid conditions. Based on this information, a Hematopoietic Cell Transplant-Specific Comorbidity Index (HCT-CI) is calculated [40]. In addition to the comorbidity evaluations, patients undergo a social and psychological assessment to confirm they can follow transplant procedures and have enough support for weeks to months after the procedure.

Once a patient is determined to be a candidate for HCT based on their disease and clinical status, the following will occur:

1. *Donor identification*: Hematopoietic progenitor cells are immature cells that can form all of the mature hematopoietic cells and lead to long-term persistent functioning of the bone marrow. In autologous HCT, the donor is the patient. In allogeneic HCT, potential sources of hematopoietic stem cells are human leukocyte antigen (HLA)-matched siblings or unrelated donors versus alternative donors, including partially matched family members or umbilical cord blood. The period for obtaining the hematopoietic cell source ranges from several weeks to several months. This process is frequently initiated during the time that the patient is undergoing initial therapy and physiologic assessments.
2. *Hematopoietic cell collection:* Collection for autologous HCT occurs once the patient is approved for transplant based on their physiologic performance status and response to prior treatment. In general, patients proceeding to autologous HCT for hematologic malignancies should have chemotherapy-sensitive disease. In the modern era, hematopoietic cells are collected from the peripheral blood through a process called "stem cell mobilization." This process starts with patients receiving either chemotherapy, growth factors, or other agents, leading to increased circulation of hematopoietic cells in the peripheral blood. Then, patients are connected to an apheresis machine and cells are collected daily for several hours over 1–4 days until sufficient stem cells are collected. These cells are cryopreserved until the day of transplant.
3. *Hematopoietic cell collection*: In allogeneic HCT, the collection is generally initiated while patients are undergoing the conditioning therapy; however, there are instances where this may occur before the start of conditioning. Hematopoietic cells may be cryopreserved and stored until needed. Allogeneic hematopoietic cells may be collected either by peripheral blood mobilization or a bone marrow harvest, depending on the specifics of the transplant.
4. *Conditioning regimen*: The initiation of the conditioning regimen marks the beginning of the transplant period. Conditioning includes chemotherapy but may also include total body irradiation or other forms of radiation. In autologous HCT for hematologic malignancies, the conditioning treatment is most commonly high-dose chemotherapy targeting the underlying malignancy. In allogeneic HCT, the conditioning regimen must effectively target the patient's immune system to prevent rejection of the donor cells and may or may not include high-dose chemoradiation to target the underlying disease. Allogeneic HCT preparative regimens range from myeloablative regimens to reduced-intensity regimens to nonmyeloablative regimens, which are the least intensive conditioning therapies aimed at suppressing the recipient's immune system. How well the patient tolerates the conditioning therapy generally correlates with the intensity of the regimen.
5. *Transplantation*: On the day of transplant (Day 0), hematopoietic cells are administered by intravenous infusion after completing the conditioning regimen. The time between the hematopoietic cell infusion and the end of the conditioning regimen is usually 1–2 days.
6. *Recovery and engraftment*: The recovery-and-engraftment period follows hematopoietic cell infusion. During this time, most patients will develop pancytopenia and other short-term chemotherapy effects, including mucositis, enteritis, fever, and infections. The duration of this period can be highly variable and depends on several factors. HCT from bone marrow, umbilical cord blood, and from haploidentical transplant donors recover more slowly. The time that the cells demonstrate recovery is called "engraftment."
7. *Immune recovery—autologous*: Immune recovery in autologous HCT is marked by the recovery of neutrophils within weeks of the HCT; however, patients remain susceptible to opportunistic infections for months following the transplant. At 90 days after transplant, patients will start a re-immunization protocol for all of their childhood vaccinations.

8. *Immune recovery—allogeneic*: Immune recovery in allogeneic HCT is much more complex and requires the use of immunosuppressive medications to support the development of immune tolerance for months. These patients have a more prolonged and variable period of risk for opportunistic infections. This period is also the period that patients may develop acute or chronic graft-versus-host disease.

## Autologous HCT

Autologous HCT success for malignant diseases depends on chemotherapy sensitivity. The use of hematopoietic cells is to facilitate recovery from high-dose chemotherapy. The treatment-related mortality for autologous HCT is markedly lower than allogeneic HCT. The therapeutic effect of autologous HCT is dependent on the presence of some degree of chemotherapy-sensitive disease. CIBMTR reported outcomes for 2007–2017 are described below [39]:

- Hodgkin lymphoma: Autologous HCT is indicated in relapsed disease after response to salvage chemotherapy. The 3-year probability of survival is 86% for patients with chemosensitive disease versus 74% for chemoresistant disease.
- Follicular lymphoma: Transplants in this setting are non-curative but are expected to increase remission duration. HCT is utilized in patients at relapse with chemosensitive disease with 3-year probabilities of survival of 80% in chemosensitive disease versus 66% for patients with chemoresistant disease.
- Diffuse large b-cell lymphoma: HCT is indicated at first relapse best with chemosensitive disease. The 3-year probabilities of survival are 67% for chemosensitive disease versus 47% in the setting chemoresistant disease. Autologous HCT is sometimes used in the first remission as consolidation; however, the value of autologous HCT in this setting is debated.
- Mantle cell lymphoma: Transplants in this setting are non-curative but expected to increase remission duration. Autologous HCT is used most effectively in the first remission as consolidation. The 3-year probability of survival is reported to be 82%.
- Plasma cell disorders: Transplants in this setting are non-curative but expected to increase remission duration. The 5-year survival after autologous HCT is 77% in AL amyloidosis, 66% in multiple myeloma, and 28% in plasma cell leukemia.
- Peripheral T-cell lymphoma: Transplants in this setting are a potentially curable depending of International Prognostic Index score and risk group. In highly select patients, post-HCT 3-year overall survival rates are as high as 85%, and 5-year survival rates near 30% [41, 42].
- Acute leukemia: rarely used.

## Allogeneic HCT

Allogeneic HCT permits two potential effective strategies for disease control. The preparative regimen can have anti-tumor activity in the setting of high-dose chemotherapy or total body irradiation-based regimens. Importantly, allogeneic HCT provides a new immune system to the patient, with the potential for improved immune surveillance and improved graft-versus-tumor effect. Unfortunately, this immune process is also accompanied by serious and potentially life-threatening complications, including an increased rate of opportunistic infections, graft-versus-host disease, interstitial lung disease, and diffuse endothelial injury-associated complications such as veno-occlusive disease (VOD) and atypical hemolytic uremic syndrome. These types of complications substantially increase the treatment-related mortality for allogeneic transplants. Despite these risks, the most common cause of death after allogeneic HCT is the primary disease relapse. CIBMTR reported outcomes for allogeneic HCT between 2007 and 2017 are described below [39]:

- Acute myelogenous leukemia: Predictors for posttransplant survival are disease status at the transplant and the donor type. After HLA-matched sibling transplant, the 3-year probabilities of survival are 59%, 53%, and 29% for patients with early, intermediate, and advanced disease, respectively. In comparison, after an unrelated donor transplant, the probabilities of survival are 53%, 50%, and 27% for patients with early, intermediate, and advanced disease, respectively.
- Myelodysplastic syndrome: The 3-year survival outcomes are 52% and 49% for recipients of sibling and unrelated donor transplants for early MDS, respectively. Among patients with advanced MDS, corresponding probabilities are 46% and 42%.
- Myeloproliferative neoplasms: The 3-year probabilities of survival are 55% for myelofibrosis and 48% for other MPNs. Among HLA-matched sibling donor recipients for MPNs, the corresponding probabilities are 61% and 51%, respectively.
- Chronic myelogenous leukemia: Three-year probabilities of survival for HLA-matched siblings transplants are 65%, 48%, and 33% for patients transplanted in chronic phase, in accelerated phase, and in blast phase, respectively. In the setting of unrelated donor transplants, the 3-year probabilities for survival were 61%, 49%, and 33%

for patients in chronic phase, accelerated phase, and blast phase, respectively.

- Acute lymphoblastic leukemia: The 3-year survival probabilities are 62%, 40%, and 31% for patients with early, intermediate, and advanced disease, respectively. For recipients of unrelated donor HCT, the 3-year survival probabilities are 60%, 40%, and 28% for early, intermediate, and advanced disease, respectively.
- Hodgkin lymphoma: The 3-year probabilities of survival are 61% and 59% after sibling and unrelated donor transplants, respectively.
- Follicular lymphoma: The 3-year probabilities of survival are 74% and 56% for patients with chemotherapy-sensitive and chemotherapy-resistant disease, respectively. The corresponding probabilities for patients receiving unrelated donor transplants were 67% and 52% for chemotherapy-sensitive and chemotherapy-resistant disease.
- Diffuse large b-cell lymphoma: The 3-year probabilities of survival are 54% and 27% for patients with chemotherapy-sensitive and chemotherapy-resistant disease, respectively.
- Mantle cell lymphoma: Three-year probabilities of survival are 54%.

While survival after allogeneic HCT has continued to improve, early severe morbidity and substantial premature mortality can impact over 50% of the patients. As opposed to other patient populations approaching the end of life, transplant recipients frequently undergo the transplant in relatively good health, accepting high early treatment-related mortality as a necessary risk to achieve long-term cure. Approximately 50% of patients who die from allogeneic HCT will do so within 5 months and 66% within 14 months. About 30% of patients who succumb to the effects of allogeneic HCT cannot be discharged home after transplant, and two-thirds of these patients undergo invasive procedures, including advanced life support at the end of life. As a result of specific transplant-associated effects and end of life experiences associated with hematologic malignancies, the support of HCT-patients with severe complications and at the end of life is challenging.

## Long-Term Impact of Transplant on Patient-Reported Outcomes

The long-term effects in survivors of HCT are well recognized but are particularly underappreciated as patients initially contemplate HCT. While most allogeneic and autologous HCT survivors experience improvement of transplant-associated symptoms over time and return to their pre-HCT status by 1 year, many survivors report ongoing residual deficits including chronic fatigue, sleep disturbance, psychological distress, sexual dysfunction, cognitive dysfunction, financial toxicity, and the consequences of chronic graft-versus-host disease.

Interventions to improve patient-centered outcomes have been predominantly tested in the early post-HCT period. The most frequently tested interventions in randomized clinical trials include exercise [43], cognitive behavioral therapy [44], and mind-body practices with stress management [45]. Multiple randomized trials of these interventions have shown small to moderate benefits in improving quality of life, fatigue, and psychological distress in HCT recipients. However, higher-intensity interventions are associated with more substantial benefits. Most transplant patients will return to their communities and local doctors within months of transplant with little guidance or opportunity for follow-up and management of these complications.

## Conclusion

In summary, patients with hematologic malignancies and patients undergoing HCT have unique and rapidly evolving therapeutic and supportive care needs. Patients are commonly faced with the need to proceed with intensive and high-risk therapies rapidly. While there have been promising improvements in treatment-related outcomes, the number of patients who are faced with a complex treatment course and the potentially life-threatening and life-altering risks remains high. Providing comprehensive support of the whole patient and directing therapy toward patient-centered outcomes requires multidisciplinary support that should be considered at diagnosis in most patients.

## References

1. Swerdlow SH, Campo E, Pileri SA, Harris NL, Stein H, Siebert R, et al. The 2016 revision of the World Health Organization classification of lymphoid neoplasms. Blood. 2016;127(20):2375–90.
2. Tan D, Horning SJ, Hoppe RT, Levy R, Rosenberg SA, Sigal BM, et al. Improvements in observed and relative survival in follicular grade 1-2 lymphoma during 4 decades: the Stanford University experience. Blood. 2013;122(6):981–7.
3. Casulo C, Byrtek M, Dawson KL, Zhou X, Farber CM, Flowers CR, et al. Early relapse of follicular lymphoma after rituximab plus cyclophosphamide, doxorubicin, vincristine, and prednisone defines patients at high risk for death: an analysis from the National LymphoCare study. J Clin Oncol. 2015;33(23):2516.
4. Zell JA, Cinar P, Mobasher M, Ziogas A, Meyskens FL Jr, Anton-Culver H. Survival for patients with invasive cutaneous melanoma among ethnic groups: the effects of socioeconomic status and treatment. J Clin Oncol Off J Am Soc Clin Oncol. 2008;26(1):66–675.
5. Solal-Céligny P, Roy P, Colombat P, White J, Armitage JO, Arranz-Saez R, et al. Follicular lymphoma international prognostic index. Blood. 2004;104(5):1258–65.

6. Morschhauser F, Fowler NH, Feugier P, Bouabdallah R, Tilly H, Palomba ML, et al. Rituximab plus lenalidomide in advanced untreated follicular lymphoma. N Engl J Med. 2018;379(10):934–47.
7. Hans CP, Weisenburger DD, Greiner TC, Gascoyne RD, Delabie J, Ott G, et al. Confirmation of the molecular classification of diffuse large B-cell lymphoma by immunohistochemistry using a tissue microarray. Blood. 2004;103(1):275–82.
8. Villano J, Koshy M, Shaikh H, Dolecek T, McCarthy B. Age, gender, and racial differences in incidence and survival in primary CNS lymphoma. Br J Cancer. 2011;105(9):1414–8.
9. Ferreri AJ, Blay J-Y, Reni M, Pasini F, Spina M, Ambrosetti A, et al. Prognostic scoring system for primary CNS lymphomas: the International Extranodal Lymphoma Study Group experience. J Clin Oncol. 2003;21(2):266–72.
10. Abrey LE, Ben-Porat L, Panageas KS, Yahalom J, Berkey B, Curran W, et al. Primary central nervous system lymphoma: the Memorial Sloan-Kettering Cancer Center prognostic model. J Clin Oncol. 2006;24(36):5711–5.
11. Mendez JS, Ostrom QT, Gittleman H, Kruchko C, DeAngelis LM, Barnholtz-Sloan JS, et al. The elderly left behind—changes in survival trends of primary central nervous system lymphoma over the past 4 decades. Neuro-Oncology. 2018;20(5):687–94.
12. DeAngelis LM, Seiferheld W, Schold SC, Fisher B, Schultz CJ. Combination chemotherapy and radiotherapy for primary central nervous system lymphoma: radiation therapy oncology group study 93-10. J Clin Oncol. 2002;20(24):4643–8.
13. Gavrilovic IT, Hormigo A, Yahalom J, DeAngelis LM, Abrey LE. Long-term follow-up of high-dose methotrexate-based therapy with and without whole brain irradiation for newly diagnosed primary CNS lymphoma. J Clin Oncol. 2006;24(28):4570–4.
14. Nelson DF, Martz KL, Bonner H, Nelson JS, Newall J, Kerman HD, et al. Non-Hodgkin's lymphoma of the brain: can high dose, large volume radiation therapy improve survival? Report on a prospective trial by the Radiation Therapy Oncology Group (RTOG): RTOG 8315. Int J Radiat Oncol Biol Physics. 1992;23(1):9–17.
15. Reni M, Ferreri A, Villa E. Second-line treatment for primary central nervous system lymphoma. Br J Cancer. 1999;79(3–4):530.
16. Oyama T, Yamamoto K, Asano N, Oshiro A, Suzuki R, Kagami Y, et al. Age-related EBV-associated B-cell lymphoproliferative disorders constitute a distinct clinicopathologic group: a study of 96 patients. Clin Cancer Res. 2007;13(17):5124–32.
17. Aladily TN, Mansour A, Alsughayer A, Sughayer M, Medeiros LJ. The utility of CD83, fascin and CD23 in the differential diagnosis of primary mediastinal large B-cell lymphoma versus classic Hodgkin lymphoma. Ann Diagn Pathol. 2019;40:72–6.
18. Green MR, Monti S, Rodig SJ, Juszczynski P, Currie T, O'Donnell E, et al. Integrative analysis reveals selective 9p24. 1 amplification, increased PD-1 ligand expression, and further induction via JAK2 in nodular sclerosing Hodgkin lymphoma and primary mediastinal large B-cell lymphoma. Blood. 2010;116(17):3268–77.
19. Chadburn A, Said J, Gratzinger D, Chan JK, de Jong D, Jaffe ES, et al. HHV8/KSHV-positive lymphoproliferative disorders and the spectrum of plasmablastic and plasma cell neoplasms 2015 SH/EAHP workshop report—part 3. Am J Clin Pathol. 2017;147(2):171–87.
20. Sukswai N, Lyapichev K, Khoury JD, Medeiros LJ. Diffuse large B-cell lymphoma variants: an update. Pathology. 2020;52(1):53–67.
21. Okada S, Goto H, Yotsumoto M. Current status of treatment for primary effusion lymphoma. Intract Rare Diseases Res. 2014;3(3):65–74.
22. Dunleavy K. Approach to the diagnosis and treatment of adult Burkitt's lymphoma. J Oncol Pract. 2018;14(11):665–71.
23. Criscione VD, Weinstock MA. Incidence of cutaneous T-cell lymphoma in the United States, 1973-2002. Arch Dermatol. 2007;143(7):854–9.
24. Foss FM, Zinzani PL, Vose JM, Gascoyne RD, Rosen ST, Tobinai K. Peripheral T-cell lymphoma. Blood. 2011;117(25):6756–67.
25. Willemze R, Cerroni L, Kempf W, Berti E, Facchetti F, Swerdlow SH, et al. The 2018 update of the WHO-EORTC classification for primary cutaneous lymphomas. Blood. 2019;133(16):1703–14.
26. Barlogie B. Plasma cell dyscrasias. J Am Med Assoc. 1992;268(20):2946.
27. Siegel RL, Miller KD, Fuchs HE, Jemal A. Cancer statistics, 2022. CA Cancer J Clin. 2022;72(1):7–33.
28. Kyle RA, Gertz MA, Witzig TE, Lust JA, Lacy MQ, Dispenzieri A, et al. Review of 1027 patients with newly diagnosed multiple myeloma. Mayo Clin Proc. 2003;78(1):21–33.
29. Rajkumar SV, Dimopoulos MA, Palumbo A, Blade J, Merlini G, Mateos M-V, et al. International myeloma working group updated criteria for the diagnosis of multiple myeloma. Lancet Oncol. 2014;15(12):e538–e48.
30. van de Donk NW, Lokhorst HM, Anderson KC, Richardson PG. How I treat plasma cell leukemia. Blood. 2012;120(12):2376–89.
31. Usmani S, Rodriguez-Otero P, Bhutani M, Mateos M, Miguel J. Defining and treating high-risk multiple myeloma. Leukemia. 2015;29(11):2119–25.
32. Badros A, Barlogie B, Siegel E, Roberts J, Langmaid C, Zangari M, et al. Results of autologous stem cell transplant in multiple myeloma patients with renal failure. Br J Haematol. 2001;114(4):822–9.
33. Yin X, Tang L, Fan F, Jiang Q, Sun C, Hu Y. Allogeneic stem-cell transplantation for multiple myeloma: a systematic review and meta-analysis from 2007 to 2017. Cancer Cell Int. 2018;18(1):1–17.
34. Sonneveld P, Avet-Loiseau H, Lonial S, Usmani S, Siegel D, Anderson KC, et al. Treatment of multiple myeloma with high-risk cytogenetics: a consensus of the International Myeloma Working Group. Blood. 2016;127(24):2955–62.
35. Treon SP, Xu L, Yang G, Zhou Y, Liu X, Cao Y, et al. MYD88 L265P somatic mutation in Waldenström's macroglobulinemia. N Engl J Med. 2012;367(9):826–33.
36. Brandefors L, Melin B, Lindh J, Lundqvist K, Kimby E. Prognostic factors and primary treatment for Waldenström macroglobulinemia—a Swedish Lymphoma Registry study. Br J Haematol. 2018;183(4):564–77.
37. Palladini G, Kastritis E, Maurer MS, Zonder J, Minnema MC, Wechalekar AD, et al. Daratumumab plus CyBorD for patients with newly diagnosed AL amyloidosis: safety run-in results of ANDROMEDA. Blood. 2020;136(1):71–80.
38. Dispenzieri A, Seenithamby K, Lacy MQ, Kumar SK, Buadi FK, Hayman SR, et al. Patients with immunoglobulin light chain amyloidosis undergoing autologous stem cell transplantation have superior outcomes compared with patients with multiple myeloma: a retrospective review from a tertiary referral center. Bone Marrow Transplant. 2013;48(10):1302–7.
39. Shah NN, Ahn KW, Litovich C, Fenske TS, Ahmed S, Battiwalla M, et al. Outcomes of Medicare-age eligible NHL patients receiving RIC allogeneic transplantation: a CIBMTR analysis. Blood Adv. 2018;2(8):933–40.
40. Sorror ML, Maris MB, Storb R, Baron F, Sandmaier BM, Maloney DG, et al. Hematopoietic cell transplantation (HCT)-specific comorbidity index: a new tool for risk assessment before allogeneic HCT. Blood. 2005;106(8):2912–9.
41. Rodríguez J, Caballero MD, Gutiérrez A, Marín J, Lahuerta JJ, Sureda A, et al. High-dose chemotherapy and autologous stem cell transplantation in peripheral T-cell lymphoma: the GEL-TAMO experience. Ann Oncol. 2003;14(12):1768–75.

42. Numata A, Miyamoto T, Ohno Y, Kamimura T, Kamezaki K, Tanimoto T, et al. Long-term outcomes of autologous PBSCT for peripheral T-cell lymphoma: retrospective analysis of the experience of the Fukuoka BMT group. Bone Marrow Transplant. 2010;45(2):311–6.
43. Wiskemann J, Huber G. Physical exercise as adjuvant therapy for patients undergoing hematopoietic stem cell transplantation. Bone Marrow Transplant. 2008;41(4):321–9.
44. DuHamel KN, Mosher CE, Winkel G, Labay LE, Rini C, Meschian YM, et al. Randomized clinical trial of telephone-administered cognitive-behavioral therapy to reduce post-traumatic stress disorder and distress symptoms after hematopoietic stem-cell transplantation. J Clin Oncol. 2010;28(23):3754.
45. Duong N, Davis H, Robinson PD, Oberoi S, Cataudella D, Culos-Reed SN, et al. Mind and body practices for fatigue reduction in patients with cancer and hematopoietic stem cell transplant recipients: a systematic review and meta-analysis. Crit Rev Oncol Hematol. 2017;120:210–6.

# 3 Hematopoietic Cell Transplantation

Effie Wang Petersdorf

## Overview

Since the first bone marrow transplant performed by E Donnall Thomas in 1957, blood and marrow transplantation has cured individuals suffering from life-threatening blood disorders [1]. The one millionth transplant was performed in December 2012 [2] and reflects the tremendous advances worldwide in clinical and basic research that have substantially improved the safety, efficacy, and availability of this therapeutic modality [3]. Current activities in the United States show continued increase in both autologous and allogeneic transplantation, with over 14,000 autologous and 8000 allogeneic transplants having been performed in 2017 alone [4]. The most common indications for autologous transplantation are lymphoproliferative disorders with plasma cell disorders, Hodgkin and non-Hodgkin lymphoma being the primary diseases (85%) [2]. Among allogeneic transplantations, the vast majority (72%) are performed for leukemia [2].

The overall approach to an individual's transplant is influenced by the disease, disease stage, type of conditioning, and stem cell source. In turn, the potential immediate and late effects of a given transplant are highly dependent on those same factors, as well as non-medical circumstances that can affect the overall sense of well-being and quality of life after transplantation [5]. It has been increasingly recognized that transplant recipients and their caregivers are as much in need of palliative and supportive care, as they are the specialized care aimed at eradicating the underlying disease and the prevention of the organ toxicity post-transplant. This chapter is dedicated to a description of the transplantation procedure itself and of the palliative and supportive care required to ensure a successful transplant.

## Safety, Efficacy, and Availability of Transplantation

The safety and efficacy of transplantation have significantly improved over the past several decades [6] with the results of unrelated donor transplantation similar to that after matched sibling donor transplantation [7]. In a single center study, comparison of clinical outcomes after allogeneic transplantations performed between 2003–2007 and 2013–2017 illustrated substantial reductions in complications and improvement in overall survival. Specific reductions in organ toxicity included jaundice, renal insufficiency, requirement for mechanical ventilation, cytomegalovirus (CMV) viremia, gram-negative bacteremia, invasive mold infection, acute and chronic graft-versus-host disease (GVHD), and requirement for corticosteroid therapy. The study identified relapse to be the major complication after transplantation. The overall lowering of mortality was observed following myeloablative (MA) and reduced-intensity conditioning (RIC) and in those who received transplants from related or unrelated donors. The development of RIC and non-myeloablative (NMA) conditioning regimens has significantly extended the range of patient age [8], and despite an increased number of patients aged over 70 years, overall survival continues to increase. (Table 3.1).

The availability of transplantation has been extended through the development of registries of unrelated volunteer donors and cord blood banks worldwide. Currently, there are over 37 million registered donors and cord blood units available for clinical use [9]. Coordination of unrelated donors and cord blood units is through transplant centers, donor registries, and cord blood banks under the auspices of the World Marrow Donor Association (WMDA) [10].

E. W. Petersdorf (✉)
Division of Hematology and Oncology, University of Washington, Seattle, WA, USA

Division of Translational Science and Therapeutics, Fred Hutchinson Cancer Center, Seattle, WA, USA
e-mail: epetersd@fredhutch.org


C. K. Ullrich, E. J. Roeland (eds.), *Palliative Care in Hematologic Malignancies and Serious Blood Disorders*, https://doi.org/10.1007/978-3-031-38058-7_3

**Table 3.1** Common terminology in transplantation

| Term | Abbreviation |
|---|---|
| Co-morbidity index | CI |
| Stem cell source | |
| Autologous | "Auto" |
| Allogeneic | "Allo" |
| Related | |
| Unrelated donor | URD |
| Cord blood | CB |
| Product | |
| Bone marrow | BM |
| Peripheral blood stem cells | PBSC |
| Cord blood units | CBU |
| Conditioning regimen | |
| Myeloablative | MA |
| Reduced intensity | RIC |
| Non-myeloablative | NMA |
| GVHD prevention | |
| T-replete | |
| T-cell depletion | TCD |
| Outcomes | |
| Graft-versus-host disease | GVHD |
| Transplant-related mortality | TRM |
| Relapse | |
| Disease-free survival | DFS |
| Minimal residual disease | MRD |
| Graft-versus-leukemia | GVL |
| Long-term follow-up | LTFU |

## Indications and Timing of Transplantation

The American Society for Transplantation and Cellular Therapy, ASTCT (formerly American Society for Blood and Marrow Transplantation, ASBMT) convened a task force in 2014 to provide guidance on the indications and timing of transplantation based on the best evidence to date [11]. The task force evaluated hematologic and non-hematologic malignant and non-malignant disorders including solid tumors (e.g., germ cell, Ewing sarcoma, breast and renal cancer) and non-malignant diseases (e.g., severe aplastic anemia, Fanconi anemia, thalassemia, sickle cell disease, multiple sclerosis, rheumatoid arthritis, Crohn disease). The task force provided recommendations for five broad categories: (1) standard of care with strong, well-defined evidence, involving randomized trials with validation across large multi-center databases; (2) standard of care based on clinical evidence including single center large datasets but needing future clinical trials; (3) standard of care for rare diseases for which trials are not feasible (due to the rarity of the disorder); (4) developmental based on encouraging pre-clinical and/or early phase trials; and (5) not generally recommended in which the available evidence does not currently support the routine use of transplantation. As an example, for acute myeloid leukemia, the task force identified transplantation as standard of care when the disease is in the first complete remission with intermediate or high-risk features, and when in the second complete remission. Additionally, there is strong available evidence for the use of transplantation for third or more advanced complete remission and when the disease is in relapse. Transplantation is not recommended for low-risk acute myeloid leukemia in first complete remission, where the risks of the transplant procedure itself outweigh the potential benefits. The major goal of pre-transplant assessment is to define the risks and benefits of transplantation for the individual in order to reduce morbidity and mortality after transplantation. Transplantation is optimal when the benefits of the procedure outweigh the risks. Several tools have been developed to aid in the assessment of a patient's activities of daily living and their transplant eligibility. The best known tools for patient performance status are the Karnovsky Performance Scale Index [12], the Eastern Cooperative Cancer Group (ECOG) Performance Status [13], and European Group for Blood and Marrow Transplantation (EBMT) Risk Score [2]. Most recently, the Co-Morbidity Index (CI) has been developed and validated in large, multi-institutional prospective studies [14]. The CI is informative for both autologous and allogeneic transplant recipients and provides prognostic information for transplant outcomes for non-relapse mortality and overall mortality. The index is calculated based on organ-specific laboratory findings. Many transplant centers rely on a score or index and supplement pre-transplant assessment with screening tests including, but not limited to, cardiac echocardiography for left-ventricular ejection fraction, pulmonary function tests, renal and hepatic function, and psychosocial health and well-being. The specific eligibility of a given patient for transplantation may depend on the overall score or index as an estimate of potential organ toxicity and mortality. The optimal timing of the transplant may be influenced by the patient's overall health balanced with the disease stage and urgency of the transplant for the control of the underlying disease.

## Clinical Algorithms and Characteristics

### Stem Cell Source

Stem cells for transplantation may derive from the patient (autologous, "auto") or from a source other than the patient (allogeneic, "allo"). Allogeneic stem cell sources include family members, unrelated volunteers, and cord blood units. Since 2008, the use of unrelated volunteer donors has steadily increased and the transplantation of mismatched-related donors surpassed the number of cord blood transplantations in 2014 [4]. The optimal allogeneic stem cell source is often defined by the degree of histocompatibility between the recipient and the candidate donors. Histocompatibility is defined by the gene products of the human leukocyte antigen (HLA) system encoded on human chromosome 6 [15]. Among family members, siblings who have inherited the same chromosome six haplotypes are identical-by-descent ("HLA genotypically-identical siblings") and represent the optimal donor, as they are generally associated with very low rates of graft rejection and severe acute and chronic GVHD. Family members who share one HLA haplotype but who differ for the second haplotype ("haploidentical") represent an important potential pool of donors [16–18].

The demonstration of the immunosuppressive qualities of post-transplant cyclophosphamide (PTCy) propelled the use of haploidentical family members as donors for HCT [16–18]. PTCy selectively depletes proliferating alloantigen-stimulated donor and host T cells and non-specifically kills T cells *in vivo*. It takes advantage of the higher sensitivity of proliferating alloreactive T cells to cyclophosphamide at this time after conditioning and graft infusion. Cyclophosphamide facilitates the development of peripheral tolerance, possibly through clonal deletion, suppression of T regulatory cells, and anergy. PTCy suppresses both graft rejection and GVHD and can be used in concert with standard immunosuppression. Immunosuppression is delayed until the completion of cyclophosphamide to avoid blocking the beneficial tolerance-inducing effects of cyclophosphamide. The application of PTCy for immunosuppression in haploidentical transplantation has led to extensive clinical experience, with survival after haploidentical related donor transplantation now achieving similar rates as those seen for genotypically matched sibling donor transplantation with an added advantage of lower overall rates of chronic GVHD [17, 19].

Outside of the family, transplantation from unrelated volunteer donors and cord blood units provides curative therapy [20–23]. The relative advantages of each source of stem cells are well described and include availability, donor risk, and associated risks of engraftment and GVHD (Table 3.2).

**Table 3.2** Comparison of stem cell sources for transplantation

| Feature | Unrelated donor | Haploidentical related donor | Cord blood unit |
|---|---|---|---|
| Time to identification | Fast–slow | Fast | Fast |
| Flexibility in scheduling | Lower | Lower | Higher |
| Stringency of HLA matching | High | Moderate | Low |
| Risks to donor | Yes | Yes | No |
| Rate of neutrophil/ platelet engraftment | Faster | Faster | Slower |
| Risk of graft rejection | Low | Low | Higher |
| Risk of GVHD | Low–high | Low–high | Lower |
| Possibility of DLI | Yes | Yes | No |

*DLI* donor lymphocyte infusion; *GVHD* graft-versus-host disease; *HLA* "Hu Locus A"

The choice of stem cell source may be transplant center-specific, notably when clinical trials define the use of specific products. A worldwide network of donor registries and cord blood banks link HLA tissue types of over 37 million registered donors and cord blood units [9, 10]. A search for the best HLA-matched unrelated donor or cord blood unit is conducted by the transplant center, and a primary and secondary source are identified. Unrelated donors undergo health assessments, and the donor stem cell product is procured through the donor registry and transported to the transplant center to coincide with the transplant date. Cord blood units are previously collected and are shipped to transplant centers prior to the start of conditioning.

Donor-recipient HLA mismatching is a major risk factor for GVHD, and the criteria for the selection of unrelated donors and cord blood units are based on the degree of HLA matching. A minimal level of compatibility for unrelated donors is DNA-level matching for alleles at HLA-A, -B, -C, -DRB1 [24]; however, many transplant centers strive to match for ten determinants at five genes, HLA-A, -B, -C, -DRB1, -DQB1. Donors who match the recipient at all ten determinants are referred to as HLA 10/10-matched. When no HLA 10/10-matched donor is available, use of donors with one mismatch may be considered [25]. Use of donors with multi-locus mismatches is associated with significantly increased risks of GVHD [25].

The probability of identifying HLA-matched unrelated donors depends on patient ancestry and HLA tissue type. Whereas patients of Caucasian ancestry have better than 80% probability of identifying HLA-matched donors, patients of other ancestries have substantial difficulty, particularly African American patients [26]. The use of unrelated donors with selected mismatches has permitted patients to benefit from life-saving transplantation. The identification of HLA mismatch combinations that are better tolerated is an active area of clinical and basic research [25].

Further options among allogeneic donors are the use of peripheral blood stem cells (PBSC) and bone marrow (BM). Marrow is a preferred stem sell product for those with non-malignant life-threatening blood disorders, including severe aplastic anemia, in whom the goal is to minimize the negative impact of GVHD and the consequential requirements for immunosuppressive therapy that contribute to transplant-related mortality (TRM) and overall mortality [27]. PBSCs are apheresed after mobilization with growth factor, a process that is well-tolerated in donors [28]. Bone marrow is directly harvested from the posterior iliac crest of donors most commonly with general anesthesia. Compared to PBSC, marrow is associated with lower chronic GVHD and related to the number of alloreactive T cells in marrow products [20]. Longitudinal assessment of recipients of marrow and PBSC products indicates better patient-reported psychological outcomes and greater likelihood of returning to work in individuals who received marrow grafts [29].

An advantage of cord blood transplantation is the lower level of stringency required for HLA matching due to the lower numbers of mature alloreactive donor T cells in naïve cord blood grafts [21–23]. General criteria include assessment of HLA-A, -B, and -DRB1 ("HLA 6/6"), with many centers striving to achieve matching for HLA-A, -B, -C, -DRB1 ("HLA 8/8") [24]. The major clinical course of CBT is slower immunologic recovery due to the small numbers of infused cells, particularly for adults in whom the cells dose per kilogram body weight may mandate the use of two cord blood units. To address the cell-dose requirements, in vitro cord blood expansion has been successfully used [30].

## Conditioning Regimen

The conditioning or preparative regimen consists of chemotherapy with or without radiation therapy delivered prior to the infusion of the stem cells on the transplant day (i.e., "day zero"). In autologous transplantation, patients may receive chemotherapy to mobilize stem cells for collection and may receive their autologous stem cells at any time after collection. In allogeneic transplantation, the conditioning regimen is delivered in the days prior to day zero infusion of the related, unrelated, or cord blood stem cell product.

The purpose of the conditioning regimen depends on the goal of the transplant: complete marrow ablation or partial suppression with reliance of graft-versus-tumor (GVT) effects. As such, conditioning regimens differ from one another regarding the "intensity" of the regimen and the specific agent(s) used to achieve the desired degree of ablation or suppression (Table 3.3).

"Myeloablative" conditioning (MAC) regimens consist of combinations of high-dose chemotherapy with or without radiation therapy and lead to ablation of stem cell regeneration; the transplantation of stem cells in this scenario can be considered a "rescue" to restore hematopoiesis. Patients who benefit from ablative regimens generally have high-risk diseases and are medically fit to tolerate the intense therapy. "Reduced-intensity" (reduced-intensity conditioning, RIC) and "non-myeloablative" (NMA) regimens provide lower intensity myelosuppression and are ideal for patients whose medical comorbidities or older age may place them at higher risk for regimen-related toxicities. The degree of myelosuppression associated with RIC and NMA regimens is a continuum [31]. RIC and NMA regimens rely primarily on (GVT) effects to eradicate the underlying malignancy. The reduced intensity of the conditioning necessitates immunosuppressive therapy to establish the graft and to prevent GVHD. RIC and MAC regimens span a range of immunosuppressive and myelosuppressive potential.

Differences in myelosuppression across various RIC and NMA regimens affect the degree of marrow aplasia and the tempo of complete donor engraftment. The degree of donor engraftment is expressed as a percent chimerism. Chimerism is the state in which donor cells have durably engrafted in the recipient. Full donor chimerism implies that 100% of bone marrow and blood cells are of donor origin. Regimens that are more myelosuppressive generally result in severe hypoplasia before restoration of graft function. Complete donor engraftment occurs rapidly. Blood counts may be moderately depressed with less myelosuppressive regimens, and most recipients of RIC or NMA regimens are mixed donor and host chimeras that require up to 6–12 months to establish complete donor engraftment. Notable examples of the clinical applications of RIC and NMA procedures in HCT are summarized in Table 3.4:

## GVHD Prophylaxis

The prevention of acute and chronic GVHD remains an active area of clinical research. GVHD is a clinical syndrome that arises from the recognition of disparities between the graft (donor) and host (patient) tissues. The choice of specific immunosuppressive agents is directly tied into the spe-

**Table 3.3** Comparison of conditioning regimens

| Ablative | Reduced intensity | Non-myeloablative |
|---|---|---|
| Cyclophosphamide (CY) with total body irradiation (TBI) given as a single dose >500 centigray (cGY) or as fractionated TBI >800 cGY total | TBI less than 500 cGY single dose | TBI 200 cGY |
| CY/etoposide (VP16)/TBI | TBI less than 800 cGY fractionated | Fludarabine (FLU)/TBI 200 cGY |
| Busulfan (BU)/CY | Melphalan 150 mg/m$^2$ or less | FLU/CY |
| TBI 500 cGY or greater single dose | BU 9 mg/kg or less | FLU/cytosine arabinoside (ARA-C) |
| TBI 800 cGY or greater fractionated | Carmustine (BCNU)/VP16/ cytarabine/melphalan [BEAM] | |
| Melphalan greater than 150 mg/m$^2$ | CY/BCNU/VP16 [CBV] | |
| BU greater than 9 mg/kg | VP16/CY | |
| BU/melphalan | | |

**Table 3.4** RIC and NMA conditioning for disease control

| Role | Purpose | Study |
|---|---|---|
| Stand-alone RIC/NMA HCT | Lower morbidity and regimen-related toxicity in patients who cannot tolerate intense conditioning | [32] |
| Tandem autologous-allogeneic HCT | Pre-plan the allogeneic HCT as "consolidation" after the autologous HCT; leverage graft-versus-tumor (GVT) and graft-versus-leukemia effects (GVLE) for high-risk malignancies in allogeneic HCT | [33] |
| Second allogeneic HCT | Salvage therapy to induce remission after unsuccessful first high-dose HCT | [34, 35] |

cific conditioning regimen. In T cell-replete transplantation, the use of immunosuppressive agents is mandatory. Specific classes of agents include post-transplant cyclophosphamide, calcineurin inhibitors, antimetabolites, sirolimus, and mycophenolate mofetil [36, 37]. Early investigation demonstrated the superiority of multi-agent immunosuppressive regimens to the use of a single immunosuppressive agent [38, 39]. The duration of immunosuppressive therapy depends on the development of clinical GVHD in the patient and is correlated with the degree of HLA compatibility and corresponding risk of GVHD [40].

The removal of alloreactive T cells (T-cell depletion, TCD) with the use of agents such as anti-thymocyte globulin (ATG) or alemtuzumab is an effective approach for mitigating acute GVHD [41–43]. More recently, depletion of naïve T cell in vitro with anti-CD45RA, expressed by more naïve T cells, has been used to reduce both severe acute and chronic GVHD [44].

PTCy administered on days three and four following RIC with tacrolimus, and mycophenolate mofetil is associated with low rates of acute and chronic GVHD after transplantation from haploidentical related, HLA-matched related, HLA-matched and mismatched unrelated donor marrow and PBSC donors, and after myeloablative and RIC conditioning [17–19, 45, 46]. The mechanisms of PTCy involve the targeting of rapidly proliferating alloreactive T cells while quiescent cells involved in immune reconstitution are spared [47].

## The Early Post-transplant Course

Supportive care in the post-transplant time period is focused on engraftment and the prevention and treatment of GVHD infection and the prevention of organ toxicity. Patients in the early post-transplant period require multi-faceted support to ensure safe blood counts, to maintain and promote healthy tissues, and to minimize infection. The need for red cell and platelet transfusions depends on the intensity of marrow ablation and individual responses to chemotherapy. Screened, irradiated blood products are used to sustain patients until donor engraftment [48]. The intensity and specific organ toxicities associated with the conditioning regimen mandate excellent nutrition, [49] which may include total parenteral nutrition when prolonged oral nutrition is not feasible. Supportive care includes the use of anti-bacterial, anti-viral, and anti-fungal agents to prevent infection [50–52]. The specific selection of anti-microbial agents may depend on the local transplant center demographics, but all are aimed at comprehensive coverage of the most common organisms that are typically observed in immunocompromised hosts, including CMV.

## Engraftment

The kinetics of engraftment are directly related to the intensity of the conditioning regimen and degree of myeloablation. The formal definition of engraftment is based on the absolute neutrophil count (ANC) (Table 3.5).

Failure to achieve an ANC after ablative conditioning may be due to any one of a number of factors: quantitative (e.g., low CD34+ cell yield); qualitative (e.g., marrow fibrosis, extensive pre-transplant therapy); immunological (e.g., HLA mismatching, anti-HLA antibodies, viral infection). The term "graft rejection" specifically refers to an immunologically mediated rejection of the allogeneic donor graft due to genetic disparity between the donor and the transplant patient. The diagnosis of graft rejection is made through chimerism testing to confirm the absence or loss of donor cells.

Chimerism testing entails the use of genetic markers that are donor-specific and host-specific to quantify the percent of donor and host cells. Chimerism testing can be performed on a marrow or peripheral blood specimen. Patients undergoing MAC, unmanipulated grafts, and standard GVHD prophylaxis generally have uneventful recovery of the complete blood count and 100% full donor chimerism. In this setting, chimerism testing may be forgone if the ANC recovers uneventfully.

Patients who receive RIC require chimerism testing because there is incomplete eradication of host hematopoie-

**Table 3.5** Definition of engraftment

| Early (primary) | Late (secondary) |
|---|---|
| • Failure of ANC to meet $0.5 \times 10^9$/L by day 28, or<br>• Platelet recovery: first day when the platelet count reaches 20, 50, or $100 \times 10^9$/L for 3 consecutive days without transfusion in the prior 7 days | • Primary engraftment was reached, but subsequent loss of graft: at least two lines of cytopenia on three lab values |

sis. Full or complete donor chimerism is defined as 95–100% replacement of the host by the donor. Mixed chimerism describes presence of both donor and host cells, ranging from 5 to 95% donor type.

The treatment of graft failure depends on the etiology. Treatment options for graft failure after autologous transplantation include infusion of a previously cryopreserved autologous back-up product, growth factor support and, if appropriate, allogeneic transplantation. Approaches for graft failure following allogeneic transplantation include infusion of previously stored autologous stem cells, growth factor support, donor lymphocyte infusion to convert falling chimerism to full donor chimerism and a second transplant.

## Relapse

Relapse remains the chief cause of mortality before and after day 100 after HLA-matched sibling transplantation and after day 100 after unrelated donor transplantation [4]. The risk of recurrence of disease after transplantation depends on the features of the underlying malignancy and presence of minimal residual disease (MRD). The molecular features that characterize high-risk leukemias have significantly shaped the practice of transplantation, with the integration of transplantation earlier in the disease process for high-risk diseases [11]. MRD is defined as the presence of small amounts of leukemia cells without overt morphologic evidence of disease [53–55]. The mechanisms that lead to relapse include loss of the HLA haplotype in host leukemia cells; this completely abrogates the recognition of the leukemia by donor T cells [56, 57]. The choice of specific conditioning and stem cell source for any given individual is shaped by the disease stage, molecular features of the underlying disease, and presence of MRD [54, 55].

The graft-versus-leukemia (GVL) effect is a term that describes an inverse correlation between clinical GVHD and relapse in which transplant recipients who experience clinical GVHD have a lower overall rate of post-transplant relapse compared to those who do not have GVHD [58–60]. The anti-leukemic effect of an allogeneic transplant is abolished with the depletion of donor T cells, and relapse rates are highest for patients receiving identical twin transplants. These critical clinical observations provided early evidence of a role of donor T cells and the recognition of host disparities as integral to a robust GVL effect.

## GVHD

In HLA-matched sibling transplantation, 8% of deaths occurring before day 100 and 10% of deaths occurring after day 100 are due to GVHD; conversely, in unrelated donor transplantation, those incidences are 11% and 12%, respectively [4]. Acute GVHD is a clinical triad of dermatitis, hepatitis, and enteritis. It is classically defined as the development of any of these clinical symptoms within the first 100 days after an allogeneic transplant. With the increasing use of RIC and NMA regimens, the clinical signs and symptoms may present after 100 days. The diagnosis is based on clinical findings. Often, pathology may be helpful to confirm clinical suspicion.

The risk of acute GVHD is influenced by the degree of donor HLA compatibility, patient age, and transplantation from female donors for male recipients [61]. GVHD risk increases with increasing numbers of donor HLA disparities in the graft-versus-host vector of incompatibility, defined as recipient HLA tissue types not present in the donor [25]. Of the five classic loci currently tested, a single HLA-DQB1 mismatch is tolerated better than mismatches at HLA-A, B, C or DRB1. Mismatching for the sixth genetic locus, HLA-DP, increases GVHD, and HLA-12/12 matching is routinely performed at many centers [62, 63].

Chronic GVHD is a major cause of morbidity and mortality after allogeneic transplantation [64–66]. Chronic GVHD is classically defined as clinical signs and symptoms occurring after day 100 of transplantation, with 50% of all patients developing chronic GVHD within the first 6 months after transplantation [66]. The risk factors for chronic GVHD include a prior history of acute GVHD, older patient age, female donors for male patients, HLA-mismatched graft sources, and use of growth factor-mobilized peripheral blood stem cell grafts compared to bone marrow grafts. The strategies that lower acute GVHD rates have not reliably reduced chronic GVHD rates. Increasing immunosuppression is the primary treatment strategy for acute GVHD, with corticosteroids being the mainstay of therapy.

The clinical manifestations of chronic GVHD may be restricted to one organ but typically involve two or three organ systems and may be dynamic. The diagnosis is based on the presence of at least one diagnostic feature that is highly suggestive and confirmed by biopsy or other relevant test(s). Eighty-five percent of transplant recipients who develop chronic GVHD and survive beyond 5 years are ultimately able to discontinue systemic therapy [40]. Corticosteroids are effective in approximately 50% of patients, although prolonged therapy may be required for some [66]. New regimens for the treatment of chronic GVHD offer promise [67]. Because of the range of tissues and organs that may be involved, a multidisciplinary team including transplant clinicians, pulmonologists, ophthalmologists, dermatologist, gynecologists, dentists, and physical therapists, among others, are often needed to care for patients with chronic GVHD.

## Infection and Organ Toxicity

In HLA-matched sibling transplantation, 19% of deaths before day 100 and 11% of deaths after day 100 are due to infectious complications; those rates in unrelated donor transplants are 21% and 13% [4]. Infectious complications after transplantation stem from the immunosuppressive consequences of the conditioning regimen, GVHD prophylaxis, and the need for immunosuppressive therapy of established clinical GVHD. Fever of unknown origin (FUO) is multifactorial and includes infections due to CMV, central venous catheter, occult sinusitis, hepatosplenic candidiasis, pulmonary or disseminated aspergillosis; additionally, acute GVHD may present as an FUO. Specific bacterial organisms that cause infections may differ in the pre- and post-engraftment periods [68].

There has been significantly lower incidence of severe liver disease and gastrointestinal toxicity with the use of RIC and NMA conditioning regimens and the use of prophylactic agents to prevent cholestatic liver injury associated with GVHD [69]. One of the more serious potential complications is sinusoidal obstructive syndrome (SOS, formerly veno-occlusive disease), which most commonly arises in the setting of sinusoidal toxicity due to myeloablative conditioning. SOS presents with the triad of tender hepatomegaly, fluid retention, and elevated serum bilirubin and is associated with portal hypertension. A recent international consensus conference for the diagnosis, grading, and treatment of SOS for pediatric and young adults provides the most comprehensive guidelines to date [70].

Idiopathic pneumonia syndrome (IPS) is an important non-infectious pulmonary complication associated with poor prognosis [71]. Prevention of IPS includes avoidance of drugs with pulmonary toxicity for conditioning and GVHD prevention and treatment. In-depth presentation of infectious complications and organ toxicity is beyond the scope of this chapter, and the reader is directed to outstanding review articles in these subjects [72–77].

## Late Effects

With the substantial improvements in early post-transplant support and management of transplant recipients, long-term survivorship is increasing and continued longitudinal preventive and treatment measures are required to maintain the health and quality of life of transplant survivors [78, 79]. It is estimated that by 2030, the number of transplant survivors may surpass 500,000 and represent all age groups [80]. Patients may be cured of their original malignancy, but remain at risk for potentially significant late effects including the development of secondary malignancies, chronic GVHD, and infection [81–85]. Cooperative research groups have provided consensus guidelines for the prevention, screening, and treatment of late effects [86–94].

Transplant recipients have nearly twice the risk of developing a subsequent neoplasm after transplantation than the general population, estimated to reach 15% at 25 years after transplantation with no evidence to date of a plateau [95]. The major cancer types include therapy-related myelodysplastic syndrome and acute leukemia, lymphoma, malignant melanoma, and solid tumors. The risk factors include receipt of chemotherapy and radiation therapy prior to transplantation, use of total body irradiation with the transplant conditioning regimen, HLA-mismatched transplantation, requirements for GVHD therapy, and viral infections (e.g., Epstein–Barr virus, EBV). Current recommendations for screening for post-transplant malignancies follow general guideline for breast, colorectal, cervical cancers; however, continued investigation into transplant-directed screening is a priority [91].

## Role of Palliative and Supportive Care in Transplantation

### Evidence for the Role of Palliative and Supportive Care in the Management of Patients and Caregivers

The psychological and social sequelae of transplantation are well described, and recently emphasis has been placed on the integration of palliative and supportive care into the long-term management of individuals who have received a transplant. Anxiety, depression, and somatization are well-recognized sequelae in transplant survivors and negatively impact long-term health and quality of life [96–100].

The burden of unmet psychological needs include anxiety, depression, and psychological distress that revolve around uncertainty and fear of disease recurrence, treatment-related financial burden, and may manifest as post-traumatic stress disorder and cognitive impairment [101–107]. The transplant process may significantly impact the patient's career goals and life priorities [108–115]. Suicidal ideation among transplant survivors is more frequent than in healthy caregivers and may require inpatient management [99, 116, 117].

Integral to the success of a transplant is the immeasurable support from caregivers. Evidence that related transplant donors and caregivers experience very complex emotions that may have long-lasting effects showcases the importance of supporting the entire family through the transplant process and beyond [118]. In many ways, caregivers may be impacted emotionally as much as the patient him/herself, if not perhaps more [119].

Evidence for the beneficial effects of palliative and supportive care in the management of transplant patients is available and broadly applicable to patients of all ages and diseases and all forms of transplantation procedures [120]. In an early study of patient and physician perceptions, physicians were less optimistic of the curative potential of transplantation than were patients [121]. A recent study by the ASTCT further sheds light on transplant physicians' perceptions on the role of palliative and supportive care [122]. Designed as a cross-sectional survey of transplant physicians, the questionnaire probed physician attitudes and access to palliative care services in their practice. The majority of transplant physicians trust palliative care clinicians but identified roadblocks to prescribing these services including a concern for the level of understanding needed to counsel transplant-specific medical issues and the negative connotation that the name "palliative care" has for clinicians. Female clinicians, clinicians in practice for less than 10 years, and clinicians with positive perceptions of the quality of palliative care services had more positive attitudes toward palliative care.

Taken together, substantial clinical experience to date provides strong rationale for the early integration of palliative and support care into the management of all transplant recipients and their caregivers. The specific interventions mandate multidisciplinary collaboration between transplantation, palliative care clinicians, and support teams.

## Goals

The goals of supportive care of patients and caregivers are to ease symptoms and psychological stress, aid clarification of treatment goals, and improve the quality of life [5, 123, 124]. Collaboration among palliative care and transplant clinicians ensures smooth communication between clinicians, patients and caregivers, and coordination of therapies [125]. Palliative care specialists serve an important role to support the patient and family in grief and with difficult decisions [5, 126].

Integration of palliative and supportive care for patients and caregivers early in the trajectory of the transplant offers patients, caregivers, and clinicians invaluable opportunities to assess individual needs for advanced care decisions and goals of care [127, 128]. Specific guidelines for symptom relief of fatigue [129], neuro-cognitive dysfunction [130], sleep disruption [131], nutritional compromise [132], mood disturbance and psychological distress [133] provide a foundation for clinical care. The importance of longitudinal follow-up cannot be overstated [81].

## Conclusions

A successful transplant is one that restores a patient's health and quality of life consistent with her or his life goals. It can be achieved through a multidisciplinary approach that encompasses disease eradication and achievement of immunological tolerance while preserving the physical and emotional well-being of the patient.

## References


1. Thomas ED. A history of haemopoietic cell transplantation. Br J Haematol. 1999;105(2):330–9. https://doi.org/10.1111/j.1365-2141.1999.01337.x.
2. Gratwohl A, Pasquini MC, Aljurf M, Atsuta Y, Baldomero H, Foeken L, Gratwohl M, Bouzas LF, Confer D, Frauendorfer K, Gluckman E, Greinix H, Horowitz M, Iida M, Lipton J, Madrigal A, Mohty M, Noel L, Novitzky N, Nunez J, Oudshoorn M, Passweg J, van Rood J, Szer J, Blume K, Appelbaum FR, Kodera Y, Niederwieser D, et al. One million haemopoietic stem-cell transplants: a retrospective observational study. Lancet Haematol. 2015;2(3):e91–100. https://doi.org/10.1016/S2352-3026(15)00028-9.
3. Gooley TA, Chien JW, Pergam SA, Hingorani S, Sorror ML, Boeckh M, Martin PJ, Sandmaier BM, Marr KA, Appelbaum FR, Storb R, McDonald GB. Reduced mortality after allogeneic hematopoietic-cell transplantation. N Engl J Med. 2010;363(22):2091–101. https://doi.org/10.1056/NEJMoa1004383.
4. D'Souza A, Fretham C. Current uses and outcomes of Hematopoietic Cell Transplantation (HCT): CIBMTR summary slides. 2019. https://www.cibmtr.org.
5. Tierney DK, Passaglia J, Jenkins P. Palliative care of hematopoietic cell transplant recipients and families. Semin Oncol Nurs. 2014;30(4):253–61. https://doi.org/10.1016/j.soncn.2014.08.007.
6. McDonald GB, Sandmaier BM, Mielcarek M, Sorror M, Pergam SA, Cheng G-S, Hingorani S, Boeckh M, Flowers MD, Lee SJ, Appelbaum FR, Storb R, Martin PJ, Deeg HJ, Schoch G, Gooley TA. Survival, nonrelapse mortality, and relapse-related mortality after allogeneic hematopoietic cell transplantation: comparing 2003–2007 versus 2013–2017 cohorts. Ann Intern Med. 2020;172(4):229–39. https://doi.org/10.7326/M19-2936.
7. Saber W, Opie S, Rizzo JD, Zhang MJ, Horowitz MM, Schriber J. Outcomes after matched unrelated donor versus identical sibling hematopoietic cell transplantation in adults with acute myelogenous leukemia. Blood. 2012;119(17):3908–16. https://doi.org/10.1182/blood-2011-09-381699.
8. Muffly L, Pasquini MC, Martens M, Brazauskas R, Zhu X, Adekola K, Aljurf M, Ballen KK, Bajel A, Baron F, Battiwalla M, Beitinjaneh A, Cahn JY, Carabasi M, Chen YB, Chhabra S, Ciurea S, Copelan E, D'Souza A, Edwards J, Foran J, Freytes CO, Fung HC, Gale RP, Giralt S, Hashmi SK, Hildebrandt GC, Ho V, Jakubowski A, Lazarus H, Luskin MR, Martino R, Maziarz R, McCarthy P, Nishihori T, Olin R, Olsson RF, Pawarode A, Peres E, Rezvani AR, Rizzieri D, Savani BN, Schouten HC, Sabloff M, Seftel M, Seo S, Sorror ML, Szer J, Wirk BM, Wood WA, Artz A. Increasing use of allogeneic hematopoietic cell transplantation in patients aged 70 years and older in the United States. Blood. 2017;130(9):1156–64. https://doi.org/10.1182/blood-2017-03-772368.
9. WorldMarrow.org. Total number of donors and cord blood units. 2020. https://statistics.wmda.info. Accessed 11 Mar 2020.
10. Petersdorf EW. The World Marrow Donor Association: 20 years of international collaboration for the support of unrelated donor and cord blood hematopoietic cell transplantation. Bone Marrow Transplant. 2010;45(5):807–10. https://doi.org/10.1038/bmt.2010.10.
11. Majhail NS, Farnia SH, Carpenter PA, Champlin RE, Crawford S, Marks DI, Omel JL, Orchard PJ, Palmer J, Saber W, Savani BN, Veys PA, Bredeson CN, Giralt SA, LeMaistre CF. Indications

for autologous and allogeneic hematopoietic cell transplantation: guidelines from the American Society for Blood and Marrow Transplantation. Biol Blood Marrow Transplant. 2015;21(11):1863–9. https://doi.org/10.1016/j.bbmt.2015.07.032.

12. Karnofsky DA, Abelmann WH, Craver LF, Burchenal JH. The use of the nitrogen mustards in the palliative treatment of carcinoma. With particular reference to bronchogenic carcinoma. Cancer. 1948;1(4):634–56. https://doi.org/10.1002/1097-0142(194811)1:4<634::AID-CNCR2820010410>3.0.CO;2-L.
13. Oken MM, Creech RH, Tormey DC, Horton J, Davis TE, McFadden ET, Carbone PP. Toxicity and response criteria of the Eastern Cooperative Oncology Group. Am J Clin Oncol. 1982;5(6):649–55.
14. Sorror ML, Logan BR, Zhu X, Rizzo JD, Cooke KR, McCarthy PL, Ho VT, Horowitz MM, Pasquini MC. Prospective validation of the predictive power of the hematopoietic cell transplantation comorbidity index: a center for International Blood and Marrow Transplant Research study. Biol Blood Marrow Transplant. 2015;21(8):1479–87. https://doi.org/10.1016/j.bbmt.2015.04.004.
15. Forman SJ, Negrin R, Antin JH, Appelbaum FR. Histocompatibility. In: Forman SJ, Antin JH, Appelbaum FR, editors. Thomas' hematopoietic cell transplantation. 5th ed. Wiley Blackwell; 2016. https://doi.org/10.1002/9781118416426.ch10.
16. Luznik L, O'Donnell PV, Fuchs EJ. Post-transplantation cyclophosphamide for tolerance induction in HLA-haploidentical bone marrow transplantation. Semin Oncol. 2012;39(6):683–93. https://doi.org/10.1053/j.seminoncol.2012.09.005.
17. Bashey A, Zhang X, Jackson K, Brown S, Ridgeway M, Solh M, Morris LE, Holland HK, Solomon SR. Comparison of outcomes of hematopoietic cell transplants from T-replete haploidentical donors using post-transplantation cyclophosphamide with 10 of 10 HLA-A, -B, -C, -DRB1, and -DQB1 allele-matched unrelated donors and HLA-identical sibling donors: a multivariable analysis including disease risk index. Biol Blood Marrow Transplant. 2016;22(1):125–33. https://doi.org/10.1016/j.bbmt.2015.09.002.
18. Luznik L, O'Donnell PV, Symons HJ, Chen AR, Leffell MS, Zahurak M, Gooley TA, Piantadosi S, Kaup M, Ambinder RF, Huff CA, Matsui W, Bolanos-Meade J, Borrello I, Powell JD, Harrington E, Warnock S, Flowers M, Brodsky RA, Sandmaier BM, Storb RF, Jones RJ, Fuchs EJ. HLA-haploidentical bone marrow transplantation for hematologic malignancies using nonmyeloablative conditioning and high-dose, posttransplantation cyclophosphamide. Biol Blood Marrow Transplant. 2008;14(6):641–50. https://doi.org/10.1016/j.bbmt.2008.03.005.
19. Ghosh N, Karmali R, Rocha V, Ahn KW, DiGilio A, Hari PN, Bachanova V, Bacher U, Dahi P, de Lima M, D'Souza A, Fenske TS, Ganguly S, Kharfan-Dabaja MA, Prestidge TD, Savani BN, Smith SM, Sureda AM, Waller EK, Jaglowski S, Herrera AF, Armand P, Salit RB, Wagner-Johnston ND, Fuchs E, Bolanos-Meade J, Hamadani M. Reduced-intensity transplantation for lymphomas using haploidentical related donors versus HLA-matched sibling donors: a Center for International Blood and Marrow Transplant Research Analysis. J Clin Oncol. 2016;34(26):3141–9. https://doi.org/10.1200/JCO.2015.66.3476.
20. Anasetti C, Logan BR, Lee SJ, Waller EK, Weisdorf DJ, Wingard JR, Cutler CS, Westervelt P, Woolfrey A, Couban S, Ehninger G, Johnston L, Maziarz RT, Pulsipher MA, Porter DL, Mineishi S, McCarty JM, Khan SP, Anderlini P, Bensinger WI, Leitman SF, Rowley SD, Bredeson C, Carter SL, Horowitz MM, Confer DL, et al. Peripheral-blood stem cells versus bone marrow from unrelated donors. N Engl J Med. 2012;367(16):1487–96. https://doi.org/10.1056/NEJMoa1203517.
21. Gluckman E, Rocha V, Boyer-Chammard A, Locatelli F, Arcese W, Pasquini R, Ortega J, Souillet G, Ferreira E, Laporte JP, Fernandez M, Chastang C. Outcome of cord-blood transplantation from related and unrelated donors. Eurocord Transplant Group and the European Blood and Marrow Transplantation Group. N Engl J Med. 1997;337(6):373–81. https://doi.org/10.1056/NEJM199708073370602.
22. Rubinstein P, Carrier C, Scaradavou A, Kurtzberg J, Adamson J, Migliaccio AR, Berkowitz RL, Cabbad M, Dobrila NL, Taylor PE, Rosenfield RE, Stevens CE. Outcomes among 562 recipients of placental-blood transplants from unrelated donors. N Engl J Med. 1998;339(22):1565–77. https://doi.org/10.1056/nejm199811263392201.
23. Wagner JE, Broxmeyer HE, Byrd RL, Zehnbauer B, Schmeckpeper B, Shah N, Griffin C, Emanuel PD, Zuckerman KS, Cooper S, et al. Transplantation of umbilical cord blood after myeloablative therapy: analysis of engraftment. Blood. 1992;79(7):1874–81.
24. Dehn J, Spellman S, Hurley CK, Shaw BE, Barker JN, Burns LJ, Confer DL, Eapen M, Fernandez-Vina M, Hartzman R, Maiers M, Marino SR, Mueller C, Perales MA, Rajalingam R, Pidala J. Selection of unrelated donors and cord blood units for hematopoietic cell transplantation: guidelines from the NMDP/CIBMTR. Blood. 2019;134(12):924–34. https://doi.org/10.1182/blood.2019001212.
25. Petersdorf EW, Carrington M, O'hUigin C, Bengtsson M, De Santis D, Dubois V, Gooley T, Horowitz M, Hsu K, Madrigal JA, Maiers MJ, Malkki M, McKallor C, Morishima Y, Oudshoorn M, Spellman SR, Villard J, Stevenson P, International Histocompatibility Working Group in Hematopoietic Cell T. Role of HLA-B exon 1 in graft-versus-host disease after unrelated haemopoietic cell transplantation: a retrospective cohort study. Lancet Haematol. 2020;7(1):e50–60. https://doi.org/10.1016/S2352-3026(19)30208-X.
26. Gragert L, Eapen M, Williams E, Freeman J, Spellman S, Baitty R, Hartzman R, Rizzo JD, Horowitz M, Confer D, Maiers M. HLA match likelihoods for hematopoietic stem-cell grafts in the U.S. registry. N Engl J Med. 2014;371(4):339–48. https://doi.org/10.1056/NEJMsa1311707.
27. Killick SB, Bown N, Cavenagh J, Dokal I, Foukaneli T, Hill A, Hillmen P, Ireland R, Kulasekararaj A, Mufti G, Snowden JA, Samarasinghe S, Wood A, Marsh JC, British Society for Standards in H. Guidelines for the diagnosis and management of adult aplastic anaemia. Br J Haematol. 2016;172(2):187–207. https://doi.org/10.1111/bjh.13853.
28. Pulsipher MA, Chitphakdithai P, Logan BR, Shaw BE, Wingard JR, Lazarus HM, Waller EK, Seftel M, Stroncek DF, Lopez AM, Maharaj D, Hematti P, O'Donnell PV, Loren AW, Leitman SF, Anderlini P, Goldstein SC, Levine JE, Navarro WH, Miller JP, Confer DL. Acute toxicities of unrelated bone marrow versus peripheral blood stem cell donation: results of a prospective trial from the National Marrow Donor Program. Blood. 2013;121(1):197–206. https://doi.org/10.1182/blood-2012-03-417667.
29. Lee SJ, Logan B, Westervelt P, Cutler C, Woolfrey A, Khan SP, Waller EK, Maziarz RT, Wu J, Shaw BE, Confer D, Horowitz MM, Anasetti C. Comparison of patient-reported outcomes in 5-year survivors who received bone marrow vs peripheral blood unrelated donor transplantation: long-term follow-up of a randomized clinical trial. JAMA Oncol. 2016;2(12):1583–9. https://doi.org/10.1001/jamaoncol.2016.2520.
30. Delaney C, Heimfeld S, Brashem-Stein C, Voorhies H, Manger RL, Bernstein ID. Notch-mediated expansion of human cord blood progenitor cells capable of rapid myeloid reconstitution. Nat Med. 2010;16(2):232–6. https://doi.org/10.1038/nm.2080.
31. Storb R, Sandmaier BM. Nonmyeloablative allogeneic hematopoietic cell transplantation. Haematologica. 2016;101(5):521–30. https://doi.org/10.3324/haematol.2015.132860.

32. Storb R, Gyurkocza B, Storer BE, Sorror ML, Blume K, Niederwieser D, Chauncey TR, Pulsipher MA, Petersen FB, Sahebi F, Agura ED, Hari P, Bruno B, McSweeney PA, Maris MB, Maziarz RT, Langston AA, Bethge W, Vindelov L, Franke GN, Laport GG, Yeager AM, Hubel K, Deeg HJ, Georges GE, Flowers ME, Martin PJ, Mielcarek M, Woolfrey AE, Maloney DG, Sandmaier BM. Graft-versus-host disease and graft-versus-tumor effects after allogeneic hematopoietic cell transplantation. J Clin Oncol. 2013;31(12):1530–8. https://doi.org/10.1200/jco.2012.45.0247.
33. Krishnan A, Pasquini MC, Logan B, Stadtmauer EA, Vesole DH, Alyea E 3rd, Antin JH, Comenzo R, Goodman S, Hari P, Laport G, Qazilbash MH, Rowley S, Sahebi F, Somlo G, Vogl DT, Weisdorf D, Ewell M, Wu J, Geller NL, Horowitz MM, Giralt S, Maloney DG, Blood Marrow Transplant Clinical Trials N. Autologous haemopoietic stem-cell transplantation followed by allogeneic or autologous haemopoietic stem-cell transplantation in patients with multiple myeloma (BMT CTN 0102): a phase 3 biological assignment trial. Lancet Oncol. 2011;12(13):1195–203. https://doi.org/10.1016/S1470-2045(11)70243-1.
34. Baron F, Storb R, Storer BE, Maris MB, Niederwieser D, Shizuru JA, Chauncey TR, Bruno B, Forman SJ, McSweeney PA, Maziarz RT, Pulsipher MA, Agura ED, Wade J, Sorror M, Maloney DG, Sandmaier BM. Factors associated with outcomes in allogeneic hematopoietic cell transplantation with nonmyeloablative conditioning after failed myeloablative hematopoietic cell transplantation. J Clin Oncol. 2006;24(25):4150–7. https://doi.org/10.1200/jco.2006.06.9914.
35. Gyurkocza B, Deeg HJ. Allogeneic hematopoietic cell transplantation for MDS: for whom, when and how? Blood Rev. 2012;26(6):247–54. https://doi.org/10.1016/j.blre.2012.08.002.
36. Chao NJ, Chen BJ. Prophylaxis and treatment of acute graft-versus-host disease. Semin Hematol. 2006;43(1):32–41. https://doi.org/10.1053/j.seminhematol.2005.09.007.
37. Ferrara JL, Levine JE, Reddy P, Holler E. Graft-versus-host disease. Lancet (London, England). 2009;373(9674):1550–61. https://doi.org/10.1016/s0140-6736(09)60237-3.
38. Marks DI, Hughes TP, Szydlo R, Kelly S, Cullis JO, Schwarer AP, Mackinnon S, Apperley J, Barrett AJ, Hows JM, et al. HLA-identical sibling donor bone marrow transplantation for chronic myeloid leukaemia in first chronic phase: influence of GVHD prophylaxis on outcome. Br J Haematol. 1992;81(3):383–90. https://doi.org/10.1111/j.1365-2141.1992.tb08244.
39. Ringden O, Pihlstedt P, Markling L, Aschan J, Baryd I, Ljungman P, Lonnqvist B, Tollemar J, Janossy G, Sundberg B. Prevention of graft-versus-host disease with T cell depletion or cyclosporin and methotrexate. A randomized trial in adult leukemic marrow recipients. Bone Marrow Transplant. 1991;7(3):221–6.
40. Stewart BL, Storer B, Storek J, Deeg HJ, Storb R, Hansen JA, Appelbaum FR, Carpenter PA, Sanders JE, Kiem HP, Nash RA, Petersdorf EW, Moravec C, Morton AJ, Anasetti C, Flowers ME, Martin PJ. Duration of immunosuppressive treatment for chronic graft-versus-host disease. Blood. 2004;104(12):3501–6. https://doi.org/10.1182/blood-2004-01-0200.
41. Kroger N, Solano C, Wolschke C, Bandini G, Patriarca F, Pini M, Nagler A, Selleri C, Risitano A, Messina G, Bethge W, Perez de Oteiza J, Duarte R, Carella AM, Cimminiello M, Guidi S, Finke J, Mordini N, Ferra C, Sierra J, Russo D, Petrini M, Milone G, Benedetti F, Heinzelmann M, Pastore D, Jurado M, Terruzzi E, Narni F, Volp A, Ayuk F, Ruutu T, Bonifazi F. Antilymphocyte globulin for prevention of chronic graft-versus-host disease. N Engl J Med. 2016;374(1):43–53. https://doi.org/10.1056/NEJMoa1506002.
42. Marmont AM, Gale RP, Butturini A, Goldman JM, Martelli MF, Prentice HG, Slavin S, Storb R, Truitt RL, Van Bekkum DW. T-cell depletion in allogeneic bone marrow transplantation: progress and problems. Haematologica. 1989;74(3):235–48.
43. Marmont AM, Horowitz MM, Gale RP, Sobocinski K, Ash RC, van Bekkum DW, Champlin RE, Dicke KA, Goldman JM, Good RA, et al. T-cell depletion of HLA-identical transplants in leukemia. Blood. 1991;78(8):2120–30.
44. Bleakley M, Heimfeld S, Loeb KR, Jones LA, Chaney C, Seropian S, Gooley TA, Sommermeyer F, Riddell SR, Shlomchik WD. Outcomes of acute leukemia patients transplanted with naive T cell-depleted stem cell grafts. J Clin Invest. 2015;125(7):2677–89. https://doi.org/10.1172/JCI81229.
45. Kasamon YL, Ambinder RF, Fuchs EJ, Zahurak M, Rosner GL, Bolanos-Meade J, Levis MJ, Gladstone DE, Huff CA, Swinnen LJ, Matsui WH, Borrello I, Brodsky RA, Jones RJ, Luznik L. Prospective study of nonmyeloablative, HLA-mismatched unrelated BMT with high-dose posttransplantation cyclophosphamide. Blood Adv. 2017;1(4):288–92. https://doi.org/10.1182/bloodadvances.2016002766.
46. Mielcarek M, Furlong T, O'Donnell PV, Storer BE, McCune JS, Storb R, Carpenter PA, Flowers ME, Appelbaum FR, Martin PJ. Posttransplantation cyclophosphamide for prevention of graft-versus-host disease after HLA-matched mobilized blood cell transplantation. Blood. 2016;127(11):1502–8. https://doi.org/10.1182/blood-2015-10-672071.
47. Luznik L, Fuchs EJ. High-dose, post-transplantation cyclophosphamide to promote graft-host tolerance after allogeneic hematopoietic stem cell transplantation. Immunol Res. 2010;47(1–3):65–77. https://doi.org/10.1007/s12026-009-8139-0.
48. Schrezenmeier H, Korper S, Hochsmann B, Weinstock C. Transfusion Support. In: Carreras E, Dufour C, Mohty M, Kroger N, editors. The EBMT handbook: hematopoietic stem cell transplantation and cellular therapies. Springer; 2019. p. 163–9. https://doi.org/10.1007/978-3-030-02278-5_23.
49. Lipkin AC, Lenssen P, Dickson BJ. Nutrition issues in hematopoietic stem cell transplantation: state of the art. Nutr Clin Pract. 2005;20(4):423–39. https://doi.org/10.1177/0115426505020004423.
50. Bays DJ, Thompson GR 3rd. Fungal infections of the stem cell transplant recipient and hematologic malignancy patients. Infect Dis Clin N Am. 2019;33(2):545–66. https://doi.org/10.1016/j.idc.2019.02.006.
51. Boeckh M, Murphy WJ, Peggs KS. Recent advances in cytomegalovirus: an update on pharmacologic and cellular therapies. Biol Blood Marrow Transplant. 2015;21(1):24–9. https://doi.org/10.1016/j.bbmt.2014.11.002.
52. Neofytos D. Antimicrobial prophylaxis and preemptive approaches for the prevention of infections in the stem cell transplant recipient, with analogies to the hematologic malignancy patient. Infect Dis Clin N Am. 2019;33(2):361–80. https://doi.org/10.1016/j.idc.2019.02.002.
53. Balsat M, Renneville A, Thomas X, de Botton S, Caillot D, Marceau A, Lemasle E, Marolleau JP, Nibourel O, Berthon C, Raffoux E, Pigneux A, Rodriguez C, Vey N, Cayuela JM, Hayette S, Braun T, Coude MM, Terre C, Celli-Lebras K, Dombret H, Preudhomme C, Boissel N. Postinduction minimal residual disease predicts outcome and benefit from allogeneic stem cell transplantation in acute myeloid leukemia with NPM1 mutation: a study by the Acute Leukemia French Association Group. J Clin Oncol. 2017;35(2):185–93. https://doi.org/10.1200/JCO.2016.67.1875.
54. Gilleece MH, Labopin M, Yakoub-Agha I, Volin L, Socie G, Ljungman P, Huynh A, Deconinck E, Wu D, Bourhis JH, Cahn JY, Polge E, Mohty M, Savani BN, Nagler A. Measurable residual disease, conditioning regimen intensity, and age predict outcome of allogeneic hematopoietic cell transplantation for acute myeloid leukemia in first remission: a registry analysis of 2292 patients by

the Acute Leukemia Working Party European Society of Blood and Marrow Transplantation. Am J Hematol. 2018;93(9):1142–52. https://doi.org/10.1002/ajh.25211.
55. Milano F, Gooley T, Wood B, Woolfrey A, Flowers ME, Doney K, Witherspoon R, Mielcarek M, Deeg JH, Sorror M, Dahlberg A, Sandmaier BM, Salit R, Petersdorf E, Appelbaum FR, Delaney C. Cord-blood transplantation in patients with minimal residual disease. N Engl J Med. 2016;375(10):944–53. https://doi.org/10.1056/NEJMoa1602074.
56. Crucitti L, Crocchiolo R, Toffalori C, Mazzi B, Greco R, Signori A, Sizzano F, Chiesa L, Zino E, Lupo Stanghellini MT, Assanelli A, Carrabba MG, Marktel S, Marcatti M, Bordignon C, Corti C, Bernardi M, Peccatori J, Bonini C, Fleischhauer K, Ciceri F, Vago L. Incidence, risk factors and clinical outcome of leukemia relapses with loss of the mismatched HLA after partially incompatible hematopoietic stem cell transplantation. Leukemia. 2015;29(5):1143–52. https://doi.org/10.1038/leu.2014.314.
57. Vago L, Perna SK, Zanussi M, Mazzi B, Barlassina C, Stanghellini MT, Perrelli NF, Cosentino C, Torri F, Angius A, Forno B, Casucci M, Bernardi M, Peccatori J, Corti C, Bondanza A, Ferrari M, Rossini S, Roncarolo MG, Bordignon C, Bonini C, Ciceri F, Fleischhauer K. Loss of mismatched HLA in leukemia after stem-cell transplantation. N Engl J Med. 2009;361(5):478–88. https://doi.org/10.1056/NEJMoa0811036.
58. Horowitz MM, Gale RP, Sondel PM, Goldman JM, Kersey J, Kolb HJ, Rimm AA, Ringden O, Rozman C, Speck B, et al. Graft-versus-leukemia reactions after bone marrow transplantation. Blood. 1990;75(3):555–62.
59. Kolb HJ, Schattenberg A, Goldman JM, Hertenstein B, Jacobsen N, Arcese W, Ljungman P, Ferrant A, Verdonck L, Niederwieser D, van Rhee F, Mittermueller J, de Witte T, Holler E, Ansari H. Graft-versus-leukemia effect of donor lymphocyte transfusions in marrow grafted patients. Blood. 1995;86(5):2041–50.
60. Weiden PL, Flournoy N, Thomas ED, Prentice R, Fefer A, Buckner CD, Storb R. Antileukemic effect of graft-versus-host disease in human recipients of allogeneic-marrow grafts. N Engl J Med. 1979;300(19):1068–73. https://doi.org/10.1056/nejm197905103001902.
61. Holler E, Greinix H, Zeiser R. Acute graft-versus-host disease. In: The EBMT handbook: hematopoietic stem cell transplantation and cellular therapies. 7th ed. Springer; 2019.
62. Fleischhauer K, Shaw BE, Gooley T, Malkki M, Bardy P, Bignon JD, Dubois V, Horowitz MM, Madrigal JA, Morishima Y, Oudshoorn M, Ringden O, Spellman S, Velardi A, Zino E, Petersdorf EW. Effect of T-cell-epitope matching at HLA-DPB1 in recipients of unrelated-donor haemopoietic-cell transplantation: a retrospective study. Lancet Oncol. 2012;13(4):366–74. https://doi.org/10.1016/s1470-2045(12)70004-9.
63. Petersdorf EW, Malkki M, O'hUigin C, Carrington M, Gooley T, Haagenson MD, Horowitz MM, Spellman SR, Wang T, Stevenson P. High HLA-DP expression and graft-versus-host disease. N Engl J Med. 2015;373(7):599–609. https://doi.org/10.1056/NEJMoa1500140.
64. Horwitz ME, Sullivan KM. Chronic graft-versus-host disease. Blood Rev. 2006;20(1):15–27. https://doi.org/10.1016/j.blre.2005.01.007.
65. Carpenter PA, Kitko CL, Elad S, Flowers ME, Gea-Banacloche JC, Halter JP, Hoodin F, Johnston L, Lawitschka A, McDonald GB, Opipari AW, Savani BN, Schultz KR, Smith SR, Syrjala KL, Treister N, Vogelsang GB, Williams KM, Pavletic SZ, Martin PJ, Lee SJ, Couriel DR. National Institutes of Health Consensus Development Project on Criteria for Clinical Trials in Chronic Graft-versus-Host Disease: V. The 2014 Ancillary Therapy and Supportive Care Working Group Report. Biol Blood Marrow Transplant. 2015;21(7):1167–87. https://doi.org/10.1016/j.bbmt.2015.03.024.
66. Flowers ME, Martin PJ. How we treat chronic graft-versus-host disease. Blood. 2015;125(4):606–15. https://doi.org/10.1182/blood-2014-08-551994.
67. Hill L, Alousi A, Kebriaei P, Mehta R, Rezvani K, Shpall E. New and emerging therapies for acute and chronic graft versus host disease. Ther Adv Hematol. 2018;9(1):21–46. https://doi.org/10.1177/2040620717741860.
68. Leather H, Wingard J. Bacterial infections. In: Thomas' hematopoietic cell transplantation; 2016. p. 1038–62. https://doi.org/10.1002/9781118416426.ch85.
69. McDonald GB. Advances in prevention and treatment of hepatic disorders following hematopoietic cell transplantation. Best Pract Res Clin Haematol. 2006;19(2):341–52. https://doi.org/10.1016/j.beha.2005.11.008.
70. Mahadeo KM, Bajwa R, Abdel-Azim H, Lehmann LE, Duncan C, Zantek N, Vittorio J, Angelo J, McArthur J, Schadler K, Chan S, Tewari P, Khazal S, Auletta JJ, Choi SW, Shoberu B, Kalwak K, Harden A, Kebriaei P, Abe JI, Li S, Moffet JR, Abraham S, Tambaro FP, Kleinschmidt K, Richardson PG, Corbacioglu S. Diagnosis, grading, and treatment recommendations for children, adolescents, and young adults with sinusoidal obstructive syndrome: an international expert position statement. Lancet Haematol. 2020;7(1):e61–72. https://doi.org/10.1016/s2352-3026(19)30201-7.
71. Vande Vusse LK, Madtes DK. Early onset noninfectious pulmonary syndromes after hematopoietic cell transplantation. Clin Chest Med. 2017;38(2):233–48. https://doi.org/10.1016/j.ccm.2016.12.007.
72. Dhar R. Neurologic complications of transplantation. Neurocrit Care. 2018;28(1):4–11. https://doi.org/10.1007/s12028-017-0387-6.
73. Gargiulo G, Orlando L, Alberani F, Crabu G, Di Maio A, Duranti L, Errico A, Liptrott S, Pitrone R, Santarone S, Soliman C, Trunfio A, Selleri C, Bruno B, Mammoliti S, Pane F. Haemorrhagic cystitis in haematopoietic stem cell transplantation (HSCT): a prospective observational study of incidence and management in HSCT centres within the GITMO network (Gruppo Italiano Trapianto Midollo Osseo). Ecancermedicalscience. 2014;8:420. https://doi.org/10.3332/ecancer.2014.420.
74. Kemmner S, Verbeek M, Heemann U. Renal dysfunction following bone marrow transplantation. J Nephrol. 2017;30(2):201–9. https://doi.org/10.1007/s40620-016-0345-y.
75. Kendler DL, Body JJ, Brandi ML, Broady R, Cannata-Andia J, Cannata-Ortiz MJ, El Maghraoui A, Guglielmi G, Hadji P, Pierroz DD, de Villiers TJ, Rizzoli R, Ebeling PR. Bone management in hematologic stem cell transplant recipients. Osteoporosis Int. 2018;29(12):2597–610. https://doi.org/10.1007/s00198-018-4669-4.
76. Majorana A, Schubert MM, Porta F, Ugazio AG, Sapelli PL. Oral complications of pediatric hematopoietic cell transplantation: diagnosis and management. Support Care Cancer. 2000;8(5):353–65. https://doi.org/10.1007/s005200050003.
77. Rotz SJ, Leino D, Szabo S, Mangino JL, Turpin BK, Pressey JG. Severe cytokine release syndrome in a patient receiving PD-1-directed therapy. Pediatr Blood Cancer. 2017;64(12). https://doi.org/10.1002/pbc.26642.
78. Inamoto Y, Lee SJ. Late effects of blood and marrow transplantation. Haematologica. 2017;102(4):614–25. https://doi.org/10.3324/haematol.2016.150250.
79. Majhail NS. Long-term complications after hematopoietic cell transplantation. Hematol Oncol Stem Cell Ther. 2017;10(4):220–7. https://doi.org/10.1016/j.hemonc.2017.05.009.
80. Majhail NS, Rizzo JD. Surviving the cure: long term followup of hematopoietic cell transplant recipients. Bone Marrow Transplant. 2013;48(9):1145–51. https://doi.org/10.1038/bmt.2012.258.

81. Clark CA, Savani M, Mohty M, Savani BN. What do we need to know about allogeneic hematopoietic stem cell transplant survivors? Bone Marrow Transplant. 2016;51(8):1025–31. https://doi.org/10.1038/bmt.2016.95.
82. Majhail NS, Rizzo JD, Lee SJ, Aljurf M, Atsuta Y, Bonfim C, Burns LJ, Chaudhri N, Davies S, Okamoto S, Seber A, Socie G, Szer J, Van Lint MT, Wingard JR, Tichelli A, Center for International B, Marrow Transplant R, American Society for B, Marrow T, European Group for B, Marrow T, Asia-Pacific B, Marrow Transplantation G, Bone Marrow Transplant Society of A, New Z, East Mediterranean B, Marrow Transplantation G, Sociedade Brasileira de Transplante de Medula O. Recommended screening and preventive practices for long-term survivors after hematopoietic cell transplantation. Biol Blood Marrow Transplant. 2012b;18(3):348–71. https://doi.org/10.1016/j.bbmt.2011.12.519.
83. Majhail NS, Tao L, Bredeson C, Davies S, Dehn J, Gajewski JL, Hahn T, Jakubowski A, Joffe S, Lazarus HM, Parsons SK, Robien K, Lee SJ, Kuntz KM. Prevalence of hematopoietic cell transplant survivors in the United States. Biol Blood Marrow Transplant. 2013;19(10):1498–501. https://doi.org/10.1016/j.bbmt.2013.07.020.
84. Savani BN, Griffith ML, Jagasia S, Lee SJ. How I treat late effects in adults after allogeneic stem cell transplantation. Blood. 2011;117(11):3002–9. https://doi.org/10.1182/blood-2010-10-263095.
85. Syrjala KL, Martin PJ, Lee SJ. Delivering care to long-term adult survivors of hematopoietic cell transplantation. J Clin Oncol. 2012;30(30):3746–51. https://doi.org/10.1200/JCO.2012.42.3038.
86. Armenian SH, Chemaitilly W, Chen M, Chow EJ, Duncan CN, Jones LW, Pulsipher MA, Remaley AT, Rovo A, Salooja N, Battiwalla M. National Institutes of Health Hematopoietic Cell Transplantation Late Effects Initiative: the Cardiovascular Disease and Associated Risk Factors Working Group Report. Biol Blood Marrow Transplant. 2017;23(2):201–10. https://doi.org/10.1016/j.bbmt.2016.08.019.
87. Battiwalla M, Tichelli A, Majhail NS. Reprint of: long-term survivorship after hematopoietic cell transplantation: roadmap for research and care. Biol Blood Marrow Transplant. 2017;23(3S):S1–9. https://doi.org/10.1016/j.bbmt.2017.01.001.
88. Bevans M, El-Jawahri A, Tierney DK, Wiener L, Wood WA, Hoodin F, Kent EE, Jacobsen PB, Lee SJ, Hsieh MM, Denzen EM, Syrjala KL. National Institutes of Health Hematopoietic Cell Transplantation Late Effects Initiative: the Patient-Centered Outcomes Working Group Report. Biol Blood Marrow Transplant. 2017;23(4):538–51. https://doi.org/10.1016/j.bbmt.2016.09.011.
89. Gea-Banacloche J, Komanduri KV, Carpenter P, Paczesny S, Sarantopoulos S, Young JA, El Kassar N, Le RQ, Schultz KR, Griffith LM, Savani BN, Wingard JR. National Institutes of Health Hematopoietic Cell Transplantation Late Effects Initiative: the Immune Dysregulation and Pathobiology Working Group Report. Biol Blood Marrow Transplant. 2017;23(6):870–81. https://doi.org/10.1016/j.bbmt.2016.10.001.
90. Hashmi SK, Bredeson C, Duarte RF, Farnia S, Ferrey S, Fitzhugh C, Flowers MED, Gajewski J, Gastineau D, Greenwald M, Jagasia M, Martin P, Rizzo JD, Schmit-Pokorny K, Majhail NS. National Institutes of Health Blood and Marrow Transplant Late Effects Initiative: the Healthcare Delivery Working Group Report. Biol Blood Marrow Transplant. 2017;23(5):717–25. https://doi.org/10.1016/j.bbmt.2016.09.025.
91. Majhail NS, Rizzo JD, Lee SJ, Aljurf M, Atsuta Y, Bonfim C, Burns LJ, Chaudhri N, Davies S, Okamoto S, Seber A, Socie G, Szer J, Van Lint MT, Wingard JR, Tichelli A. Recommended screening and preventive practices for long-term survivors after hematopoietic cell transplantation. Biol Blood Marrow Transplant. 2012a;18(3):348–71. https://doi.org/10.1016/j.bbmt.2011.12.519.
92. Morton LM, Saber W, Baker KS, Barrett AJ, Bhatia S, Engels EA, Gadalla SM, Kleiner DE, Pavletic S, Burns LJ. National Institutes of Health Hematopoietic Cell Transplantation Late Effects Initiative: the Subsequent Neoplasms Working Group Report. Biol Blood Marrow Transplant. 2017;23(3):367–78. https://doi.org/10.1016/j.bbmt.2016.09.005.
93. Rizzo JD, Wingard JR, Tichelli A, Lee SJ, Van Lint MT, Burns LJ, Davies SM, Ferrara JL, Socie G. Recommended screening and preventive practices for long-term survivors after hematopoietic cell transplantation: joint recommendations of the European Group for Blood and Marrow Transplantation, the Center for International Blood and Marrow Transplant Research, and the American Society of Blood and Marrow Transplantation. Biol Blood Marrow Transplant. 2006;12(2):138–51. https://doi.org/10.1016/j.bbmt.2005.09.012.
94. Shaw BE, Hahn T, Martin PJ, Mitchell SA, Petersdorf EW, Armstrong GT, Shelburne N, Storer BE, Bhatia S. National Institutes of Health Hematopoietic Cell Transplantation Late Effects Initiative: the Research Methodology and Study Design Working Group Report. Biol Blood Marrow Transplant. 2017;23(1):10–23. https://doi.org/10.1016/j.bbmt.2016.08.018.
95. Bhatia S, Bhatia R. Subsequent malignant neoplasms after hematopoietic cell transplantation. In: Thomas' hematopoietic cell transplantation. Wiley-Blackwell; 2016. p. 1275–89. https://doi.org/10.1002/9781118416426.ch104.
96. Bevans MF, Mitchell SA, Barrett JA, Bishop MR, Childs R, Fowler D, Krumlauf M, Prince P, Shelburne N, Wehrlen L, Yang L. Symptom distress predicts long-term health and well-being in allogeneic stem cell transplantation survivors. Biol Blood Marrow Transplant. 2014;20(3):387–95. https://doi.org/10.1016/j.bbmt.2013.12.001.
97. Esser P, Kuba K, Scherwath A, Johansen C, Schwinn A, Schirmer L, Schulz-Kindermann F, Kruse M, Koch U, Zander AR, Kroger N, Gotze H, Mehnert A. Stability and priority of symptoms and symptom clusters among allogeneic HSCT patients within a 5-year longitudinal study. J Pain Symptom Manag. 2017a;54(4):493–500. https://doi.org/10.1016/j.jpainsymman.2017.07.012.
98. Esser P, Kuba K, Scherwath A, Schirmer L, Schulz-Kindermann F, Dinkel A, Balck F, Koch U, Kroger N, Gotze H, Mehnert A. Posttraumatic stress disorder symptomatology in the course of allogeneic HSCT: a prospective study. J Cancer Surviv. 2017b;11(2):203–10. https://doi.org/10.1007/s11764-016-0579-7.
99. Sun CL, Francisco L, Baker KS, Weisdorf DJ, Forman SJ, Bhatia S. Adverse psychological outcomes in long-term survivors of hematopoietic cell transplantation: a report from the Bone Marrow Transplant Survivor Study (BMTSS). Blood. 2011;118(17):4723–31. https://doi.org/10.1182/blood-2011-04-348730.
100. Syrjala KL, Langer SL, Abrams JR, Storer B, Sanders JE, Flowers ME, Martin PJ. Recovery and long-term function after hematopoietic cell transplantation for leukemia or lymphoma. JAMA. 2004;291(19):2335–43. https://doi.org/10.1001/jama.291.19.2335.
101. Abel GA, Albelda R, Khera N, Hahn T, Salas Coronado DY, Odejide OO, Bona K, Tucker-Seeley R, Soiffer R. Financial hardship and patient-reported outcomes after hematopoietic cell transplantation. Biol Blood Marrow Transplant. 2016;22(8):1504–10. https://doi.org/10.1016/j.bbmt.2016.05.008.
102. Barata A, Wood WA, Choi SW, Jim HS. Unmet needs for psychosocial care in hematologic malignancies and hematopoietic cell transplant. Curr Hematol Malig Rep. 2016;11(4):280–7. https://doi.org/10.1007/s11899-016-0328-z.
103. El-Jawahri AR, Vandusen HB, Traeger LN, Fishbein JN, Keenan T, Gallagher ER, Greer JA, Pirl WF, Jackson VA, Spitzer TR, Chen YB, Temel JS. Quality of life and mood predict posttraumatic stress disorder after hematopoietic stem cell transplanta-

tion. Cancer. 2016b;122(5):806–12. https://doi.org/10.1002/cncr.29818.
104. Epstein AS, Goldberg GR, Meier DE. Palliative care and hematologic oncology: the promise of collaboration. Blood Rev. 2012;26(6):233–9. https://doi.org/10.1016/j.blre.2012.07.001.
105. Khera N, Chang YH, Hashmi S, Slack J, Beebe T, Roy V, Noel P, Fauble V, Sproat L, Tilburt J, Leis JF, Mikhael J. Financial burden in recipients of allogeneic hematopoietic cell transplantation. Biol Blood Marrow Transplant. 2014;20(9):1375–81. https://doi.org/10.1016/j.bbmt.2014.05.011.
106. Kim W, McNulty J, Chang YH, Weise M, Hashmi S, Ailawadhi S, Khera N. Financial burden after allogeneic hematopoietic cell transplantation: a qualitative analysis from the patient's perspective. Bone Marrow Transplant. 2015;50(9):1259–61. https://doi.org/10.1038/bmt.2015.128.
107. Rueda-Lara M, Lopez-Patton MR. Psychiatric and psychosocial challenges in patients undergoing haematopoietic stem cell transplants. Int Rev Psychiatry. 2014;26(1):74–86. https://doi.org/10.3109/09540261.2013.866075.
108. Hamilton JG, Wu LM, Austin JE, Valdimarsdottir H, Basmajian K, Vu A, Rowley SD, Isola L, Redd WH, Rini C. Economic survivorship stress is associated with poor health-related quality of life among distressed survivors of hematopoietic stem cell transplantation. Psychooncology. 2013;22(4):911–21. https://doi.org/10.1002/pon.3091.
109. Jeon M, Yoo IY, Kim S, Lee J. Post-traumatic growth in survivors of allogeneic hematopoietic stem cell transplantation. Psychooncology. 2015;24(8):871–7. https://doi.org/10.1002/pon.3724.
110. Kirchhoff AC, Leisenring W, Syrjala KL. Prospective predictors of return to work in the 5 years after hematopoietic cell transplantation. J Cancer Surviv. 2010;4(1):33–44. https://doi.org/10.1007/s11764-009-0105-2.
111. Morrison EJ, Ehlers SL, Bronars CA, Patten CA, Brockman TA, Cerhan JR, Hogan WJ, Hashmi SK, Gastineau DA. Employment status as an indicator of recovery and function one year after hematopoietic stem cell transplantation. Biol Blood Marrow Transplant. 2016;22(9):1690–5. https://doi.org/10.1016/j.bbmt.2016.05.013.
112. Nelson AM, Juckett MB, Coe CL, Costanzo ES. Illness perceptions predict health practices and mental health following hematopoietic stem cell transplantation. Psychooncology. 2019;28(6):1252–126.
113. Nenova M, DuHamel K, Zemon V, Rini C, Redd WH. Posttraumatic growth, social support, and social constraint in hematopoietic stem cell transplant survivors. Psychooncology. 2013;22(1):195–202. https://doi.org/10.1002/pon.2073.
114. Norkin M, Hsu JW, Wingard JR. Quality of life, social challenges, and psychosocial support for long-term survivors after allogeneic hematopoietic stem-cell transplantation. Semin Hematol. 2012;49(1):104–9. https://doi.org/10.1053/j.seminhematol.2011.10.004.
115. Prince P, Mitchell SA, Wehrlen L, Childs R, Savani B, Yang L, Bevans M. Spiritual well-being in hispanic and non-hispanic survivors of allogeneic hematopoietic stem cell transplantation. J Psychosoc Oncol. 2015;33(6):635–54. https://doi.org/10.1080/07347332.2015.1082167.
116. Flowers ME, Traina F, Storer B, Maris M, Bethge WA, Carpenter P, Appelbaum F, Storb R, Sandmaier BM, Martin PJ. Serious graft-versus-host disease after hematopoietic cell transplantation following nonmyeloablative conditioning. Bone Marrow Transplant. 2005;35(3):277–82. https://doi.org/10.1038/sj.bmt.1704767.
117. Tichelli A, Labopin M, Rovo A, Badoglio M, Arat M, van Lint MT, Lawitschka A, Schwarze CP, Passweg J, Socie G. Increase of suicide and accidental death after hematopoietic stem cell transplantation: a cohort study on behalf of the Late Effects Working Party of the European Group for Blood and Marrow Transplantation (EBMT). Cancer. 2013;119(11):2012–21. https://doi.org/10.1002/cncr.27987.
118. Hutt D, Nehari M, Munitz-Shenkar D, Alkalay Y, Toren A, Bielorai B. Hematopoietic stem cell donation: psychological perspectives of pediatric sibling donors and their parents. Bone Marrow Transplant. 2015;50(10):1337–42. https://doi.org/10.1038/bmt.2015.152.
119. Posluszny DM, Bovbjerg DH, Syrjala KL, Agha M, Dew MA. Correlates of anxiety and depression symptoms among patients and their family caregivers prior to allogeneic hematopoietic cell transplant for hematological malignancies. Support Care Cancer. 2019;27(2):591–600. https://doi.org/10.1007/s00520-018-4346-3.
120. Ehrlich KB, Miller GE, Scheide T, Baveja S, Weiland R, Galvin J, Mehta J, Penedo FJ. Pre-transplant emotional support is associated with longer survival after allogeneic hematopoietic stem cell transplantation. Bone Marrow Transplant. 2016;51(12):1594–8. https://doi.org/10.1038/bmt.2016.191.
121. Lee SJ, Loberiza FR, Rizzo JD, Soiffer RJ, Antin JH, Weeks JC. Optimistic expectations and survival after hematopoietic stem cell transplantation. Biol Blood Marrow Transplant. 2003;9(6):389–96. https://doi.org/10.1016/s1083-8791(03)00103-4.
122. El-Jawahri A, LeBlanc TW, Burns LJ, Denzen E, Meyer C, Mau LW, Roeland EJ, Wood WA, Petersdorf E. What do transplant physicians think about palliative care? A national survey study. Cancer. 2018;124(23):4556–66. https://doi.org/10.1002/cncr.31709.
123. Ferrell BR, Temel JS, Temin S, Alesi ER, Balboni TA, Basch EM, Firn JI, Paice JA, Peppercorn JM, Phillips T, Stovall EL, Zimmermann C, Smith TJ. Integration of palliative care into standard oncology care: American Society of Clinical Oncology Clinical Practice guideline update. J Clin Oncol. 2017;35(1):96–112. https://doi.org/10.1200/JCO.2016.70.1474.
124. Smith TJ, Temin S, Alesi ER, Abernethy AP, Balboni TA, Basch EM, Ferrell BR, Loscalzo M, Meier DE, Paice JA, Peppercorn JM, Somerfield M, Stovall E, Von Roenn JH. American Society of Clinical Oncology provisional clinical opinion: the integration of palliative care into standard oncology care. J Clin Oncol. 2012;30(8):880–7. https://doi.org/10.1200/jco.2011.38.5161.
125. Chung HM, Lyckholm LJ, Smith TJ. Palliative care in BMT. Bone Marrow Transplant. 2009;43(4):265–73. https://doi.org/10.1038/bmt.2008.436.
126. Vergo MT, Cullinan AM. Joining together to improve outcomes: integrating specialty palliative care into the care of patients with cancer. J Natl Compr Cancer Netw. 2013;11(Suppl 4):S38–46. https://doi.org/10.6004/jnccn.2013.0220.
127. El-Jawahri A, LeBlanc T, VanDusen H, Traeger L, Greer JA, Pirl WF, Jackson VA, Telles J, Rhodes A, Spitzer TR, McAfee S, Chen YA, Lee SS, Temel JS. Effect of inpatient palliative care on quality of life 2 weeks after hematopoietic stem cell transplantation: a randomized clinical trial. JAMA. 2016a;316(20):2094–103. https://doi.org/10.1001/jama.2016.16786.
128. Mitchell SA. Palliative care during and following allogeneic hematopoietic stem cell transplantation. Curr Opin Support Palliat Care. 2018;12(1):58–64. https://doi.org/10.1097/SPC.0000000000000327.
129. Jafari H, Jannati Y, Nesheli HM, Hassanpour S. Effects of non-pharmacological interventions on reducing fatigue after hematopoietic stem cell transplantation. J Res Med Sci. 2017;22:13. https://doi.org/10.4103/1735-1995.199094.
130. Kelly DL, Buchbinder D, Duarte RF, Auletta JJ, Bhatt N, Byrne M, DeFilipp Z, Gabriel M, Mahindra A, Norkin M, Schoemans H, Shah AJ, Ahmed I, Atsuta Y, Basak GW, Beattie S, Bhella S, Bredeson C, Bunin N, Dalal J, Daly A, Gajewski J, Gale RP, Galvin J, Hamadani M, Hayashi RJ, Adekola K, Law J, Lee CJ,

Liesveld J, Malone AK, Nagler A, Naik S, Nishihori T, Parsons SK, Scherwath A, Schofield HL, Soiffer R, Szer J, Twist I, Warwick A, Wirk BM, Yi J, Battiwalla M, Flowers ME, Savani B, Shaw BE. Neurocognitive dysfunction in hematopoietic cell transplant recipients: expert review from the Late Effects and Quality of Life Working Committee of the Center for International Blood and Marrow Transplant Research and Complications and Quality of Life Working Party of the European Society for Blood and Marrow Transplantation. Biol Blood Marrow Transplant. 2018;24(2):228–41. https://doi.org/10.1016/j.bbmt.2017.09.004.

131. Jim HS, Evans B, Jeong JM, Gonzalez BD, Johnston L, Nelson AM, Kesler S, Phillips KM, Barata A, Pidala J, Palesh O. Sleep disruption in hematopoietic cell transplantation recipients: prevalence, severity, and clinical management. Biol Blood Marrow Transplant. 2014;20(10):1465–84. https://doi.org/10.1016/j.bbmt.2014.04.010.

132. Fuji S, Einsele H, Savani BN, Kapp M. Systematic nutritional support in allogeneic hematopoietic stem cell transplant recipients. Biol Blood Marrow Transplant. 2015;21(10):1707–13. https://doi.org/10.1016/j.bbmt.2015.07.003.

133. Baliousis M, Rennoldson M, Snowden JA. Psychological interventions for distress in adults undergoing haematopoietic stem cell transplantation: a systematic review with meta-analysis. Psychooncology. 2016;25(4):400–11. https://doi.org/10.1002/pon.3925.

# Serious Blood Disorders: A Focus on Sickle Cell Disease and Hemophilia

4

Sharl S. Azar and Srila Gopal

## Introduction to Inherited Nonmalignant Blood Disorders

Nonmalignant hematologic disorders impact the building blocks of coagulation, platelet and red cell structure and function, and the intricacies of cellular immunity. These congenital disorders affect patients from birth, coloring their childhood, challenging the transitions of adolescence, shaping the foundations of adulthood, and impacting the quality and quantity of life. Based on the pattern of genetic inheritance, they can often impact an entire family who may face more than one affected member while attempting to impose lifestyle changes in the home, school, and workplace. This chapter will focus on two of the most common congenital nonmalignant blood disorders: sickle cell disease and hemophilia. It is our hope that the models for the consideration and management of these disorders can be extended and tailored to the needs of their rarer counterparts and that this can become a rich area of investigation and development for patient populations that have often stood in the shadows of hematologic research.

S. S. Azar
Division of Hematology, Department of Medicine, Massachusetts General Hospital, Harvard Medical School, Boston, MA, USA
e-mail: sazar1@mgh.harvard.edu

S. Gopal (✉)
Division of Hematology/Oncology, Department of Medicine, University of California San Diego, La Jolla, CA, USA
e-mail: srgopal@health.ucsd.edu

## Sickle Cell Disease

### Overview

#### Epidemiology and Patterns of Inheritance

Sickle cell disease (SCD) is an inherited, life-threatening blood disorder, affecting nearly 100,000 Americans [1, 2]. In the United States (US) alone, 4000–5000 pregnancies annually result in some variant of SCD. The disease is most commonly seen in the African American population where the gene frequency for sickle hemoglobin (HbS) is 4% [3]. The disease is largely diagnosed at birth by newborn screening in the developed world, which is mandated in all 50 states in the US [4].

SCD is inherited in an autosomal recessive pattern and is characterized by the presence of an abnormal hemoglobin, also known as HbS [5]. HbS formation is the result of a single missense mutation in the gene encoding the beta globin chain (HBB) of the hemoglobin molecule that replaces a glutamic acid with a valine in the final polypeptide. If an HbS allele is paired with another HbS allele, this homozygous genotype (HbSS) confers sickle cell anemia (SCA), the most severe form of SCD. The HbS allele can also combine with other mutations in the HBB gene such as HbC or $HbSB^0$/$HbB^+$ alleles to form other SCD variants such as HbSC or HbS/$Beta^0$ or HbS/$Beta^+$ thalassemia [4]. HbS/$Beta^0$ thalassemia may be clinically indistinguishable from HbSS disease, while HbSC and HbS/$B^+$ thalassemia tend to be less severe forms.

#### Disease Manifestations, Signs, and Symptoms

The hallmark of SCD is the formation of sickle shaped red blood cells (RBCs) under conditions of stress due to polymerization of HbS. Unlike normal RBCs, sickle RBCs have altered rheological properties because of their abnormal shape, higher density and decreased distensibility and attract inflammatory cells, causing microvascular occlusion [5, 6]. Clinical manifestations of SCD are not apparent at birth due


C. K. Ullrich, E. J. Roeland (eds.), *Palliative Care in Hematologic Malignancies and Serious Blood Disorders*,
https://doi.org/10.1007/978-3-031-38058-7_4

to the higher percentage of fetal hemoglobin (HbF). It is only within the first few months of life as HbF levels wane that HbS levels begin to rise that the first signs and symptoms of disease become apparent. Dactylitis, a severe inflammation of the digits, is the most common initial symptom in SCD and occurs in 40% of the population overall [7]. As the spleen attempts to filter the aberrant sickled red cells, splenic sequestration will eventually manifest in 20% of patients and in 33% of patients who are symptomatic by 2 years of age [8]. In later years, the disease is characterized by episodes of blood vessel occlusion also known as vaso-occlusive crises (VOCs), which can cause widespread complications and affect nearly every organ system.

## Vaso-occlusive Crises

### Overview of Pain Crises

Of all the forms that VOCs can take, acute pain crisis remains the most recognizable complication for which patients seek medical attention. The frequency of acute pain crises peaks between 19 and 39 years of age and more frequent episodes over the age of 19 has been associated with increased mortality [9, 10]. In general, think of the incidence of VOCs in thirds: up to one-third of patients with SCD will rarely face a pain crisis, another one-third will experience pain crises with two to six hospitalizations annually, while the final third will be hospitalized more than six times per year. Triggers for pain crisis can vary widely from patient to patient. Both a higher hemoglobin concentration of >8.5 g/dL and low levels of HbF have both independently been shown to increase the risk of frequent pain crises [11]. Change in humidity or temperature, dehydration, infection, initiation of menses, alcohol consumption, and psychosocial stressors have been demonstrated to induce a pain crisis. An average pain crisis will last between 2 and 7 days and affect any part of the body, but most patients note pain in their bones [9]. Approximately 50% of episodes are accompanied with an additional finding like fever, swelling, tenderness, hypertension, or nausea and vomiting. Notably, there is no lab test that can definitively diagnose a pain crisis. A peripheral blood smear may indicate sickle cells, but this is not diagnostic of a crisis. Similarly, increased levels of acute phase reactants and inflammatory markers like C-reactive protein, fibrinogen, and lactate dehydrogenase can be seen as well as intriguing research evaluating levels of interleukin-1 and TNF but there has been no conclusive correlation between these values and the manifestation of an event [12–14].

### Overview of VOCs

VOCs can affect any and all organ systems in SCD. Common complications include acute chest syndrome (ACS), acute hepatopathy, fat necrosis and more chronically, avascular necrosis of the bones [7]. ACS refers to the collective acute pulmonary complications of SCD and occurs in 30–50% of patients with SCD, accounting for the second leading cause of hospitalization and the leading cause of death in adults [15]. Clinically, ACS is defined by the new appearance of an infiltrate on imaging with accompanying respiratory symptoms. This is often accompanied by fever, chest pain, cough, and hypoxia. ACS often will follow or occur in tandem with another VOC [16].

Patients with SCD are at an increased risk for infections, particularly by encapsulated organisms, due to functional asplenia from repeated splenic infarction [17, 18]. Augmenting this further is the inherent impact on the immune system itself with patients with SCD having irregular IgG and IgM antibody responses and defects in the alternative complement pathway. Bacteremia can be associated with aplastic or hypo-proliferative crises from marrow suppression or disseminated intravascular coagulopathy (DIC) leading to a mortality rate of 20–50% [19].

Approximately 24% of patients with SCD will experience a stroke by age 45, and 25% of children will have a silent ischemic lesion that may lead to impaired neurocognitive development [20–22]. Epilepsy is two to three times more common in individuals with SCD when compared to healthy controls and the development of dactylitis in childhood along with male sex have both been independently associated with an increased risk of developing a seizure syndrome [20]. As patients with SCD age, they are ultimately at an increased risk of neurocognitive decline and intracranial hemorrhage.

Cardiac complications of the disease also remain a major cause of death in adult patients. Myocardial infarction can occur in patients with SCD even in the absence of atherosclerotic or obstructive disease and is driven by increased oxygen supply demand mismatch [23, 24]. Chronic anemia impacts the cardiovascular system and can cause cardiac compromise and cardiomyopathy. SCD can also cause nephropathy, causing chronic kidney disease and sometimes end-stage renal disease [25]. Painful erections, also known as priapism, can occur in young boys and men, causing significant pain and distress. Recurrent priapism can lead to infertility and sexual dysfunction [26, 27].

Microvascular thromboses can cause infarction of the bone trabeculae and marrow cells in patients with SCD resulting in osteonecrosis [28]. Bone infarcts are worsened by increased rates of vitamin D deficiency and osteoporosis in the population. Such osseous abnormalities can give rise to fractures or deformities of the vertebrae that can lead to spinal instability [28].

## Treatment Options

Despite recent advances, SCD has limited effective treatment options. From a historical and contemporary perspective, hydroxyurea remains the cornerstone for the management of the disease and is strongly recommended by the National Heart Lung and Blood Institute guidelines for management of SCD [29]. The Multicenter Study of Hydroxyurea was a 2-year, multicenter double-blind, randomized, placebo-controlled trial in 300 patients with SCD that demonstrated a 50% reduction in VOC and 40% reduction in mortality with the use of hydroxyurea [30]. Hydroxyurea stimulates the production of HbF, possibly by augmenting HbF mRNA synthesis [31]. It has also been posited to increase the release of nitric oxide which in turn modulates the genetic regulation of HbF transcription and translation [32]. In addition, hydroxyurea may have anti-inflammatory effects at the sites of VOC, possibly by decreasing neutrophil counts [29]. Hydroxyurea is indicated for patients with frequent painful episodes (≥3 episodes within a 12-month period), with a history of ACS, other severe VOCs, or in severe symptomatic anemia [33]. The therapy is continued as long as it remains well tolerated and the dose is titrated to achieve a HbF level of around 15%. Adherence can be measured using the RBC mean corpuscular volume (MCV), which typically rises upon treatment with hydroxyurea. Despite recommendations for use, hydroxyurea is often poorly tolerated in adult patients and therapy adherence, unfortunately, is low [34].

RBC transfusions also play a significant role in the treatment of SCD. Transfusions have benefit both in the acute setting, in the treatment of life-threatening complications, and chronically, in prophylaxis [35]. Transfusions decrease HbS levels by dilution, decreasing blood viscosity, improving oxygen carrying capacity of the blood, and chronically by suppressing the hematopoietic drive and thereby decreasing the production of HbS. It must be stated that transfusions in SCD are not used to correct anemia in the absence of complications as this strategy poses more risks than benefits. In the acute setting, a clear benefit for transfusions has been seen in the management of acute strokes and severe ACS and to a lesser extent in multi-organ failure [36–38]. In the chronic setting, transfusions are effective in the secondary prevention of stroke and for prophylaxis against recurrent ACS and VOCs and in pregnancy [39]. The use of transfusions in the perioperative period has been shown to reduce the risk of surgery complications [40]. When available, automated or manual RBC exchange may be considered as an alternative to simple transfusions. Exchange transfusions, where a portion of the patient's blood volume is removed and replaced with donor blood, can be done in the acute setting and also every 4–6 weeks to maintain a goal HbS percentage of less than 30%. This strategy helps decrease HbS levels more efficiently while keeping blood viscosity low and also decreases the risk for iron overload. Selecting an exchange transfusion over a simple transfusion can be a practical matter of resources; however, exchange transfusions are preferred over simple transfusions where available [36, 37].

The risks and benefits of ongoing transfusion therapy should be reassessed frequently with the patient, especially given the high rates of transfusion-related complications, particularly RBC alloimmunization and iron overload. Iron overload is particularly problematic in this population as it threatens further organ damage [41]. Each unit of RBCs transfused introduces 200–250 mg of elemental iron to the patient and over time, this can lead to iron overload and deposition in the visceral organs. Iron chelation therapy is, thus, an important adjunct to any RBC transfusion program [42]. Liver biopsy or quantitative magnetic resonance imaging can be used to assess liver iron concentration, and chelation therapy should be considered when liver iron concentration is ≥7 mg Fe/g dry weight [43, 44]. Three iron chelators are currently commercially available in the US. No head-to-head trial has been completed to compare the efficacy or safety of these medications but one of the three agents, deferoxamine requires a daily, slow, subcutaneous injection. As a result, the two oral agents, deferiprone and deferasirox are more easily administered but have adverse effects and need frequent monitoring resulting in poor adherence [42, 45].

In the last few years, recognizing the need for additional therapeutics in SCD, the Food and Drug Administration (FDA) has fast tracked and approved three new therapeutic agents: L-Glutamine, voxelotor, and crizanlizumab (Table 4.1). L-Glutamine has been shown to decrease hospitalizations in SCD, especially when used in combination with hydroxyurea and was approved by the FDA in 2017 [46]. In November 2019, the FDA also approved voxelotor as the first modulator of hemoglobin oxygen affinity and as a hemoglobin stabilizer. In the HOPE trial, a randomized, double-blind, placebo-controlled study of 274 patients with SCD, voxelotor increased hemoglobin concentrations while reducing hemolysis but the trial failed to demonstrate an improvement in VOCs and this remains an area of future study [47]. The FDA also recently approved crizanlizumab for the prevention of VOCs in SCD [48]. Crizanlizumab is a P-selectin antagonist that reduces the adhesion of red cells to inflammatory cells and platelets during a VOC. In a phase 2 study of 198 patients with SCD and a history of VOCs, patients who received crizanlizumab experienced an average of 1.63 pain episodes annually with 35% of patients experiencing no episodes [49]. Patients in the placebo arm experienced 2.98 pain episodes annually while only 17% had no episodes at all [49].

The only potentially curative option in SCD is a hematopoietic cell transplant [50]. Several studies have demonstrated excellent results, even up to 80–90% sickle cell free 5-year survival coupled with a 90–97% overall survival. The complication rates of conditioning, post-transplant adverse events, and lack of matched donors, however, have markedly limited the wide use of hematopoietic stem cell transplants, especially in adult patients [51–53].

**Table 4.1** Therapeutic agents in sickle cell disease and their use

| Medication | Mechanism of action | Indications | Dose | Selected adverse reactions | Notes | Reference |
|---|---|---|---|---|---|---|
| Hydroxyurea | Exact mechanism unknown; increased HgF possibly through stimulation of HgF mRNA or regulation of transcription through nitric oxide release | ≥3 episodes within a 12-month period, history of ACS, history of other severe VOC, severe symptomatic anemia | 15–35 mg/kg/dose PO qd | Myelosuppression<br>Nail and skin hyperpigmentation<br>Nail and skin atrophy<br>Mucositis<br>Hepatotoxicity | Approved for patients 2 years and older | [29, 31–33] |
| L-Glutamine | Exact mechanism unknown; improved NAD redox potential preventing oxidative damage | If hydroxyurea is not well tolerated or VOCs persist despite hydroxyurea | **<30 kg:**<br>5 g PO bid<br>**30–65 kg:**<br>10 g PO bid<br>**>65 kg:**<br>15 g PO bid | Hypersplenism<br>Constipation<br>Chest and extremity Pain<br>Hot Flashes | Approved for patients 5 years and older | [46] |
| Voxelotor | Binds to the alpha chain of HbS increasing oxygen affinity and reducing polymerization | If hydroxyurea is not well tolerated or VOCs persist despite hydroxyurea | 1500 mg PO qd | Headache<br>Diarrhea<br>Abdominal pain | Approved for patients 12 years and older | [47] |
| Crizanlizumab | Inhibits P-selectin reducing interactions between endothelial cells and circulating blood cells | Persistent VOCs unresponsive to hydroxyurea, L-Glutamine, or both | 5 mg/kg IV on weeks 0 and 2; q4 weeks thereafter | Arthralgias<br>Fever<br>Infusion site reaction | Approved for patients 16 years and older | [48, 49] |

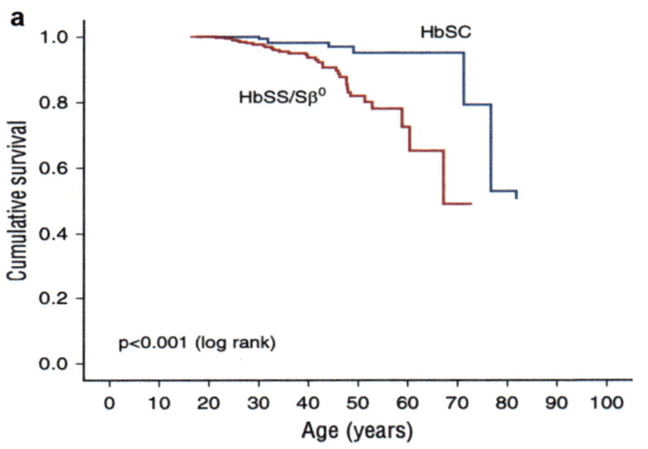


**Fig. 4.1** Survival curves for SCD by genotype (**a**) and for HbSS/HbSB by number of hospitalizations (**b**). Adult patients with SCD ($n$ = 712, 16–80 years of age) at King's College Hospital (London, United Kingdom) were observed over 10 years (2004–2013 inclusive) and mortality outcome was identified. Paulukonis S et al. [189]

Lastly, gene therapy offers tremendous promise in the management of SCD and may be a potential curative option for decades [54]. Currently, gene addition techniques, gene editing techniques, and induction of HbF synthesis are under investigation in pre-clinical models and in ongoing clinical trials. Gene therapy offers potential for cure and is an area of intense and rigorous study, but are yet to enter routine clinical practice [55].

## Prognosis and Lifespan Considerations

As a result of newborn screening, immunizations, treatment of infections, disease-modifying agents like hydroxyurea, and improved supportive care, the survivability of SCD has markedly improved over the last 10 years, but continues to be lower than that of the general population [4] (Fig. 4.1). However, in many parts of the world, particularly in sub-Saharan Africa, death in childhood remains an unfortunate reality. In the US, the greatest impact on mortality has occurred in pediatric patients with a steady decline in mortality rate over the last 20 years, particularly in children aged 0–3 years, where a 68% reduction in mortality has been observed [1]. It is now estimated that 94% of children with SCD in this country will survive into adulthood. Despite these improvements, patients with SCD die at a younger age than matched peers. A recent study projected life expectancy of 54 years for patients with SCD vs 76 years for a matched non-SCD cohort [56]. Adults with SCD face complications that involve nearly every organ including pulmonary hypertension, congestive heart failure, sickle nephropathy, sickle retinopathy, and sickle hepatopathy. Recent population-based studies suggest that SCD-related deaths in adults are more likely to be related to acute cardiac, pulmonary, and cerebrovascular complications; acute infections; and chronic cardiac and pulmonary complications and renal disorders [191].

## Transitions of Care

### Pediatric to Adult Transitions

As described above, a comprehensive approach to the care of patients with SCD is key to reduce morbidity and improve mortality in countries where such advances have been possible [57, 58]. As a result, the care of patients with SCD is best delivered through a multidisciplinary treatment center where patients can be followed longitudinally. Comprehensive SCD centers can help to empower and educate both the patients and their families while allowing them access to psychosocial and financial support [59]. Pediatric patients and their families can be followed by genetic counselors and social workers during important developmental milestones while being educated on the importance of infection control, complication reduction, and administration of disease-modifying agents. As patients approach adulthood, adolescents can be given tools and resources to detect complications of their disease early while learning to treat their symptoms and seek care independently [60–62].

### Challenges in Providing Comprehensive Adult Care

As the prognosis of SCD has shifted within the last several years with the majority of patients now reaching adulthood, the emergence of adult treatment centers has not risen quickly enough to absorb the new patients. Many patients with SCD remain under the care of their pediatric hematologists or fail to transition to an adult clinician, simply because they are unable to find an adult-trained physician with experience or expertise in SCD [57]. Despite the improvements in mortality and morbidity, young adults in the second and third decade of life suffer higher rates of disease-related complications and higher healthcare costs overall, possibly because of lack of access to standard measures such as transfusions and therapeutics [62]. Such findings stress the need for improved comprehensive adult care of patients with SCD and the urgent need for adult hematology clinicians interested in the management of this disease.

## Acute and Chronic Pain Management

### Opioid and Multimodality Therapy Plans

Pain management is an integral part of sickle cell therapy. Pain crises remain one of the costliest complications of SCD to both the patients and the healthcare systems [63]. Frequent hospital admissions are associated with school absenteeism and academic challenges in pediatric patients with similar occupational absenteeism as adults with diminished quality of life. Efforts to empower patients to live with their disease rather than live by the consequences of their disease are stifled by recurrent hospitalizations. An analysis in the US found that the lifetime cost of care for a patient with SCD was $460,151 per patient with 80.5% of that cost associated with hospital admissions [64]. A similar evaluation in the United Kingdom demonstrated that 91% of costs were dedicated to hospitalizations [65].

At the same time, VOCs can be extremely distressing to patients and their families and even maximal efforts to manage pain as an outpatient can falter requiring patients to seek more intensive treatment. Ultimately, the approach to managing a patient with SCD's pain, like all aspects of their care, is best done through a comprehensive and multidisciplinary approach [66]. Individual pain management plans have been developed to tailor management to each patient's needs. These plans layout strategies for managing both acute and chronic visceral and neuropathic pain, and not only provide guidance to the patient and their caregivers at home, but also standardize and normalize treatment when they present to the hospital for clinicians during an era when opioid prescribing has come under increased scrutiny [67–71]. Outpatient components of pain management plans can include the use of non-steroidal anti-inflammatory drugs along with long-acting and short-acting opioids. Inpatient plans can help direct clinicians to early initiation of opioids at effective doses and set titration schedules via continuous infusion and bolus dosing. Additional neuropathic therapeutics including ketamine and lidocaine infusions have also been studied for inpatient use and have demonstrated reduced opioid use during hospitalizations along with improved pain scores [72, 73].

Data regarding the impact of individualized pain management plans on hospitalizations is unfortunately limited but the use of such plans in the emergency department (ED) does improve pain control [68]. One study demonstrated that a coordinated multidisciplinary effort to develop individualized pain led to 88% of eligible patients having a plan in place with a concomitant reduction in ED visits for uncomplicated SCD-related pain [74]. These plans can also help overcome bias and discrimination that these patients often suffer when they access medical care, where they can often be mislabeled as "drug seekers" and denied appropriate pain control. For example, a 5-year quality improvement project at Yale New Haven Children's Hospital demonstrated the value of incorporating multiple modalities for the treatment of pain. In their study published in 2019, the researchers explored the role of a multidisciplinary team with representatives from pediatric hematology, child psychology, child psychiatry, adolescent medicine, pain medicine, pediatric emergency medicine, nursing, social work, child life, and quality improvement [66]. Their coordinated interventions yielded a 61% reduction in hospitalizations, a decreased hospital stay, reduction in readmission rates from 33.9% to 19.4%, and decreased direct hospital costs [66].

The development and utilization of a "day hospital" has also been demonstrated to reduce admission rates and augment quality of life for patients. Day hospitals act as monitored units that allow patients' pain crises to be managed with hydration, intravenous pain medications, and transfusions as needed over the course of several hours [75]. In one study, a 2-bed monitored day hospital that operated between the hours of 8 am and 5 pm 5 days per week for the evaluation and treatment of acute uncomplicated SCD-related pain demonstrated a marked reduction in hospital admissions [76]. Mean hospital cost and average length of stay for patients who ultimately did get admitted were also reduced with the day hospital [76–78].

Ultimately, improving the management of acute and chronic pain for patients with SCD requires buy in and education across the healthcare system. Teaching and empowering patients to care for their pain at home and recognizing when it is no longer safe to do so is only part of the solution. It is equally important to educate clinicians caring for patients with SCD long before the hematologist may be involved to assure that appropriate care is not delayed and that the patient is safe and comfortable.

### Optimizing Pain Management through Technology

As the electronic medical record (EMR) becomes a standard component of hospital systems and outpatient clinics across the US, utilization of the various systems to improve the care of patients with SCD has been of increasing interest. The development of individual pain management plans as described in the previous section is largely made possibly by EMR [74]. Some systems create alerts for clinicians in the ED that the patient has an individualized pain management plan in place and directs them to a location in the patient's chart where this plan can be found. Other systems have integrated safeguards to assure that the outpatient hematology team is contacted and involved early in the patient's care through the use of secure messaging or a virtual pager system. Order sets also standardize care across environments with curated options for pain control and symptom support along with preferred diagnostic lab and imaging choices [66]. While each patient's symptoms and management are dictated by their individual disease manifestations, such standards allow a framework for clinicians who may not be comfortable with the management of the disease. Additionally, the use of smart phone apps has been explored as a secure means of communication between patients and their clinicians, as a reminder for patients to remain vigilant about their disease modifying and pain regimens as well as a record keeping tool to track pain crises, other symptoms, and barriers to care [79–83].

### Integrative Medicine Approaches

The use of complementary and alternative medicine for the support of patients with SCD has been of increasing interest with one study observing that 92% of patients with SCD use some form of integrative medicine approach [84]. Unfortunately, data on the efficacy of these treatments in the SCD population is limited. Small studies have demonstrated that acupuncture and massage therapy may be effective in reducing pain [85–88]. While patients have individually reported use of massage, relaxation techniques, prayer, and other modalities as part of their treatment, no comprehensive evaluations of these interventions have been done to date.

## Considerations in Psychosocial Support

### Mental Health Considerations

As with any chronic disease starting in childhood, SCD is plagued with mental health issues. In addition, this disorder afflicts a minority population, often belonging to lower socio-economic strata which poses additional psychosocial challenges. In one study, 27.6% of patients with SCD had undiagnosed depression with 6.5% of patients having a previously undiagnosed anxiety disorder [89]. Patients noted to have depression recorded pain on significantly more days than non-depressed patients with higher distress from their pain and an increased interference in their activities of daily living. When assessed for overall functionality, patients with SCD and anxiety or depression had poorer overall function and anxious patients reported more opioid use [90–93]. Studies outside the US have demonstrated similar findings [94]. Moreover, the rise of the opioid epidemic in the US has made the management of SCD-related pain even more challenging for patients and clinicians alike. Adults with SCD report difficulties in obtaining prescriptions, inadequate dosing, and stigmatization that pose significant barriers in their treatment [95].

### Cognitive Impairment and the Impact of Silent Cerebral Infarctions

Patients with SCD can develop silent or overt cerebral infarctions, which over time, lead to neurocognitive impairment

[21]. SCD adults score worse than their healthy siblings on objective cognitive testing. Patients with SCD have reduced working memory, an integral component of language comprehension, learning, and reasoning [96]. Other studies show that these patients have reduced attention and selective visual scanning than age-matched healthy unrelated controls. These cognitive deficits can often impact their ability to care for themselves and their adherence with medications. Educating patients about these anticipated changes over time can allow identification and delivery of educational and occupational support in school and the workplace.

## Quality of Life Estimation Tools

### Adult Sickle Cell Quality of Life Measurement Information System

The Adult Sickle Cell Quality of Life Measurement Information System (ASCQ-Me) is a patient-reported outcome measurement system that evaluates the physical, social, and emotional impacts of living with SCD [97]. The questionnaire uses five items in each of six categories including emotional, pain episodes, pain impact, sleep impact, social functioning, and stiffness. It also incorporates nine questions about the patient's individual medical history. The reliability of this tool has been well demonstrated, and patients can fill out the questions themselves, however, the length of questionnaire often precludes its routine use in the clinic setting [98–100].

### Patient-Reported Outcome Measurement Information System

The Patient-Reported Outcome Measurement Information System (PROMIS) is a comprehensive tool that evaluates the physical, mental, and social health of patients across multiple disease states including patients with SCD [101, 102]. Specific tools are directed for pediatric patients with accompanying parent or guardian questionnaires with a separate tool tailored for adult patients [101, 103]. With four to six item questionnaires across a variety of domains, the individual components of PROMIS can be used independently to evaluate a single domain or can be collectively used with a common metric score that has been weighed against the mean US general population. The PROMIS has also been studied in conjunction with other tools including the ASCQ-Me [100, 104].

## Palliative Care and Sickle Cell Disease

The utilization of the palliative care team as an advocate for the SCD patient or as a facilitator for improved communication around symptom management has been proposed [105, 106]. Because of the physical, psychological, and emotional toll that the disease can take on patients and their families, initiating and building an open dialog that encourages and empowers patients to express how their disease plays into their daily activities and relationships can be an important tool in their treatment [107]. Palliative care providers can help young patients and their caregivers set goals and expectations while allowing them to revise these goals as they enter adulthood and become more independent. At the same time, integration of the palliative care team can help provide additional guidance on pain management and additional symptoms that can accompany VOCs. Finally, while advances in the disease are allowing patients to live a more full and robust life, the considerable morbidities of SCD along with its mortality warrant ongoing discussions about goals of care at the end of life and advance care planning. Our palliative care colleagues should be cognizant of the unique relationship that is forged between a patient and their medical team when they have faced a disease that has been present since childhood and that may impact other members of their families. Some patients have seen older family members suffer from comorbidities or die from the disease with those experiences playing a critical role in their own decision-making. At the same time, the fact that SCD primarily impacts people of color lends itself to important questions about health disparities and social determinants of health that call for an ongoing reevaluation of how we establish and build trust. These imperative discussions in the care of patients with SCD will only benefit further from the additional perspectives of our palliative care colleagues.

## Hemophilia A and B

## Overview

### Epidemiology and Patterns of Inheritance

Hemophilia A and B are X-linked bleeding diatheses defined by the absence or reduced production of coagulation Factor VIII and Factor IX, respectively [108]. Hemophilia A occurs in 1 in every 5000 live male births, and Hemophilia B occurs in 1 in every 30,000 live male births [109]. A vast number of point mutations, frameshift mutations, or missense mutations in the factor VIII or factor IX genes have been identified. Being X-linked, hemophilia affects males predominantly, female carriers can have varying degrees of symptoms rarely augmented by lyonization [110].

### Disease Manifestations, Signs, and Symptoms

Hemophilia A and B are categorized as mild, moderate, or severe based on the degree to which factor activity is reduced. Patients with undetectable factor activity (<1%) have severe disease, while those with a factor VIII activity of 1–5% or

>5% have moderate or mild disease, respectively [108]. Patients with severe hemophilia bleed spontaneously into their joints and muscles, while mild and moderate hemophiliacs have less severe bleeding patterns. Repeated bleeding into joints leads to the development of "target joints" and hemophilic arthropathy (HA), characterized by synovial proliferation along with bone and cartilage destruction [111]. Arthropathy can occur during childhood, and joint status can worsen with increasing age. The primary manifestation of HA is pain, but many patients will also describe a sense of fullness or swelling in the joint along with overlying erythema. On physical examination, the joint may appear edematous or boggy or may have no outward signs of injury aside from pain to palpation or with passive or active motion. Similar to joint bleeds, muscle bleeds can occur spontaneously or with injury. In addition to pain and swelling in the muscle, compartment syndrome can occur if bleeding is unabated, especially if the bleed occurs in the muscles of the arm or leg [112]. While less prone to occur spontaneously, intracranial bleeds after a traumatic event can be potentially devastating as can bleeds in the thoracic or abdominal cavities after injury [113].

## Treatment Options

In 1973, the National Hemophilia Foundation launched a campaign aimed at providing comprehensive services to patients with bleeding disorders at a single site [114, 115]. The goal of these comprehensive Hemophilia Treatment Centers (HTCs) was to meet the medical, physical, psychological, emotional, and social needs of patients with hemophilia [116]. Today, there are 141 federally funded HTCs in the US which manage both acute and preventative aspects of this disease, where the patient is evaluated and treated by each member of the multidisciplinary team. A federally funded HTC mandates that patients have access to a hematologist with experience in the management of bleeding disorders in addition to nurses, social work, and physical therapists with special expertise with this patient population [116]. Some centers will manage patients from infancy into adulthood while others manage only pediatric patients and then transition them to nearest adult centers. Pediatric centers often provide patients and their families access to genetic counselors, child life specialists, educational counselors, and nutritionists. Whereas many adult centers have integrated pharmacists, dental care, and primary care providers into their teams. HTCs also allow patients access to ongoing national and international clinical trials focused on improving the diagnosis and treatment of hemophilia.

HTCs remain the primary site for the acute treatment and prophylaxis of bleeding episodes. The treatment and prevention of bleeding episodes involve replacement of the missing clotting factor, which may be achieved using fresh frozen plasma (FFP), plasma derived or recombinant factor concentrates, and other novel therapies. Administration of FFP at 20–40 mL/kg (the equivalent of 4–6 units in an adult) will raise the levels of deficient factor by approximately 20% [117]. FFP however also carries the risks associated with blood product transfusions coupled with the additional volume of 250 mL with each unit.

The development of plasma-derived coagulation factor concentrates in the 1970s and 1980s allowed patients a treatment with markedly reduced fluid volume and the capacity to self-manage symptoms via an intravenous infusion at home [114]. Proprietary methods of viral inactivation have allowed these plasma-derived products to become increasingly safe. In 1992, the FDA approved the first recombinant factor VIII product and subsequently many recombinant factor VIII and factor IX products have been produced and are now standard of care in the management of hemophilia [115]. Modification of these recombinant products through PEGylation or the addition of an immunoglobulin chain (Fc) component has extended the product half-life allowing patients to dose less frequently or use lower doses [118].

Within the past 5 years, hemophilia management has dramatically shifted with the first introduction of non-factor treatment options [119]. In 2017, the FDA approved the bispecific monoclonal antibody, emicizumab for patients with hemophilia A. Emicizumab has binding sites for factor IX and activated factor X, and plays the role that factor VIII ordinarily would in the coagulation cascade [120]. The advantage of this medication over traditional factor replacement is that it can be injected subcutaneously rather than intravenously, sparing patients the need to access their own veins. After a weekly loading dose for 4 weeks, the medication can then be injected weekly, every 2 weeks, or even every 4 weeks, thus liberating patients from infusing factor two or three times weekly as is required in most prophylactic regimens.

Additionally, the advent of molecularly directed nucleic acid-targeting therapies is poised to further revolutionize the management of hemophilia [120, 121]. Ribonucleic acid inhibitor (RNAi)-based treatments treat hemophilia without replacing the absent or reduced protein. By targeting anticoagulant proteins like tissue factor pathway inhibitor (TFPI) or activated protein C (APC), these treatments aim to adjust the "hemostatic teeter-totter" that is off-balance through the endogenous absence of clotting factor [119, 120, 122]. Gene therapy aimed at increasing endogenous production of factor via hepatotropic vectors poses a potentially exciting approach to the management of hemophilia [123]. While prior attempts gave rise to mild augmentation of native factor production at best, newer approaches currently in clinical trials aim to transition patients with severe hemophilia to moderate or mild disease [123, 124]. While early data in this field is very promising, the practical limitations in adopting this into routine clinical practice remain.

### Disease Complications: Inhibitor Formation and Treatment

A considerable challenge in treating patients with hemophilia is the development of antibodies or "inhibitors" that neutralize infused clotting factor. These inhibitors are at greatest risk of occurring in the first 30–50 days after exposure to exogenous factor and as a result, are most often first detected in childhood [125, 126]. Eradication of an inhibitor can be achieved through use of immune tolerance induction (ITI) therapy [127]. This approach utilizes high doses of exogenous factor infused daily over several months in an effort to tolerize the immune system to the absent factor protein. This treatment is expensive and burdensome for patients, and the only has an efficacy of 50% [127]. The presence of an inhibitor not only prevents the continued use of exogenous factor but also necessitates a change in the treatment plan. Bypassing agents such as recombinant factor VIIa (rFVIIa), factor eight inhibitor bypassing agent (FEIBA), and emicizumab are potential treatment options for patients with inhibitors [127, 128]. Each of these approaches has its own limitations, rFVIIa and FEIBA are expensive, breakthrough bleeds can still occur, have unfavorable pharmacokinetics requiring more frequent dosing (every 2–4 h in the case of rFVIIa) for an active bleed, and lack a laboratory measure for monitoring their efficacy.

In the absence of bypassing agents, plasma-derived or recombinant factor products can be used at two to four times standard dosing temporarily in the setting of an acute bleed [128]. This will likely augment the inhibitor titer but should be restricted to emergency settings. Emicizumab has been approved by the FDA to treat congenital hemophilia A with inhibitors based on favorable clinical trial data with a significant decrease in bleeds [121, 129].

Notably, the development of alloantibodies against exogenous factor in patients with congenital hemophilia is biologically different from the autoantibodies that can develop in otherwise healthy individuals and induce acquired hemophilia. The long-term management of the two phenomena is different even though similar medications can be employed to treat acute bleeding in both settings.

### Prognosis and Lifespan Considerations

Prior to the introduction of plasma-derived and recombinant factor products, most patients with hemophilia would struggle to survive into adulthood. With these developments and with the introduction of the HTC comprehensive care model described above, most patients with hemophilia are now able to lead a full life [130, 131]. Significant strides have been made in the improvement of disease mortality sparking new discussions about the management of hemophilia in the aging population, including management of complications such as heart disease and high blood pressure [130–132]. The approach to maintaining patients with hemophilia on anticoagulants or antiplatelet agents after suffering thrombotic events, myocardial infarctions, or cerebrovascular accidents poses significant clinical conundrums [133]. Likewise managing patients with hemophilia in the setting of platelet altering chemotherapeutic regimens has become an emerging challenge as these patients develop malignancies often seen only in the last decades of life. As the current generation of patients with hemophilia age, identification of the best practices is required in managing joint pathology that developed over a full lifespan of bleeds [132].

## Transitions of Care

### Pediatric to Adult Transitions

With patients with hemophilia now able to live well into adulthood, the transition from pediatric to adult care has become an important priority of national hemophilia organizations for the last several years [134, 135]. In childhood, patients will have the support of parents or guardians who can help them detect and treat a bleed, bring them to appointments at the HTC, and inform schools about management considerations. As they age and become more independent, patients must learn to acquire many of these disease-management skills [136]. Many HTCs have established formal transition programs to help patients achieve milestones on their way to adult care [137]. Transition programs often begin by introducing the patient to the adult clinician and her or his team, if separate from the team caring for the patient in the pediatric setting. Many lifespan centers who see patients from infancy into adulthood will have the same social workers, nurses, or physical therapists who can provide valuable continuity for these patients.

Nursing and physician team members can coach patients on how to recognize the signs and symptoms of a bleed and how to reconstitute and infuse factor [135, 136]. Social workers are imperative in assisting patients with changes in insurance as they shift from their parents' plans onto their own. At the same time, social work can provide vocational or education guidance as adolescent patients plan for their future [134, 136]. It is critical to assure patients that their bleeding disorder does not prevent them from attending college or starting a job and that the HTC can provide resources and support to assure that the symptoms of the disease do not impact the quality of their studying or work. Physical therapy and athletic training can help improve strengthening and balance while initiating healthy lifestyle habits that can support them for decades to come.

### Inpatient to Outpatient Transitions and Perioperative Management

Despite the innovations in the management of patients with hemophilia, acute bleeds that necessitate inpatient management, and surgical interventions and procedures continue to occur. In the era of the aging hemophilia population with significant and debilitating arthropathy, joint replacement surgeries have become very common and require extensive coordination between the surgeons, anesthesiologists, inpatient and outpatient teams, physical therapists, social workers, and financial staff [138]. The HTC plays a central role in setting a factor support plan and coordinating care across specialties. HTCs also develop mechanisms to support patients who need help adjusting to a new and more vigorous factor infusion schedule after discharge, manage intravenous access, obtain insurance authorization for prescription coverage, and ensure access to clotting factor [139–141]. Efforts to improve and standardize these processes remain the subject of study and quality improvement interventions at HTCs across the country. At the center of all of this communication, it is imperative that the patient feel comfortable and confident that their hemophilia will not be a barrier to their safe and timely recovery.

## Hemophilic Arthropathy and Pain Management

### Overview and Factor Prophylaxis

As described above, HA remains one of the hallmarks of the disease and one of its most life-altering complications [111] (Fig. 4.2). Injury to the joint space through the recurrent deposition of blood over time leads to changes in the architecture and integrity of the joint and can give rise to crippling pain, reduced mobility, and decreased function [142]. At the same time, factor VIII may play a role in bone health and development overall and thus the combination of factor deficiency and recurrent joint bleeds can cause long-term skeletal damage [143, 144].

In her seminal work, Dr. Marilyn Manco-Johnson and colleagues identified that the integration of routine prophylaxis with exogenous factor could slow the development of HA and reduce the number of bleeds overall [145]. This pediatric study paved the way for prophylaxis to become the standard of care in patients with frequent bleeds [146]. Today, patients with severe hemophilia A or B or patients with mild or moderate disease that still manifest frequent bleeds are initiated on factor prophylaxis. However, maintaining a strict prophylaxis regimen can be taxing for even the most diligent patient and even a flawlessly followed prophylactic regimen will still give rise to intermittent bleeds and hence these patients often need therapy managed closely by the HTC.

### Integration of Physical Therapy

The role of physical therapy in the acute and long-term management of patients with hemophilia cannot be overstated. Physical therapy has been shown to reduce pain in the setting of an acute bleed and more rapidly restore joint function after a bleed has resolved [147, 148]. Beyond this, the inte-

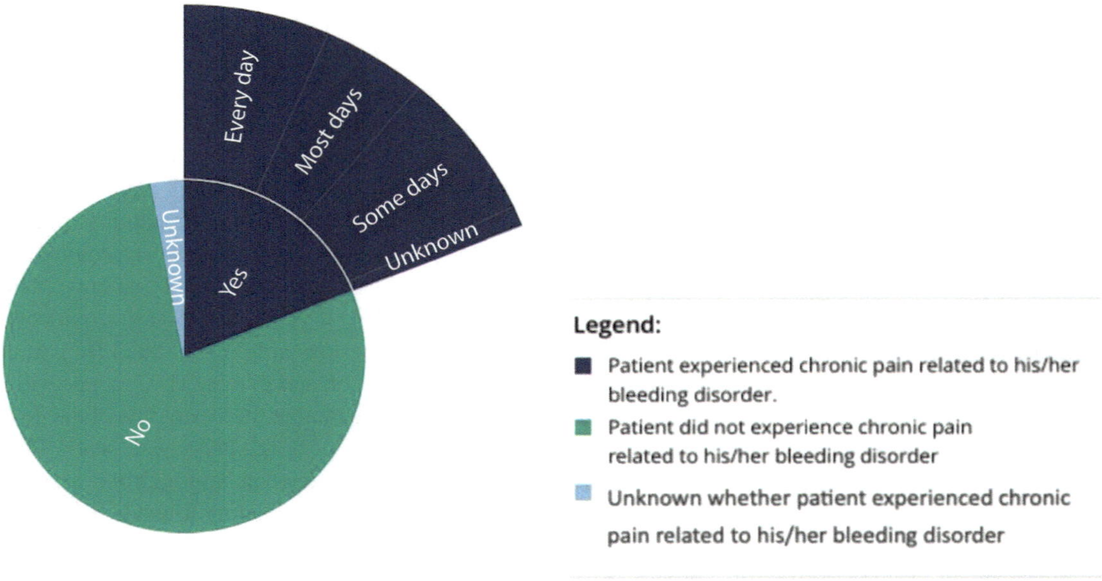


**Fig. 4.2** According to data from Centers for Disease Control (CDC) Registry for Bleeding disorders, this figure describes the distribution of chronic pain due to bleeding disorder among participants in the hemophilia registry over 12 months. The data reveal that 24.46% of patients with hemophilia reported chronic pain, of which a third reported that they had it every day. Registry data include unique participants enrolled since December 2013 as reported at the time of enrollment [190]

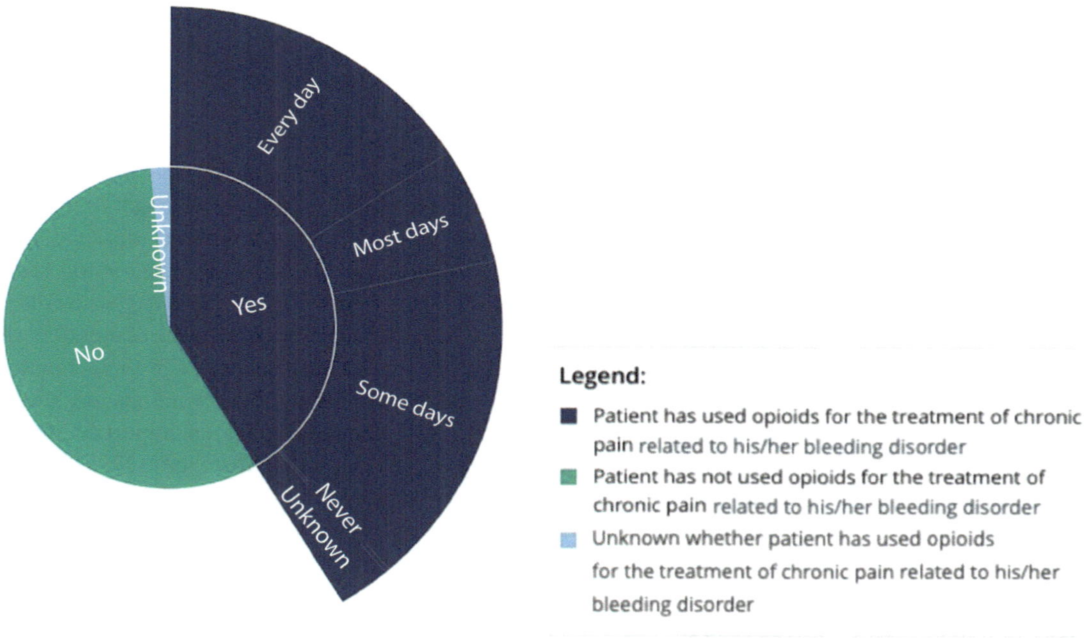


**Fig. 4.3** Frequency of opioid use in the treatment of chronic pain in patients with hemophilia per the CDC Community Counts registry over 12 months. Of the available responses, 10% of patients with hemophilia reported opioid use with most using opioids some days [190]

gration of physical therapy has been shown to improve balance and strength while improving overall joint outcomes as patients age [148–150]. The National Hemophilia Foundation's Physical Therapy Working Group has developed guidelines specifically for physical therapy assessment and management of patients with hemophilia in various settings. Current recommendations suggest these patients be evaluated by a hemophilia-trained physical therapist at least once annually.

### Nonsteroidal Anti-inflammatory Drugs (NSAIDs) and Opioids

NSAIDs are commonly used for the management of arthritis; however, their use in HA has been limited because of the propensity to induce upper gastrointestinal bleeding, a risk made that much more challenging with an underlying bleeding diathesis [151]. The selective cyclooxengase-2 (COX-2) inhibitors offer a more promising alternative for patients with hemophilia [151–153]. While providing a comparable analgesic effect, these agents also offer a reduced risk of upper gastrointestinal bleeding. A multicenter case-control study in patients with hemophilia assessed rates of upper gastrointestinal bleeds and determined that the risk increased in the first month of NSAID use but did not increase in patients who were using a COX-2 inhibitor over the same period [154]. Current evaluations of the COX-2 inhibitor, rofecoxib for the treatment of HA are underway [155].

Limited data guide the use of opioids in the long-term pain management of patients with hemophilia [156] (Fig. 4.3). In their 2005 recommendations, the World Federation of Hemophilia discouraged the use of opioids in the management of HA and subsequently, anecdotal data and expert advice have suggested approaching patient's risks and benefits individually.

In one small cohort of 183 adult patients from two HTCs, about half of the patients used chronic pain medication, defined as the use of analgesic drugs for more than 3 months consecutively [157]. Of those, 21% were on a opioid-containing regimen and severity of disease was a predictor of opioid exposure odds ratio 3.14 [95% CI, 1.6–6.2]; $P < 0.001$) [157]. In a similar cohort of 135 pediatric patients, 10% required chronic pain medication but none of the patients used an opioid-containing regimen. The same study demonstrated that HTCs prescribed only a minority of the opioid prescriptions [157]. Indeed, providers at HTCs are often not well versed in the utility of opioids in the management of non-cancer pain and opioid prescribing is often deferred to primary care providers or pain specialists.

### Intervention-Based Pain Management

The utilization of intraarticular corticosteroid joint injections has long been a controversial intervention for the treatment of acute and chronic joint pain in hemophilia and remains a topic of ongoing research [158]. While a single center study in 2017 of 25 patients demonstrated a promising reduction in pain, a larger 2018 review demonstrated only low-level evidence for short-term pain relief with a high cost; ultimately, the investigators did not recommend intraarticular joint injections even with point-of-care ultrasound guidance [159, 160]. Additional small studies have demonstrated modest reductions in pain with injections of hyaluronic acid or platelet-rich plasma [161].

Chronic and unremitting pain, with progressive HA may eventually require surgical intervention. Many HTCs form partnerships with experienced orthopedic surgeons who are well versed in the management of patients with bleeding disorders and who can provide patients with information to aid their decision-making as they consider invasive interventions. Less invasive procedures like joint synovectomy can reduce chronic pain but they are not as effective in patients with advanced disease [162]. Total joint replacements are increasingly more common with increasing surgical expertise and clotting factor availability [163]. The impact of joint replacement is long lasting with follow-up studies showing similar observations over 10 years [164, 165]. When joint replacements are not feasible, joint fusions may reduce pain and joint instability.

Beyond procedural or surgery-based approaches to pain, recent interest has increased in the incorporation of integrative medicine approaches. These include exercise and fitness programs, acupuncture, biofeedback, and transcutaneous electrical neurostimulation (TENS) [166–168]. Hydrotherapy and therapeutic massage are also emerging modalities that may further treat pain without medications or surgery [169].

## Considerations in Psychosocial Support

### Historical Caveats and Patient Trust

The history of hemophilia treatment is tainted by the HIV epidemic that afflicted a large proportion of this population due to the use of contaminated blood products [170]. In 1982, the CDC began to receive reports of an increased incidence of pneumocystis pneumonia in patients with hemophilia. Between 1981 and 1984, it is estimated that over 50% of patients with hemophilia were infected with HIV as a result of their treatment [170].

Survivors of the HIV outbreak in the 1980s describe the tragic losses experienced around them [171, 172]. Many patients lost family members or friends with hemophilia to advanced HIV while others faced the challenge of another unwanted viral infection—hepatitis C. This generation of patients with hemophilia remains cautious about new developments in the management of their disease and may lack trust in their physicians and other clinicians [171–173]. Today, identifying the viral status of patients with hemophilia patients remains an integral aspect of initial assessment in clinic and partnerships with infectious disease specialists and hepatologists are key in managing infection-related complications.

### Mental Health Considerations

Patients with hemophilia experience high levels of anxiety and depression, which often affects treatment adherence and pain. In 2019, a study of 200 adults with hemophilia A and B using the 9-item Patient Health Questionnaire (PHQ-9) [174] and the 7-item Generalized Anxiety Disorder (GAD-7) [175] scales demonstrated that more than half of patients had moderate to severe depression without a prior diagnosis [176]. Patients with more anxiety and depression reported lower levels of social support as well as higher levels of pain and lack of treatment adherence. Both depression and generalized anxiety are underdiagnosed in the hemophilia population suggesting targeted interventions for diagnosing and treating patients might have an important impact on pain, quality of life, and factor adherence [177, 178]. Consequently, social workers, psychologists, and psychiatrists are an integral clinician of the comprehensive HTC team. Further research is required to measure the impacts of mental health interventions in assessing and educating patients regarding depression. Clinicians should routinely screen for depression and anxiety and optimize treatment.

### Financial Challenges in Hemophilia Management

Despite the availability of recombinant factor products for nearly three decades with plasma-derived products available even longer, the cost of these medications remains staggering [179, 180]. HTCs in the US are funded by a federal grant to provide factor at a reduced price when billing insurance. The profit margin is then mandatorily translated directly into patient resources and often pays for the comprehensive care team and research team. Patients without insurance however are often left with limited resources to access expensive factor products, and HTCs may be subject to institutional regulations regarding the care of uninsured patients [179, 181]. Patients with limited medicaid-based insurance programs may have access to HTC care and factor but may face barriers in acquiring coverage for newer therapies like emicizumab and gene therapy [123, 124].

## Quality of Life Estimation Tools

### Hemophilia Activities List

The Hemophilia Activities List (HAL) is a 42-question survey used to measure the impact of hemophilia on self-perceived functional abilities in adults [182]. The questions are all multiple choice and query patients about aspects of their lives in seven domains. The first three of these domains address aspects of physical function: lying, kneeling, sitting, and standing along with functions of the legs and functions of the arms. The additional domains focus on the use of transportation, self-care, household activities, and the ability to participate in sports and other leisure activities. The HAL is easy to administer and is estimated to take only 5–10 min to complete. It can provide a snapshot into how patients perceive that their disease is impacting their lives and describe a baseline evaluation of quality of life. However, the HAL has not yet been validated in the longitudinal evaluation of patients with hemophilia and thus it cannot be used to measure change over time [183, 184].

#### The Quality of Life Assessment Instrument for Children and Adolescents with Hemophilia

The Quality of Life Assessment Instrument for Children and Adolescents with Hemophilia (Haemo-Qol) is a collection of tools developed by six European countries that measure quality of life from both the patient and parent perspectives [185, 186]. The Haemo-Qol is tailored for three age groups: children aged 4–7 (16–21 items), children aged 8–12, and adolescents aged 13–18 (35–77 items). Both and long and short versions of the questionnaires exist [187]. Unlike the HAL, the Haemo-Qol has been validated for longitudinal assessment that can be used to assess for changes in each of the surveyed domains; yet, it requires more time to complete and has a more complex scoring system [188].

### Advance Care Planning

There is very little data on the integration of advance care planning conversations and documentation in patients with hemophilia. While advances in disease management have allowed patients to live longer, the risk for traumatic and spontaneous life-threatening bleeds remains. It is also important to understand the thoughts and feelings of members of the bleeding disorders community on advance care planning, to determine what they know about the process, and to ascertain what their feelings are about integrating advance care planning into their comprehensive care. Please see Chap. 11 for more details regarding advance care planning.

### Palliative Care and Hemophilia Management

There is a dearth of data regarding the role of palliative care in the management of hemophilia, and palliative care providers have not traditionally been integrated into the comprehensive, multidisciplinary hemophilia treatment team. While this may be because of the fact that most patients with hemophilia are able to live a nearly normal lifespan, this only undercuts the valuable ways that palliative care could be integrated into a patient with hemophilia's care. Our considerations regarding the role of palliative care in SCD are echoed here again as hemophilia also encompasses the physical, psychological, and emotional considerations that accompany a chronic, congenital disease. The development of gene therapy raises important questions about patient choice and identity that may be better explored through a facilitated discussion with patients and their families about the role their disease plays in their life. Palliative care can become central to these discussions while also helping patients set goals and expectations around quality of life, pain management, the desire to pursue potentially invasive joint surgeries, and the way by which their disease impacts their families. Much like in SCD, our palliative care colleagues should always remember that most patients with hemophilia have lived with their disease since childhood. It is a constant part of their daily decision-making impacting everything from how they exercise to how they chop vegetables. These patients have a unique relationship with the health care system and their medical team that relies on a keenly developed partnership. By better integrating palliative care into hemophilia management, patients can begin to see these providers as another important part of their team.

## References


1. Kato GJ, Piel FB, Reid CD, Gaston MH, Ohene-Frempong K, Krishnamurti L, et al. Sickle cell disease. Nat Rev Dis Primers. 2018;4:18010.
2. Piel FB, Steinberg MH, Rees DC. Sickle cell disease. N Engl J Med. 2017;376(16):1561–73.
3. Pinto VM, Balocco M, Quintino S, Forni GL. Sickle cell disease: a review for the internist. Intern Emerg Med. 2019;14(7):1051–64.
4. Azar S, Wong TE. Sickle cell disease: a brief update. Med Clin North Am. 2017;101(2):375–93.
5. Sundd P, Gladwin MT, Novelli EM. Pathophysiology of sickle cell disease. Annu Rev Pathol. 2019;14:263–92.
6. Connes P, Alexy T, Detterich J, Romana M, Hardy-Dessources MD, Ballas SK. The role of blood rheology in sickle cell disease. Blood Rev. 2016;30(2):111–8.
7. Shah N, Bhor M, Xie L, Paulose J, Yuce H. Sickle cell disease complications: prevalence and resource utilization. PLoS One. 2019;14(7):e0214355.
8. Brousse V, Buffet P, Rees D. The spleen and sickle cell disease: the sick(led) spleen. Br J Haematol. 2014;166(2):165–76.
9. Ballas SK, Darbari DS. Review/overview of pain in sickle cell disease. Complement Ther Med. 2020;49:102327.
10. Darbari DS, Sheehan VA, Ballas SK. The vaso-occlusive pain crisis in sickle cell disease: definition, pathophysiology, and management. Eur J Haematol. 2020.
11. Fiocchi J, Urits I, Orhurhu V, Orhurhu MS, Giacomazzi S, Hoyt B, et al. A comprehensive review of the treatment and management of pain in sickle cell disease. Curr Pain Headache Rep. 2020;24(5):17.
12. Alagbe AE, Olaniyi JA, Aworanti OW. Adult sickle cell anaemia patients in bone pain crisis have elevated pro-inflammatory cytokines. Mediterr J Hematol Infect Dis. 2018;10(1):e2018017.
13. Hu X, Jhun EH, Yao Y, He Y, Molokie RE, Wilkie DJ, et al. IL1A rs1800587 associates with chronic noncrisis pain in sickle cell disease. Pharmacogenomics. 2016;17(18):1999–2006.
14. Sarray S, Saleh LR, Lisa Saldanha F, Al-Habboubi HH, Mahdi N, Almawi WY. Serum IL-6, IL-10, and TNFα levels in pediatric sickle cell disease patients during vasoocclusive crisis and steady state condition. Cytokine. 2015;72(1):43–7.

15. Farooq S, Abu Omar M, Salzman GA. Acute chest syndrome in sickle cell disease. Hosp Pract (1995). 2018;46(3):144–51.
16. Jain S, Bakshi N, Krishnamurti L. Acute chest syndrome in children with sickle cell disease. Pediatr Allergy Immunol Pulmonol. 2017;30(4):191–201.
17. Navalkele P, Özgönenel B, McGrath E, Lephart P, Sarnaik S. Invasive pneumococcal disease in patients with sickle cell disease. J Pediatr Hematol Oncol. 2017;39(5):341–4.
18. Yee ME, Bakshi N, Graciaa SH, Lane PA, Jerris RC, Wang YF, et al. Incidence of invasive Haemophilus influenzae infections in children with sickle cell disease. Pediatr Blood Cancer. 2019;66(6):e27642.
19. Morrissey BJ, Bycroft TP, Almossawi O, Wilkey OB, Daniels JG. Incidence and predictors of bacterial infection in febrile children with sickle cell disease. Hemoglobin. 2015;39(5):316–9.
20. Galadanci AA, DeBaun MR, Galadanci NA. Neurologic complications in children under five years with sickle cell disease. Neurosci Lett. 2019;706:201–6.
21. Hirtz D, Kirkham FJ. Sickle cell disease and stroke. Pediatr Neurol. 2019;95:34–41.
22. Noubiap JJ, Mengnjo MK, Nicastro N, Kamtchum-Tatuene J. Neurologic complications of sickle cell disease in Africa: a systematic review and meta-analysis. Neurology. 2017;89(14):1516–24.
23. Ofori-Acquah SF. Sickle cell disease as a vascular disorder. Expert Rev Hematol. 2020:1–9.
24. Astadicko I, Dresse MF, Seghaye MC. [Cardiac complications of sickle cell disease in children]. Rev Med Leiege. 2018;73(11):550–6.
25. Drawz P, Ayyappan S, Nouraie M, Saraf S, Gordeuk V, Hostetter T, et al. Kidney disease among patients with sickle cell disease, Hemoglobin SS and SC. Clin J Am Soc Nephrol. 2016;11(2):207–15.
26. Arduini GAO, Trovó de Marqui AB. Prevalence and characteristics of priapism in sickle cell disease. Hemoglobin. 2018;42(2):73–7.
27. Chinegwundoh FI, Smith S, Anie KA. Treatments for priapism in boys and men with sickle cell disease. Cochrane Database Syst Rev. 2017;9:CD004198.
28. Adesina OO, Neumayr LD. Osteonecrosis in sickle cell disease: an update on risk factors, diagnosis, and management. Hematology Am Soc Hematol Educ Program. 2019;2019(1):351–8.
29. Nevitt SJ, Jones AP, Howard J. Hydroxyurea (hydroxycarbamide) for sickle cell disease. Cochrane Database Syst Rev. 2017;4:CD002202.
30. Moore RD, Charache S, Terrin ML, Barton FB, Ballas SK. Cost-effectiveness of hydroxyurea in sickle cell anemia. Investigators of the Multicenter Study of Hydroxyurea in Sickle Cell Anemia. Am J Hematol. 2000;64(1):26–31.
31. McGann PT, Ware RE. Hydroxyurea therapy for sickle cell anemia. Expert Opin Drug Saf. 2015;14(11):1749–58.
32. McMahon TJ, Shan S, Riccio DA, Batchvarova M, Zhu H, Telen MJ, et al. Nitric oxide loading reduces sickle red cell adhesion and vaso-occlusion in vivo. Blood Adv. 2019;3(17):2586–97.
33. Tisdale JF, Thein SL, Eaton WA. Treating sickle cell anemia. Science. 2020;367(6483):1198–9.
34. Creary SE, Modi AC, Stanek JR, Chisolm DJ, O'Brien SH, Nwankwo C, et al. Allocation of treatment responsibility and adherence to hydroxyurea among adolescents with sickle cell disease. J Pediatr Psychol. 2019;44(10):1196–204.
35. Boulat C. [Transfusion and sickle cell disease]. Transfus Clin Biol. 2013;20(2):68–71.
36. Ballas SK. Indications for RBC exchange transfusion in patients with sickle cell disease: revisited. Ann Clin Lab Sci. 2019;49(6):836–7.
37. Biller E, Zhao Y, Berg M, Boggio L, Capocelli KE, Fang DC, et al. Red blood cell exchange in patients with sickle cell disease-indications and management: a review and consensus report by the therapeutic apheresis subsection of the AABB. Transfusion. 2018;58(8):1965–72.
38. Chou ST, Alsawas M, Fasano RM, Field JJ, Hendrickson JE, Howard J, et al. American Society of Hematology 2020 guidelines for sickle cell disease: transfusion support. Blood Adv. 2020;4(2):327–55.
39. Estcourt LJ, Hopewell S, Trivella M, Hambleton IR, Cho G. Regular long-term red blood cell transfusions for managing chronic chest complications in sickle cell disease. Cochrane Database Syst Rev. 2019;2019(10).
40. Khurmi N, Gorlin A, Misra L. Perioperative considerations for patients with sickle cell disease: a narrative review. Can J Anaesth. 2017;64(8):860–9.
41. Coates TD, Wood JC. How we manage iron overload in sickle cell patients. Br J Haematol. 2017;177(5):703–16.
42. Sridharan K, Sivaramakrishnan G. Efficacy and safety of iron chelators in thalassemia and sickle cell disease: a multiple treatment comparison network meta-analysis and trial sequential analysis. Expert Rev Clin Pharmacol. 2018;11(6):641–50.
43. Puri L, Flanagan JM, Kang G, Ding J, Bi W, McCarville BM, et al. *GSTM1* and liver iron content in children with sickle cell anemia and iron overload. J Clin Med. 2019;8(11):1878.
44. Yassin M, Soliman A, De Sanctis V, Nashwan A, Abusamaan S, Moustafa A, et al. Liver Iron Content (LIC) in Adults with Sickle Cell Disease (SCD): correlation with Serum Ferritin and Liver Enzymes Concentrations in Trasfusion Dependent (TD-SCD) and Non-Transfusion Dependent (NT-SCD) Patients. Mediterr J Hematol Infect Dis. 2017;9(1):e2017037.
45. Binding A, Ward R, Tomlinson G, Kuo KHM. Deferiprone exerts a dose-dependent reduction of liver iron in adults with iron overload. Eur J Haematol. 2019;103(2):80–7.
46. Niihara Y, Miller ST, Kanter J, Lanzkron S, Smith WR, Hsu LL, et al. A phase 3 trial of l-glutamine in sickle cell disease. N Engl J Med. 2018;379(3):226–35.
47. Vichinsky E, Hoppe CC, Ataga KI, Ware RE, Nduba V, El-Beshlawy A, et al. A phase 3 randomized trial of voxelotor in sickle cell disease. N Engl J Med. 2019;381(6):509–19.
48. Ataga KI, Kutlar A, Kanter J, Liles D, Cancado R, Friedrisch J, et al. Crizanlizumab for the prevention of pain crises in sickle cell disease. N Engl J Med. 2017;376(5):429–39.
49. Kutlar A, Kanter J, Liles DK, Alvarez OA, Cançado RD, Friedrisch JR, et al. Effect of crizanlizumab on pain crises in subgroups of patients with sickle cell disease: a SUSTAIN study analysis. Am J Hematol. 2019;94(1):55–61.
50. Gardner RV. Sickle cell disease: advances in treatment. Ochsner J. 2018;18(4):377–89.
51. Dalle JH. Hematologist and transplant physicians: how and where to meet for the best of sickle cell disease patients? Hematol Oncol Stem Cell Ther. 2020;13(2):58–60.
52. Faulkner L. How to setup a successful transplant program for hemoglobinopathies in developing countries: the Cure2Children approach. Hematol Oncol Stem Cell Ther. 2020;13(2):71–5.
53. Gluckman E, Cappelli B, Scigliuolo GM, De la Fuente J, Corbacioglu S. Alternative donor hematopoietic stem cell transplantation for sickle cell disease in Europe. Hematol Oncol Stem Cell Ther. 2020;13(4):181–8.
54. Leonard A, Tisdale J, Abraham A. Curative options for sickle cell disease: haploidentical stem cell transplantation or gene therapy? Br J Haematol. 2020;189(3):408–23.
55. Ikawa Y, Miccio A, Magrin E, Kwiatkowski JL, Rivella S, Cavazzana M. Gene therapy of hemoglobinopathies: progress and future challenges. Hum Mol Genet. 2019;28(R1):R24–30.
56. Lubeck D, Agodoa I, Bhakta N, Danese M, Pappu K, Howard R, et al. Estimated life expectancy and income of patients with sickle

cell disease compared with those without sickle cell disease. JAMA Netw Open. 2019;2(11):e1915374.
57. Howard J, Thein SL. Optimal disease management and health monitoring in adults with sickle cell disease. Hematology Am Soc Hematol Educ Program. 2019;2019(1):505–12.
58. Inusa BPD, Stewart CE, Mathurin-Charles S, Porter J, Hsu LL, Atoyebi W, et al. Paediatric to adult transition care for patients with sickle cell disease: a global perspective. Lancet Haematol. 2020;7(4):e329–e41.
59. Smith WR, Sisler IY, Johnson S, Lipato TJ, Newlin JS, Owens ZS, et al. Lessons learned from building a pediatric-to-adult sickle cell transition program. South Med J. 2019;112(3):190–7.
60. Allemang B, Allan K, Johnson C, Cheong M, Cheung P, Odame I, et al. Impact of a transition program with navigator on loss to follow-up, medication adherence, and appointment attendance in hemoglobinopathies. Pediatr Blood Cancer. 2019;66(8):e27781.
61. Colinart-Thomas M, Noël V, Roques G, Gordes-Grosjean S, Abely M, Pluchart C. [From pediatric care to adult medicine: transition of sickle cell patients, a French monocentric study]. Arch Pediatr. 2018;25(3):199–206.
62. Molter BL, Abrahamson K. Self-efficacy, transition, and patient outcomes in the sickle cell disease population. Pain Manag Nurs. 2015;16(3):418–24.
63. Peterson EE, Salemi JL, Dongarwar D, Salihu HM. Acute care utilization in pediatric sickle cell disease and sickle cell trait in the USA: prevalence, temporal trends, and cost. Eur J Pediatr. 2020.
64. Kauf TL, Coates TD, Huazhi L, Mody-Patel N, Hartzema AG. The cost of health care for children and adults with sickle cell disease. Am J Hematol. 2009;84(6):323–7.
65. Pizzo E, Laverty AA, Phekoo KJ, AlJuburi G, Green SA, Bell D, et al. A retrospective analysis of the cost of hospitalizations for sickle cell disease with crisis in England, 2010/11. J Public Health (Oxf). 2015;37(3):529–39.
66. Balsamo L, Shabanova V, Carbonella J, Szondy MV, Kalbfeld K, Thomas DA, et al. Improving care for sickle cell pain crisis using a multidisciplinary approach. Pediatrics. 2019;143(5).
67. Matthie N, Jenerette C. Sickle cell disease in adults: developing an appropriate care plan. Clin J Oncol Nurs. 2015;19(5):562–7.
68. Krishnamurti L, Smith-Packard B, Gupta A, Campbell M, Gunawardena S, Saladino R. Impact of individualized pain plan on the emergency management of children with sickle cell disease. Pediatr Blood Cancer. 2014;61(10):1747–53.
69. Mager A, Pelot K, Koch K, Miller L, Hubler C, Ndifor A, et al. Opioid management strategy decreases admissions in high-utilizing adults with sickle cell disease. J Opioid Manag. 2017;13(3):143–56.
70. Schefft MR, Swaffar C, Newlin J, Noda C, Sisler I. A novel approach to reducing admissions for children with sickle cell disease in pain crisis through individualization and standardization in the emergency department. Pediatr Blood Cancer. 2018;65(10):e27274.
71. Tanabe P, Freiermuth CE, Cline DM, Silva S. A prospective emergency department quality improvement project to improve the treatment of vaso-occlusive crisis in sickle cell disease: lessons learned. Jt Comm J Qual Patient Saf. 2017;43(3):116–26.
72. Hagedorn JM, Monico EC. Ketamine infusion for pain control in acute pediatric sickle cell painful crises. Pediatr Emerg Care. 2019;35(1):78–9.
73. Puri L, Morgan KJ, Anghelescu DL. Ketamine and lidocaine infusions decrease opioid consumption during vaso-occlusive crisis in adolescents with sickle cell disease. Curr Opin Support Palliat Care. 2019;13(4):402–7.
74. Crosby LE, Simmons K, Kaiser P, Davis B, Boyd P, Eichhorn T, et al. Using quality improvement methods to implement an electronic medical record (EMR) supported individualized home pain management plan for children with sickle cell disease. J Clin Outcomes Manag. 2014;21(5):210–7.
75. Karkoska K, Appiah-Kubi A, Rocker J, Stoffels G, Aygun B. Management of vaso-occlusive episodes in the day hospital decreases admissions in children with sickle cell disease. Br J Haematol. 2019;186(6):855–60.
76. Adewoye AH, Nolan V, McMahon L, Ma Q, Steinberg MH. Effectiveness of a dedicated day hospital for management of acute sickle cell pain. Haematologica. 2007;92(6):854–5.
77. Cline DM, Silva S, Freiermuth CE, Thornton V, Tanabe P. Emergency Department (ED), ED observation, day hospital, and hospital admissions for adults with sickle cell disease. West J Emerg Med. 2018;19(2):311–8.
78. Han J, Saraf SL, Kavoliunaite L, Jain S, Hassan J, Hsu LL, et al. Program expansion of a day hospital dedicated to manage sickle cell pain. Am J Hematol. 2018;93(1):E20–E1.
79. Frost JR, Cherry RK, Oyeku SO, Faro EZ, Crosby LE, Britto M, et al. Improving sickle cell transitions of care through health information technology. Am J Prev Med. 2016;51(1 Suppl 1):S17–23.
80. Jonassaint CR, Kang C, Abrams DM, Li JJ, Mao J, Jia Y, et al. Understanding patterns and correlates of daily pain using the Sickle cell disease Mobile Application to Record Symptoms via Technology (SMART). Br J Haematol. 2018;183(2):306–8.
81. Leonard S, Anderson LM, Jonassaint J, Jonassaint C, Shah N. Utilizing a novel mobile health "selfie" application to improve compliance to iron chelation in pediatric patients receiving chronic transfusions. J Pediatr Hematol Oncol. 2017;39(3):223–9.
82. Shah N, Jonassaint J, De Castro L. Patients welcome the Sickle Cell Disease Mobile Application to Record Symptoms via Technology (SMART). Hemoglobin. 2014;38(2):99–103.
83. Virella Pérez YI, Medlow S, Ho J, Steinbeck K. Mobile and web-based apps that support self-management and transition in young people with chronic illness: systematic review. J Med Internet Res. 2019;21(11):e13579.
84. Majumdar S, Thompson W, Ahmad N, Gordon C, Addison C. The use and effectiveness of complementary and alternative medicine for pain in sickle cell anemia. Complement Ther Clin Pract. 2013;19(4):184–7.
85. Mahmood LA, Reece-Stremtan S, Idiokitas R, Martin B, Margulies S, Hardy SJ, et al. Acupuncture for pain management in children with sickle cell disease. Complement Ther Med. 2020;49:102287.
86. Tsai SL, Bombacie M, Licursi M, Qian Y, Stiles GM, Lee MT. Acupuncture for pediatric sickle cell pain management: a promising non-opioid therapy. Complement Ther Med. 2020;49:102314.
87. Oliver-Carpenter G, Barach I, Crosby LE, Valenzuela J, Mitchell MJ. Disease management, coping, and functional disability in pediatric sickle cell disease. J Natl Med Assoc. 2011;103(2):131–7.
88. Sanchez HC, Karlson CW, Hsu JH, Ostrenga A, Gordon C. Complementary and alternative medicine use in pediatric hematology/oncology patients at the University of Mississippi Medical Center. J Altern Complement Med. 2015;21(11):660–6.
89. Levenson JL, McClish DK, Dahman BA, Bovbjerg VE, et al. Depression and anxiety in adults with sickle cell disease: the PiSCES project. Psychosom Med. 2008;70(2):192–6.
90. Graves JK, Hodge C, Jacob E. Depression, anxiety, and quality of life in children and adolescents with sickle cell disease. Pediatr Nurs. 2016;42(3):113–9, 44.
91. Reader SK, Rockman LM, Okonak KM, Ruppe NM, Keeler CN, Kazak AE. Systematic review: pain and emotional functioning in pediatric sickle cell disease. J Clin Psychol Med Settings. 2020;27(2):343–65.
92. Robbins MA, Carroll CP, North CS. Psychological symptom screening in an adult sickle cell disease clinic and predictors of treatment follow up. Psychol Health Med. 2020:1–9.

93. Valrie C, Floyd A, Sisler I, Redding-Lallinger R, Fuh B. Depression and anxiety as moderators of the pain-social functioning relationship in youth with sickle cell disease. J Pain Res. 2020;13:729–36.
94. Raji SO, Lawani AO, James BO. Prevalence and correlates of major depression among Nigerian adults with sickle cell disease. Int J Psychiatry Med. 2016;51(5):456–66.
95. Sanders KA, Labott SM, Molokie R, Shelby SR, Desimone J. Pain, coping and health care utilization in younger and older adults with sickle cell disease. J Health Psychol. 2010;15(1):131–7.
96. Smith KE, Schatz J. Working memory in children with neurocognitive effects from sickle cell disease: contributions of the central executive and processing speed. Dev Neuropsychol. 2016;41(4):231–44.
97. Bulgin D, Douglas C, Tanabe P. A pilot test of the Adult Sickle Cell Quality of Life Measurement Information System (ASCQ-Me) and the Jenerette Self-Care Assessment (J-SAT) Tools in adults with sickle cell disease. Pilot Feasibility Stud. 2019;5:85.
98. Cooper O, McBain H, Tangayi S, Telfer P, Tsitsikas D, Yardumian A, et al. Psychometric analysis of the adult sickle cell quality of life measurement information system (ACSQ-Me) in a UK population. Health Qual Life Outcomes. 2019;17(1):74.
99. Esham KS, Rodday AM, Smith HP, Noubary F, Weidner RA, Buchsbaum RJ, et al. Assessment of health-related quality of life among adults hospitalized with sickle cell disease vaso-occlusive crisis. Blood Adv. 2020;4(1):19–27.
100. Hanmer J, Jensen RE, Rothrock N, Team H. A reporting checklist for HealthMeasures' patient-reported outcomes: ASCQ-Me, Neuro-QoL, NIH Toolbox, and PROMIS. J Patient Rep Outcomes. 2020;4(1):21.
101. Cox ED, Connolly JR, Palta M, Rajamanickam VP, Flynn KE. Reliability and validity of PROMIS® pediatric family relationships short form in children 8-17 years of age with chronic disease. Qual Life Res. 2020;29(1):191–9.
102. Reeve BB, Edwards LJ, Jaeger BC, Hinds PS, Dampier C, Gipson DS, et al. Assessing responsiveness over time of the PROMIS. Qual Life Res. 2018;27(1):249–57.
103. Singh A, Panepinto JA. Clinical meaning of PROMIS pain domains for children with sickle cell disease. Blood Adv. 2019;3(15):2244–9.
104. Keller S, Yang M, Treadwell MJ, Hassell KL. Sensitivity of alternative measures of functioning and wellbeing for adults with sickle cell disease: comparison of PROMIS® to ASCQ-Me℠. Health Qual Life Outcomes. 2017;15(1):117.
105. Wilkie DJ, Johnson B, Mack AK, Labotka R, Molokie RE. Sickle cell disease: an opportunity for palliative care across the life span. Nurs Clin North Am. 2010;45(3):375–97.
106. Ajayi TA, Edmonds KP, Thornberry K, Atayee RA. Palliative care teams as advocates for adults with sickle cell disease. J Palliat Med. 2016;19(2):195–201.
107. Benjamin L. Pain management in sickle cell disease: palliative care begins at birth? Hematology Am Soc Hematol Educ Program. 2008:466–74.
108. Zimmerman B, Valentino LA. Hemophilia: in review. Pediatr Rev. 2013;34(7):289–94; quiz 95.
109. Franchini M, Mannucci PM. Hemophilia A in the third millennium. Blood Rev. 2013;27(4):179–84.
110. Kasper CK, Buzin CH. Mosaics and haemophilia. Haemophilia. 2009;15(6):1181–6.
111. Nacca CR, Harris AP, Tuttle JR. Hemophilic arthropathy. Orthopedics. 2017;40(6):e940–e6.
112. Donaldson J, Goddard N. Compartment syndrome in patients with haemophilia. J Orthop. 2015;12(4):237–41.
113. Zanon E, Pasca S. Intracranial haemorrhage in children and adults with haemophilia A and B: a literature review of the last 20 years. Blood Transfus. 2019;17(5):378–84.
114. Franchini M, Mannucci PM. The history of hemophilia. Semin Thromb Hemost. 2014;40(5):571–6.
115. Schramm W. The history of haemophilia—a short review. Thromb Res. 2014;134(Suppl 1):S4–9.
116. Page D. Comprehensive care for hemophilia and other inherited bleeding disorders. Transfus Apher Sci. 2019;58(5):565–8.
117. Afifi OAH, Abdelsalam EMN, Makhlouf AAEA, Ibrahim MAM. Evaluation of coagulation factors activity in different types of plasma preparations. Indian J Hematol Blood Transfus. 2019;35(3):551–6.
118. Malec LM, Cheng D, Witmer CM, Jaffray J, Kouides PA, Haley KM, et al. The impact of extended half-life factor concentrates on prophylaxis for severe hemophilia in The United States. Am J Hematol. 2020;95(8):960–5.
119. Pelland-Marcotte MC, Carcao MD. Hemophilia in a changing treatment landscape. Hematol Oncol Clin North Am. 2019;33(3):409–23.
120. Spadarella G, Di Minno A, Milan G, Franco N, Polimeno M, Castaldo F, et al. Paradigm shift for the treatment of hereditary haemophilia: towards precision medicine. Blood Rev. 2020;39:100618.
121. Nogami K, Shima M. New therapies using nonfactor products for patients with hemophilia and inhibitors. Blood. 2019;133(5):399–406.
122. Lillicrap D, Fijnvandraat K, Young G, Mancuso ME. Patients with hemophilia A and inhibitors: prevention and evolving treatment paradigms. Expert Rev Hematol. 2020;13(4):313–21.
123. Batty P, Lillicrap D. Advances and challenges for hemophilia gene therapy. Hum Mol Genet. 2019;28(R1):R95–R101.
124. Arruda VR, Doshi BS, Samelson-Jones BJ. Novel approaches to hemophilia therapy: successes and challenges. Blood. 2017;130(21):2251–6.
125. Tieu P, Chan A, Matino D. Molecular mechanisms of inhibitor development in hemophilia. Mediterr J Hematol Infect Dis. 2020;12(1):e2020001.
126. Cormier M, Batty P, Tarrant J, Lillicrap D. Advances in knowledge of inhibitor formation in severe haemophilia A. Br J Haematol. 2020;189(1):39–53.
127. Merlin S, Follenzi A. Escape or fight: inhibitors in hemophilia A. Front Immunol. 2020;11:476.
128. Lacroix-Desmazes S, Voorberg J, Lillicrap D, Scott DW, Pratt KP. Tolerating factor VIII: recent progress. Front Immunol. 2019;10:2991.
129. Young G, Liesner R, Chang T, Sidonio R, Oldenburg J, Jiménez-Yuste V, et al. A multicenter, open-label phase 3 study of emicizumab prophylaxis in children with hemophilia A with inhibitors. Blood. 2019;134(24):2127–38.
130. Angelini D, Konkle BA, Sood SL. Aging among persons with hemophilia: contemporary concerns. Semin Hematol. 2016;53(1):35–9.
131. Mannucci PM, Iacobelli M. Progress in the contemporary management of hemophilia: the new issue of patient aging. Eur J Intern Med. 2017;43:16–21.
132. Shapiro S, Makris M. Haemophilia and ageing. Br J Haematol. 2019;184(5):712–20.
133. Sousos N, Gavriilaki E, Vakalopoulou S, Garipidou V. Understanding cardiovascular risk in hemophilia: a step towards prevention and management. Thromb Res. 2016;140:14–21.
134. Brand B, Dunn S, Kulkarni R. Challenges in the management of haemophilia on transition from adolescence to adulthood. Eur J Haematol. 2015;95(Suppl 81):30–5.
135. Valentino LA, Santagostino E, Blanchette V, van den Berg M. Managing the pediatric patient and the adolescent/adult transition. Semin Thromb Hemost. 2006;32(Suppl 2):28–31.
136. Quon D, Reding M, Guelcher C, Peltier S, Witkop M, Cutter S, et al. Unmet needs in the transition to adulthood: 18- to 30-year-

old people with hemophilia. Am J Hematol. 2015;90(Suppl 2):S17–22.
137. Sun HL, Breakey VR, Straatman L, Wu JK, Jackson S. Outcomes indicators and processes in transitional care in adolescents with haemophilia: a Delphi survey of Canadian haemophilia care providers. Haemophilia. 2019;25(2):296–305.
138. Lison S, Spannagl M. [Perioperative management of patients with hemophilia]. Anaesthesist. 2014;63(1):6–15.
139. Hart DP, Hay CRM, Liesner R, Tobaruela G, Du-Mont B, Makris M. Perioperative laboratory monitoring in congenital haemophilia patients with inhibitors: a systematic literature review. Blood Coagul Fibrinolysis. 2019;30(7):309–23.
140. Kobayashi K, Imagama S, Ando K, Ito K, Tsushima M, Morozumi M, et al. Perioperative management of patients with hemophilia during spinal surgery. Asian Spine J. 2018;12(3):442–5.
141. Odonkor P, Srinivas A, Strauss E, Williams B, Mazzeffi M, Tanaka KA. Perioperative coagulation management of a hemophilia A patient during cardiac surgery. Semin Cardiothorac Vasc Anesth. 2017;21(4):312–20.
142. Melchiorre D, Manetti M, Matucci-Cerinic M. Pathophysiology of hemophilic arthropathy. J Clin Med. 2017;6(7).
143. Gay ND, Lee SC, Liel MS, Sochacki P, Recht M, Taylor JA. Increased fracture rates in people with haemophilia: a 10-year single institution retrospective analysis. Br J Haematol. 2015;170(4):584–6.
144. Kempton CL, Antoniucci DM, Rodriguez-Merchan EC. Bone health in persons with haemophilia. Haemophilia. 2015;21(5):568–77.
145. Manco-Johnson MJ, Abshire TC, Shapiro AD, Riske B, Hacker MR, Kilcoyne R, et al. Prophylaxis versus episodic treatment to prevent joint disease in boys with severe hemophilia. N Engl J Med. 2007;357(6):535–44.
146. Moreno MM, Cuesta-Barriuso R. A history of prophylaxis in haemophilia. Blood Coagul Fibrinolysis. 2019;30(2):55–7.
147. Guodemar-Pérez J, Ruiz-López M, Rodríguez-López E, García-Fernández P, Hervás-Pérez JP. Physiotherapy treatments in musculoskeletal pathologies associated with haemophilia. Hamostaseologie. 2018;38(3):141–9.
148. Stephensen D, Bladen M, McLaughlin P. Recent advances in musculoskeletal physiotherapy for haemophilia. Ther Adv Hematol. 2018;9(8):227–37.
149. Timmer MA, Veenhof C, de Kleijn P, de Bie RA, Schutgens REG, Pisters MF. Movement behaviour patterns in adults with haemophilia. Ther Adv Hematol. 2020;11:2040620719896959.
150. Wagner B, Krüger S, Hilberg T, Ay C, Hasenoehrl T, Huber DF, et al. The effect of resistance exercise on strength and safety outcome for people with haemophilia: a systematic review. Haemophilia. 2020;26(2):200–15.
151. Arachchillage DRJ, Makris M. Choosing and using non-steroidal anti-inflammatory drugs in haemophilia. Haemophilia. 2016;22(2):179–87.
152. Boban A, Lambert C, Hermans C. Is the cardiovascular toxicity of NSAIDS and COX-2 selective inhibitors underestimated in patients with haemophilia? Crit Rev Oncol Hematol. 2016;100:25–31.
153. Rattray B, Nugent DJ, Young G. Celecoxib in the treatment of haemophilic synovitis, target joints, and pain in adults and children with haemophilia. Haemophilia. 2006;12(5):514–7.
154. Riley RR, Witkop M, Hellman E, Akins S. Assessment and management of pain in haemophilia patients. Haemophilia. 2011;17(6):839–45.
155. Ross JS, Krumholz HM. Bringing Vioxx back to market. BMJ. 2018;360:k242.
156. Holstein K, Klamroth R, Richards M, Carvalho M, Pérez-Garrido R, Gringeri A, et al. Pain management in patients with haemophilia: a European survey. Haemophilia. 2012;18(5):743–52.
157. Peltier SJ, Mazepa MA, Freese RL, Nelson SF, Kearney SL, Reding MT. Opioid exposure in haemophilia patients is common and underreported. Haemophilia. 2020;26(2):251–6.
158. Buccheri E, Avola M, Vitale N, Pavone P, Vecchio M. Haemophilic arthropathy: a narrative review on the use of intra-articular drugs for arthritis. Haemophilia. 2019;25(6):919–27.
159. Martin EJ, Cooke EJ, Ceponis A, Barnes RF, Moran CM, Holle S, et al. Efficacy and safety of point-of-care ultrasound-guided intra-articular corticosteroid joint injections in patients with haemophilic arthropathy. Haemophilia. 2017;23(1):135–43.
160. Rodriguez-Merchan EC. Intra-articular corticosteroid injections in haemophilic arthropathy: are they recommended? Hosp Pract (1995). 2018;46(1):1–4.
161. Rodriguez-Merchan EC, Valentino LA. Joint lavage followed by intra-articular injection of hyaluronic acid and/or corticosteroids in patients with severe hemophilic arthropathy of the knee: is this intervention really effective? Expert Rev Hematol. 2018;11(6):449–54.
162. Rodriguez-Merchan EC. Surgical approaches to hemophilic arthropathy. Blood Coagul Fibrinolysis. 2019;30(1S Suppl 1):S11–3.
163. Liddle AD, Rodriguez-Merchan EC. Evidence-based management of the knee in hemophilia. JBJS Rev. 2017;5(8):e12.
164. Rodríguez-Merchán EC. The role of orthopaedic surgery in haemophilia: current rationale, indications and results. EFORT Open Rev. 2019;4(5):165–73.
165. Parsa A, Azizbaig Mohajer M, Mirzaie M. Hip arthroplasty in haemophilia: a systematic review. Hip Int. 2018;28(5):459–67.
166. Rodriguez-Merchan EC. Treatment of musculo-skeletal pain in haemophilia. Blood Rev. 2018;32(2):116–21.
167. Lambing A, Kohn-Converse B, Hanagavadi S, Varma V. Use of acupuncture in the management of chronic haemophilia pain. Haemophilia. 2012;18(4):613–7.
168. Wallny TA, Brackmann HH, Gunia G, Wilbertz P, Oldenburg J, Kraft CN. Successful pain treatment in arthropathic lower extremities by acupuncture in haemophilia patients. Haemophilia. 2006;12(5):500–2.
169. Neelapala YVR, Attal R, Tandale S. Aquatic exercise for persons with haemophilia: a review of literature. Complement Ther Clin Pract. 2019;34:195–200.
170. Aledort LM, Evatt BL, Lusher JM, Brownstein AP. HIV and hemophilia. J Thromb Haemost. 2007;5(3):607–10.
171. Mannucci PM. Viral safety of coagulation factor concentrates: memoirs from an insider. J Thromb Haemost. 2018;16(4):630–3.
172. Poon MC, Shedden N, Card RT. Healthcare professionals in the 'tainted blood' era in Canada: their forgotten emotions. Haemophilia. 2019;25(4):651–5.
173. Page D. Setting the scene: historical overview of challenges and what led to advances in comprehensive care in developed countries, the Canadian experience. Haemophilia. 2020;26(Suppl 3):4–5.
174. Kroenke K, Spitzer RL, Williams JB. The PHQ-9: validity of a brief depression severity measure. J Gen Intern Med. 2001;16(9):606–13.
175. Spitzer RL, Kroenke K, Williams JB, Löwe B. A brief measure for assessing generalized anxiety disorder: the GAD-7. Arch Intern Med. 2006;166(10):1092–7.
176. Witkop ML, Lambing A, Nichols CD, Munn JE, Anderson TL, Tortella BJ. Interrelationship between depression, anxiety, pain, and treatment adherence in hemophilia: results from a US cross-sectional survey. Patient Prefer Adherence. 2019;13:1577–87.
177. Al-Huniti A, Reyes Hernandez M, Ten Eyck P, Staber JM. Mental health disorders in haemophilia: systematic literature review and meta-analysis. Haemophilia. 2020.

178. Palareti L, Melotti G, Cassis F, Nevitt SJ, Iorio A. Psychological interventions for people with hemophilia. Cochrane Database Syst Rev. 2020;3:CD010215.
179. Chen SL. Economic costs of hemophilia and the impact of prophylactic treatment on patient management. Am J Manag Care. 2016;22(5 Suppl):s126–33.
180. Tencer T, Friedman HS, Li-McLeod J, Johnson K. Medical costs and resource utilization for hemophilia patients with and without HIV or HCV infection. J Manag Care Pharm. 2007;13(9):790–8.
181. Thorat T, Neumann PJ, Chambers JD. Hemophilia burden of disease: a systematic review of the cost-utility literature for hemophilia. J Manag Care Spec Pharm. 2018;24(7):632–42.
182. van Genderen FR, van Meeteren NL, van der Bom JG, Heijnen L, de Kleijn P, van den Berg HM, et al. Functional consequences of haemophilia in adults: the development of the Haemophilia Activities List. Haemophilia. 2004;10(5):565–71.
183. van Genderen FR, Westers P, Heijnen L, de Kleijn P, van den Berg HM, Helders PJ, et al. Measuring patients' perceptions on their functional abilities: validation of the Haemophilia Activities List. Haemophilia. 2006;12(1):36–46.
184. Timmer MA, Gouw SC, Feldman BM, Zwagemaker A, de Kleijn P, Pisters MF, et al. Measuring activities and participation in persons with haemophilia: a systematic review of commonly used instruments. Haemophilia. 2018;24(2):e33–49.
185. Bullinger M, von Mackensen S, Fischer K, Khair K, Petersen C, Ravens-Sieberer U, et al. Pilot testing of the 'Haemo-QoL' quality of life questionnaire for haemophiliac children in six European countries. Haemophilia. 2002;8(Suppl 2):47–54.
186. von Mackensen S, Bullinger M, Group H-Q. Development and testing of an instrument to assess the Quality of Life of Children with Haemophilia in Europe (Haemo-QoL). Haemophilia. 2004;10(Suppl 1):17–25.
187. Pollak E, Mühlan H, Von Mackensen S, Bullinger M, GROUP H-Q. The Haemo-QoL Index: developing a short measure for health-related quality of life assessment in children and adolescents with haemophilia. Haemophilia. 2006;12(4):384–92.
188. Trindade GC, Viggiano LGL, Brant ER, Lopes CAO, Faria ML, Ribeiro PHNS, et al. Evaluation of quality of life in hemophilia patients using the WHOQOL-bref and Haemo-A-Qol questionnaires. Hematol Transfus Cell Ther. 2019;41(4):335–41.
189. Gardner K, Douiri A, Drasar E, Allman M, Mwirigi A, Awogbade M, et al. Survival in adults with sickle cell disease in a high-income setting. Blood. 2016;128(10):1436–8.
190. Centers for Disease Control and Prevention. 2014 Community Counts Registry Report. 2018. https://www.cdc.gov/ncbddd/hemophilia/communitycounts/registry-report/index.html. Accessed 14 May 2020.
191. Payne AB, Mehal JM, Chapman C, Haberling DL, Richardson LC, Bean CJ, Hooper WC. Trends in sickle cell disease-related mortality in the United States, 1979 to 2017. Ann Emerg Med. 2020;76(3S):S28–36.

# Cellular Therapies: A Description of the Types of Existing Cellular Therapies and Associated Toxicities

5

Gopi S. Mohan, Daniel J. Kats, Samantha D. Martin, and Pietro Miozzo

## Introduction

The idea that cells can be used as living drugs to treat disease has captured the imagination of biomedical scientists since the first investigations into blood transfusion hundreds of years ago. In the second half of the twentieth century, hematopoietic cell transplantation (HCT) demonstrated the power of adoptive cellular therapies to fight cancer, control infection, and permanently cure a number of hematologic, immunologic, and metabolic disorders. In many ways, engineered cellular therapies represent the evolution of these early non-engineered therapies and seek to rationally harness the power of the immune system to treat intractable malignancies and infections. The last two decades have seen an explosion in cellular therapy research, and several novel agents for both benign and malignant hematologic conditions have demonstrated great promise in clinical trials. The coming decade will likely see many cellular therapies transition from experimental agents to the standard of care. It will be increasingly important for all clinicians caring for these patients to become well-versed in the available therapies, their benefits, and their toxicities. Here, we will introduce the most important available engineered cellular therapies, including chimeric antigen receptor CAR T-cells, hematopoietic gene therapy, and antiviral cytotoxic T-lymphocytes (CTLs).

G. S. Mohan (✉)
Department of Pediatrics, Pediatric Critical Care, Massachusetts General Hospital, Boston, MA, USA

Division of Hematology-Oncology, Boston Children's Hospital, Boston, MA, USA

Harvard Medical School, Boston, MA, USA

Department of Pediatrics, Pediatric Critical Care, The University of Texas MD Anderson Cancer Center, Houston, TX, USA
e-mail: gmohan@mdanderson.org

D. J. Kats · S. D. Martin · P. Miozzo
Harvard Medical School, Boston, MA, USA

Department of Pediatrics, Massachusetts General Hospital, Boston, MA, USA

## Chimeric Antigen Receptor T-Cell (CAR-T) Therapy

CAR T- cells represent the culmination of decades of immunotherapy research. They are the most widely used and studied engineered cellular immunotherapy today. Inspired by older biologic cancer immunotherapeutic agents such as rituximab (anti-CD20 for B-cell lymphomas) and trastuzumab (anti-HER2 for breast cancer), CAR-T cells are a "living drug" that leverage the antigen specificity and "engineerability" of monoclonal antibodies while harnessing the cytotoxicity and *in vivo* proliferative power of T-cells [1, 2].

Conventional T-cells recognize their cognate antigen as a processed peptide bound to a Major Histocompatibility Complex (MHC) molecule expressed on the target cell surface (Fig. 5.1). This interaction results in the activation of T-cells, which then release cytotoxic mediators such as perforin and granzyme, killing the target cell. Unsurprisingly, the alteration of antigen processing and presentation is a major mechanism of immune evasion by many cancers [3]. CARs are generated by fusing an engineered antigen-binding portion of an antibody called a "single-chain variable fragment" (scFv) with transmembrane and intracellular domains of the T-cell receptor complex (Fig. 5.2). This approach allows CAR-T cells to recognize native unprocessed antigens in the same manner as an antibody and then specifically kill target cells that express those antigens (Fig. 5.1) [2, 4, 5].

Early-generation CAR-T products were composed of a scFv linked to CD3ζ (an intracellular component of the T-cell receptor complex responsible for signal transduction) (Fig. 5.2). While such constructs demonstrated anti-tumor activity, they were unable to effect a sustained T-cell response. These first-generation constructs gave way to second-generation constructs, which incorporated intracel-


C. K. Ullrich, E. J. Roeland (eds.), *Palliative Care in Hematologic Malignancies and Serious Blood Disorders*,
https://doi.org/10.1007/978-3-031-38058-7_5

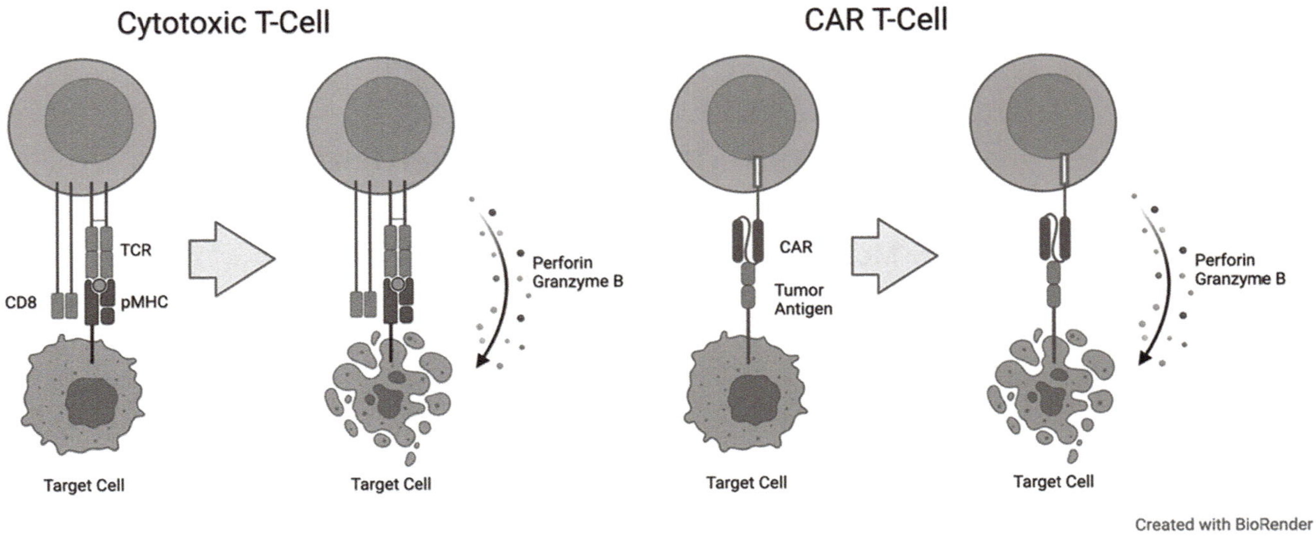


**Fig. 5.1** Target cell recognition and killing by classical cytotoxic T-cells versus CAR T-cells. *TCR* T-cell receptor, *pMHC* peptide-MHC complex, *CAR* chimeric antigen receptor. Created with BioRender.com

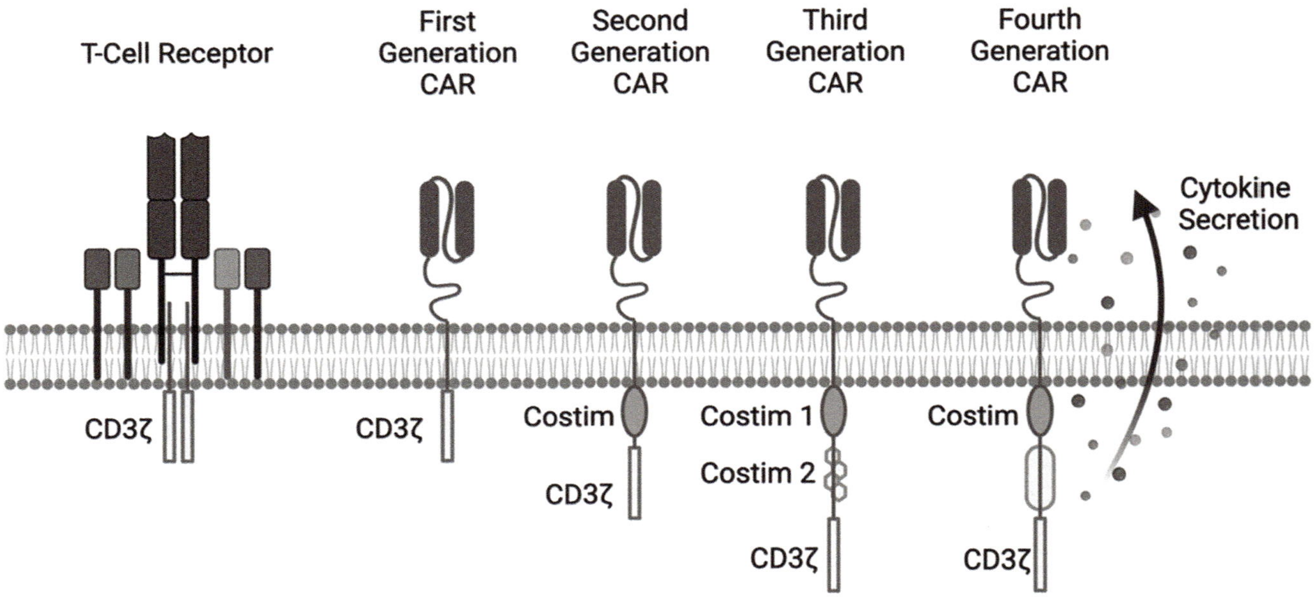


**Fig. 5.2** Comparison of T-cell receptor and different generations of CARs. Costim = costimulatory domain (CD28 and/or 4-1BB). Created with BioRender.com

lular costimulatory domains (either CD28 or 4-1BB) to augment proliferation and promote the persistence of expanded CAR T-cells *in vivo*. These products yielded more promising clinical results, and all FDA-approved CAR-T products to date use this design [4, 6]. More recently, third and fourth-generation CAR-T constructs are being investigated, which incorporate additional costimulatory domains, and even direct cytokine production to further augment anticancer activity in the context of an immunosuppressive tumor microenvironment [1, 7]. Notably, the complexity and range of application of CAR-T products and similar engineered cellular immunotherapies are expected to expand dramatically over the coming decade.

## Patient Selection and CAR-T Production

Currently B-cell and plasma cell malignancies are the only diseases for which there are FDA-approved CAR T-cell products (Table 5.1). For each CAR-T product and indica-

**Table 5.1** FDA-approved CAR T-cell products (as of 2022). *B-ALL* B-cell acute lymphoblastic leukemia; *DLBCL* diffuse large B-cell lymphoma; *R/R* relapsed/refractory; *BCMA* B-cell maturation antigen

| Drug (brand name) | Manufacturer | Target | Indication | FDA approval |
|---|---|---|---|---|
| Tisagenlecleucel (*Kymriah*) | Novartis | CD19 | Pediatric (<26 y/o) R/R B-ALL | 2017 |
| | | | Adult R/R DLBCL | 2018 |
| Axicabtagene Ciloleucel (*Yescarta*) | Kite | CD19 | Adult R/R large B-cell lymphoma | 2017 |
| | | | Adult R/R follicular lymphoma | 2021 |
| Brexucabtagene Autoleucel (*Tecartus*) | Kite | CD19 | Mantle cell lymphoma | 2020 |
| Lisocabtagene Maraleucel (*Breyanzi*) | Juno | CD19 | R/R large B-cell lymphoma | 2021 |
| Idecabtagene Vicleucel (*Abecma*) | Bristol Myers Squibb/Bluebird | BCMA | R/R multiple myeloma | 2021 |
| Ciltacabtagene Autoleucel (*Carvykti*) | Janssen | BCMA | R/R multiple myeloma | 2022 |

tion, specific patient criteria and cytogenetic/molecular features of the malignancy must be met to qualify for treatment [8].

CAR-T therapy is not currently included in the primary treatment regimen for any cancer and is generally reserved for patients with multiply relapsed/refractory disease. Though this may change as CAR-T becomes more widely used and its safety and efficacy profiles better characterized, most patients must have undergone at least two rounds of "standard" therapy with cancer relapse before being considered for CAR-T [8].

Numerous patient factors are also considered when evaluating an individual for CAR-T therapy including disease burden, age (adult vs. pediatric), physiologic reserve, chronic viral infections (HIV, viral hepatitides, and herpesvirus infections), and active graft-versus-host disease (GVHD) from a prior HCT. Various hematologic and biochemical parameters are also considered, which are covered elsewhere [8, 9]. Importantly, patients must have an adequate absolute lymphocyte count (preferably >500/uL) to ensure efficient leukapheresis for product manufacture.

Finally, the patient's cancer must express the appropriate CAR-T cognate antigen (e.g., B-lymphoblasts from a patient with B-ALL must express CD-19 if the patient is being considered for Tisagenlecleucel [Kymriah®], an anti-CD-19 CAR construct). Antigen expression is generally confirmed by flow cytometry on blood/tissue specimens.

From a palliative care perspective, CAR T-cell therapy represents an exciting new option for patients with advanced malignant disease who may not previously have had further curative options. As palliative care clinicians, special attention should be paid to the prognostic uncertainty associated with these therapies. Although remission is possible, it is not guaranteed, nor is the long-term durability of these outcomes known [10, 11]. Thus, clinicians should seek to understand their patients' expectations of this novel therapeutic approach and assist with contextualizing and framing their understanding. As with all novel and experimental therapeutics, careful consideration of a patient's goals, the potential risks and benefits of a given therapy, and the expected disease trajectory should be discussed with patients and caregivers.

## CAR-T Product Manufacture

Manufacturing CAR T-cells is a complex, time-intensive, and expensive process. After patients have been screened, CAR-T preparation involves collecting the patient's own leukocytes from their peripheral blood (leukapheresis), isolation of target T-cells (enrichment), transduction of these cells with the CAR, expansion of transduced CAR T-cells, and re-infusion back into the patient. The entire process can take several weeks for a single patient from leukapheresis to infusion.

*Leukapheresis*: Patients undergo whole blood removal using a large bore peripheral or central intravenous catheter, which can take several hours. Of note, the extracorporeal tubing requires priming and anticoagulation to prevent intra-procedure thrombosis. The anticoagulation used is generally not systemic and thus does not increase the risk of bleeding for patients undergoing this procedure [8].

The patient's whole blood is run through an apheresis device which separates blood components by density. This process allows for isolating and harvesting of white blood cells (including lymphocytes, monocytes, blasts, and granulocytes) from the remainder of the whole blood components (plasma, platelets, and red blood cells). Once the leukocytes have been removed from the patient, the remainder of the filtered products (red blood cells, plasma, and platelets) are reinfused [8].

*Enrichment*: Following leukapheresis, the peripheral blood mononuclear cell (PBMC) fraction is enriched for T-cells using one of a variety of methods such as density gradient separation, counterflow elutriation, or magnetic beads. Enrichment increases the purity of cytotoxic lymphocytes while eliminating certain cell types, such as monocytes and granulocytes, which may prevent successful T-cell expansion [8, 12].

*Transduction and expansion*: Once the PBMC product is enriched for T-cells, transduction (the process of introducing the CAR) can begin. Generally, this step utilizes lentivirus or retrovirus vectors that have been engineered to encode the CAR genes. Transduction of the CAR gene into activated patient T-cells produces CARs on the T-cell surface and creates a CAR T-cell [8]. Of note, new methods of transduction are being explored, including Clustered Regularly Interspaced Short Palindromic Repeats (CRISPR)-Cas9 technology.

Following successful transduction, the CAR T-cells then undergo expansion. There remains great variability between protocols regarding expansion methods, but generally, the CAR T-cell population is expanded using cytokines (predominantly interleukin [IL]-2), anti-CD3 antibodies, and anti-CD28 antibodies [8].

*Quality control*: Lot release testing, conducted after completion of manufacturing steps and prior to infusion of CAR T-cells into the patient, is required to evaluate the product's sterility, purity, transduction efficiency, viability, and potency. Bacterial and fungal cultures are performed to demonstrate sterility of the product. The product is also tested for persistent viral vector components capable of replication. Once sterility is confirmed, the product's purity (proportion of CAR-expressing cells) and phenotype (CD4+ vs. CD8+) are evaluated using flow cytometry. CAR T-cell viability and potency are also assessed with functional assays. Once this testing has been completed and the CAR T-cells have passed quality control, they can be cryopreserved for up to 12 months or infused fresh into the patient [8].

## Pre- and Post-infusion Care

Since CAR T-cell manufacturing is time-intensive, patients experience a "bridging" period between the initial apheresis and the infusion of CAR T-cells, during which they may experience disease progression or sequelae of untreated malignancy. Thus, they may receive cancer-directed therapy to prevent disease progression while waiting.

Separate from "bridging" chemotherapy, patients undergo chemotherapeutic lymphodepletion several days prior to infusion in order to enhance CAR T-cell engraftment and activation [8]. The rationale here is to eliminate host lymphocytes that may compete with CAR T-cells for homeostatic signals and survival niches [13]. Additionally, it is hypothesized that lymphodepleting chemotherapy may eliminate suppressive regulatory T-cells and myeloid cells [14] and may elicit an adjuvant effect by killing tumor cells and releasing tumor antigens and danger signals [15].

Before infusion, the patient usually receives pre-treatment with acetaminophen and diphenhydramine to reduce the risk of an infusion reaction. Infusion-related hypersensitivity immune reactions are characterized by hypotension, fever, urticaria, and rarely respiratory distress. These reactions are rare among the available FDA-approved CAR T-cell products [8]. Post-infusion nausea and fatigue are more common but relatively mild and are best managed with anti-emetics and rest [8].

## Complications of CAR-T Cell Therapy

Similar to other immunotherapies, complications of CAR-T therapy primarily derive from inflammatory dysregulation resulting from immune activation and tumor killing. The most common serious complications are Cytokine Release Syndrome (CRS) and Immune Effector Cell-Associated Neurotoxicity Syndrome (ICANS). Other complications, such as CAR-T associated Hemophagocytic Lymphohistiocytosis (HLH), GVHD, and B-cell aplasia, have also been described and will be reviewed here.

## Cytokine Release Syndrome

At its core, CRS is a cytokine storm caused by CAR-T activation, resulting in systemic hyperinflammation. CRS is very common, with many CAR-T trials observing over 50% incidence [16], including 77% of pediatric patients in the seminal ELIANA trial [10]. Severe CRS demonstrates many similarities with inflammatory shock states like sepsis, and its management follows many of the same principles. Several factors are associated with CRS risk and severity, including disease burden, disease type, and prior therapy (Table 5.2).

CRS begins when CAR T-cells recognize target cells expressing their cognate antigen (Fig. 5.3). The activated CAR T-cells then release cytotoxic mediators (e.g., perforin and granzyme) to kill the target cells, as well as inflammatory cytokines such as interferon gamma (IFN-γ and tumor necrosis factor alpha (TNF-α), which recruit and activate macrophages. The activated macrophages then secrete interleukin-6 (IL-6), interleukin-1 (IL-1), and more TNF-α, which results in the recruitment and activation of additional bystander T-cells These bystander T-cells then secrete more IFN-γ and TNF-α, thereby propagating a feed-forward loop promoting systemic hyperinflammation [8, 17].

**Table 5.2** Clinical risk factors associated with developing cytokine release syndrome (CRS) and immune effector cell-associated neurotoxicity syndrome (ICANS)

| Risk factor | CRS | ICANS |
|---|---|---|
| High disease burden | X | X |
| Acute lymphoblastic leukemia (primary disease) | X | X |
| Extramedullary disease/CNS involvement | | X |
| High CAR T-cell dose | X | X |
| High CAR T-cell expansion peak | X | X |
| Thrombocytopenia and endothelial activation before CAR T-cell therapy | X | X |
| Presence of CD28 costimulatory domain | X | X |
| Fludarabine and cyclophosphamide use during lymphodepletion | X | X |
| Concurrent CRS | – | X |
| Pre-existing neurologic disorder | | X |
| Elevated LDH prior to CAR T infusion | | X |

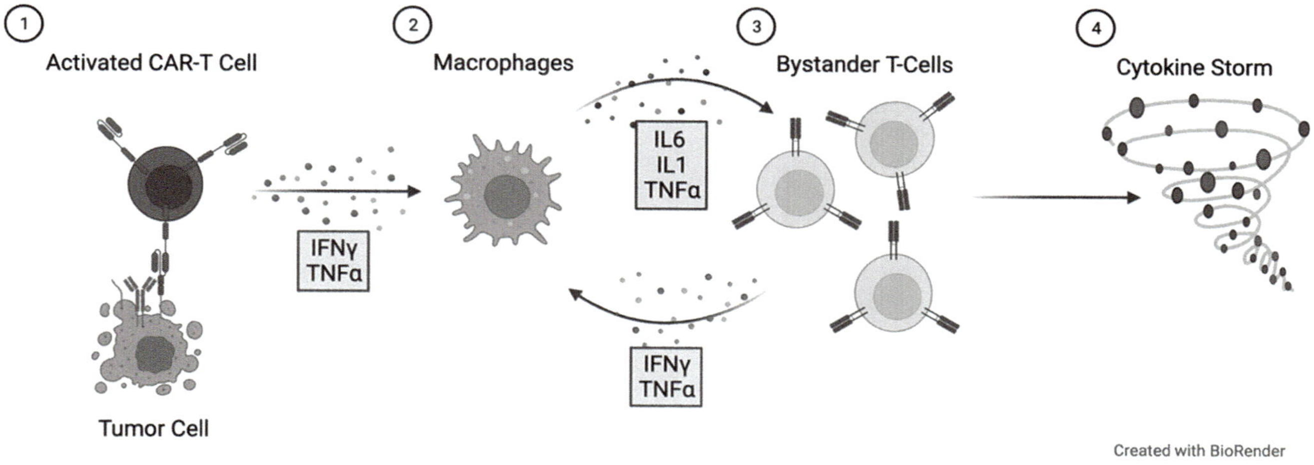


**Fig. 5.3** Pathophysiology of cytokine release syndrome (CRS). *CAR* chimeric antigen receptor; *IFN* interferon; *TNF* tumor necrosis factor; *IL* interleukin. Created with BioRender.com

**Table 5.3** Signs and symptoms of cytokine release syndrome by organ system

| Organ system | Signs/symptoms |
|---|---|
| Constitutional | Fever ≥38 °C, arthralgias, fatigue, myalgias |
| Cardiovascular | Tachycardia, hypotension, shock, myocardial dysfunction, arrhythmias |
| Respiratory | Tachypnea, hypoxemia, pulmonary edema, pleural effusions |
| Gastrointestinal | Nausea, vomiting, diarrhea, anorexia |
| Hepatic | Elevated liver transaminases, hyperbilirubinemia, liver synthetic dysfunction |
| Renal | Oliguria/anuria, acute kidney injury, elevation of serum creatinine, electrolyte derangements |
| Dermatologic | Rash |
| Rheumatologic | Elevation of inflammatory markers including C-reactive protein, ferritin, procalcitonin, and interleukins/cytokines |
| Hematologic | Bleeding, coagulopathy, disseminated intravascular coagulation |

## CRS: Clinical Presentation, Grading, and Management

CRS typically presents in the first 14 days following CAR T-cell infusion, with a median onset of 2–3 days [10, 18]. CRS can involve every major organ system (Table 5.3), and hemodynamic instability and respiratory insufficiency are the primary drivers of morbidity and mortality [8].

In 2018, the American Society of Transplantation and Cellular Therapy (ASTCT) released a consensus grading system to standardize the diagnosis, reporting, and management of CRS (Table 5.4) [19]. Fever ≥ 38 °C is required to diagnose CRS, and grading severity is based on levels of required hemodynamic and respiratory support. Fever without hypotension or hypoxemia defines Grade 1 CRS and is usually managed with antipyretics and close hemodynamic and respiratory monitoring. Because CAR-T recipients are inherently immunosuppressed and CRS is clinically difficult to differentiate from sepsis, all patients should be cultured and started on broad-spectrum antibiotics. Grade 2 CRS is defined by fluid-responsive hypotension, or by hypoxemia responding to oxygen delivered by low-flow nasal canula (LFNC). In contrast, Grades 3 and 4 are defined by persistent hypotension requiring intravenous vasopressor support and escalation of respiratory support. Typically all patients with Grade 3–4 CRS will be admitted to the ICU, while some patients with Grade 2 CRS will be transferred to the ICU based on risk factors, trajectory, and institutional protocol (Table 5.4) [20].

As with sepsis, CRS-related hemodynamic instability often involves mixed distributive and cardiogenic shock resulting from vasoplegia, capillary leak, and inflammation-related myocardial dysfunction [21, 22]. Management of shock in CRS is discussed in detail elsewhere [20, 22] and should focus on prompt restoration of end-organ perfusion through judicious fluid resuscitation, restoration of vascular tone, and appropriate myocardial support. In particular, patients with concern for myocardial dysfunction should have echocardiographic evaluation and appropriate inotropic agents used to support cardiac function [20].

Respiratory insufficiency in CRS is usually hypoxemic and falls on the acute respiratory distress syndrome (ARDS) spectrum [19, 23]. Capillary leak and inflammatory pulmonary edema result in alveolar fluid accumulation, surfactant dysfunction, and impaired lung mechanics. Management of CRS-related respiratory insufficiency should follow generally accepted ARDS management [24], focusing on restoring normal gas exchange through supplemental oxygen delivery, alveolar recruitment, and low-volume lung-protective ventilation where required. Fluid administration and diuresis must be carefully balanced to reverse pulmonary edema while

**Table 5.4** Grading and management of CRS. Adapted from ASTCT consensus grading for CRS (Lee et al. 2019). *ATG* anti-thymocyte globulin; *CAR* chimeric antigen receptor; *CPAP* continuous positive airway pressure; *BiPAP* bi-level positive airway pressure; *ICU* intensive care unit

| | | Grade 1 | Grade 2 | Grade 3 | Grade 4 |
|---|---|---|---|---|---|
| **Diagnosis** | Fever | Temperature ≥ 38 °C | | | |
| | | With | | | |
| | Hypotension | None | Hypotension responding to fluids | Hypotension requiring single vasopressor +/− vasopressin | Hypotension requiring multiple pressors |
| | | And/or | | | |
| | Hypoxemia | None | Hypoxemia responding to low-flow nasal cannula or blow-by oxygen | Hypoxemia requiring high-flow nasal cannula, facemask, or nonrebreather | Hypoxemia requiring CPAP, BiPAP, or invasive ventilation |
| **Management** | **Tocilizumab dosing:**<br><30 kg: 12 mg/kg<br>≥30 kg: 8 mg/kg (max 800 mg)<br>**Steroid dosing:**<br>Methylprednisolone IV:<br>0.5–1 mg/kg q12h<br>Dexamethasone IV:<br>0.5–1 mg/kg (max 10 mg) Q6h | – Blood cultures and broad-spectrum antibiotics<br>– Antipyretics<br>– Maintain euvolemia<br>– Frequent labs and q12h CRS grading<br>– Consider Tocilizumab q8h for 3–4 doses for prolonged fever not responding to antipyretics | – Grade 1 interventions<br>Plus<br>– Low threshold for tocilizumab<br>– Consider stress-dose corticosteroids if adrenally suppressed<br>– Consider ICU transfer depending on the patient's trajectory | – Grade 2 interventions<br>Plus<br>– ICU transfer<br>– Tocilizumab q8h for 3–4 doses<br>– Low threshold for corticosteroids, especially if symptoms do not respond by the second dose of tocilizumab | – Grade 3 interventions<br>Plus<br>– Consider third-line agents if symptoms do not respond to 2 doses of tocilizumab plus corticosteroids<br>– Third-line agents: anakinra, siltuximab, high-dose steroids<br>– CAR-T-specific "safety switches": Dasatinib, ATG |

maintaining appropriate intravascular volume and organ perfusion.

Anti-cytokine biologics have been used successfully in CRS management and are considered core pharmacologic interventions. Tocilizumab is an anti-IL-6 monoclonal antibody that has been FDA-approved for managing CRS and should be considered in any patient with protracted fevers or severe symptomatology [25]. Corticosteroids are lymphotoxic and can theoretically impair CAR-T cell function, but may be used as a second-line agent in patients with severe CRS. Other biologics targeting cytokines such as siltuximab (IL-6), anakinra (IL-1), and infliximab (TNF-α) may be considered as third-line agents in refractory patients [20]. Additional third-line agents such as high-dose corticosteroids, chemotherapeutic agents, and small molecule kinase inhibitors have been investigated. All decisions regarding immunosuppression in patients with CRS should be made in close collaboration with relevant managing and consulting clinicians.

## Immune Effector Cell-Associated Neurotoxicity Syndrome

ICANS (formerly known as cytokine release encephalopathy syndrome [CRES]) is a neuropsychiatric syndrome associated with CAR T-cell therapy and some other immunotherapies. The pathophysiology of ICANS is not fully understood but is thought to result from cytokine-mediated cerebral endothelial dysfunction resulting in neuroinflammation, encephalopathy, and cerebral edema. ICANS can occur separately from, alongside, or following CRS [26, 27].

### ICANS: Clinical Presentation, Grading, and Management

Several factors are associated with the risk and severity of ICANS, including concomitant CRS, high disease burden, and pre-existing neurologic disorders (Table 5.2) [8, 26]. Clinically, ICANS can present with a range of neurologic signs and symptoms, from mild drowsiness and confusion to seizures stroke syndromes, and coma [19]. While oftentimes transient, ICANS symptoms may be disturbing and may include dysphasia, frank aphasia, or hallucinations. Of note, while headache is an extremely common nonspecific symptom associated with ICANS, it is not part of the diagnostic criteria.

The ASTCT consensus grading system for ICANS defines Grade 1 ICANS as isolated mild mental status changes as measured by the Immune Effector Cell-Associated Encephalopathy (ICE) [19] score in patients ≥12 years old or by Cornell Assessment of Pediatric Delirium (CAPD) [28] score in patients <12 years old or with pre-existing cognitive deficits (Table 5.5) [19]. Neurologic consultation should be obtained for these patients, and close neurologic monitoring should be initiated. Antiseizure prophylaxis may be considered depending on the patient's underlying seizure risk. Progressive mental status changes without seizure constitute Grade 2 ICANS, which warrants a more involved neurologic workup including neuroimaging, EEG, fundoscopy, and possible lumbar puncture to evaluate for infection. Grade 3 ICANS is defined by severe encephalopathy or any clinical seizure and is usually the threshold at which most institutions will transfer patients to the ICU. These patients should be treated with therapeutic doses of antiepileptics (usually levetiracetam), and corticosteroids (dexamethasone or methylprednisolone) may be administered and escalated as needed. Such patients will also likely require serial neuroimaging to monitor for evolving cerebral edema and cerebrovascular insults [8, 26, 27]. Grade 4 ICANS is the most severe and is defined by coma, protracted seizure, or clinical signs of increased intracranial pressure (ICP). In addition to interventions for lower-grade ICANS, these patients often require aggressive neuroprotective measures and intensive seizure control (Table 5.5). Patients should be intubated and

**Table 5.5** Grading and management of ICANS. Adapted from ASTCT consensus grading for CRS (Lee et al. 2019). *CRS* cytokine release syndrome; *ICANS* immune effector cell-associated neurotoxicity syndrome; *ICE* immune effector cell encephalopathy; *CAPD* Cornell assessment of pediatric delirium; *EEG* electroencephalogram; *ICP* intracranial pressure; *CT* computed tomography; *ICU* intensive care unit; *$pCO_2$* partial pressure of carbon dioxide

| | | Grade 1 | Grade 2 | Grade 3 | Grade 4 |
|---|---|---|---|---|---|
| **Diagnosis** | Cognitive scoring | ICE score 7–9 (≥12 years)<br>Or<br>CAPD score 1–8 (<12 years) | ICE score 3–6 (≥12 years)<br>Or<br>CAPD score 1–8 (<12 years) | ICE score 0–2 (≥12 years)<br>Or<br>CAPD score ≥9 (<12 years) | Unable to perform ICE<br>Or<br>Unable to perform CAPD |
| | Level of consciousness | Awakens spontaneously | Awakens to voice | Awakens only to tactile stimulus | May localize noxious tactile stimulus, stupor, or coma |
| | Seizures | None | None | Any clinical seizure that resolves spontaneously<br>Or<br>Nonconvulsive seizures on EEG that respond to treatment | Prolonged seizure (>5 min) with concerning vital sign changes<br>Or<br>Status epilepticus |
| | Cerebral edema | No radiographic cerebral edema | No radiographic cerebral edema | Focal/local radiographic cerebral edema | Clinical signs/symptoms of increased ICP (e.g., Cushing triad, papilledema, etc.)<br>Or<br>Diffuse radiographic cerebral edema |
| | Weakness | None | None | None | Territorial motor weakness (hemi/paraparesis) |
| **Management** | **Methylprednisolone IV:** 0.5–1 mg/kg q12h<br>**Dexamethasone IV:** 1 mg/kg (max 20 mg) Q6h<br>**High-dose methylprednisolone IV:** 30 mg/kg daily up to 1000 mg | – Close neuro monitoring with regular ICE/CAPD scoring<br>– Fundoscopy<br>– Low threshold for cross-sectional imaging (non-contrast head CT)<br>– Consider lumbar puncture with opening pressure<br>– Low-dose lorazepam or haloperidol as needed for agitation<br>– EEG for any acute mental status changes<br>– Consider levetiracetam for seizure prophylaxis | – Grade 1 interventions<br>Plus<br>– Consider steroids if concurrent CRS<br>– For ICANS without CRS, prioritize steroids over anti-IL6 therapy | – Grade 2 interventions<br>Plus<br>– Initiate steroids<br>– Consider ICU transfer depending on the patient's trajectory<br>– Initiate levetiracetam for maintenance seizure control | – Grade 3 interventions<br>Plus<br>– ICU transfer<br>– High-dose methylprednisolone<br>– Neuroprotective measures: Head of bed 30°, normothermia, normocarbia ($pCO_2$ 35–40 mmHg) euglycemia, eunatremia<br>– Seizure management as required<br>– Increased ICP/herniation: Initiate hyperosmolar therapy, deep sedation, hyperventilate ($pCO_2$ 30–35 mmHg), stat head CT, consider neurosurgery consult |

sedated, and clinical signs of increased ICP should be managed by established critical care standards, including lowering cerebral metabolic demand, promoting cerebral venous drainage, and maintaining eunatremia, euglycemia, normocarbia, and normothermia (Table 5.5). Evidence of herniation should be addressed with prompt hyperventilation, initiation of hyperosmolar therapy, and urgent cross-sectional imaging with neurosurgical consultation. Of note, while patients with ICANS may have already received tocilizumab for concomitant CRS, tocilizumab is not indicated in primary management of ICANS because it does not cross the blood–brain barrier and can paradoxically increase intracerebral IL-6 levels [29, 30].

## Other Complications of CAR T-Cell Therapy

*CAR-T-associated HLH:* HLH has some shared features with CRS but remains a separately defined entity. Pathophysiology and management of HLH are detailed in the *HLH-2004 Diagnostic and Therapeutic Guidelines* [31]. The theoretical goal of CAR-T-associated HLH treatment is to break the macrophage-CD8$^+$ T cell hyperactivation cycle, although no targeted therapies yet exist. CAR-T HLH often resolves with first-line CRS-directed treatment (tocilizumab and/or corticosteroids) [9], and refractory HLH should be managed per HLH-2004 guidelines.

*B-cell aplasia and long-term hypogammaglobulinemia*: Anti-CD-19 and CD-22 CAR T-cells deplete nonmalignant precursor and mature B-cells leading to hypogammaglobulinemia. These effects are expected to last months to years after CAR T-cell infusion. Monitoring IgG levels allows for surveillance of these long-term effects, and intravenous immunoglobulin (IVIG) infusion may be administered as treatment [8].

*GVHD*: Because transduced CAR T-cells still express their native T-cell receptors, activated CAR T-cells whose T-cell receptors recognize self-antigens can attack host cells and cause GVHD. This phenomenon is more common in patients who have previously received an allogeneic HCT because the CAR T-cells express donor-derived TCRs. Still, GVHD has also been described in patients receiving autologous CAR-T product [32]. Treatment for CAR-T-associated GVHD includes topical corticosteroids or topical calcineurin inhibitors for lower-grade presentations, introduction of systemic corticosteroids for higher-grade presentations, and other adjunctive immunosuppression for more severe or refractory cases [33].

## The Future of CAR-T Therapy

The success of CAR T-cell therapy for hematologic malignancies has led to widespread interest in applying this technology to other cancers. Solid tumors represent a particular challenge for CAR T-cell therapies. Solid tumors often exhibit antigenic heterogeneity and rarely express a single specific tumor antigen that would serve as a suitable CAR T-cell target. Solid tumors also promote a complex tumor microenvironment that supports tumor cell proliferation and suppresses host immunity [34].

Despite these challenges, there are ongoing efforts to develop CAR T-cells targeting solid tumor-associated targets. Early in vitro efficacy data exists for CAR T-cells targeting breast, ovarian, prostate, gastric, pancreatic, lung, and liver cancers [34]. Additional efforts are underway to develop bi-specific CAR T-cells as well as CAR T-cells against universal tumor antigen targets that could transcend specific malignancy classes [4, 35].

Novel fourth-generation CAR T-cells are engineered to secrete immunomodulatory proteins such as cytokines, exerting a direct effect on the tumor microenvironment to encourage more anti-tumor immune cell activation [7]. These "armored CAR" T-cells hold great promise in overcoming the immunologic obstacles to effective solid tumor immunotherapy.

Though currently FDA approved only for treating malignancy, CAR T-cells can theoretically eliminate any unwanted cell type, including chronic viral reservoirs. Indeed, CAR-T therapy has been investigated for treating chronic HIV, hepatitis B, cytomegalovirus, and Epstein–Barr virus [36–38].

## Gene Therapy

Gene therapy refers to the introduction or editing of genes in human cells to treat disease. Gene therapy offers the possibility of a permanent cure and can replace genes with pathogenic mutations (as with inborn errors of metabolism and hemoglobinopathies) or introduce new genes to impart novel biologic functions. Indeed, CAR T-cell therapy is a gene therapy in which a patient's native T-cells are transduced to express the CAR construct to fight cancer. Gene therapy is a vibrant area of research and innovation, and there are many strategies for introducing, replacing, or silencing genes into specific cells and tissues. In this section, we will focus on *ex vivo* gene therapy for hematopoietic stem cells, in which stem cells are removed, modified, and then reinfused into the patient.

## Patient Selection, Product Manufacture, and Administration

While there have been numerous clinical trials (Table 5.6) [39–47], there are currently no FDA-approved non-CAR-T hematopoietic gene therapies. In order to be selected for a gene therapy trial, patients must meet specific criteria including prior treatment, performance status, and ability to survive the duration of product manufacture [48]. Additionally, the patient must be at an institution that can provide proper pre-administration care, manufacture and administer the product, and manage complications.

The process of *ex vivo* gene therapy starts with harvesting stem cells from bone marrow or peripheral blood. These cells are then processed and transduced to introduce the gene of interest. Most of the currently investigated gene therapies employ viral vectors (primarily retroviruses and adeno-associated viruses) to transduce hematopoietic stem cells (Fig. 5.4a, b) [49, 50]. Novel gene editing techniques such as CRISPR-Cas9 are also under investigation [49, 50]. Post-transduction quality control is performed and is generally similar to that employed for CAR-T cells discussed earlier in this chapter.

**Table 5.6** Non-exhaustive list of *ex vivo* hematopoietic gene therapy trials

| Disease target | Reference |
|---|---|
| Adenosine deaminase deficiency | Aiuti, et al. 2009 [41] |
| β-thalassemia | Cavazzana, et al. 2010 [39] |
| Wiskott-Aldrich syndrome | Aiuti, et al. 2013 [42, 47] |
| IL2R©-deficient X-SCID | De Ravin, et al. 2016 [43] |
| Sickle cell disease | Ribeil, et al. 2017 [40, 46] |
| Adrenoleukodystrophy | Eichler, et al. [45] |
| Chronic granulomatous disease | Kohn, et al. 2020 [44] |

Similar to HCTs, patients may receive a conditioning regimen before administering gene therapy to "clear" the bone marrow and improve the engraftment of the modified hematopoietic stem cells. The intensity of conditioning depends on both the product and the condition, the goal being to induce minimum toxicity while maximizing the chance of engraftment. For instance, low-intensity regimens may be employed when mixed chimerism can be tolerated, such as in immunodeficiencies where gene-corrected cells have a natural selective advantage over native cells [51]. Alternatively, a high-intensity regimen may be administered in conditions like thalassemia or lysosomal storage disorders where high-efficiency engraftment is required.

## Complications of Gene Therapy

Due to the challenge of accurately targeting gene insertion, oncogenesis and myelodysplasia are major risks of gene therapy. In an early SCID-X1 trial, four of nine successfully treated patients developed uncontrolled clonal proliferation of T-cells around 3 years following initial treatment [52, 53]. This clonal proliferation was due to retrovirus vector insertion near a proto-oncogene promoter (LMO2), leading to unregulated premalignant cell proliferation due to retrovirus enhancer activity. More recently, a promising gene therapy trial for sickle cell anemia was halted after two patients developed myelodysplastic syndrome (MDS), though the causal relationship to gene therapy is doubted [54]. Recent advances have improved targeted gene insertion and demonstrated decreased clustering of insertion sites within lymphoid proto-oncogenes [53, 55].

Another risk of gene therapy is viremia and inflammation from viral vectors [56, 57]. This risk is particularly relevant

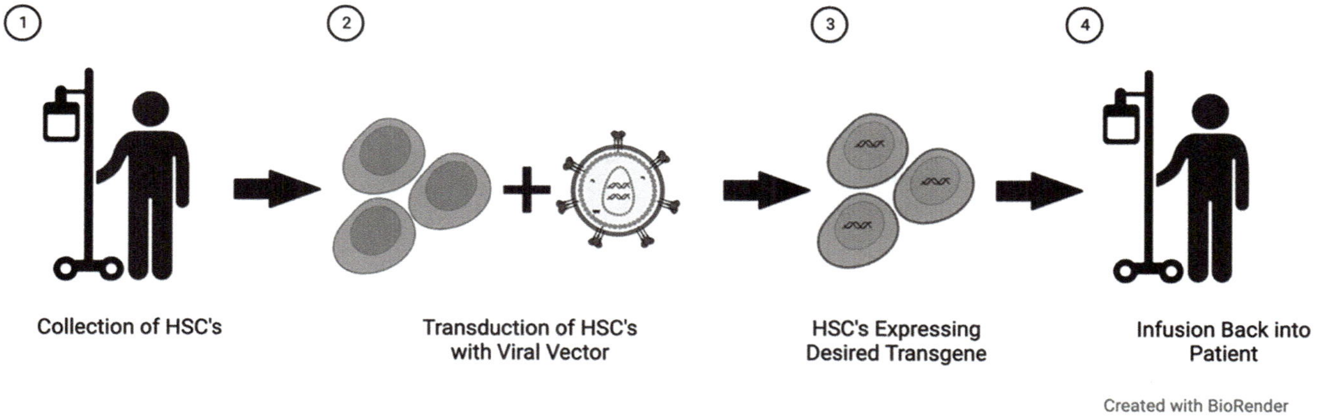


**Fig. 5.4** Process of *ex vivo* gene therapy. *HSC* hematopoietic stem cell. Created with BioRender.com

given that many gene therapy patients are intrinsically or iatrogenically immunosuppressed. Indeed, the entire field of gene therapy suffered a dramatic setback in the late 1990s when a young patient with ornithine transcarbamylase deficiency suffered overwhelming viral sepsis and died days after receiving gene therapy via an adenovirus vector [58]. An immune response against a vector can also promote clearance of the vector leading to decreased transduction efficiency with *in vivo* therapy, though this is less of a concern in *ex vivo* treatment [56, 59].

Though the above risks are real, the lack of longitudinal data coupled with the heterogeneity of gene therapy products means there is no standardized protocol for managing such complications. Gene therapy-related cancers should be managed by the same protocols employed for primary malignancies. Vector-related viremia in *ex vivo* gene therapy is theoretical, with no definitively documented cases, and treatment should be focused on suppressing viremia and inflammation with appropriate agents [56].

## Antiviral Cytotoxic T-Lymphocyte Therapy

Antiviral cytotoxic T-lymphocytes (CTLs) are an allogeneic cellular therapy in which T-cells against a particular virus are infused into a patient to treat viral infection or reactivation. The first antiviral T-cell infusions were performed in the late 1990s when patients who received an HCT also received virus-specific donor T-cell infusions for management of cytomegalovirus (CMV) and Epstein–Barr virus (EBV)-related complications [60, 61]. Since then, numerous antiviral cellular therapies have been studied for various viruses including adenovirus, BK virus, and human herpesvirus 6 [62]. While initial antiviral CTLs used expanded lymphocytes obtained from a patient's donor, more recent efforts have focused on generating pre-expanded banks of HLA-typed antiviral lymphocytes that can be quickly matched and infused on demand [63, 64]. Because of the cost and time associated with antiviral CTL therapy, it is not currently regarded as a first-line therapy. Nevertheless, antiviral CTLs represent a promising modality for managing high-morbidity viral infections for which traditional antiviral pharmacologic treatment is either ineffective or otherwise unsuitable.

## CTLs: Patient Selection, Product Matching, and Administration

Antiviral CTLs are most commonly used in post-HCT patients experiencing lymphopenia because they frequently experience viral reactivation or de novo infection from the transplant. These patients are generally either seropositive for the target virus or have received a transplant from a seropositive donor. Antiviral CTLs can also treat infection in patients with primary T-cell immunodeficiencies such as Severe Combined Immunodeficiency (SCID) or HLH [65]. Patients experiencing lymphopenia with active viral infection are typically first treated with a small molecule antiviral agent (e.g., ganciclovir or foscarnet for CMV). Antiviral immunoglobulins (e.g., CMV-IVIG) may also be used. Antiviral CTL therapy is pursued in the setting of adverse effects to these agents (e.g., myelosuppression, nephrotoxicity), insufficient response, or other contraindications (e.g., impaired renal or hepatic function).

Presently, most antiviral CTLs are derived from a single donor who is HLA-matched to the recipient. There are two ways to acquire enough cells for transfusion: purification of a large number of cells from the donor or *ex vivo* expansion after a relatively small number of cells is collected (Table 5.7). Purification is much faster but requires processing a large volume of donor blood. *Ex vivo* expansion, on the other hand, is time-intensive because of the need to culture target CTLs. Finally, third-party (taken from an individual who is not the patient's HCT donor) antiviral T-cells are being increasingly used because they are bankable and immediately available. However, these products are only available for more common human leukocyte antigen (HLA) types, and the cells may not persist as long *in vivo* as donor-derived CTLs. The administration of antiviral CTLs is similar to the procedure for CAR T-cells described earlier in this chapter, without leukodepletion. Patients are commonly premedicated with acetaminophen and diphenhydramine.

**Table 5.7** Comparison of antiviral CTL production strategies. *HSC* hematopoietic stem cell; *HLA* human leukocyte antigen

| Method | Advantages | Disadvantages |
|---|---|---|
| *Ex vivo* culture | – Expansion of low-frequency populations | – Several weeks process<br>– The donor must be seropositive<br>– Contamination with other cell populations |
| Purification | – Fast | – Requires target cells to express specific markers<br>– It may still require *ex vivo* expansion<br>– The donor must be seropositive |
| Third-party/ bulk T-cells | – Immediately available<br>– It does not depend on the seropositivity of the HCT donor | – Only available for common HLA types<br>– Shorter persistence of cells |

### CTLs: Complications

The most commonly observed complications of antiviral T-cell therapy are immediate post-infusion reactions typical of transfused blood products (e.g., itching, rash, fevers). These can be managed conservatively with antipyretics and antihistamines and are typically prevented with standard pre-medication. More serious complications include systemic inflammatory responses that begin days after infusion (e.g., CRS and HLH), which can be managed similarly as CAR-T-associated CRS and HLH. Additionally, patients can develop GVHD if the CTLs are contaminated with alloreactive lymphocytes, although this is likely very rare [66]. Lastly, in the setting of virus-driven neoplasms like EBV-driven post-transplant lymphoproliferative disorder, there is a theoretical risk of a tumor lysis-like reaction. However, there are no published accounts of this in the literature.

## Other Cellular Immunotherapies

### Donor Regulatory T-Cells

Adoptive transfer of allogeneic antigen-specific regulatory T-cells is being investigated to treat a range of immunopathologic conditions including autoimmune disease (e.g., type-1 diabetes and inflammatory bowel disease), solid organ transplantation and HCT rejection, and both treatment and prevention of acute and chronic GVHD [67, 68]. While these applications of $T_{reg}$ cells have all used cells from a single donor, there are also investigations into fabricating CAR-$T_{reg}$-cells that could be administered off the shelf [69].

### Donor Anticancer T-Cells

Similar to antiviral CTLs, tumor-infiltrating lymphocytes (TILs) against specific cancer antigens can be harvested from patients or HLA-matched donors, expanded, and therapeutically infused to fight cancer. T-cell receptors from these anti-tumor lymphocytes can also be cloned and transduced into new T-cells similarly to CAR T-cells [70]. Unlike traditional CAR T-cells, these adoptive cellular therapies recognize target cells through classical major histocompatibility complex (MCH)-peptide complexes. Early evidence suggests that they may better penetrate and survive immunosuppressive tumor microenvironments and may exhibit lower immunotoxicity [70].

### Activated Cytokine-Induced Killer Cells

Cytokine-induced killer cells are a heterogenous mixture of cytotoxic lymphocytes including T-cells, natural killer (NK) cells, and natural killer T-cells (NKT) that can be harvested, stimulated, and expanded *ex vivo* and then infused into patients to effect potent anticancer activity and a low side-effect profile [71]. Importantly, these cells appear to kill both solid and hematologic malignancies in an MHC-independent manner. As with other cellular therapies, there are ongoing investigations into generating cytokine-induced killer cells with recombinant receptors that have augmented capabilities, are not donor-dependent, and can be banked and administered quickly and with less expense.

## The Future of Cellular Therapies

Cellular therapies have tremendous potential to rationally control human biology and treat disease. While their use is relatively limited as of this publication, the development of novel cellular therapies represents an intense area of biomedical investment. Over the next decade, we can expect cell therapies to expand dramatically and for significant advancements to be made in augmenting biological function, minimizing the side-effect profiles of these agents, and prolonging recipient survival. The growth of cellular therapies is essential in the broader trend toward personalized treatment for malignant and nonmalignant conditions. Palliative care clinicians will be increasingly tasked with helping patients evaluate these novel therapies in the setting of prognostic uncertainty and a rapidly evolving drug landscape. Moving forward, it will be critical for all members of cancer treatment teams, including palliative care clinicians, to be well-versed in the benefits, limitations, and potential complications of cellular therapies so that their patients may most benefit from these powerful living drugs.

## References

1. Sterner RC, Sterner RM. CAR-T cell therapy: current limitations and potential strategies. Blood Cancer J. 2021;11(4):69.
2. June CH, O'Connor RS, Kawalekar OU, Ghassemi S, Milone MC. CAR T cell immunotherapy for human cancer. Science (1979). 2018;359(6382):1361–1365.
3. Dhatchinamoorthy K, Colbert JD, Rock KL. Cancer immune evasion through loss of MHC Class I antigen presentation. Front Immunol. 2021;12:469.

4. Larson RC, Maus MV. Recent advances and discoveries in the mechanisms and functions of CAR T cells. Nat Rev Cancer. 2021;21(3):145–61.
5. Picanço-Castro V, Swiech K, Malmegrim KCR, Covas DT. CAR-T cells for cancer treatment: current design and next frontiers. Methods Mol Biol. 2020;2086:1–10.
6. Milone MC, Fish JD, Carpenito C, Carroll RG, Binder GK, Teachey D, et al. Chimeric receptors containing CD137 signal transduction domains mediate enhanced survival of T cells and increased antileukemic efficacy in vivo. Mol Ther. 2009;17(8):1453–64.
7. Hawkins ER, D'souza RR, Klampatsa A. Armored CAR T-cells: the next chapter in T-cell cancer immunotherapy. Biologics. 2021;15:95–105.
8. Lee DW, Shah N. Chimeric antigen receptor T-cell therapies for cancer: a practical guide. 222 p.
9. Mahadeo KM, Khazal SJ, Abdel-Azim H, Fitzgerald JC, Taraseviciute A, Bollard CM, et al. Management guidelines for paediatric patients receiving chimeric antigen receptor T cell therapy. Nat Rev Clin Oncol. 2019;16(1):45–63.
10. Maude SL, Laetsch TW, Buechner J, Rives S, Boyer M, Bittencourt H, et al. Tisagenlecleucel in children and young adults with B-cell lymphoblastic leukemia. N Engl J Med. 2018;378(5):439–48.
11. Cappell KM, Sherry RM, Yang JC, Goff SL, Vanasse DA, McIntyre L, et al. Long-term follow-up of anti-CD19 chimeric antigen receptor T-cell therapy. J Clin Oncol. 2020;38(32):3805–15.
12. Stroncek DF, Ren J, Lee DW, Tran M, Frodigh SE, Sabatino M, et al. Myeloid cells in peripheral blood mononuclear cell concentrates inhibit the expansion of chimeric antigen receptor T cells. Cytotherapy. 2016;18(7):893–901.
13. Klebanoff CA, Khong HT, Antony PA, Palmer DC, Restifo NP. Sinks, suppressors and antigen presenters: how lymphodepletion enhances T cell-mediated tumor immunotherapy. Trends Immunol. 2005;26(2):111–7.
14. Wang Z, Till B, Gao Q. Chemotherapeutic agent-mediated elimination of myeloid-derived suppressor cells. Onco Targets Ther. 2017;6(7):e1331807. https://doi.org/10.1080/2162402X.2017.1331807.
15. Bracci L, Schiavoni G, Sistigu A, Belardelli F. Immune-based mechanisms of cytotoxic chemotherapy: implications for the design of novel and rationale-based combined treatments against cancer. Cell Death Differ. 2014;21(1):15–25. https://www.nature.com/articles/cdd201367
16. Grigor EJM, Fergusson D, Kekre N, Montroy J, Atkins H, Seftel MD, et al. Risks and benefits of chimeric antigen receptor T-cell (CAR-T) therapy in cancer: a systematic review and meta-analysis. Transfus Med Rev. 2019;33(2):98–110.
17. Lee DW, Kochenderfer JN, Stetler-Stevenson M, Cui YK, Delbrook C, Feldman SA, et al. T cells expressing CD19 chimeric antigen receptors for acute lymphoblastic leukaemia in children and young adults: a phase 1 dose-escalation trial. Lancet. 2015;385(9967):517–28.
18. Neelapu SS, Locke FL, Bartlett NL, Lekakis LJ, Miklos DB, Jacobson CA, et al. Axicabtagene Ciloleucel CAR T-cell therapy in refractory large B-cell lymphoma. N Engl J Med. 2017;377(26):2531–44.
19. Lee DW, Santomasso BD, Locke FL, Ghobadi A, Turtle CJ, Brudno JN, et al. ASTCT consensus grading for cytokine release syndrome and neurologic toxicity associated with immune effector cells. Biol Blood Marrow Transplant. 2019;25(4):625–38.
20. Baumeister SHC, Mohan GS, Elhaddad A, Lehmann L. Cytokine release syndrome and associated acute toxicities in pediatric patients undergoing immune effector cell therapy or hematopoietic cell transplantation. Front Oncol. 2022;12:696.
21. Burstein DS, Maude S, Grupp S, Griffis H, Rossano J, Lin K. Cardiac profile of chimeric antigen receptor T cell therapy in children: a single-institution experience. Biol Blood Marrow Transplant. 2018;24(8):1590–5.
22. Gutierrez C, McEvoy C, Munshi L, Stephens RS, Detsky ME, Nates JL, et al. Critical care management of toxicities associated with targeted agents and immunotherapies for cancer. Crit Care Med. 2020;48(1):10.
23. Fitzgerald JC, Weiss SL, Maude SL, Barrett DM, Lacey SF, Melenhorst JJ, et al. Cytokine release syndrome after chimeric antigen receptor T cell therapy for acute lymphoblastic leukemia. Crit Care Med. 2017;45(2):e124–5.
24. Dellinger RP, Levy MM, Carlet JM, Bion J, Parker MM, Jaeschke R, et al. Surviving sepsis campaign: international guidelines for management of severe sepsis and septic shock: 2008. Crit Care Med. 2008;36(1):296–327.
25. Kotch C, Barrett D, Teachey DT. Tocilizumab for the treatment of chimeric antigen receptor T cell-induced cytokine release syndrome. Expert Rev Clin Immunol. 2019;15(8):813–22.
26. Schubert ML, Schmitt M, Wang L, Ramos CA, Jordan K, Müller-Tidow C, et al. Side-effect management of chimeric antigen receptor (CAR) T-cell therapy. Ann Oncol. 2021;32(1):34–48.
27. Morris EC, Neelapu SS, Giavridis T, Sadelain M. Cytokine release syndrome and associated neurotoxicity in cancer immunotherapy. Nat Rev Immunol. 2021;22(2):85–96.
28. Traube C, Silver G, Kearney J, Patel A, Atkinson TM, Yoon MJ, et al. Cornell assessment of pediatric delirium: a valid, rapid, observational tool for screening delirium in the PICU*. Crit Care Med. 2014;42(3):656–63. https://journals.lww.com/ccmjournal/Fulltext/2014/03000/Cornell_Assessment_of_Pediatric_Delirium__A_Valid,.20.aspx.
29. Santomasso BD, Park JH, Salloum D, Riviere I, Flynn J, Mead E, et al. Clinical and biological correlates of neurotoxicity associated with CAR T-cell therapy in patients with B-cell acute lymphoblastic leukemia. Cancer Discov. 2018;8(8):958–71.
30. Nellan A, Lester McCully CM, Garcia RC, Jayaprakash N, Widemann BC, Lee DW, et al. Improved CNS exposure to tocilizumab after cerebrospinal fluid compared to intravenous administration in rhesus macaques. Blood 2018;132(6):662–6.
31. Henter JI, Horne AC, Aricó M, Egeler RM, Filipovich AH, Imashuku S, et al. HLH-2004: diagnostic and therapeutic guidelines for hemophagocytic lymphohistiocytosis. Pediatr Blood Cancer. 2007;48(2):124–31.
32. Sanber K, Savani B, Jain T. Graft-versus-host disease risk after chimeric antigen receptor T-cell therapy: the diametric opposition of T cells. Br J Haematol. 2021;195(5):660–8.
33. Dignan FL, Clark A, Amrolia P, Cornish J, Jackson G, Mahendra P, et al. Diagnosis and management of acute graft-versus-host disease. Br J Haematol. 2012;158(1):30–45.
34. Marofi F, Motavalli R, Safonov VA, Thangavelu L, Yumashev AV, Alexander M, et al. CAR T cells in solid tumors: challenges and opportunities. Stem Cell Res Ther. 2021;12(1):81.
35. Zhao J, Lin Q, Song Y, Liu D. Universal CARs, universal T cells, and universal CAR T cells. J Hematol Oncol. 2018;11(1):132.
36. Seif M, Einsele H, Löffler J. CAR T cells beyond cancer: hope for immunomodulatory therapy of infectious diseases. Front Immunol. 2019;10:2711.
37. Kuhlmann AS, Peterson CW, Kiem HP. Chimeric antigen receptor T-cell approaches to HIV cure. Curr Opin HIV AIDS. 2018;13(5):446–53.
38. Maldini CR, Claiborne DT, Okawa K, Chen T, Dopkin DL, Shan X, et al. Dual CD4-based CAR T cells with distinct costimulatory domains mitigate HIV pathogenesis in vivo. Nat Med. 2020;26(11):1776–87.
39. Cavazzana-Calvo M, Payen E, Negre O, Wang G, Hehir K, Fusil F, et al. Transfusion independence and HMGA2 activation after gene therapy of human β-thalassaemia. Nature. 2010;467(7313):318–22. https://www.nature.com/articles/nature09328.

40. Ribeil JA, Hacein-Bey-Abina S, Payen E, Magnani A, Semeraro M, Magrin E, et al. Gene therapy in a patient with sickle cell disease. N Engl J Med. 2017;376(9):848–55. https://pubmed.ncbi.nlm.nih.gov/28249145/.
41. Aiuti A, Cattaneo F, Galimberti S, Benninghoff U, Cassani B, Callegaro L, et al. Gene therapy for immunodeficiency due to adenosine deaminase deficiency. N Engl J Med. 2009;360(5):447–58. https://pubmed.ncbi.nlm.nih.gov/19179314/.
42. Aiuti A, Biasco L, Scaramuzza S, Ferrua F, Cicalese MP, Baricordi C, et al. Lentiviral hematopoietic stem cell gene therapy in patients with Wiskott-Aldrich syndrome. Science (1979). 2013;341(6148):1233151. https://doi.org/10.1126/science.1233151.
43. de Ravin SS, Wu X, Moir S, Anaya-O'Brien S, Kwatemaa N, Littel P, et al. Lentiviral hematopoietic stem cell gene therapy for X-linked severe combined immunodeficiency. Sci Transl Med. 2016;8(335):335–57. https://doi.org/10.1126/scitranslmed.aad8856.
44. Kohn DB, Booth C, Kang EM, Pai SY, Shaw KL, Santilli G, et al. Lentiviral gene therapy for X-linked chronic granulomatous disease. Nat Med. 2020;26(2):200–6. https://www.nature.com/articles/s41591-019-0735-5.
45. Eichler F, Duncan C, Musolino PL, Orchard PJ, de Oliveira S, Thrasher AJ, et al. Hematopoietic stem-cell gene therapy for cerebral Adrenoleukodystrophy. N Engl J Med. 2017;377(17):1630–8. https://doi.org/10.1056/NEJMoa1700554.
46. Esrick EB, Lehmann LE, Biffi A, Achebe M, Brendel C, Ciuculescu MF, et al. Post-transcriptional genetic silencing of BCL11A to treat sickle cell disease. N Engl J Med. 2021;384(3):205–15. https://doi.org/10.1056/NEJMoa2029392.
47. Magnani A, Semeraro M, Adam F, Booth C, Dupré L, Morris EC, et al. Long-term safety and efficacy of lentiviral hematopoietic stem/progenitor cell gene therapy for Wiskott–Aldrich syndrome. Nat Med. 2022;28(1):71–80. https://www.nature.com/articles/s41591-021-01641-x.
48. Elverum K, Whitman M. Delivering cellular and gene therapies to patients: solutions for realizing the potential of the next generation of medicine. Gene Ther. 2020;27(12):537–44.
49. Ferrari S, Vavassori V, Canarutto D, Jacob A, Castiello MC, Javed AO, et al. Gene editing of hematopoietic stem cells: hopes and hurdles toward clinical translation. Front Genome Ed. 2021;3:618378.
50. Dunbar CE, High KA, Joung JK, Kohn DB, Ozawa K, Sadelain M. Gene therapy comes of age. Science. 2018;359(6372):eaan4672.
51. Bernardo ME, Aiuti A. The role of conditioning in hematopoietic stem-cell gene therapy. Hum Gene Ther. 2016;27(10):741–8.
52. Hacein-Bey-Abina S, Von Kalle C, Schmidt M, McCormack MP, Wulffraat N, Leboulch P, et al. LMO2-associated clonal T cell proliferation in two patients after gene therapy for SCID-X1. Science. 2003;302(5644):415–9.
53. Cavazzana M, Six E, Lagresle-Peyrou C, André-Schmutz I, Hacein-Bey-Abina S. Gene therapy for X-linked severe combined immunodeficiency: where do we stand? Hum Gene Ther. 2016;27(2):108–16.
54. Hsieh MM, Bonner M, Pierciey FJ, Uchida N, Rottman J, Demopoulos L, et al. Myelodysplastic syndrome unrelated to lentiviral vector in a patient treated with gene therapy for sickle cell disease. Blood Adv. 2020;4(9):2058–63.
55. Hacein-Bey-Abina S, Pai SY, Gaspar HB, Armant M, Berry CC, Blanche S, et al. A modified γ-retrovirus vector for X-linked severe combined immunodeficiency. N Engl J Med. 2014;371(15):1407–17.
56. High KA, Roncarolo MG. Gene therapy. N Engl J Med. 2019;381(5):455–64.
57. Liu Q, Muruve DA. Molecular basis of the inflammatory response to adenovirus vectors. Gene Ther. 2003;10(11):935–40.
58. Raper SE, Chirmule N, Lee FS, Wivel NA, Bagg A, Gao GP, et al. Fatal systemic inflammatory response syndrome in a ornithine transcarbamylase deficient patient following adenoviral gene transfer. Mol Genet Metab. 2003;80(1–2):148–58.
59. Morgan RA, Gray D, Lomova A, Kohn DB. Hematopoietic stem cell gene therapy: progress and lessons learned. Cell Stem Cell. 2017;21(5):574–90.
60. Rooney CM, Smith CA, Ng CYC, Loftin SK, Sixbey JW, Gan Y, et al. Infusion of cytotoxic T cells for the prevention and treatment of Epstein-Barr virus–induced lymphoma in allogeneic transplant recipients. Blood. 1998;92(5):1549–55.
61. Walter EA, Greenberg PD, Gilbert MJ, Finch RJ, Watanabe KS, Thomas ED, et al. Reconstitution of cellular immunity against cytomegalovirus in recipients of allogeneic bone marrow by transfer of T-cell clones from the donor. N Engl J Med. 1995;333(16):1038–44.
62. Gerdemann U, Keirnan JM, Katari UL, Yanagisawa R, Christin AS, Huye LE, et al. Rapidly generated multivirus-specific cytotoxic T lymphocytes for the prophylaxis and treatment of viral infections. Mol Ther. 2012;20(8):1622–32.
63. Tzannou I, Papadopoulou A, Naik S, Leung K, Martinez CA, Ramos CA, et al. Off-the-shelf virus-specific T cells to treat BK virus, human herpesvirus 6, cytomegalovirus, Epstein-Barr virus, and adenovirus infections after allogeneic hematopoietic stem-cell transplantation. J Clin Oncol. 2017;35(31):3547–57.
64. Leen AM, Bollard CM, Mendizabal AM, Shpall EJ, Szabolcs P, Antin JH, et al. Multicenter study of banked third-party virus-specific T cells to treat severe viral infections after hematopoietic stem cell transplantation. Blood. 2013;121(26):5113–23.
65. Keller MD, Bollard CM. Virus-specific T-cell therapies for patients with primary immune deficiency. Blood. 2020;135(9):620–8.
66. Melenhorst JJ, Leen AM, Bollard CM, Quigley MF, Price DA, Rooney CM, et al. Allogeneic virus-specific T cells with HLA alloreactivity do not produce GVHD in human subjects. Blood. 2010;116(22):4700–2.
67. Brunstein CG, Miller JS, McKenna DH, Hippen KL, DeFor TE, Sumstad D, et al. Umbilical cord blood–derived T regulatory cells to prevent GVHD: kinetics, toxicity profile, and clinical effect. Blood. 2016;127(8):1044–51.
68. Whangbo J, Nikiforow S, Kim HT, Wahl J, Reynolds CG, Chamling Rai S, et al. A phase 1 study of donor regulatory T-cell infusion plus low-dose interleukin-2 for steroid-refractory chronic graft-vs-host disease. Blood Adv. 2022;6(21):5786–96.
69. MacDonald KG, Hoeppli RE, Huang Q, Gillies J, Luciani DS, Orban PC, et al. Alloantigen-specific regulatory T cells generated with a chimeric antigen receptor. J Clin Invest. 2016;126(4):1413.
70. Titov A, Zmievskaya E, Ganeeva I, Valiullina A, Petukhov A, Rakhmatullina A, et al. Adoptive immunotherapy beyond CAR T-cells. Cancers (Basel). 2021;13(4):1–23.
71. Zhang Y, Schmidt-Wolf IGH. Ten-year update of the international registry on cytokine-induced killer cells in cancer immunotherapy. J Cell Physiol. 2020;235(12):9291–303.

# Part II

# Palliative Care

# Palliative Care Approach for Patients with Hematologic Malignancies and Other Serious Blood Disorders

6

Li Mo and David Hui

## Introduction

Despite major advances in therapeutics over the past decades, patients with refractory hematologic malignancies and other serious blood disorders continue to experience a poor prognosis and often die of their disease. More than 50,000 people die annually from hematologic malignancies in the United States [1]. In hematologic malignancies, leukemia and non-Hodgkin lymphoma (NHL) were the top two contributors to absolute years of life lost [2]. The Global Burden of Disease study showed that between 2006 and 2016, the incidence of leukemia increased by 26% and the incidence of NHL increased by 45%, leading to 310,000 leukemia deaths and 240,000 NHL deaths in 2016 [2, 3]. A population-based study of 11 lymphoid and myeloid malignancies in 20 European countries demonstrated that the 5-year survival of acute myeloid leukemia (AML) was only 14.8%, precursor lymphoblastic leukemia/lymphoma was 41.1%, and multiple myeloma/plasmacytoma was 39.6% [4]. Furthermore, survival was particularly low among patients with advanced age. In elderly patients 65 years or older, the 5-year survival of acute lymphoblastic leukemia (ALL) was only 17% and AML was 13.1% in the US [5].

Cancer and its treatments can have a significant effect on the health-related quality of life during diagnosis and treatment and years after the treatment has been completed [6]. Due to the availability of new agents that significantly improve survival [7], several hematologic malignancies and other serious blood disorders (e.g., sickle cell disease) that were rapidly fatal have become chronic conditions that can be managed with continued treatment [8, 9]. Therefore, patients with hematologic malignancies or other serious blood disorders might experience more chronic symptoms and complications along the disease trajectory. Throughout the disease, patients could receive treatment with systemic therapy (e.g., chemotherapy, targeted therapy, and immunotherapy), radiotherapy, or combined modality therapy. These interventions might result in severe morbidity and cause multiple organ dysfunction and even secondary malignancies. Moreover, patients with hematologic malignancies or other serious blood disorders and their caregivers often experience significant distress and psychosocial concerns [10–17].

Similar to patients with solid tumors, patients with hematologic malignancies or other serious blood disorders have a significant symptom burden, especially at the end of life. Common symptoms include pain, fatigue, dyspnea, nausea, vomiting, anorexia, weight loss, drowsiness, night sweats, and delirium [9, 18–24]. Hochman et al. found that pain, dyspnea, nausea, and anorexia were as frequent among patients with hematologic malignancies as those with solid malignancies. Furthermore, patients with blood cancer had higher rates of clinically significant fatigue and drowsiness than solid tumor patients [22]. Similarly, Fadul et al. used the Edmonton Symptom Assessment System (ESAS) to assess the symptom burden in patients with hematologic malignancies and reported they were more likely to be drowsy and delirious compared to patients with solid tumors [24].

Patients with hematologic malignancies have significantly lower performance status and quality of life than the general population [11, 25]. They are more likely to have intensive end-of-life care and less likely to be seen by palliative care compared to patients with solid tumors [26]. Additionally, survivors also often face challenges during their recovery, including unemployment, problems obtaining new health insurance and life insurance, and difficulties

L. Mo
The Center of Gerontology and Geriatrics, National Clinical Research Center of Geriatrics, West China Hospital, Sichuan University, Chengdu, Sichuan, China

D. Hui (✉)
Department of Palliative Care, Rehabilitation, and Integrative Medicine, University of Texas MD Anderson Cancer Center, Houston, TX, USA
e-mail: DHui@mdanderson.org



C. K. Ullrich, E. J. Roeland (eds.), *Palliative Care in Hematologic Malignancies and Serious Blood Disorders*,
https://doi.org/10.1007/978-3-031-38058-7_6

applying for mortgages and continuing rehabilitation [11, 25, 27, 28]. These issues can seriously impact the quality of life of patients and survivors. Given the significantly prolonged survival of patients with hematologic malignancies, it is critical that we expand our view of the outcomes of therapy to enhance patients' physical, emotional, and social well-being during treatment and beyond [23].

It is important to highlight the significant symptom burden and supportive care needs that exist despite intensive supportive care provided by hematologic oncology teams. Recently, El-Jawahri and colleagues conducted a randomized trial comparing routine oncologic care provided by hematopoietic cell transplant (HCT) teams with or without specialist palliative care [12]. All patients reported a steep deterioration in quality of life and worsened depression as expected; however, patients randomly assigned to receive inpatient palliative care consultation had better quality of life, symptom burden, depression, and anxiety compared routine oncologic care alone [29]. Importantly, patients in the control group were already receiving high-intensity supportive care provided by their hematologic oncology team. This important study highlights the added benefits of specialist palliative care consultation for patients with hematologic malignancies.

Palliative care is "an approach that improves the quality of life of patients and their families facing the problem associated with life-threatening illness, through the prevention and relief of suffering by means of early identification and impeccable assessment and treatment of pain and other problems, physical, psychosocial and spiritual" [30]. During the last few decades, palliative care as a field has offered significant expertise in symptom management, psychosocial care, communication, complex decision-making, caregiver support, transition of care, and end-of-life care [31, 32]. Since the opening of the first palliative care unit in 1976 in Montreal, Canada, these programs have become available at a large number of acute care hospitals and cancer centers around the world [33–35].

In this chapter, we shall discuss the palliative care approach for patients with hematologic malignancies and other serious blood disorders using the World Health Organization (WHO) framework and discuss how this could potentially contribute to improved patient outcomes [30]. Specifically, palliative care:

1. Provides relief from pain and other distressing symptom
2. Affirms life and regards dying as a normal process
3. Intends neither to hasten or postpone death
4. Integrates the psychological and spiritual aspects of patient care
5. Offers a support system to help patients live as actively as possible until death
6. Offers a support system to help caregivers cope during the patients illness and in their own bereavement
7. Uses a team approach to address the needs of patients and their families, including bereavement counseling, if indicated
8. Enhances quality of life, and may also positively influence the course of illness
9. Is applicable early in the course of illness, in conjunction with other therapies that are intended to prolong life, such as chemotherapy or radiation therapy, and includes those investigations needed to better understand and manage distressing clinical complications

## Pain and Symptom Management

Symptoms are common in individuals with hematologic malignancies and other serious blood disorders and often interrelated [18–24]. Providing patients with relief from pain and other distressing symptoms is a key element of palliative care. Pain is a common symptom in cancer patients, occurring in 20–60% of patients with hematologic malignancies [36–38]. The causes of pain in patients with hematologic malignancies are complex and intertwined (Fig. 6.1) [36, 39, 40]. Although cancer progression is an important source of pain in these patients, cancer treatment, psychological factors (e.g., depression, anxiety), spiritual distress, and financial toxicity may also contribute to the experience of pain. Interaction among these factors may affect the nature, extent, and duration of pain [41]. In a pilot study of 61 patients who received a HCT, one-third of patients reported pain impaired their daily function. Anxiety and depression were associated with functional impairment due to pain [42]. Poorly controlled pain has a significant impact on patients' mobility, sleep, mood, function, and overall quality of life [43].

Specialist palliative care teams have significant symptom management expertise to optimize patients' symptom distress and are thus are well positioned to support patients from diagnosis to the end of life. The complex symptoms are often best managed with a combination of pharmacological and non-pharmacological interventions delivered by an interdisciplinary team. Interdisciplinary care coupled with an emphasis of patient/caregiver education, longitudinal monitoring, and counseling support may allow patients to achieve optimal symptom control. This comprehensive approach has been used successfully to help patients manage their pain while maximizing safe opioid use during the opioid crisis [44–47].

Polypharmacy is another major challenge for both oncologists and patients [48–52]. Due to the increased number of comorbidities, polypharmacy is particularly common in elderly cancer patients and could lead to more drug interactions, hospital admissions, adverse events, and increased mortality [53–56]. Jorgensen and colleagues reported that

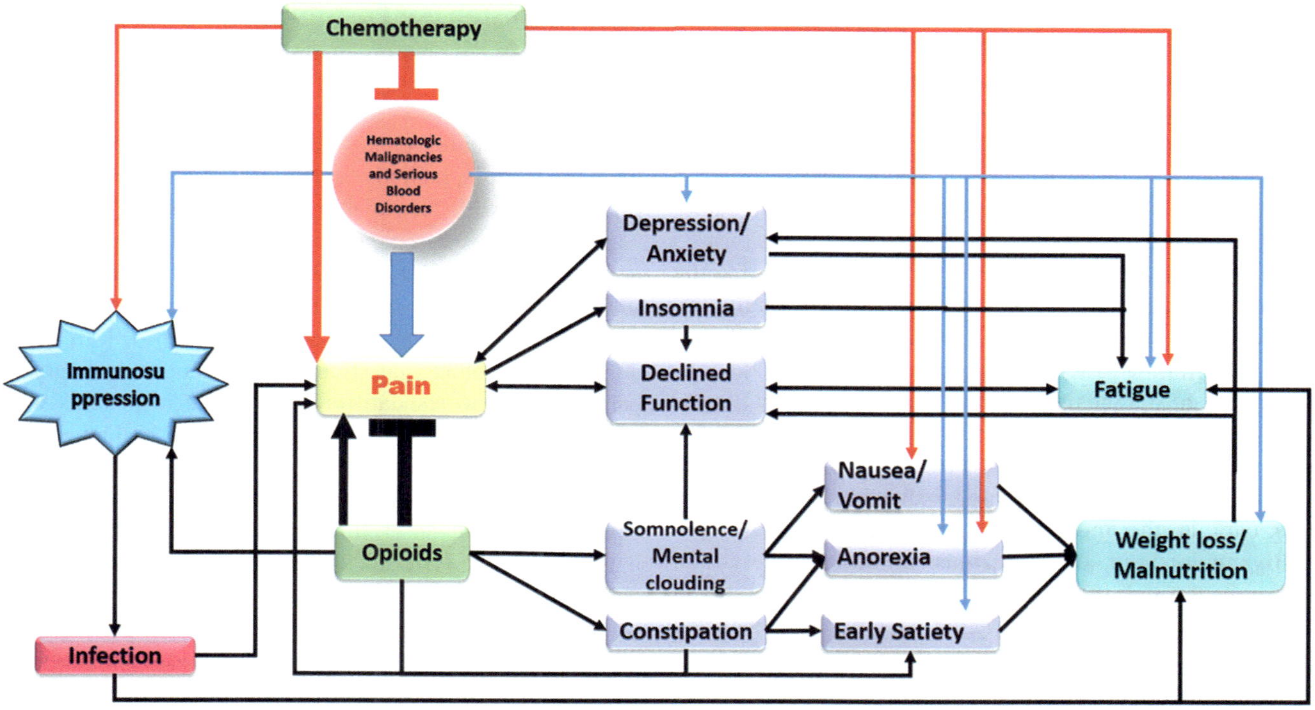


**Fig. 6.1** Interrelated symptoms in hematologic malignancies and serious blood disorders. This highly simplified example illustrates the complexity of symptom expression in an individual with hematologic malignancy. Physical pain caused by cancer may lead to depression/anxiety, insomnia, and functional decline. All symptoms can contribute to fatigue. Depression/anxiety in turn may increase pain expression and the level of fatigue. When opioids are used to treat pain, constipation and early satiety may occur, contributing to weight loss and malnutrition. Hematologic malignancy and sometimes serious blood disorders, chemotherapy, and opioids are immunosuppressive and may increase the risk of serious infection. Infection can then contribute to pain, fatigue, weight loss, and malnutrition. Changes in body image as a result of weight loss may lead to depression. Because symptoms are often interrelated and multifactorial in nature, multidimensional assessments and interventions are needed [40]. Adapted from Hui D, Bruera E. Supportive and Palliative Oncology—A New Paradigm for Comprehensive Cancer Care. Oncology & Hematology Review. 2013;9(1):68–74

35% of patients in a large, population-based cancer registry in Denmark aged 70 years or older were taking at least five drugs at any given time [49]. Furthermore, Alkan found that 35.1% of the elderly patients with cancer were exposed to severe drug interactions and it was associated with potentially inappropriate medication use [57]. Because palliative care teams often works with frail patients, the team can prioritize medication use and minimize polypharmacy through patient education, careful selection of medications, selective deprescribing, and adherence to safe prescription principles [58]. Some medications such as olanzapine can be used to treat multiple symptoms at the same time, including nausea, appetite, anxiety, and insomnia. This embodies the principle of "use a relatively small number of drugs, know them well, and use them appropriately" [58].

## Life-Affirming, Patient-Centered Care

Palliative care affirms life with an emphasis on patient-centered care. It shifts from the traditional biomedical model in favor of putting goal-concordant care at the center of clinical practice [59, 60]. Goal-concordant care, or care that aligns with patients' goals and values, is an important feature of high-quality medical treatment. It is associated with improved clinical outcomes, reduced patient distress, and healthcare costs [61–64]. Goals of care may include therapeutic goals (e.g., cancer treatments, intensive care unit (ICU) admission) and quality of life goals (e.g., living at home, maintaining relationship with loved ones, symptom management, advance care planning, and preparation for end of life). Palliative care teams have significant expertise navigating the complex discussions to address quality of life goals and can support therapeutic goals working in conjunction with the patient's hematology/oncology team [65]. Specifically, palliative care clinicians can facilitate goals of care discussions by improving patients' prognostic/illness understanding, engaging in advance care planning, and fostering realistic hope [66–68].

Death is associated with significant stigma in our society. Palliative care sees death and dying as a nature part of life. By helping patients to plan ahead proactively, palliative care can help to minimize undesired outcomes which may include emergency department visits and ICU admissions in the last days of life. Palliative care also recognizes that patients often require more intensive symptom management and psychosocial support as death approaches [69]. By engaging patients and caregivers in goals of care discussions along the disease trajectory, palliative care can have a positive impact on quality of end-of-life care [64].

Importantly, palliative care should not be limited to the end of life because patients with hematologic malignancies and other serious blood disorders have plenty of supportive/palliative care needs throughout disease trajectory from time of diagnosis [22, 24, 70]. Currently, palliative care referral for patients with hematologic malignancies patients is still mostly limited to the last weeks of life (Fig. 6.2a). An integration model that introduces palliative care at the moment of diagnosis of hematologic malignancies and other serious blood disorders and increases through the course of the disease (Fig. 6.2b and c) would allow patients to benefit from comprehensive care provided by their oncologists and palliative care teams [71, 72].

## Neither Hasten nor Postpone Death

Palliative care is designed to optimize care, support patients' goals, relieve patients' discomfort and caregivers' burden instead of hastening or postponing death. Among hematologic oncologists, palliative care is still often perceived to be synonymous with "end-of-life care" or "hospice care" [73–75] with some expressing concerns it may "take away hope" or even shorten survival by discontinuing cancer treatments. In fact, several studies found that palliative care is associated with improved survival in cancer patients [76–78]. In a randomized controlled trial, Temel et al. compared integrated palliative care to standard oncologic care in patients with metastatic non-small-cell lung cancer. The palliative care group not only had less aggressive care at the end of life but also longer survival [76]. Recently, a population-based study designed by Sullivan et al. examined 23,154 patients with lung cancer (stage IIIB and stage IV) reported that specialist palliative care received 31–365 days after cancer diagnosis was associated with increased survival compared with usual care. Receipt of palliative care was also associated with a reduced risk of death in an acute care setting [78].

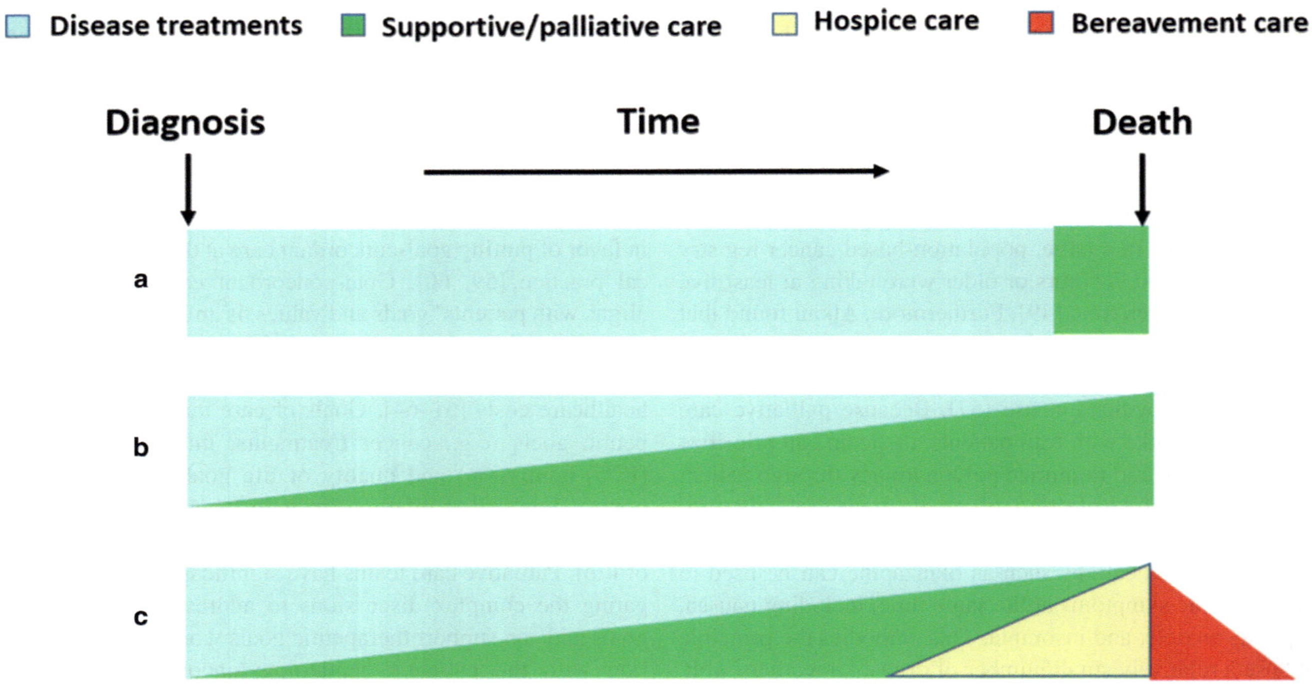


**Fig. 6.2** Time-based palliative care model. (**a**) Palliative care is introduced only when no more disease-directed treatments are possible; (**b**) palliative care is introduced from time of diagnosis and increases its involvement over time; (**c**) in addition to palliative care, this model includes hospice care and bereavement [72]. Adapted from Hui D, Bruera E. Models of integration of oncology and palliative care. Ann Palliat Med. 2015;4(3):89–98

There remains the misconception that patients may be persuaded to stop their cancer treatments once referred to palliative care. As discussed below, palliative care has the biggest impact when delivered timely and concurrent with cancer treatments. A randomized controlled trial found that although early palliative care did not reduce chemotherapy regimens use for patients with metastatic non-small-cell lung cancer, but only the timing of it. Early palliative care reduced half the odds of receiving chemotherapy within 60 days of death and a longer interval between the last dose of intravenous chemotherapy and death [79].

There are several postulated mechanisms on how palliative care may improve survival, such as improved symptom control, enhanced psychosocial support, interventions to improve nutrition and physical function, and less aggressive treatments at the end of life [31]. It should be noted that the survival benefit with palliative care has not been consistently demonstrated across randomized trials and systematic reviews [80]. Ultimately, the main goal of palliative care is to improve quality of life and quality of care.

## Integrating Psychological and Spiritual Care

Recognizing the importance of psychological and spiritual aspects of care and how much they can impact quality of life, palliative care places a strong emphasis on these domains. Previous studies have found that spiritual care provided by clergy in the community was associated with more intensive care and cost of care at the end of life among cancer patients with positive religious coping [81, 82]. In contrast, Balboni et al. reported that receipt of spiritual support from the medical team was associated with higher rates of hospice use, fewer aggressive interventions, and fewer ICU deaths among patients with advanced cancer [81]. Unique to the palliative care approach is the involvement of psychiatrist, psychologists, counselors, chaplains, and/or social workers in the interdisciplinary team who have significant expertise in these domains. Members of the palliative care team can ensure clear communication and discuss complex and sensitive topics with patients and caregivers in a unified and cohesive manner, while sharing different perspectives to ensure they can address the multidimensional aspects of suffering.

## Emphasis on Patient Function

Function is another important outcome in palliative care [70, 83]. Performance status is strongly associated with quality of life, independence, and survival. Patients with hematologic malignancies often present with reduced muscle and physical function related to underlying disease or cancer treatment [84, 85]. Fatigue caused by treatment is also a frequent and a severe problem in patients with hematologic malignancies and is associated with depressive mood and reduced physical and cognitive performance [86]. Palliative care aims at improving not only physical function but also emotional and social function by helping the patients to optimize their pain control, nutrition, depression, anxiety, and relationships [76, 87–89].

Caregivers may also benefit from palliative care interventions for emotional support, which may in turn, help them to maximize the patients' functional well-being. Specifically, palliative care teams may collaborate with rehabilitation services and involve physical therapists and occupational therapists and psychosocial professionals to maximize the patients' function. In turn, palliative physiatrists could deliver function-directed care in partnership with other disciplines and aligned with patient values to comprehensively address threats to patients' waning independence [88].

Increasing evidence suggests that physical exercise can improve functional status and quality of life in patients with hematologic malignancies. A systematic review that included nine randomized control trials (RCTs) involving 818 participants with hematologic malignancies reported that physical exercise improved quality of life, especially physical functioning, depression, and fatigue [90]. Recently, Fukushima et al. also found that low-intensity exercise therapy with high frequency significantly improved physical function, activity of daily livings, psychological distress, and quality of life among patients with hematologic malignancies undergoing chemotherapy, while maintaining muscle function, compared to low-frequency groups [91]. Because optimizing function is a desired outcome, involvement of palliative care early on from time of diagnosis may offer more opportunities for collaborative teamwork to maximize patient function and treatment tolerance [76, 87, 88].

## Caregiver Support

Palliative care not only focuses on patients but also sees family caregivers as a unit of care. Cancer as a chronic serious illness affects both patients and their caregivers. Caregivers have to confront with the possibility of losing their loved ones and a host of caregiving responsibilities [92, 93]. Moreover, the intensive nature of cancer treatment is often associated with many physical, psychological, social, logistical, and financial stressors that may add significant burden to caregivers [94, 95]. In some studies, the level of caregiver distress may be higher than patients' [95]. Sources of stress include prognostic uncertainty, anticipatory grief, juggling patients' needs with their own, and difficulties adapting to role changes [95]. These emotional burden can have an adverse effect on their post-bereavement mental health [96].

Caregivers who experience the most intense and prolonged emotional suffering near the end of life are more vulnerable in subsequent years to developing mental health diagnoses, functional disability, and potentially higher mortality [96–98]. Home-based specialized palliative and hospice care can provide logistical and healthcare supplies and staffing support aimed at reducing the caregivers' burden during the patients' illness and in their own bereavement [99]. The Domus trial, the first RCT targeting distress in patients and caregivers, found that home-based specialized palliative care with an integrated dyadic psychological intervention significantly attenuated caregiver anxiety and depression overall before and during bereavement [99–101]. Further studies confirmed the reduction of emotional distress among caregivers with early palliative care intervention [80, 102, 103]. Early palliative care involvement including psychosocial, spiritual, and bereavement support may help caregivers to better cope with grief [104]. Additionally, respite care is another good option and may be provided to further alleviate caregivers and to maximize patient safety.

## Interdisciplinary Team Model

One of the most unique and fundamental aspects of palliative care is its interdisciplinary nature, which allows the team to deliver multidimensional care addressing the complex supportive care needs of patients with advanced cancer and their families (Fig. 6.3). A multidisciplinary team is a group of domain experts working on separate parts of the same project. In this structure, each member operates as a part of a chain of responsibility. Interdisciplinary teams are different. On these teams, individuals from different fields are expected to contribute ideas to the entire project stack, not just the part they know the most about. A strength of this interdisciplinary approach within the context of palliative care is the shared decision-making, responsibility, and leadership to support patients and caregivers who are viewed from a holistic perspective. The physician, nurse, psychologist, social worker, chaplain, pharmacist, physiotherapist, occupational therapist, and other allied health professionals each contribute their unique expertise while working

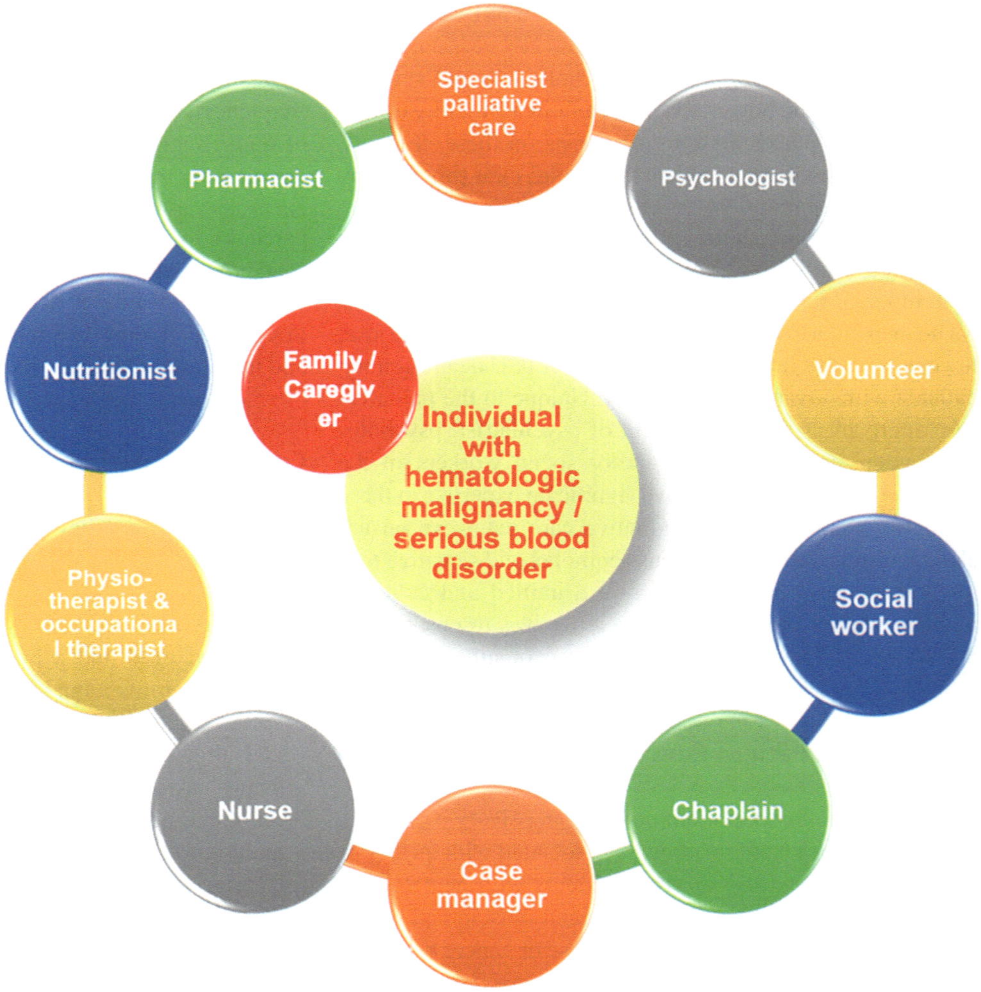


**Fig. 6.3** The interdisciplinary palliative care team. One of the most unique aspects of palliative care is its interdisciplinary nature, with different members of the team providing different expertise, thus allowing a patient's needs to be addressed in a holistic and timely fashion as well as augmenting family/caregiver(s) support. Other advantages of an interdisciplinary team include enhanced patient-clinician communication and shared responsibility, workload, decision-making, leadership, and stresses while providing care for patients with significant distress [31]. Adapted from Hui D, Hannon BL, Zimmermann C, Bruera E. Improving patient and caregiver outcomes in oncology: Team-based, timely, and targeted palliative care. CA Cancer J Clin. 2018;68(5):356–76

together in a cohesive manner to support the patient's goals through assessments, coordinated communication, and multidimensional interventions. The inter-professional approach is not only particularly useful in addressing intense care needs at the end of life, but also appropriate for patients earlier in the disease trajectory. An interdisciplinary intervention may be particularly helpful to support cancer patients with complex symptom needs and also help to reduce burnout among palliative care clinicians [31]. Interdisciplinary palliative care is particularly important given the wide array of supportive care needs in patients with hematologic malignancies [105].

In the climate of financial constraints, some leaders have advocated to do less with more. Some investigators have examined if palliative care team with limited team members can improve outcomes [106–109]. Overall, studies suggest that interdisciplinary teamwork is associated with better outcomes than single disciplinary teams such as nurse-only palliative care or physician-only palliative care [31, 107]. Consistent with this philosophy, an international Delphi study in 2015 reached consensus that, at a minimum, interdisciplinary teams should consist of a physician, nurse, and psychosocial team member [110].

## Improved Quality of Life and Patient Outcomes

Over the past decade, multiple RCTs and systematic reviews have found that specialist palliative care in conjunction with routine oncological care improved patient and caregiver outcomes compared to routine oncologic care alone [29, 68, 79, 80]. For example, EI-Jawahri et al. found that compared to those assigned to standard transplant care, patients assigned to the intervention who were seen by palliative care clinicians at least twice a week during HCT hospitalization had higher quality of life, less depression, and lower symptom burden after hospitalization for HCT [29]. Temel et al. also reported that for patients with newly diagnosed incurable lung and gastrointestinal cancer, early integrated palliative care and oncology care improved quality of life significantly from baseline to week 24 [68]. Taken together, studies suggest that timely involvement of palliative care, ideally by an interdisciplinary team, has the greatest impact on health outcomes.

Patients with hematologic malignancies often have worse quality of end-of-life care outcomes compared to those with advanced solid tumors. They were more likely to have emergency department visits, hospital admissions, intensive care unit admissions and death, chemotherapy use, and targeted-therapy use compared to patients with solid tumors, and are less likely to have palliative care unit admissions [16, 26, 111]. Clinical studies have consistently found that timely involvement of palliative care was associated with improved quality of end-of-life care for individuals with cancer [112–114]. Further studies in the hematologic populations and also other serious blood disorders are needed to determine best models of palliative care integration.

## Proactive Care through Timely Involvement

In the diagnosis and treatment of diseases, prevention always takes precedence over crisis management. Proactive approach to symptom management and care planning is better than a reactive approach. This idea has been endorsed in many chronic disease management, such as hypertension, diabetes, and cardiovascular diseases [115, 116].

Rather than giving up hope, palliative care can foster realistic hope by personalizing care decisions and engaging the patients and caregivers to plan ahead proactively [117]. For patients with incurable malignancies, palliative care can help identify and intervene early on patients' symptom, psychological and social burden, and improve patient and caregiver understanding of prognosis and survival [68, 77, 79, 87, 102, 118, 119]. Additionally, outpatient clinics have an important role to facilitate timely palliative care [119, 120]. Recently, a systematic review examined 15 RCTs of outpatient palliative care and 13 RCTs of palliative home care for patients with serious illnesses reported significant advantages with outpatient palliative care provided earlier in the disease trajectory, including improved symptoms, reduced depression, improved quality of life, reduced intensive care at the end of life, increased advance directive completion, reduced hospitalizations and length of stay, improved caregiver burden and quality of life, higher patient and family satisfaction, and reduction in the cost of medical care [119].

Because the definition of "early" palliative care differed among studies, an international Delphi panel was conducted to identify an appropriate timing for outpatient palliative care referral. The panel determined that a timely referral should occur at least 6 months before death [121]. However, it is often difficult to prognosticate. Thus, the panel also arrived at the conclusion that palliative care referral should be based on patients' supportive care needs, such as severe pain and neurological complications, rather than by prognosis alone. Systematic screening of supportive and palliative care needs, coupled with automatic triggers, can facilitate timely referral and potentially optimize resource use [31, 107, 122].

## Summary

Patients with hematologic malignancies and other serious blood disorders often have significant symptom burden and unmet supportive/palliative care needs throughout their illness. The palliative care approach focuses on providing timely, patient-centered and holistic care delivered by an interdisciplinary team. Specialist palliative care teams have significant expertise in symptom management and psychological, spiritual and caregiver care, communication, and complex decision-making that complement the expertise of hematologic oncologists to optimize symptom control, function, quality of life, and care outcomes. Further research is needed to examine how different models of integrating palliative care and hematologic oncology could optimize patient care.

## References


1. Chino F, Kamal AH, Chino J, LeBlanc TW. Disparities in place of death for patients with hematological malignancies, 1999 to 2015. Blood Adv. 2019;3(3):333–8.
2. Global Burden of Disease Cancer C, Fitzmaurice C, Akinyemiju TF, Al Lami FH, Alam T, Alizadeh-Navaei R, et al. Global, regional, and National Cancer Incidence, mortality, years of life lost, years lived with disability, and disability-adjusted life-years for 29 cancer groups, 1990 to 2016: a systematic analysis for the global burden of disease study. JAMA Oncologia. 2018;4(11):1553–68.
3. The LH. The global burden of haematological diseases. Lancet Haematol. 2018;5(1):e1.
4. Sant M, Minicozzi P, Mounier M, Anderson LA, Brenner H, Holleczek B, et al. Survival for haematological malignancies in Europe between 1997 and 2008 by region and age: results of EUROCARE-5, a population-based study. Lancet Oncol. 2014;15(9):931–42.
5. Redaniel MT, Pulte D, Jeffreys M. Survival disparities by age and country of diagnosis for patients with acute leukemia. Leuk Lymphoma. 2015;56(10):2787–92.
6. Mols F, Vingerhoets AJ, Coebergh JW, van de Poll-Franse LV. Quality of life among long-term breast cancer survivors: a systematic review. Eur J Cancer. 2005;41(17):2613–9.
7. Cortes JE, Kantarjian HM, Goldberg SL, Powell BL, Giles FJ, Wetzler M, et al. High-dose imatinib in newly diagnosed chronic-phase chronic myeloid leukemia: high rates of rapid cytogenetic and molecular responses. J Clin Oncol. 2009;27(28):4754–9.
8. Huang X, Cortes J, Kantarjian H. Estimations of the increasing prevalence and plateau prevalence of chronic myeloid leukemia in the era of tyrosine kinase inhibitor therapy. Cancer. 2012;118(12):3123–7.
9. Ajayi TA, Edmonds KP, Thornberry K, Atayee RA. Palliative care teams as advocates for adults with sickle cell disease. J Palliat Med. 2016;19(2):195–201.
10. Henry-Amar M, Joly F. Late complications after Hodgkin's disease. Ann Oncol. 1996;7(Suppl 4):115–26.
11. Mols F, Vingerhoets AJ, Coebergh JW, Vreugdenhil G, Aaronson NK, Lybeert ML, et al. Better quality of life among 10-15 year survivors of Hodgkin's lymphoma compared to 5-9 year survivors: a population-based study. Eur J Cancer. 2006;42(16):2794–801.
12. El-Jawahri AR, Traeger LN, Kuzmuk K, Eusebio JR, Vandusen HB, Shin JA, et al. Quality of life and mood of patients and family caregivers during hospitalization for hematopoietic stem cell transplantation. Cancer. 2015;121(6):951–9.
13. Zimmermann C, Yuen D, Mischitelle A, Minden MD, Brandwein JM, Schimmer A, et al. Symptom burden and supportive care in patients with acute leukemia. Leuk Res. 2013;37(7):731–6.
14. Bevans M, Sternberg EM. Caregiving burden, stress, and health effects among family caregivers of adult cancer patients. JAMA. 2012;307(4):398–403.
15. Nissim R, Zimmermann C, Minden M, Rydall A, Yuen D, Mischitelle A, et al. Abducted by the illness: a qualitative study of traumatic stress in individuals with acute leukemia. Leuk Res. 2013;37(5):496–502.
16. LeBlanc TW, El-Jawahri A. When and why should patients with hematologic malignancies see a palliative care specialist? Hematology Am Soc Hematol Educ Program. 2015;2015:471–8.
17. Rodin G, Yuen D, Mischitelle A, Minden MD, Brandwein J, Schimmer A, et al. Traumatic stress in acute leukemia. Psychooncology. 2013;22(2):299–307.
18. Ruffer JU, Flechtner H, Tralls P, Josting A, Sieber M, Lathan B, et al. Fatigue in long-term survivors of Hodgkin's lymphoma; a report from the German Hodgkin Lymphoma Study Group (GHSG). Eur J Cancer. 2003;39(15):2179–86.
19. Hjermstad MJ, Fossa SD, Oldervoll L, Holte H, Jacobsen AB, Loge JH. Fatigue in long-term Hodgkin's disease survivors: a follow-up study. J Clin Oncol. 2005;23(27):6587–95.
20. Ng AK, Li S, Recklitis C, Neuberg D, Chakrabarti S, Silver B, et al. A comparison between long-term survivors of Hodgkin's disease and their siblings on fatigue level and factors predicting for increased fatigue. Ann Oncol. 2005;16(12):1949–55.
21. Esser P, Kuba K, Mehnert A, Johansen C, Hinz A, Lordick F, et al. Quality of life in survivors of hematological malignancies stratified by cancer type, time since diagnosis and stem cell transplantation. Eur J Haematol. 2018;101(3):340–8.
22. Hochman MJ, Yu Y, Wolf SP, Samsa GP, Kamal AH, LeBlanc TW. Comparing the palliative care needs of patients with hematologic and solid malignancies. J Pain Symptom Manag. 2018;55(1):82–8 e1.
23. Cleeland CS, Williams LA. Symptom burden in hematologic malignancies. Blood. 2014;123(24):3686–7.
24. Fadul NA, El Osta B, Dalal S, Poulter VA, Bruera E. Comparison of symptom burden among patients referred to palliative care with hematologic malignancies versus those with solid tumors. J Palliat Med. 2008;11(3):422–7.
25. Mols F, Aaronson NK, Vingerhoets AJ, Coebergh JW, Vreugdenhil G, Lybeert ML, et al. Quality of life among long-term non-Hodgkin lymphoma survivors: a population-based study. Cancer. 2007;109(8):1659–67.
26. Hui D, Didwaniya N, Vidal M, Shin SH, Chisholm G, Roquemore J, et al. Quality of end-of-life care in patients with hematologic malignancies: a retrospective cohort study. Cancer. 2014;120(10):1572–8.
27. Joly F, Henry-Amar M, Arveux P, Reman O, Tanguy A, Peny AM, et al. Late psychosocial sequelae in Hodgkin's disease survivors: a French population-based case-control study. J Clin Oncol. 1996;14(9):2444–53.
28. van Tulder MW, Aaronson NK, Bruning PF. The quality of life of long-term survivors of Hodgkin's disease. Ann Oncol. 1994;5(2):153–8.
29. El-Jawahri A, LeBlanc T, VanDusen H, Traeger L, Greer JA, Pirl WF, et al. Effect of inpatient palliative care on quality of life 2 weeks after hematopoietic stem cell transplantation: a randomized clinical trial. JAMA. 2016;316(20):2094–103.
30. Organization WH. WHO definition of palliative care. World Health Organization; 2020. https://www.who.int/cancer/palliative/definition/en/.
31. Hui D, Hannon BL, Zimmermann C, Bruera E. Improving patient and caregiver outcomes in oncology: team-based, timely, and targeted palliative care. CA Cancer J Clin. 2018;68(5):356–76.
32. Bruera E, Hui D. Integrating supportive and palliative care in the trajectory of cancer: establishing goals and models of care. J Clin Oncol. 2010;28(25):4013–7.

33. Hui D, De La Rosa A, Chen J, Dibaj S, Delgado Guay M, Heung Y, et al. State of palliative care services at US cancer centers: an updated national survey. Cancer. 2020;126(9):2013–23.
34. Hui D, Cherny N, Latino N, Strasser F. The 'critical mass' survey of palliative care programme at ESMO designated centres of integrated oncology and palliative care. Ann Oncol. 2017;28(9):2057–66.
35. Hui D, Elsayem A, De la Cruz M, Berger A, Zhukovsky DS, Palla S, et al. Availability and integration of palliative care at US cancer centers. JAMA. 2010;303(11):1054–61.
36. Ma JD, El-Jawahri AR, LeBlanc TW, Roeland EJ. Pain syndromes and management in adult hematopoietic stem cell transplantation. Hematol Oncol Clin North Am. 2018;32(3):551–67.
37. Bevans MF, Mitchell SA, Marden S. The symptom experience in the first 100 days following allogeneic hematopoietic stem cell transplantation (HSCT). Support Care Cancer. 2008;16(11):1243–54.
38. Anderson KO, Giralt SA, Mendoza TR, Brown JO, Neumann JL, Mobley GM, et al. Symptom burden in patients undergoing autologous stem-cell transplantation. Bone Marrow Transplant. 2007;39(12):759–66.
39. Vanhelleputte P, Nijs K, Delforge M, Evers G, Vanderschueren S. Pain during bone marrow aspiration: prevalence and prevention. J Pain Symptom Manag. 2003;26(3):860–6.
40. Hui D, Bruera E. Supportive and palliative oncology—a new paradigm for comprehensive cancer care. Oncol Hematol Rev. 2013;9(1):68–74.
41. Syrjala KL, Jensen MP, Mendoza ME, Yi JC, Fisher HM, Keefe FJ. Psychological and behavioral approaches to cancer pain management. J Clin Oncol. 2014;32(16):1703–11.
42. Sherman AC, Coleman EA, Griffith K, Simonton S, Hine RJ, Cromer J, et al. Use of a supportive care team for screening and preemptive intervention among multiple myeloma patients receiving stem cell transplantation. Support Care Cancer. 2003;11(9):568–74.
43. Mantyh PW. Cancer pain and its impact on diagnosis, survival and quality of life. Nat Rev Neurosci. 2006;7(10):797–809.
44. Hui D, Arthur J, Bruera E. Palliative care for patients with opioid misuse. JAMA. 2019;321(5):511.
45. Arthur J, Hui D. Safe opioid use: management of opioid-related adverse effects and aberrant behaviors. Hematol Oncol Clin North Am. 2018;32(3):387–403.
46. Gaertner J, Boehlke C, Simone CB 2nd, Hui D. Early palliative care and the opioid crisis: ten pragmatic steps towards a more rational use of opioids. Ann Palliat Med. 2019;8(4):490–7.
47. Arthur JA, Haider A, Edwards T, Waletich-Flemming J, Reddy S, Bruera E, et al. Aberrant opioid use and urine drug testing in outpatient palliative care. J Palliat Med. 2016;19(7):778–82.
48. LeBlanc TW, McNeil MJ, Kamal AH, Currow DC, Abernethy AP. Polypharmacy in patients with advanced cancer and the role of medication discontinuation. Lancet Oncol. 2015;16(7):e333–41.
49. Jorgensen TL, Herrstedt J, Friis S, Hallas J. Polypharmacy and drug use in elderly Danish cancer patients during 1996 to 2006. J Geriatr Oncol. 2012;3(1):33–40.
50. Sokol KC, Knudsen JF, Li MM. Polypharmacy in older oncology patients and the need for an interdisciplinary approach to side-effect management. J Clin Pharm Ther. 2007;32(2):169–75.
51. Whitman A, DeGregory K, Morris A, Mohile S, Ramsdale E. Pharmacist-led medication assessment and deprescribing intervention for older adults with cancer and polypharmacy: a pilot study. Support Care Cancer. 2018;26(12):4105–13.
52. Leger DY, Moreau S, Signol N, Fargeas JB, Picat MA, Penot A, et al. Polypharmacy, potentially inappropriate medications and drug-drug interactions in geriatric patients with hematologic malignancy: observational single-center study of 122 patients. J Geriatr Oncol. 2018;9(1):60–7.
53. Marcum ZA, Amuan ME, Hanlon JT, Aspinall SL, Handler SM, Ruby CM, et al. Prevalence of unplanned hospitalizations caused by adverse drug reactions in older veterans. J Am Geriatr Soc. 2012;60(1):34–41.
54. Tam-McDevitt J. Polypharmacy, aging, and cancer. Oncology (Williston Park). 2008;22(9):1052–5; discussion 5, 8, 60.
55. Turner JP, Jamsen KM, Shakib S, Singhal N, Prowse R, Bell JS. Polypharmacy cut-points in older people with cancer: how many medications are too many? Support Care Cancer. 2016;24(4):1831–40.
56. Popa MA, Wallace KJ, Brunello A, Extermann M, Balducci L. Potential drug interactions and chemotoxicity in older patients with cancer receiving chemotherapy. J Geriatr Oncol. 2014;5(3):307–14.
57. Alkan A, Yasar A, Karci E, Koksoy EB, Urun M, Senler FC, et al. Severe drug interactions and potentially inappropriate medication usage in elderly cancer patients. Support Care Cancer. 2017;25(1):229–36.
58. Vrdoljak D, Borovac JA. Medication in the elderly—considerations and therapy prescription guidelines. Acta Med Acad. 2015;44(2):159–68.
59. Kogan AC, Wilber K, Mosqueda L. Person-centered care for older adults with chronic conditions and functional impairment: a systematic literature review. J Am Geriatr Soc. 2016;64(1):e1–7.
60. Lavoie M, Blondeau D, Martineau I. The integration of a person-centered approach in palliative care. Palliat Support Care. 2013;11(6):453–64.
61. Odejide OO, Uno H, Murillo A, Tulsky JA, Abel GA. Goals of care discussions for patients with blood cancers: association of person, place, and time with end-of-life care utilization. Cancer. 2020;126(3):515–22.
62. Emiloju OE, Djibo DAM, Ford JG. Association between the timing of goals-of-care discussion and hospitalization outcomes in patients with metastatic cancer. Am J Hosp Palliat Care. 2020;37(6):433–8.
63. Song MK, Ward SE, Fine JP, Hanson LC, Lin FC, Hladik GA, et al. Advance care planning and end-of-life decision making in dialysis: a randomized controlled trial targeting patients and their surrogates. Am J Kidney Dis. 2015;66(5):813–22.
64. Wright AA, Zhang B, Ray A, Mack JW, Trice E, Balboni T, et al. Associations between end-of-life discussions, patient mental health, medical care near death, and caregiver bereavement adjustment. JAMA. 2008;300(14):1665–73.
65. Ellis EM, Orehek E, Ferrer RA. Patient-provider care goal concordance: implications for palliative care decisions. Psychol Health. 2019;34(8):983–98.
66. Thomas TH, Jackson VA, Carlson H, Rinaldi S, Sousa A, Hansen A, et al. Communication differences between oncologists and palliative care clinicians: a qualitative analysis of early, integrated palliative care in patients with advanced cancer. J Palliat Med. 2019;22(1):41–9.
67. Jackson VA, Jacobsen J, Greer JA, Pirl WF, Temel JS, Back AL. The cultivation of prognostic awareness through the provision of early palliative care in the ambulatory setting: a communication guide. J Palliat Med. 2013;16(8):894–900.
68. Temel JS, Greer JA, El-Jawahri A, Pirl WF, Park ER, Jackson VA, et al. Effects of early integrated palliative care in patients with lung and GI cancer: a randomized clinical trial. J Clin Oncol. 2017;35(8):834–41.
69. Hallet J, Davis LE, Mahar AL, Isenberg-Grzeda E, Bubis LD, Myrehaug S, et al. Symptom burden at the end of life for neuroendocrine tumors: an analysis of 2579 prospectively collected patient-reported outcomes. Ann Surg Oncol. 2019;26(9):2711–21.
70. LeBlanc TW, Smith JM, Currow DC. Symptom burden of haematological malignancies as death approaches in a community pallia-

tive care service: a retrospective cohort study of a consecutive case series. Lancet Haematol. 2015;2(8):e334–8.
71. Vidal M, Hui D, Bruera E. Palliative care in patients with leukemia: when and how? Curr Oncol Rep. 2018;20(12):95.
72. Hui D, Bruera E. Models of integration of oncology and palliative care. Ann Palliat Med. 2015;4(3):89–98.
73. Parikh RB, Kirch RA, Smith TJ, Temel JS. Early specialty palliative care—translating data in oncology into practice. N Engl J Med. 2013;369(24):2347–51.
74. Public opinion research on palliative care: a report based on research by public opinion strategies. New York: Center to Advance Palliative Care; 2011.
75. Hui D, Park M, Liu D, Reddy A, Dalal S, Bruera E. Attitudes and beliefs toward supportive and palliative care referral among hematologic and solid tumor oncology specialists. Oncologist. 2015;20(11):1326–32.
76. Temel JS, Greer JA, Muzikansky A, Gallagher ER, Admane S, Jackson VA, et al. Early palliative care for patients with metastatic non-small-cell lung cancer. N Engl J Med. 2010;363(8):733–42.
77. Bakitas MA, Tosteson TD, Li Z, Lyons KD, Hull JG, Li Z, et al. Early versus delayed initiation of concurrent palliative oncology care: patient outcomes in the ENABLE III randomized controlled trial. J Clin Oncol. 2015;33(13):1438–45.
78. Sullivan DR, Chan B, Lapidus JA, Ganzini L, Hansen L, Carney PA, et al. Association of early palliative care use with survival and place of death among patients with advanced lung cancer receiving care in the Veterans Health Administration. JAMA Oncol. 2019;5(12):1702–9.
79. Greer JA, Pirl WF, Jackson VA, Muzikansky A, Lennes IT, Heist RS, et al. Effect of early palliative care on chemotherapy use and end-of-life care in patients with metastatic non-small-cell lung cancer. J Clin Oncol. 2012;30(4):394–400.
80. Kavalieratos D, Corbelli J, Zhang D, Dionne-Odom JN, Ernecoff NC, Hanmer J, et al. Association between palliative care and patient and caregiver outcomes: a systematic review and meta-analysis. JAMA. 2016;316(20):2104–14.
81. Balboni TA, Balboni M, Enzinger AC, Gallivan K, Paulk ME, Wright A, et al. Provision of spiritual support to patients with advanced cancer by religious communities and associations with medical care at the end of life. JAMA Intern Med. 2013;173(12):1109–17.
82. Balboni T, Balboni M, Paulk ME, Phelps A, Wright A, Peteet J, et al. Support of cancer patients' spiritual needs and associations with medical care costs at the end of life. Cancer. 2011;117(23):5383–91.
83. Guo Y, Shin KY, Hainley S, Bruera E, Palmer JL. Inpatient rehabilitation improved functional status in asthenic patients with solid and hematologic malignancies. Am J Phys Med Rehabil. 2011;90(4):265–71.
84. Fukushima T, Nakano J, Ishii S, Natsuzako A, Kawachi H, Sakamoto J, et al. Influence of hemoglobin level on muscle and physical functions, activities of daily living, and quality of life in patients with hematological malignancies. Integr Cancer Ther. 2019;18:1534735419842196.
85. Xiao DY, Luo S, O'Brian K, Ganti A, Riedell P, Sanfilippo KM, et al. Impact of sarcopenia on treatment tolerance in United States veterans with diffuse large B-cell lymphoma treated with CHOP-based chemotherapy. Am J Hematol. 2016;91(10):1002–7.
86. Dimeo F, Schmittel A, Fietz T, Schwartz S, Kohler P, Boning D, et al. Physical performance, depression, immune status and fatigue in patients with hematological malignancies after treatment. Ann Oncol. 2004;15(8):1237–42.
87. Zhuang H, Ma Y, Wang L, Zhang H. Effect of early palliative care on quality of life in patients with non-small-cell lung cancer. Curr Oncol. 2018;25(1):e54–e8.
88. Cheville AL, Morrow M, Smith SR, Basford JR. Integrating function-directed treatments into palliative care. PM R. 2017;9(9S2):S335–46.
89. Lee CH, Kim JK, Jun HJ, Lee DJ, Namkoong W, Oh JH. Rehabilitation of advanced cancer patients in palliative care unit. Ann Rehabil Med. 2018;42(1):166–74.
90. Bergenthal N, Will A, Streckmann F, Wolkewitz KD, Monsef I, Engert A, et al. Aerobic physical exercise for adult patients with haematological malignancies. Cochrane Database Syst Rev. 2014;(11):CD009075.
91. Fukushima T, Nakano J, Ishii S, Natsuzako A, Sakamoto J, Okita M. Low-intensity exercise therapy with high frequency improves physical function and mental and physical symptoms in patients with haematological malignancies undergoing chemotherapy. Eur J Cancer Care (Engl). 2018;27(6):e12922.
92. Eldredge DH, Nail LM, Maziarz RT, Hansen LK, Ewing D, Archbold PG. Explaining family caregiver role strain following autologous blood and marrow transplantation. J Psychosoc Oncol. 2006;24(3):53–74.
93. Wilson ME, Eilers J, Heermann JA, Million R. The experience of spouses as informal caregivers for recipients of hematopoietic stem cell transplants. Cancer Nurs. 2009;32(3):E15–23.
94. Abbasnezhad M, Rahmani A, Ghahramanian A, Roshangar F, Eivazi J, Azadi A, et al. Cancer care burden among primary family caregivers of Iranian hematologic cancer patients. Asian Pac J Cancer Prev. 2015;16(13):5499–505.
95. Beattie S, Lebel S. The experience of caregivers of hematological cancer patients undergoing a hematopoietic stem cell transplant: a comprehensive literature review. Psychooncology. 2011;20(11):1137–50.
96. Grosse J, Treml J, Kersting A. Impact of caregiver burden on mental health in bereaved caregivers of cancer patients: a systematic review. Psychooncology. 2018;27(3):757–67.
97. Stroebe M, Schut H, Stroebe W. Health outcomes of bereavement. Lancet. 2007;370(9603):1960–73.
98. Christakis NA, Allison PD. Mortality after the hospitalization of a spouse. N Engl J Med. 2006;354(7):719–30.
99. von Heymann-Horan A, Bidstrup P, Guldin MB, Sjogren P, Andersen EAW, von der Maase H, et al. Effect of home-based specialised palliative care and dyadic psychological intervention on caregiver anxiety and depression: a randomised controlled trial. Br J Cancer. 2018;119(11):1307–15.
100. Nordly M, Benthien KS, Von Der Maase H, Johansen C, Kruse M, Timm H, et al. The DOMUS study protocol: a randomized clinical trial of accelerated transition from oncological treatment to specialized palliative care at home. BMC Palliat Care. 2014;13:44.
101. von Heymann-Horan AB, Puggaard LB, Nissen KG, Benthien KS, Bidstrup P, Coyne J, et al. Dyadic psychological intervention for patients with cancer and caregivers in home-based specialized palliative care: the domus model. Palliat Support Care. 2018;16(2):189–97.
102. Hoerger M, Cullen BD. Early integrated palliative care and reduced emotional distress in cancer caregivers: reaching the "hidden patients". Oncologist. 2017;22(12):1419–20.
103. El-Jawahri A, Greer JA, Pirl WF, Park ER, Jackson VA, Back AL, et al. Effects of early integrated palliative care on caregivers of patients with lung and gastrointestinal cancer: a randomized clinical trial. Oncologist. 2017;22(12):1528–34.
104. Osman H, Shrestha S, Temin S, Ali ZV, Corvera RA, Ddungu HD, et al. Palliative care in the global setting: ASCO resource-stratified practice guideline. J Glob Oncol. 2018;4:1–24.
105. McCaughan D, Roman E, Smith AG, Garry AC, Johnson MJ, Patmore RD, et al. Palliative care specialists' perceptions concerning referral of haematology patients to their services: findings from a qualitative study. BMC Palliat Care. 2018;17(1):33.

106. Bakitas M, Lyons KD, Hegel MT, Balan S, Brokaw FC, Seville J, et al. Effects of a palliative care intervention on clinical outcomes in patients with advanced cancer: the project ENABLE II randomized controlled trial. JAMA. 2009;302(7):741–9.
107. Hui D, Bruera E. Models of palliative care delivery for patients with cancer. J Clin Oncol. 2020;38(9):852–65.
108. Grudzen CR, Shim DJ, Schmucker AM, Cho J, Goldfeld KS, Investigators EM. Emergency Medicine Palliative Care Access (EMPallA): protocol for a multicentre randomised controlled trial comparing the effectiveness of specialty outpatient versus nurse-led telephonic palliative care of older adults with advanced illness. BMJ Open. 2019;9(1):e025692.
109. Reiser V, Rosenzweig M, Welsh A, Ren D, Usher B. The support, education, and advocacy (SEA) program of care for women with metastatic breast cancer: a nurse-led palliative care demonstration program. Am J Hosp Palliat Care. 2019;36(10):864–70.
110. Hui D, Bansal S, Strasser F, Morita T, Caraceni A, Davis M, et al. Indicators of integration of oncology and palliative care programs: an international consensus. Ann Oncol. 2015;26(9):1953–9.
111. LeBlanc TW, O'Donnell JD, Crowley-Matoka M, Rabow MW, Smith CB, White DB, et al. Perceptions of palliative care among hematologic malignancy specialists: a mixed-methods study. J Oncol Pract. 2015;11(2):e230–8.
112. Pellizzari M, Hui D, Pinato E, Lisiero M, Serpentini S, Gubian L, et al. Impact of intensity and timing of integrated home palliative cancer care on end-of-life hospitalization in northern Italy. Support Care Cancer. 2017;25(4):1201–7.
113. de Oliveira Valentino TC, Paiva CE, Hui D, de Oliveira MA, Ribeiro Paiva BS. Impact of palliative care on quality of end-of-life care among Brazilian patients with advanced cancers. J Pain Symptom Manag. 2020;59(1):39–48.
114. Hui D, Kim SH, Roquemore J, Dev R, Chisholm G, Bruera E. Impact of timing and setting of palliative care referral on quality of end-of-life care in cancer patients. Cancer. 2014;120(11):1743–9.
115. Campbell NR, Khalsa T, World Hypertension League E, Lackland DT, Niebylski ML, Nilsson PM, et al. High blood pressure 2016: why prevention and control are urgent and important. The World Hypertension League, International Society of Hypertension, World Stroke Organization, International Diabetes Foundation, International Council of Cardiovascular Prevention and Rehabilitation, International Society of Nephrology. J Clin Hypertens (Greenwich). 2016;18(8):714–7.
116. Fox CS, Golden SH, Anderson C, Bray GA, Burke LE, de Boer IH, et al. Update on prevention of cardiovascular disease in adults with type 2 diabetes mellitus in light of recent evidence: a scientific statement from the American Heart Association and the American Diabetes Association. Circulation. 2015;132(8):691–718.
117. Covinsky KE. Palliative care = hope. JAMA Intern Med. 2014;174(1):14.
118. Temel JS, Greer JA, Admane S, Gallagher ER, Jackson VA, Lynch TJ, et al. Longitudinal perceptions of prognosis and goals of therapy in patients with metastatic non-small-cell lung cancer: results of a randomized study of early palliative care. J Clin Oncol. 2011;29(17):2319–26.
119. Davis MP, Temel JS, Balboni T, Glare P. A review of the trials which examine early integration of outpatient and home palliative care for patients with serious illnesses. Ann Palliat Med. 2015;4(3):99–121.
120. Shamieh O, Khamash O, Khraisat M, Jbouri O, Awni M, Al-Hawamdeh A, et al. Impact of outpatient palliative care (PC) on symptom burden in patients with advanced cancer at a tertiary cancer center in Jordan. Support Care Cancer. 2017;25(1):177–83.
121. Hui D, Mori M, Watanabe SM, Caraceni A, Strasser F, Saarto T, et al. Referral criteria for outpatient specialty palliative cancer care: an international consensus. Lancet Oncol. 2016;17(12):e552–e9.
122. Hui D, Anderson L, Tang M, Park M, Liu D, Bruera E. Examination of referral criteria for outpatient palliative care among patients with advanced cancer. Support Care Cancer. 2019;28(1):295–301.

# Hematology/Oncology and Palliative Care Collaboration

7

Courtney W. Johnson, Deborah A. Lafond, Steven J. Hardy, Elizabeth Hardesty, and Shana S. Jacobs

## Palliative Care Consultation Within Hematology/Oncology

### Palliative Care Consultation Within Malignant Hematology

Collaboration between malignant hematology and palliative care improves both patient and caregiver quality of life [1–3]. Palliative care delivered alongside cancer directed therapy is essential for disease control and therapy-related symptom burden reduction [4]. This presents one strong rationale for why a collaborative model of care between hematologists and palliative care physicians is particularly important for complicated cases with uncertain outcomes.

The early involvement of palliative care for patients with malignant hematologic conditions is crucial as it allows relationships between palliative care clinicians, patients and their families to develop. This early involvement may facilitate end-of-life conversations, as the family already has a well-established relationship with the palliative care team, who often facilitates such discussions. Symptom management may also improve, and patients and their families have additional advocates so clinicians may better understand their personal values. Early involvement of palliative care also makes patient transitions to hospice easier and logistically less complicated for both the primary and hospice clinicians. The American Society of Clinical Oncology (ASCO) and other leading cancer organizations support early integration of palliative care as the standard of care for patients with hematologic malignancies, with the consultativ e model currently the most common. However, barriers remain to full integration [5].

Patients with hematological malignancies may have many unmet needs that palliative care could address. These needs include the management of physical and emotional symptom burden which will improve quality of life [6]. There are several common misconceptions hematologists/oncologists may have regarding palliative care, including the idea that palliative care is synonymous with hospice care and requires a terminal diagnosis [7] or that patients receiving palliative care can no longer receive therapies with curative or disease-directed intent. Hematologist/oncologists may believe that involvement of palliative care signals to their patients that they have "given up" on cure. Compared to solid tumor oncologists, hematologic oncologists are also more likely to feel a sense of failure if their patient's disease progresses [8, 9]. They are also less likely to refer patients to hospice, feel less comfortable talking about death and dying and are more likely to prescribe therapy in the last month of life for patients with limited physical functioning at baseline (Eastern Cooperative Oncology Group [ECOG] performance scale <4) [6, 8]. In addition, patients with hematologic malignancies are less likely to receive concurrent palliative care if admitted to the intensive care unit [6, 7]. These results were found regardless of hematology/oncology subspecialty [8].

C. W. Johnson (✉)
Department of Hospitalist Medicine, Children's National Health System, Washington, DC, USA

D. A. Lafond
PANDA Education Consultants, PLLC, Lakeland, FL, USA
e-mail: dlafond@pandaedcon.org

S. J. Hardy
Divisions of Hematology and Oncology, Children's National Hospital, Washington, DC, USA

Department of Psychiatry and Behavioral Sciences, George Washington University School of Medicine and Health Sciences, Washington, DC, USA
e-mail: sjhardy@childrensnational.org

E. Hardesty
Department of Oncology, Children's National Medical Center, Washington, DC, USA
e-mail: ehardest@childrensnational.org

S. S. Jacobs
Department of Oncology, Children's National Hospital, Washington, DC, USA
e-mail: SSJacobs@childrensnational.org


C. K. Ullrich, E. J. Roeland (eds.), *Palliative Care in Hematologic Malignancies and Serious Blood Disorders*,
https://doi.org/10.1007/978-3-031-38058-7_7

## Integration of Palliative Care in Hematology/Oncology: Models of Palliative Care-Including Specialty Clinics and Specialty Palliative Care Clinicians

Models for how palliative care can be integrated into hematology/oncology care include a multi-disciplinary inpatient palliative care consult service, integration into outpatient clinics, and educational opportunities about what palliative care can provide for primary teams and other pertinent hospital staff. There are nuances in how palliative care may be delivered to different subsets within hematology/oncology such as those with hematologic malignancy (including hematopoietic cell transplant [HCT] recipients (see Chap. 3), sickle cell disease (SCD), other serious blood disorders, and bone marrow failure) (Chaps. 2 and 4).

## Models of Palliative Care Integration for Malignant Hematology

Several models have been created to address the palliative care needs of patients with hematological malignancies. In some centers, a palliative care team member is embedded within the primary team and rounds regularly with the team. In other centers, the palliative care team is separate and may be associated with either the pain team or the integrative therapies team. Some centers leave the decision for palliative care referral to individual clinicians, while others have set triggers for seeking palliative care involvement. A few examples of each are listed below [10].

## Primary Palliative Care Integration Model

One method of addressing palliative care needs within the hematology/oncology population includes hematology/oncology clinician training in the tenets of primary palliative care. Primary palliative care is defined as infusing basic palliative care principles into patient care provided by primary (non-palliative care specialist) clinicians [11, 12], Clinicians with subspecialty training in palliative care, if available, may consult in situations such as those involving particularly complex symptoms management or communication.

The most common barrier to integration of primary palliative care is clinicians feeling they do not have adequate skills or access to appropriate specialty palliative care services when an advanced skill set is needed, or that there is inadequate time to attend to the unique and often lengthy goals of care conversations [12]. Published psychosocial standards for children with cancer mandate that clinicians have education and mentoring in the essential skills of palliative care to facilitate decision-making and provide support for children with cancer and their families [5]. Multiple educational and training programs (Table 7.1) are available to address the attitudes, skills, and knowledge of primary hematology/oncology clinicians [11, 13].

Several programs across the United States (US) have employed a primary palliative care model of care delivery to enhance access to care for individuals with cancer and blood disorders. One such program at a large urban hospital in the Northeast US, trained 56 interprofessional direct care clinicians in a primary pediatric palliative care educational and mentoring program over a 4-year period. Of these 56 clinicians, 2 advanced practice providers/clinicians (APPs) had a primary practice in hematologic malignancies, 3 APPs in HCT, and 44 clinicians cross all hematology/oncology care, including attending physicians, fellows, registered nurses, patient care technicians, and art therapists. The remaining 7 clinicians practiced in other hematology/oncology specialty areas. This year-long educational program consisted of didactic and mentoring opportunities based in the Education in Palliative and End-of Life Care: Pediatric (EPEC-Peds and End of Life Nursing Education Curriculum-Pediatrics (ELNEC-Pediatric) curriculums [13, 14]. Each clinician participating in the program worked on a palliative care quality improvement (QI) project to integrate what is learned into practice and to facilitate improved patient and family outcomes. Outcomes of this program demonstrated a significant increase in advance care planning for adolescents and young adults, increased specialty palliative care referrals (78% increase over 4-year period), and increased confidence of primary oncology clinicians in integrating primary palliative care into their practice (increase from 54% at baseline to 98% at 1 year post completion; $p < 0.001$). In addition, this model resulted in integration of a 4-h pediatric palliative care class for all new nurse hires as part of their orientation.

The model of primary pediatric palliative care integrated throughout a cancer, and blood disorders program can be a powerful tool promoting culture change and care focused on comfort and quality of life for patients and families. Primary palliative care can empower bedside clinicians to advocate for specialty palliative care services when needed, promote clinician resiliency, and to improve access to palliative care services. Engaging champions from within hematology/oncology in collaboration with the specialty palliative team in designing, implementing, and evaluating the program can facilitate success.

**Table 7.1** Sample of palliative care interprofessional education opportunities

| Name of program | Description | Website |
|---|---|---|
| American Association of Hospice and Palliative Medicine/Hospice and Palliative Nurses Association Annual Assembly | This annual convening of palliative and hospice care professionals from across all disciplines offers a wide variety of educational and interactive opportunities addressing the state of the science in caring for children, adolescents and adults with serious, advanced illness. Pediatric specific sessions are available | http://apps.aahpm.org/meeting?productid=30925426 |
| Education in Palliative and End-of-Life Care—Adult and Pediatric Tracks | EPEC is a comprehensive curriculum designed to address the needs of adults, children, their families, and including hematology/oncology clinicians and other interprofessional clinicians. It was developed by and continues to receive input from experts in several disciplines as well as patient/family/parent advocate advisors. It consists of 24 modules in pain and symptom management in palliative care. These topics are taught as a combination of 20 distance learning modules and 6 in-person conference sessions. This in-person conference is offered annually | https://www.bioethics.northwestern.edu/education/epec.html |
| End-of-Life Nursing Education Curriculum—Adult and Pediatric Tracks | The End-of-Life Nursing Education Consortium (ELNEC) project is a national and international education initiative to improve palliative care. Since 2000, the ELNEC project, administered by City of Hope, provides undergraduate and graduate nursing faculty, CE providers, staff development educators, specialty nurses in pediatrics, oncology, critical care and geriatrics, and other nurses with training in palliative care so they can teach this essential information to nursing students, practicing nurses and other healthcare professionals | https://www.aacnnursing.org/ELNEC/About/ELNEC-Curricula |
| Palliative Care Education and Practice (PCEP) | A comprehensive course delivered in two parts on an adult or pediatric track. PCEP provides physicians, nurses, and social workers a structure in which to efficiently acquire the competencies necessary to influence our current changing healthcare environment. Held in two parts, this course uses experiential learning, training, and consolidation | https://pallcare.hms.harvard.edu/courses |
| Pediatric Pain Master Class | The pediatric pain master class offers state of the art education in pain management for the pediatric patient from a holistic and interdisciplinary perspective. The program covers pharmacological, medical, psychosocial and integrative therapies in the management of children's acute, procedural, and complex/chronic pain. The master class is primarily designed for physicians and advanced practice nurses to develop their expertise in the field of pediatric pain medicine in a highly interactive seminar format. This course is also open to other individuals who work within the field of pediatric pain | https://www.childrensmn.org/events/12th-annual-pediatric-pain-master-class/ |
| Shiley Institute for Palliative Care | Interactive, engaging, and up-to-date courses for professionals ensure healthcare professionals have the skills needed to provide great patient care. All of our courses offer continuing education hours and some offer BRN, BBS, and CME hours. Choose from instructor-led or self-paced courses.<br>Nurses, social workers, chaplains and other healthcare professionals can get the discipline specific skills they need in palliative care through a wide range of courses | https://csupalliativecare.org/ |
| University of Washington Graduate Certificate in Palliative Care—Adult and Pediatric Tracks | This interprofessional curriculum is designed for practicing healthcare professionals from nursing, medicine, social work, spiritual care, and other disciplines seeking specialty training in palliative care. The 9-month graduate certificate includes three 5-credit courses taken sequentially in the autumn, winter, and spring quarters. This is a hybrid program that includes both online and in-person instruction. The online instruction includes self-paced online modules and monthly live webinars. There is a required 2.5 day workshop each quarter of the course | https://www.pce.uw.edu/certificates/palliative-care |
| Vital Talk | VitalTalk's virtual mastering tough conversations course consists of two elements: self-paced online modules that introduce VitalTalk's signature talking maps and relevant skills; and virtual live classes that put the skills learned into practice with simulated patients | https://www.vitaltalk.org/ |

## Trigger-Based Model

Some palliative care teams have a list of diagnoses and conditions that automatically trigger a palliative care consult. For example, El-Jawahri et al. suggest a "trigger-based" model for patients who undergo HCT [15]. In this model, every patient admitted to the HCT service automatically triggers a palliative care consult. Palliative care involvement for all HCT patients is a logical trigger point as patients undergoing transplant experience many difficulties (physical, emotional, mental, and spiritual) throughout the transplant process [2, 15–18]. Advantages of the trigger approach may include improved psychosocial support and symptom management; reaching all who may benefit so decreasing perceived stigma of palliative care as end-of-life care only; and optimizes resources to those who may benefit the most (trigger versus universal consult for all HCT) [3, 18, 19]. Disadvantages of a trigger approach may include the often unpredictable trajectory of HCT, a long-standing relationship between the hematology/oncology/HCT teams, patients' and families' potential role confusion with the integration of the palliative care team, and restriction of palliative care involvement due to continuation of curative/disease-directed therapies [3, 19].

## Embedded Model

Another successful model of palliative care is integration of a specialty palliative care clinician within a hematology/oncology multispecialty clinic or service [20, 21]. In several major pediatric cancer centers, palliative care is integrated within a neuro-oncology clinic [22–24]. In one large free-standing children's hospital in the northeast, a specialty pediatric palliative care clinician is embedded in the weekly multi-disciplinary neuro-oncology clinic [25, 26]. This model could be extended to hematologic malignancies as well.

Importantly, similar to the primary palliative care training model, the embedded model also demonstrated changes in attitudes. Prior to implementation, many families indicated that they were uncomfortable or very uncomfortable with discussing palliative care (43.5%), that palliative care meant "giving up" (31.3%), and that palliative care was for end-of-life care only (31.3%). Post-implementation, 75% of families indicated that they felt comfortable or very comfortable in discussing palliative care, no families indicated that palliative care meant "giving up" or that palliative care was for end-of-life care only. Integration of a palliative care clinician within multi-disciplinary hematology/oncology clinics is feasible and desired by families. In this example, families felt that it was important to offer palliative care services (100%), that they were likely to recommend palliative care to other families (93.8%), and that integration of palliative care services would influence their recommendation of the hospital to other families (68.8%) [23]. Approaches such as this could be translated into clinics or inpatient services for hematologic malignances and other serious blood disorders. Selvaggi et al. describe a collaboration between hematologic malignancy-bone marrow transplant units and palliative care services [27]. The collaboration, which included needs assessments, didactic lectures, palliative care consultations, and the presence of the palliative care team on rounds, resulted in patients reporting lower pain scores, increased hospice referrals, and greater satisfaction among hematology/oncology providers [27]. In addition, a proposed Nurse Practitioner Early Palliative Care for hematopoietic cell transplant (HCT) patients (NEST) algorithm has been used to foster a better relationship between the malignant hematology/HCT and palliative care teams [28].

Examples of other innovative ways that have been used for the integration of palliative care include the creative use of palliative care office hours for hematology/oncology advanced practice providers, palliative care rotations during residency and fellowship training, pamphlets to educate patients and caregivers, and an algorithm to evaluate patient's needs and creating a platform within electronic medical records (EMR) [29, 30].

## Sickle Cell Disease as a Model of Palliative Care Integration for Serious Blood Disorders

Any intervention to reduce suffering and improve functioning in SCD must first be grounded in the development of understanding and trust. In the US, SCD primarily occurs in Black individuals of African and Caribbean ancestry, a group historically exploited and mistreated in many contexts, including medicine and medical research [31–33]. However, it would be naïve to think that these are purely historical accounts; contemporary reports suggest that racism in healthcare settings persists is perceived to affect healthcare delivery by individuals with SCD and influences health behavior and outcomes [34, 35]. As such, palliative care clinicians, who may not have long-standing relationships with patients, must first prepare by reviewing the patient's medical and psychosocial history, communicating with the patient's healthcare team, and demonstrating a willingness to listen to the patient and earn their trust.

In pediatric settings, patients with SCD have often been cared for by the same team of clinicians since birth and have developed a strong bond with this team. In our own experience, it is common for patients to describe their hematology clinician as a second mother or father. Therefore, working to establish more than a superficial relationship with the patient's primary hematology team can not only lead to disclosures of unrecorded information essential to an adequate case formulation, but also to an invaluable endorsement from the patient's most trusted team members. Palliative care clinicians may also find it helpful to include questions about the patient's experience within the medical system in their assessment (e.g., "I know that for some people with SCD, they face challenges in the Emergency Department and don't always feel heard. I am wondering what it is like for you when you come into the ED to get help because you are having a pain crisis. Can you help me understand what that looks like?"). Simply asking such questions can quickly align the clinician and patient by acknowledging the injustices they have likely faced and conveying a commitment to helping advocate on their behalf.

In building a relationship with patients, palliative care clinicians should also consider the social context in which patients live by asking questions about important people (e.g., nuclear family, extended family, friends, religious and spiritual supports), perceived social standing and socioeconomic status, educational and occupational history, and values and preferred activities, among others. Some of this information may already be known from a review of the medical record, but it is still wise to empower patients to describe themselves to clinicians in their own words. This experience not only assures patients that clinicians know important details about them, but also conveys that the clinician cares enough to ask. This also creates an opportunity for patients to exert some agency over the interaction and choose the information that they want to highlight or prioritize for palliative care clinicians.

Pain is the most common symptom reported by individual with SCD, and it is likely to be the primary cause for referral to palliative care clinicians [36, 37]. Broadly speaking, pain is a complex subjective phenomenon that can be challenging to assess and treat [38]. In SCD, pain can be especially challenging because a myriad of underlying problems can generate pain (e.g., vaso-occlusion, chronic neuropathic pain, acute chest syndrome, priapism, avascular necrosis, to name a few) [39]. Clinicians must also consider how layers of developmental, psychological, neurocognitive, social, and cultural factors interact with biological mechanisms to affect pain perception and pain behavior [40]. To do so, palliative care clinicians must rely on a thorough review of the medical record, a comprehensive interview with patients and family members as appropriate, and discussions with the primary team and consulting services.

Coordinating with medical team members and support staff is an essential component of providing targeted symptom management interventions for patients with SCD. Given the long-standing relationship that many patients with SCD will have with their hematology clinicians and potentially with other consulting services (e.g., pain medicine, physical therapy, neurology, psychology), it is important to carefully consider how to integrate with the existing team. Palliative care clinicians may also want to observe relationships that exist within teams and between teams and reflect on how those relationships directly impact patient functioning and also shape referral questions. Although clinicians who have known a patient for a long time will have a base of shared experiences to draw on that affords trust and guides decisions, it is also possible that that same history contributes to a repetitive pattern of interactions and interferes with objective assessment of certain situations. In these instances, a palliative care team may represent a new space for patients and families to share questions and concerns. Palliative care teams serving this role must do so with care and respect for the existing relationships with other clinicians/teams.

Referrals for the SCD population for palliative care services may include for pain management, non-pain management, additional family support, and/or assistance with coping with chronic illness. The impact of beliefs, expectations, and team dynamics should be explored and examined for how they contribute to the referral process. Moreover, it may be useful to conceptualize the "patient" to which the palliative care clinician is providing services as both the actual patient and the referring team. In some cases, helping to identify and remedy team issues can be as effective and beneficial as treating patient issues.

Children's National, a large free-standing children's hospital in Washington, D.C., has an Integrative Medicine Clinic for SCD designed to offer complementary therapies for pain management. Integrated medicine has been defined as "the practice of medicine that reaffirms the importance of the relationship between practitioner and patient, focuses on the whole person, is informed by evidence, and makes use of all appropriate therapeutic approaches, healthcare professionals and disciplines to achieve optimal health and healing" [41]. Integrative Medicine for SCD patients is based on "the four principles of pain management and attention to psychological, social and spiritual issues." [41] There is evidence that incorporating integrative medicine to standard care for pain in SCD patients is effective. Acupuncture has had perceived clinical benefit for both patients with SCD and their families [42]. A 2016 review of nonpharmacological approaches for pain in SCD showed a significant reduction in pain with both acupuncture and massage treatment in four different studies, two of which involved children [43].

The Integrative Medicine Clinic for SCD described above includes hematologists, palliative care clinicians, an anesthesiologist trained in acupuncture, psychologists, a physical therapist, and a clinical nurse specialist who is trained in multiple integrative medicine techniques. In this setting, psychologists provide cognitive-behavioral and acceptance-based therapies to teach patients and their caregivers about how the brain perceives pain and help them build skills for improving mood, reducing stress, and sleeping better to help cope with pain. The clinical nurse specialist provides aromatherapy, healing touch, and mindfulness to support pain control. A retrospective study at this institution evaluated 12 patients who received a total of 33 acupuncture sessions between 2016 and 2018. Eleven patients reported they had a good experience with 73% stating they had improved pain or felt good after the session [44]. This integrated clinic gives these SCD patients additional ways to cope with their chronic pain other than taking opioids which will serve them as they get older and inevitably experience more symptoms due to the progression of their SCD.

## Barriers to Access of Palliative Care

Palliative care involvement with both adult and pediatric hematology/oncology patients is becoming more and more frequent as the field of palliative care becomes more established. There are however; some barriers that still exist [45]. One recent study showed that involvement of the pediatric palliative care service was accompanied with emotional distress for the primary team [45]. Also, many hematologists/oncologists believe they do not require palliative care involvement for their patients as they already have the necessary palliative care skills. There is worry that palliative care involvement will increase the family's anxiety as palliative care involvement is both symbolic of the end of life and has an emotional toll on everyone involved in the care of the patient [45]. Increased education about the role of palliative care for these patients is essential to address these barriers, see Table 7.2 below.

## Psychosocial Role Confusion

Psychosocial care is paramount to both hematology/oncology and palliative care. Social workers offer a unique and broader perspective to patient care with their expertise in communications and systems of care. As major clinicians of mental health services in the US, social work involvement in palliative care can offer support to an already vulnerable and highly stressed population. Their services can include anticipatory guidance, supportive counseling, problem-solving tools, and coping strategies. Additionally, with knowledge of both medical and social systems, they can connect families with resources to aid with stressors or barriers that are likely compounding a patient and family's distress and possibly influencing their decision-making.

Professional collaboration between the health care team, palliative care team, and social workers is central in achieving better patient outcomes, improving patient satisfaction, and reducing length of stays. To have optimal collaboration,

**Table 7.2** Strategies for addressing common challenges and misperceptions in palliative care

| Common challenges and misperceptions | Suggested strategies to address challenges | Rationale for this strategy |
|---|---|---|
| 1. Palliative care is only for the dying | Ask the surprise question. "Would it be surprising to you if [this patient] died within the next 6–12 months?" [16, 57–59]<br>Make patients/families and providers aware of how the palliative care team can help with both symptom management and support for patients and families | Brings an awareness of the seriousness of the underlying illness and provides an opportunity to begin advance care planning |
| 2. Patient and family perceptions of palliative care, e.g., the team is giving up [59] | Introduce palliative care as a standard of care for all patients with similar conditions.<br>Assessment of and focus on optimizing quality of life throughout the trajectory of the illness | This may normalize care as part of the approach to good supportive care and lessen the associated stigma |
| 3. All disease-directed therapies must be exhausted | Concurrent care is assured by federal law for children under the age of 21 years<br>Have conversations with both patients, families and providers that both disease-directed therapy and palliative care can be administered at the same time | Disease-directed therapies can continue simultaneously with palliative care interventions |
| 4. Clinicians are too busy to address palliative care needs in the midst of a busy clinic or inpatient service | Provide interdisciplinary palliative care training to primary clinicians at all levels of practice<br>Utilize the specialty palliative care service for complex needs of patients and families | Tenets of primary palliative care can be integrated from the time of diagnosis through long-term follow-up or into death and bereavement by medical and psychosocial professionals |
| 5. The trajectory of the underlying disease is less predictable, and often requires intensive disease-directed therapies, such as transfusions [3] | While many hematologic illnesses may be chronic in nature, there also exists the possibility of rapid decline and potential death. Palliative care can be presented as excellence in supportive care, from the time of diagnosis of serious illness | Continuing to provide appropriate disease-directed care is expected of patients and families. Early integration and normalization of palliative care may avoid the perception of abandonment to the palliative care team as the underlying condition declines |

**Table 7.2** (continued)

| Common challenges and misperceptions | Suggested strategies to address challenges | Rationale for this strategy |
|---|---|---|
| 6. The name "palliative care" can be off putting to some patients and families | See #2 above. Consider changing name to something more family friendly. Engage patients and families in planning palliative care supportive care service structure, including the name | A name can conjure up negative or positive connotations |
| 7. The primary hematology team is abandoning the patient and family, if they refer to palliative care | Build relationships between hematology and palliative care teams. Hematology team introduces palliative care clinicians to family. Communication between teams is paramount<br>Conduct family meetings and patient updates with both the primary hematology and palliative care teams present | Builds trust and rapport between all teams and family. Communication must be open and honest to support trusting relationships |
| 8. Lack of knowledge about palliative care | Palliative care education sessions for clinicians and families [60]<br>Consider requiring palliative care rotations for residents and fellows<br>Provide pamphlets to patients/families on admission to the hospital | Address potential misperceptions and allow participants to ask questions to dispel fears |
| 9. Lack of resources | Consider primary palliative care model.<br>Consider sharing of resources across teams, e.g., psychosocial resources | |
| 10. When to introduce palliative care | Build relationships with hematology team | |

team members must have trust, information sharing, and role negotiation. Altogether, their collaboration allows for various disciplines to solve a common set of problems that ultimately benefits the patient and their family.

## Palliative Care Training for Hematologists/Oncologists

Primary palliative care provided by the hematology/oncology team is an important model of providing palliative care. Hematologists/oncologists are already familiar with many aspects of symptom management and discussions about prognosis and end of life. A 2018 survey of 105 hematology/oncology fellows reported that after their palliative care rotation they felt better equipped to manage symptoms (98%), provide opioid prescriptions (89%), communicate with patients and families (91%), and discuss advance care planning (88%) [46]. Training primary clinicians in both pain control and emotional issues at the end of life is imperative for patients with serious hematologic illness to improve not only their physical symptoms, but their entire quality of life. This, in turn, can dramatically affect the lives of these patient's loved ones, who will have to deal with the loss indefinitely.

There are a growing number of clinicians who are trained in both hematology/oncology and palliative care. These clinicians include physicians, nurse practitioners, registered nurses, social workers, psychologists, chaplains, and pharmacists. These clinicians represent a unique model of providing palliative care. Duel-trained clinicians bring additional skills and can influence care from within the hematology/oncology culture in a meaningful way [47].

## Pearls and Pitfalls of Palliative Care Integration

Integration of palliative care for individuals with serious illness is well established in a variety of settings, including adults and children with complex medical conditions [19, 48, 49] and in the ICU [50–52]. A recent systemic review describes the psychosocial standards for children with cancer supports access to palliative care throughout the trajectory of disease [3]. Integration of palliative care for those with hematologic malignancies and serious blood disorders can be accomplished in several different ways as illustrated in the previous sections. One size does not fit all. Some institutions may have a robust palliative care team where access to services is routine. Other institutions may have access to a palliative care specialist who can be embedded within a hematology/oncology specialty clinic, while others may not have any access to palliative care specialists. Use of a primary palliative care education model may serve as a model for care delivery in these settings [12, 13, 53, 54].

## Pearls

The readiness for change and the culture of the institution must be assessed prior to program development. Considering the five C's (Collaboration, Communication, Consensus, Compromise, and Community) will aid in successful integration.

- **Collaboration** is essential for success. Engaging the hematology/oncology specialists in planning, implementation, and program evaluation will help in establishing shared goals and realistic expectations. Find out what is most important to both specialties, as well as families, and build the integrated program to address these.
- **Communication** must be open, honest, and timely. Exquisite communication between families, hematology/oncology specialists, and palliative care clinicians is paramount.
- **Consensus** of the goals of the program, setting realistic expectations, and understanding the roles of each of the teams contributes to a shared vision for palliative care integration.
- **Compromise** by building integration over time. Small successes one at a time can lead to program sustainability. Think strategically and engage families in assessing what is most important to them. Establish metrics to measure success and provide an impetus for revisions and adaptations along the way. Dream big and start small.
- **Community** in shared goals brings a sense of support and empowerment for clinicians to speak up when palliative care is appropriate. Building a shared community between hematology/oncology and palliative care clinicians allows for sharing of resources, promotion of resiliency, and building in self-care strategies for support.

## Pitfalls

- **Not establishing a shared vision** for the program may lead to role confusion, dissatisfaction, and lack of continuity in communication with families [5].
- **Lack of concise and regular communication** leads to potential errors and lack of consistency in care.
- **Building a program with lofty goals** may be difficult to implement and may lead to feelings of frustration due to lack of palliative care resources. Establish a priority for which patients should be seen and what the roles are in collaboration in care.
- **Isolation and exclusion of palliative care services** that are not integrated within hematology/oncology specialty services may lead to families feeling that palliative care is not valued or desired. Families may feel they have to choose between hematology/oncology and palliative care, when in reality strategies allowing for both disease-directed therapies and palliative care may be possible within the plan of care.
- **Lack of knowledge and education in palliative care** leads to misconceptions and misinformation about the goals. This may perpetuate the myth that palliative care is for end-of-life care only [13, 55]. There are several well-established programs of education for non-palliative care clinicians which may widen their view of what palliative care is, and when it can benefit patients and families (Table 7.1).

In summary, integration of palliative care for individuals with hematologic malignancies and serious blood disorders is feasible. It is established as a standard of psychosocial care [5, 53] and desired by families [21, 54]. Educational resources in palliative care are readily available for the interprofessional team (Table 7.1). Thinking strategically about what model of palliative care delivery best meets the needs of patients and families, specialty clinicians and the institution will promote success. Integration of palliative care services for individuals with hematologic malignancies will contribute to a high reliability organization (HRO) [56]. Examples of how integration of palliative care supports HROs include the following:

- **HRO principle 2 (Sensitivity to operations)**
  - Access to resources
  - Knowing who to go to for support as needed
- **HRO principle 3 (Reluctance to simplify interpretations)**
  - Listening carefully to patients and families; listening to other clinicians, other subspecialties, other disciplines
- **HRO principle 4 (Commitment to resilience)**
  - Opportunities for training to improve confidence and competence in palliative care with decreased moral distress
  - Building community dedicated to caring for patients with serious illness

    Relying on one another for support and advice
- **HRO principle 5 (Deference to expertise)**
  - Providing resources for staff to obtain expert assistance when something unprecedented occurs that they don't know or don't feel confident in how to handle
  - People are committed to excellence in caring for individuals with serious illness
  - Value the expertise of all

All patients deserve the same access to palliative care services, including those with hematologic malignancies and serious blood disorders. No one should be denied access to high quality palliative care for their unique needs. All patients with serious illness and their families are entitled to care that attends to suffering in all dimensions, physical, psychosocial, spiritual, and environmental. This care should be provided by trained interprofessional (defined as health care professionals from diverse disciplines using their unique knowledge, skills, and talents toward a common goal), palliative care clinicians who can address the unique needs of adults and pediatric patients with serious illness, and their families.

## References


1. Ferrell BR, Temel JS, Temin S, Alesi ER, Balboni TA, Basch EM, et al. Integration of palliative care into standard oncology care: American Society of Clinical Oncology clinical practice guideline update. J Clin Oncol. 2017;35(1):96–112.
2. El-Jawahri A, LeBlanc TW, Burns LJ, Denzen E, Meyer C, Mau L-W, et al. What do transplant physicians think about palliative care? A national survey study. Cancer. 2018;124(23):4556–66.
3. McCaughan D, Roman E, Smith AG, Garry AC, Johnson MJ, Patmore RD, et al. Palliative care specialists' perceptions concerning referral of haematology patients to their services: findings from a qualitative study. BMC Palliat Care. 2018;17(1):1–11.
4. Humphrey L, Kang TI. Palliative care in pediatric patients with hematologic malignancies. Hematol Am Soc Hematol Educ Program. 2015;2015(1):490–5.
5. Weaver MS, Heinze KE, Bell CJ, Wiener L, Garee AM, Kelly KP, et al. Establishing psychosocial palliative care standards for children and adolescents with cancer and their families: an integrative review. Palliat Med. 2016;30(3):212–23.
6. Kaye EC, Jerkins J, Gushue CA, DeMarsh S, Sykes A, Lu Z, et al. Predictors of late palliative care referral in children with cancer. J Pain Symptom Manag. 2018;55(6):1550–6.
7. LeBlanc TW, El-Jawahri A. When and why should patients with hematologic malignancies see a palliative care specialist? Hematology. 2015;2015(1):471–8.
8. Hui D, Bansal S, Park M, Reddy A, Cortes J, Fossella F, et al. Differences in attitudes and beliefs toward end-of-life care between hematologic and solid tumor oncology specialists. Ann Oncol. 2015;26(7):1440–6.
9. Healio. How oncologists can deal with palliative and end-of-life care: Healio; 2008. https://www.healio.com/hematology-oncology/practice-management/news/print/hemonc-today/{b84a0b5e-a3ba-4338-9d8b-8f10069e8b70}/how-oncologists-can-deal-with-palliative-and-end-of-life-care.
10. Weaver MS, Rosenberg AR, Tager J, Wichman CS, Wiener L. A summary of pediatric palliative care team structure and services as reported by centers caring for children with cancer. J Palliat Med. 2018;21(4):452–62.
11. Lafond DA, Bowling S, Fortkiewicz JM, Reggio C, Hinds PS. Integrating the comfort theory™ into pediatric primary palliative care to improve access to care. J Hosp Palliat Nurs. 2019;21(5):382–9.
12. Szekendi MK, Vaughn J, McLaughlin B, Mulvenon C, Porter-Williamson K, Sydenstricker C, et al. Integrating palliative care to promote earlier conversations and to increase the skill and comfort of nonpalliative care clinicians: lessons learned from an interventional field trial. Am J Hosp Palliat Care. 2018;35(1):132–7.
13. Friedrichsdorf SJ, Remke S, Hauser J, Foster L, Postier A, Kolste A, et al. Development of a pediatric palliative care curriculum and dissemination model: education in palliative and end-of-life care (EPEC) pediatrics. J Pain Symptom Manag. 2019;58(4):707–20.e3.
14. Lin J, Supiano KP, Madden C, McLeskey N. The impact of the end-of-life nurse education consortium on attitudes of undergraduate nursing students toward care of dying patients. J Hosp Palliat Nurs. 2018;20(4):340–8.
15. El-Jawahri A, LeBlanc T, VanDusen H, Traeger L, Greer JA, Pirl WF, et al. Effect of inpatient palliative care on quality of life 2 weeks after hematopoietic stem cell transplantation: a randomized clinical trial. JAMA. 2016;316(20):2094–103.
16. Ruiz M, Reynolds P, Marranzini R, Khan A, Ketterer J, Brahim A. Role of early palliative care interventions in hematological malignancies and bone marrow transplant patients: barriers and potential solutions. Am J Hosp Palliat Care. 2018;35(11):1456–60.
17. Levine DR, Van Noy K, Talleur AC, Snyder A, Kaye EC, Baker JN. Thoughts from the threshold: patient and family hopes, fears, values, and goals at the onset of pediatric hematopoietic cell transplantation. Bone Marrow Transplant. 2020;55(6):1103–13.
18. LeBlanc TW, Ritchie CS, Friedman F, Bull J, Kutner JS, Johnson KS, et al. Adherence to measuring what matters items when caring for patients with hematologic malignancies versus solid tumors. J Pain Symptom Manag. 2016;52(6):775–82.
19. Levine DR, Baker JN, Wolfe J, Lehmann LE, Ullrich C. Strange bedfellows no more: how integrated stem-cell transplantation and palliative care programs can together improve end-of-life care. J Oncol Pract. 2017;13(9):569–77.
20. Brock KE, Steineck A, Twist CJ. Trends in end-of-life care in pediatric hematology, oncology, and stem cell transplant patients. Pediatr Blood Cancer. 2016;63(3):516–22.
21. Hendricks-Ferguson VL, Haase JE. Parent perspectives of receiving early information about palliative and end-of-life care options from their child's pediatric providers. Cancer Nurs. 2019;42(4):E22–e30.
22. Abdel-Baki MS, Hanzlik E, Kieran MW. Multidisciplinary pediatric brain tumor clinics: the key to successful treatment? CNS Oncol. 2015;4(3):147–55.
23. Lafond D, Hancock L. Impact of integrating palliative care into a neuro-oncology clinic. [Oral Presentation]. 2018.
24. Manning M, Larach M, Boyles S, Stern A. Measuring the impact of integrating palliative care into a multidisciplinary brain and spine oncology clinic. J Clin Oncol. 2015;33(29_suppl):163.
25. Hancock L, Lafond D. NURS-10 IMPACT OF INTEGRATING PALLIATIVE CARE INTO A NEURO-ONCOLOGY CLINIC. Neuro-Oncology. 2018;20(Suppl 2):i152.
26. Lafond D, Hancock L, Rodriquez Y. NU-03 OVERCOMING BARRIERS AND CHALLENGES IN INTEGRATING PALLIATIVE CARE FOR CHILDREN BRAIN TUMORS: A PRIMARY PALLIATIVE CARE APPROACH. Neuro-Oncology. 2016;18(suppl_3):iii135.
27. Selvaggi KJ, Vick JB, Jessell SA, Lister J, Abrahm JL, Bernacki R. Bridging the gap: a palliative care consultation service in a hematological malignancy-bone marrow transplant unit. J Community Support Oncol. 2014;12(2):50–5.
28. Lewis EA. Optimizing the delivery of early palliative care for hematology patients receiving a stem cell transplant: a role for a nurse practitioner. Can Oncol Nurs J. 2020;30(4):239–45.
29. Foxwell AM, Moyer ME, Casarett DJ, O'Connor NR. Palliative care office hours for patients with hematologic malignancies: an innovative model for symptom management and education. J Palliat Med. 2017;20(10):1148–51.
30. Franjul Sánchez A, Fuentes Armesto AM, Briones Chávez C, Ruiz M. Revisiting early palliative care for patients with hematologic malignancies and bone marrow transplant: why the delay? Cureus. 2020;12(9):e10504.
31. Katz RV, Green BL, Kressin NR, Kegeles SS, Wang MQ, James SA, et al. The legacy of the Tuskegee syphilis study: assessing its impact on willingness to participate in biomedical studies. J Health Care Poor Underserved. 2008;19(4):1168–80.

32. Stevens EM, Patterson CA, Li YB, Smith-Whitley K, Barakat LP. Mistrust of pediatric sickle cell disease clinical trials research. Am J Prev Med. 2016;51(1 Suppl 1):S78–86.
33. Gamble VN. Under the shadow of Tuskegee: African Americans and health care. Am J Public Health. 1997;87(11):1773–8.
34. Nelson SC, Hackman HW. Race matters: perceptions of race and racism in a sickle cell center. Pediatr Blood Cancer. 2013;60(3):451–4.
35. Williams DR, Rucker TD. Understanding and addressing racial disparities in health care. Health Care Financ Rev. 2000;21(4):75–90.
36. Ballas SK. Pain management of sickle cell disease. Hematol Oncol Clin North Am. 2005;19(5):785–802, v.
37. Prevention CfDCa. Data & Statistics on Sickle Cell Disease: Centers for Disease Control and Prevention; 2019. https://www.cdc.gov/ncbddd/sicklecell/data.html.
38. Coghill RC. Individual differences in the subjective experience of pain: new insights into mechanisms and models. Headache. 2010;50(9):1531–5.
39. Ballas SK. Current issues in sickle cell pain and its management. Hematology. 2007;2007(1):97–105.
40. Edwards CL, Scales MT, Loughlin C, Bennett GG, Harris-Peterson S, De Castro LM, et al. A brief review of the pathophysiology, associated pain, and psychosocial issues in sickle cell disease. Int J Behav Med. 2005;12(3):171–9.
41. Medicine CoAHCfI. Consortium of Academic Health Centers for Integrative Medicine; 2020. www.imconsortium.org/cahcim/about/home.html.
42. Bhushan D, Conner K, Ellen JM, Sibinga EM. Adjuvant acupuncture for youth with sickle cell pain: a proof of concept study. Med Acupunct. 2015;27(6):461–6.
43. Williams H, Tanabe P. Sickle cell disease: a review of nonpharmacological approaches for pain. J Pain Symptom Manag. 2016;51(2):163–77.
44. Mahmood LA, Reece-Stremtan S, Idiokitas R, Martin B, Margulies S, Hardy SJ, et al. Acupuncture for pain management in children with sickle cell disease. Complement Ther Med. 2020;49:102287.
45. Szymczak JE, Schall T, Hill DL, Walter JK, Parikh S, DiDomenico C, et al. Pediatric oncology providers' perceptions of a palliative care service: the influence of emotional esteem and emotional labor. J Pain Symptom Manag. 2018;55(5):1260–8.
46. Reddy SK, Tanco K, Yennu S, Liu DD, Williams JL, Wolff R, et al. Integration of a mandatory palliative care education into hematology-oncology fellowship training in a comprehensive cancer center: a survey of hematology oncology fellows. J Oncol Pract. 2019;15(11):e934–e41.
47. Hui D, Finlay E, Buss MK, Prommer EE, Bruera E. Palliative oncologists: specialists in the science and art of patient care. J Clin Oncol. 2015;33(20):2314.
48. Liberman D, Song E, Radbill L, Pham P, Derrington S. Early introduction of palliative care and advanced care planning for children with complex chronic medical conditions: a pilot study. Child Care Health Dev. 2016;42(3):439–49.
49. Salins N, Ghoshal A, Hughes S, Preston N. How views of oncologists and haematologists impacts palliative care referral: a systematic review. BMC Palliat Care. 2020;19(1):1–19.
50. Morrison WE, Gauvin F, Johnson E, Hwang J. Integrating palliative care into the ICU: from core competency to consultative expertise. Pediatr Crit Care Med. 2018;19(8S):S86–91.
51. Wysham NG, Hua M, Hough CL, Gundel S, Docherty SL, Jones DM, et al. Improving intensive care unit-based palliative care delivery: a multi-center, multidisciplinary survey of critical care clinician attitudes and beliefs. Crit Care Med. 2017;45(4):e372.
52. Ma J, Chi S, Buettner B, Pollard K, Muir M, Kolekar C, et al. Early palliative care consultation in the medical ICU: a cluster randomized crossover trial. Crit Care Med. 2019;47(12):1707–15.
53. Hui D, Hannon BL, Zimmermann C, Bruera E. Improving patient and caregiver outcomes in oncology: team-based, timely, and targeted palliative care. CA Cancer J Clin. 2018;68(5):356–76.
54. Brown CR, Hsu AT, Kendall C, Marshall D, Pereira J, Prentice M, et al. How are physicians delivering palliative care? A population-based retrospective cohort study describing the mix of generalist and specialist palliative care models in the last year of life. Palliat Med. 2018;32(8):1334–43.
55. Cuviello A, Raisanen JC, Donohue PK, Wiener L, Boss RD. Defining the boundaries of palliative care in pediatric oncology. J Pain Symptom Manag. 2020;59(5):1033–42. e1
56. Gaw M, Rosinia F, Diller T. Quality and the health system: becoming a high reliability organization. Anesthesiol Clin. 2018;36(2):217–26.
57. Downar J, Goldman R, Pinto R, Englesakis M, Adhikari NK. The "surprise question" for predicting death in seriously ill patients: a systematic review and meta-analysis. CMAJ. 2017;189(13):E484–e93.
58. Yen Y-F, Lee Y-L, Hu H-Y, Sun W-J, Ko M-C, Chen C-C, et al. Early palliative care: the surprise question and the palliative care screening tool—better together. BMJ Support Palliat Care. 2020;12(2):211–7.
59. Booker R, Dunn S, Earp MA, Sinnarajah A, Biondo PD, Simon JE. Perspectives of hematology oncology clinicians about integrating palliative care in oncology. Curr Oncol. 2020;27(6):313–20.
60. Andrews CE, Ford K. Clinical facilitator learning and development needs: exploring the why, what and how. Nurse Educ Pract. 2013;13(5):413–7.

# Hematologic Malignancy and Palliative Care Integration in the Outpatient Setting

8

Heather A. Carlson and Angela Sousa

## Defining the Outpatient Population

Over recent years, palliative care (PC) presence in outpatient cancer centers has grown. Many large cancer centers across the country have begun to recognize the contributions that PC can make when caring for patients with advanced or incurable malignancies. A PC survey developed by National Comprehensive Cancer Network (NCCN) reported that a total of 22 major cancer centers endorsed an inpatient PC consult service, and that 91% of the respondents endorsed a clinic-based PC service [1]. This growth is encouraging and is supported by The American Society of Clinical Oncology (ASCO). ASCO has repeatedly reaffirmed the need for outpatient PC presence, and even went so far as to integrate comprehensive PC as part of their formal "vision" when approaching cancer care. PC is appropriate for any patient facing serious illness. Given that patients with advanced cancer have significant physical and emotional symptom burden it makes sense that PC be embedded as an integral part of the culture of a cancer center.

Let's start by reviewing the basic structure for Outpatient PC clinics. They generally function in one of two modalities, either consultative only or following a co-management model. In the consultative-only model, PC clinicians act as consultants giving recommendations back to the primary team managing the patient's care. In a co-management model, PC clinicians jointly manage a patient's care including writing prescriptions, being available for direct phone triage with the patient, and conducting joint visits with oncology. Typically, most oncologists and PC clinicians prefer a co-management model, but occasionally limitations of resources make the consultative model the only feasible and sustainable approach.

As we start to explore the role of outpatient palliative care for those with HM, we must first reflect on the current practices. Starting with the logistics, there are some barriers to scheduling patients within PC clinics. The majority of patients with advanced cancers, including those with hematologic malignancies (HM), are seen frequently by their oncology teams, and this usually makes for opportunities for collaboration and co-management. PC recognizes that most patients prioritize their oncology appointments and schedules; therefore, PC clinicians often link their visits with already scheduled oncology appointments to make coordination of care easier for the patient and the referring hematologist/oncologist. One would imagine that patients with HM would be able to connect easily with their PC providers, however this is not often the case.

Despite every attempt to coordinate patient appointments, given the variability in clinical status of an individual with, appointments are often changed last minute, added on suddenly to accommodate the need for a transfusion or canceled when patients require hospitalization. For this reason, it can be difficult for PC to have continuity with their patients, which is obviously not ideal, resulting in lack of connection for the patient and at times the providers.

Interestingly, increased presence of PC has not necessarily correlated with increased referrals from certain disease groups. One recent study found that patients with gynecologic, breast, or gastrointestinal cancers were significantly more likely to receive referral to PC than those with hematologic or genitourinary malignancies [2]. The majority of individuals diagnosed with a HM do not access PC and, if they do, PC consultation occurs at a median of 0.4 months before death [2]. This data is consistent with other studies that demonstrate patients with HM are most likely to receive intensive therapy at the end of life (Fig. 8.1).

H. A. Carlson (✉)
Division of Palliative Care, Massachusetts General Hospital, Boston, MA, USA
e-mail: HACARLSON@mgb.org

A. Sousa
Division of Palliative Care, Newton-Wellesley Hospital, Newton, MA, USA
e-mail: asousa2@mgb.org


C. K. Ullrich, E. J. Roeland (eds.), *Palliative Care in Hematologic Malignancies and Serious Blood Disorders*, https://doi.org/10.1007/978-3-031-38058-7_8

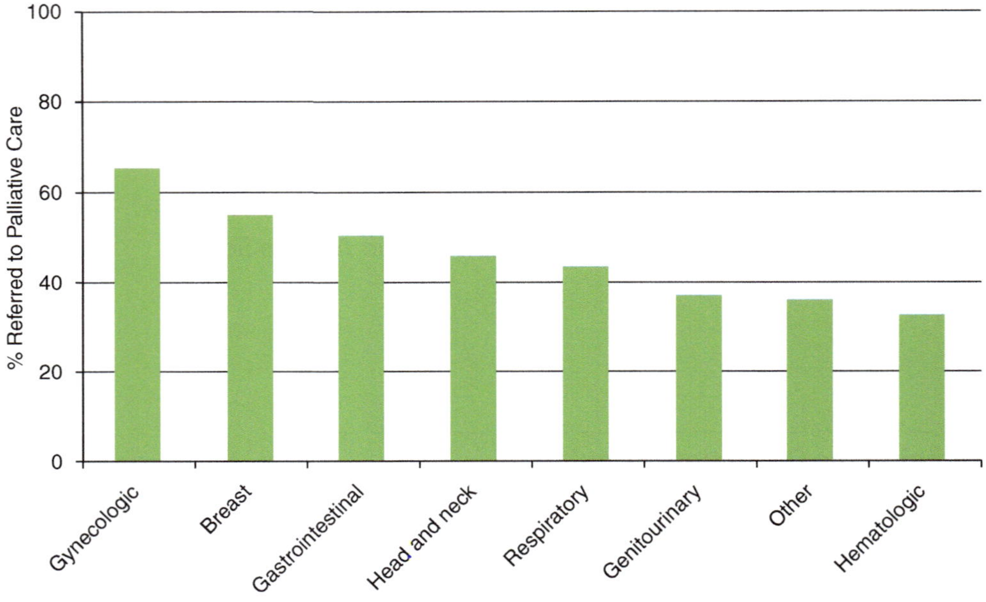


**Fig. 8.1** Significant differences in PC access by tumor type ($p < 0.001$). [Hui D, Kim S-H, Kwon JH, Tanco KC, Zhang T, et al. Access to Palliative Care Among Patients Treated at a Comprehensive Cancer Center. The Oncologist (2012) 17:1574–1580]

It is unclear what contributes to the reduced frequency of PC referrals from HM; it appears that the culture of this specific disease group is less amenable to referral than others such as gynecologic or breast. It is thought that some contributing factors that reduce frequency of PC referral or very late in disease referral include the lack of a clear definition of what constitutes "advanced disease" in the HM population, an often unpredictable disease course, and sudden physical deterioration, requiring rapid change in the therapeutic approach in an end-of-life situation [3].

Within HM, the most likely patient population to receive a PC referral are those patients with a diagnosis of multiple myeloma (MM). This is because unlike many HM, MM is characterized by the predominance of pain, with a reported pain prevalence of 80% and an incidence rate of 100% [3]. Even though many HM do not have pain as a predominant feature, any number of symptoms (examples include nausea, anxiety, insomnia) or simply having to face an incurable illness qualifies a patient to receive access to PC.

## Access to Early Intervention Palliative Care

### What Defines Early Palliative Care?

Given that late access to palliative care has been felt to be suboptimal, we would like to attempt to discern the difference between late accesses to palliative care and earlier referrals to PC. Early PC refers to accessing resources earlier in a patient's disease course, rather than waiting until end of life to start addressing things like a patient's understanding of illness, pain, and goals of care.

According to the World Health Organization, PC "… should be delivered early in the course of the disease, not just in the final stages" [4]. "Early integration of PC with oncologic care improves patients' symptoms, quality of life, satisfaction with care, and illness understanding, and can increase survival. It also reduces patients' needs for emergency and intensive care, while increasing the use of hospice for those at the end of life. By promoting treatment that is concordant with the patient's values and goals, [PC] also reduces costs" [5].

As discussed above, early PC often happens in the outpatient clinic setting. Patients meet with PC clinicians on a regular basis to review symptom management and disease understanding.

Over the course of time, as rapport is built with repeated visits, the PC clinician is able to begin to explore more in-depth topics such as patient values, hopes, and worries. This information becomes essential when patients and oncologists are faced with treatment decision-making, especially as the patient progresses through lines of therapies and approaches end of life. As Ruiz et al. [6] discovered, "early integration of PC for hematopoietic cell therapy (HCT) recipients helps to clarify goals of care, and increase occurrence of advance care planning (ACP) and improves quality of life (QOL) for both recipients and families. Early PC intervention also leads to improved outcomes in relapsed disease after [HCT]."

Much research over the past decade has evaluated the impact of early PC in patients with solid tumors. Several studies have demonstrated that early PC improves QOL, mood and decreases symptom burden in patients with solid tumors [7–9]. The landmark study by Temel et al. showed that patients with metastatic non-small cell lung cancer who received PC had lower anxiety and depression, and remarkably lived longer than their counterparts who did not receive PC [8]. Historically, research involving early PC in patients with HM has been lacking, but one could propose that this is becoming an essential area of study. Porta-Salas et al. acknowledge that "PC interventions in patients with [HM] are often administered late (and thus sub-optimally) in the disease course" [10]. As LeBlanc and El-Jawahri [11] explained, PC "emphasizes well-being at any point along the disease trajectory, regardless of prognosis." Thus, early access to PC along with simultaneous cancer-directed care has become the standard of care for many cancer patients and will hopefully become the same for patients with HM.

## Content of Palliative Care Visits

The structure of PC visits can vary, but typically start with providing patients an explanation of what PC is, and specifically clarifying any misconceptions that PC means the same as hospice care. At the beginning of the consultation, it is imperative to assess the patient's understanding of their illness and disease trajectory. The PC clinician obtains symptom assessment from the patient as well as addresses any questions they may have about their illness or what symptoms to expect. Over repeated visits, patients begin to build rapport and trust with their PC clinician, making it easier to discuss goals and priorities, which may evolve during the illness trajectory. PC clinicians foster open and honest communication, aligning with the patient as well as the treating team. Reviewing ACP is an essential role of PC as it helps patients to direct the care they receive based on their values and priorities. The cumulative effect of ongoing discussions as described above result in improved QOL of the patient.

Some palliative programs use a more structured format for outpatient PC visits. Desai et al. [5] described a program intended to systematize PC for all patients with cancer, specifically including myelodysplastic syndrome in the outpatient clinic setting. This program had a specific structure of what information should be covered during each visit. Visit one occurred as the first follow-up visit after diagnosis. The hematologist/oncologist explained PC as a routine part of the patient's cancer care. As pictured in the table below, symptom assessment occurred at every visit. The initial visit focused on gathering information on patient decision-making to help with supporting goal-concordant care. The PC clinician assessed who the patient looked to for help in making medical decisions, whether they already had elected a health care proxy and assisted the patient in completing one if needed. The second visit involved exploration of the patient's understanding of their course of illness and intent of treatment. This was also revisited quarterly. Visit 3 was spent discussing core values including the patient's sense of personhood and also incorporated patient preferences for specific care goals. Finally, structured visit 4 involved assessing the patient's caregiver and utilized tools to assess their well-being (Fig. 8.2).

Desai et al. [5] concluded that a "structured, scheduled and systemic approach is feasible to deliver PC to newly diagnosed patients with cancer at any stage and throughout their illness trajectory."

Porta-Sales et al. [10] described another such program that has prioritized early PC for their patients in Spain with HM. The hospital-based comprehensive cancer center created a combined MM and PC clinic [MM-PAL]. This patient population typically has many physical symptoms, specifically pain and fatigue, and has a long-standing history of inpatient PC involvement, but prior to this MM-PAL program had not routinely had access to outpatient PC. Porta-Sales et al. conducted a retrospective study over 11 months at

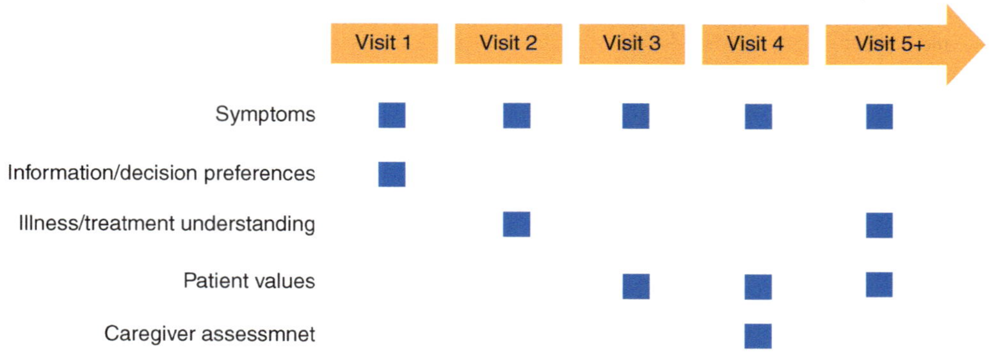


**Fig. 8.2** This figure shows an example of a visit-based protocol for assessment of key PC needs [5]. These assessments are scheduled for specific clinic visits beginning with the first (Visit 1) after confirmation of the cancer diagnosis. Understanding of the illness and discussion of patient's values are re-addressed on a quarterly basis and with important changes in patients' clinical status (e.g., an unscheduled hospitalization or progression of disease through treatment). [Desai AV, Klimek VM, Chow K, Epstein AS, Bernal C, Anderson K, Okpako M, Rawlins-Duell R, Kramer D, Romano D, Goldberg JI, Nelson JE. 1-2-3 Project: A Quality Improvement Initiative to Normalize and Systematize Palliative Care for All. Patients With Cancer in the Outpatient Clinic Setting. Journal of Oncology Practice (2018) 14:12, e775-e785]

a single institution, reviewing a total of 67 patients. The MM-PAL assessed baseline symptoms at initial visit followed by assessments at three follow-up visits. They used the modified Edmonton Symptom Assessment Scale [12] to assess presence and severity of pain, anorexia, constipation, insomnia, nausea/vomiting, dyspnea, anxiety, and sadness in patients with MM. They also used the Edmonton Classification System-Cancer Pain [13] and the Palliative Care Performance Score [14] to evaluate physical and emotional symptom burden. Most of the patients with MM were initially referred to MM-PAL for assistance with pain control; however, a large portion (42%) were also referred for shared follow-up, including " …patients without specific problems at referral but who are expected to develop complex symptoms or psychosocial problems that would warrant an early multidimensional assessment and follow-up" [10].

Porta-Salas et al. [10] study helped reveal that patients reported a significant decrease in pain with early PC involvement. These findings suggested that symptoms "improved quickly, leading to a rapid decrease in the interference of the symptoms with general activity, sleep, and mood, all of which are key factors (together with good adherence) influencing patient QOL." These findings are highly suggestive that early PC has a powerful impact on the care of patients with MM and could potentially be applicable to other types of HM (Fig. 8.3).

## Barriers to Earlier Palliative Care in HM

Despite the results of the above studies suggesting that early PC is beneficial to patients with various HM, there are several barriers that inhibit more widespread use of palliative resources. According to LeBlanc and El-Jawahri, "many hematologists/oncologists who treat HM do not have experience partnering with PC clinicians in the care of their patients, or may harbor mistrust or misconceptions about PC [11]." Literature has shown several recurrent themes that hematologist/oncologists have identified as barriers to involving PC in the care of their patients which impacts the outpatient setting. Many worry that involving PC will result in their patients perceiving a lack of hope regarding their prognosis, or that PC's agenda is to obtain a do-not-resuscitate (DNR) order on every patient. When viewing PC through that lense, one can imagine that when things are stable for a patient with HM, it can be even harder for their hematologist/oncologist to suggest referring to a palliative care clinic. Furthermore, many hematologist/oncologist clinicians do an excellent job of managing their patient's symptoms and feel that they are capable of providing their own PC to their patients without needing to introduce new clinicians to the patient's care team. Finally, for those working outside of large teaching institutions, there may not be sufficient access to PC, especially in the outpatient setting. Even those with adequate PC resources may not have PC clinicians well versed in the care of patients with HM [11].

To complicate things further, recent advances in treatment of HM have led to patients and treating clinicians focusing "singularly on curative treatment, even when the patient has advanced disease" [11]. Things can change quickly in advanced HM. For instance, patients with Acute Myeloid Leukemia (AML) are diagnosed quickly and often require hospital admission at time of diagnosis for acute care, thus not having an opportunity to meet palliative care earlier on in the outpatient setting. The high-risk nature of treatment in AML can lead to increased patient and clinician distress.

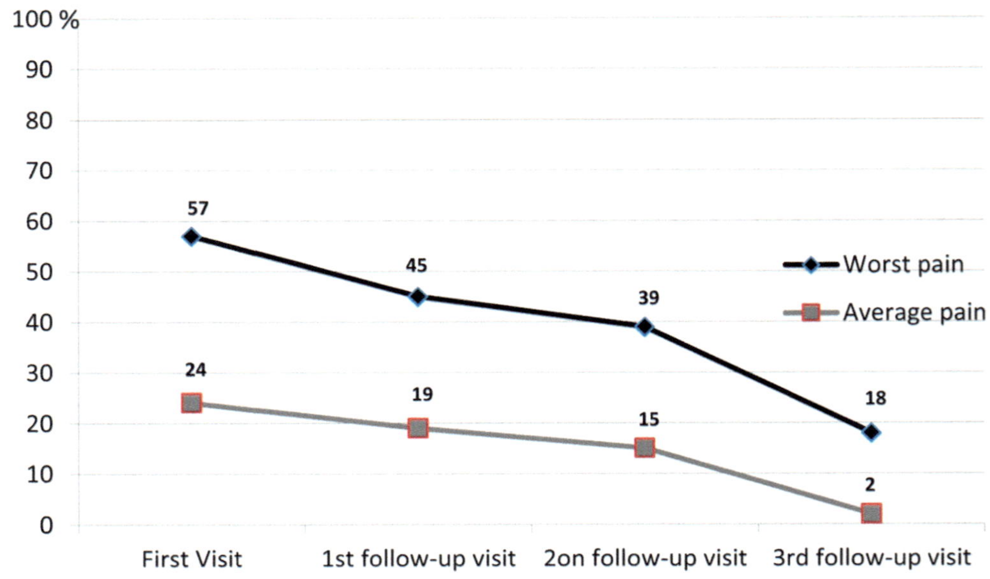


**Fig. 8.3** Changes in the proportion of patients with MM with moderate-to-severe (visual analog scale ≥5) worst and average pain over the course of the follow-up period. [Porta-Sales J, Guerrero-Torrelles M, Moreno-Alonso D, et al. Is Early Palliative Care Feasible in Patients With Multiple Myeloma? *J Pain Symptom Manage*. 2017;54(5):692–700]

This intricate dynamic leaves even PC clinicians wondering how to best approach discussions related to ACP while simultaneously discussing potential cure. This can be a challenge for PC clinicians who may be more familiar with having goals-of-care conversations with patients who do not have an option of cure. It can also be difficult for outpatient PC clinicians who are more comfortable when they can gently approach these conversations over several clinic visits. "The course of disease in patients with HM is often unpredictable, and physical deterioration can occur suddenly, requiring a rapid change in the therapeutic approach in an end-of-life situation". Consequently, patients with HM can quickly pass from stable to late-stage disease in a difficult-to-predict manner. Another often overlooked reason for delayed referral to PC is that many hematologists/oncologists erroneously equate PC with end-of-life care. LeBlanc et al. further reported a study on barriers for early PC in HM and found that "in general, there is a reluctance to utilize PC services or engage in ACP among hematologists/oncologists. Transplant teams may be so focused on cure that the usefulness and need for early PC are underestimated" [15].

So how does one overcome these barriers? It starts with a thorough explanation of the role of PC within the patient's team and the goal of having this specialized team involved. It is essential to also explain what PC is not. Patients will have a clearer understanding and may feel reassured to hear that PC is not hospice. Reviewing that the intention of consulting outpatient PC for assistance with symptom management may help patients gain clearer insight into benefits of having PC part of their oncology team. This in turn will also help foster relationships with the palliative clinic provider and the referring hematology/oncology team.

Patients with HM often experience numerous symptoms associated with induction and their treatment regimens. Controlling these symptoms, providing education regarding their disease and treatment plan, reviewing pertinent lab results as well as addressing emotional distress, complex psychosocial needs, and spiritual concerns can be overwhelming for a single hematology clinician during a 30-min follow-up visit. This is where having an outpatient PC clinician can be essential. For example, Ruiz et al. states that "recent reviews have established that physical and emotional symptoms among other psychological, social, or spiritual concerns are not addressed thoroughly in busy outpatient and inpatient oncology practices. Moreover, this situation is even worse in the setting of [HM] and [HCT]" bone [6].

## Collaboration Between Palliative Care and Hematology Oncology Clinicians

### Communication

Close collaboration and communication are imperative to providing optimal patient care in this vulnerable patient population. With ever-changing new treatment options, varying chemotherapy regimens, frequent transfusion needs, clinical trials, and difficult prognostic scenarios, the care of patients with HM is extremely complicated. PC clinicians welcome all dialogue with their hematology/oncology counterparts and consider this interaction as a necessity to provide safe and effective care. As an initial effort at information sharing, when considering a referral to a PC clinic, it is advised that the referring clinician at a minimum provide the patient's diagnosis and a reason for referral (e.g., mood, pain, coping, etc.). Optimal communication includes a "warm sign out," such as a phone call or in-person discussion regarding the patient's case and anticipated needs. PC typically aims to align with the hematology/oncology team so that a unified message is delivered to the patient and PC can avoid sending any mixed messages, especially around complicated issues such as prognostication. It is also helpful when oncology shares with PC what prior conversations regarding prognosis have occurred.

During a warm sign out between hematology and PC, there are several pieces of information that are important for the hematology/oncology clinician to share. As mentioned, patient and disease-specific education is helpful to discuss. Breaking down and explaining prior therapies a patient has already received, what therapy the patient is currently receiving, and what disease-directed treatment options remain are all useful points of information. When reviewing remaining treatment options, it is particularly helpful if discussions around the outcomes with each potential option are reviewed. This information is then used when considering prognostication for patients with HM.

During this discussion, the PC clinician frequently encourages the hematologist/oncologist to share their specific worries for the patient under discussion. These worries are typically at the core of why a referral is placed and can give important insight into what the patient's experience and help prepare for the future. Sharing details regarding previous conversations around prognosis and end-of-life care helps PC to align and pick up where the conversation may have left off or even or perhaps even stalled. One recent study noted that in older patients with AML, 90% of patients reported that they were "somewhat" or "very likely" to be cured of their disease, whereas their hematologists/oncologists estimated this chance of cure for only 31% [16]. It is important to identify when these gaps exist. Once we are aware of a patient's estimated prognosis and how it may differ from the treating hematologist/oncologist, PC can begin to address the disparity.

The palliative care clinician may also want to consider the possibility of a joint visit with the hematologist/oncologist. We have found that conducting a joint can lessen any hesitation or concerns that a patient may have around incorporating PC into their care. These visits also foster a great collaborating relationship between both providers and provides an opportunity to share insight into the patient's care in real-time. There are some barriers to joint visits, primarily logistical ones if one provider is running late and the other has to get to their next clinic patient. It can also be uncomfortable at first to have another professional sitting in on your patient visit, but as joint visits happen more frequently the benefits will likely take precedence.

Symptomatology is different in individuals with HM than in those with solid tumors. With the exception of MM in HM, pain is not a frequently reported symptom. Clarification around expected symptoms with each person with HM will help guide the PC clinician in the management of reported symptoms. For example, if the hematologist/oncologist does not expect a particular disease or patient to experience malignant pain and communicates this clearly to PC, this could prevent the misuse or overuse of opioids. If the hematology/oncology clinician is considering a patient for a clinical trial, this information should be shared, especially if PC will be prescribing for the patient. Clinical trials often have lengthy lists of medications that are contraindicated (e.g., methadone), and mistakes can be avoided by knowing this information prior to prescribing.

## Collaboration Challenges

Given the nature of how challenging and complex management is for this particular patient population, it is common for some barriers to collaboration to occur. Logistics can be difficult. Appointments can run longer than expected, patients can decide they do not want to stay for additional visits, or unexpected clinical changes requiring immediate attention may preclude an additional PC appointment. Taken together the primary barriers to collaboration can be broken down into three categories including illness specific barriers, system-based barriers, and cultural barriers [17].

Cultural barriers play a large part in the reduced access patients with HM have to PC. In a recent survey of transplantation physicians, 52% reported that PC is synonymous with end-of-life care and 66% felt it can decrease hope in patients and families. Data also supports that hematologists/oncologists who care for patients with HM also have a strong sense of ownership and feel it is their responsibility to manage all symptoms through end of life [17]. By recognizing this clinician-patient dynamic, PC can be respectful of these feelings and mindful when co-managing patients together.

Occasionally, the primary issue presenting a barrier to PC involvement is the illness itself. Often patients with HM initially pursue curative-intent intervention, such is the case for HCT. This can make it difficult to know when a patient's outlook and treatment has shifted from being curative in nature. There are no clear guidelines defining when treatment intent should shift, leaving that decision to the individual clinician. This can cause confusion in patients, caregivers, and PC clinicians when trying to provide and process accurate prognostic information and detemine the best way forward. In addition to the difficulty with prognosticating, patients with HM have unique needs at the end of life, typically including blood product support and potentially intravenous antibiotics, which can further complicate the delivery of end-of-life care out of the hospital [17]. Hospice agencies are typically unable to enroll patients still receiving blood products or intravenous antibiotics given financial limitations, but it is important to note that neither of these interventions exclude a patient from accessing PC. This is a common misconception shared by many patients and oncologists which deserves clarification.

Finally, patients themselves may present a barrier to referral. Given the high association of PC with end of life, patients may be fearful of a PC referral thus delaying access to this specialty service until the very end of their disease process. It is important to note that data gathered on patients receiving PC during prolonged hospital admission for curative-intent HCT demonstrated clinically significant improvements in their QOL, symptom burden, depression, and anxiety symptoms [15]. This is worth noting to patients and caregivers who are apprehensive regarding PC involvement; it is an educational point that PC is not just helpful at the end of life, but across all stages of illness. Study participants continued to endorse positive effects at both the 3- and 6-month intervals, which supports the lasting impacts of PC [15].

## Outpatient Symptom Management

Patients with HM experience a physical and psychological symptom burden that is comparable to or exceeding that of patients with advanced solid tumors, including pain, mucositis, dyspnea, fatigue, nausea, constipation, and diarrhea [18]. Fadul et al. reported similar severity of symptoms in both tumor groups, though discovered that "hematologic patients had increased delirium and drowsiness" [18] than their solid tumor counterparts. Understandably, symptom burden is often greater in patients undergoing active treatment as well as those with poor performance status. Please refer to Chaps. 12 and 13 regarding symptom management in patients with HM.

Once symptom management recommendations are made by PC clinicians, the outpatient PC clinic is typically responsible for their follow-up. Clinic follow-up can take place in the form of office visits, telephone calls, or virtual visits. Office visits are the gold standard for follow-up; physically seeing and speaking with the patient fosters trust and collaboration and allows the clinician to perform necessary physical exam elements. Virtual visits are sufficient and still allow the clinician to "see" their patient and assess symptom burden or response to medications recommendations. Phone follow-up is appropriate for low stake interventions, such as small medication adjustments in a fairly stable patient, and allow immunocompromised patients to remain in protective isolation at home. Some PC clinics opt rely on nurse navigators to assist with follow-up phone calls. Nurse navigators help to triage phone calls, address some symptom management questions, and allow billing providers to practice to the top of their license.

How frequently patients are seen in follow-up varies greatly depending on patient acuity and the clinic's bandwidth for accommodating close follow-up. For stable patients, follow-up is typically monthly. If a patient is experiencing an increase in symptom burden, or has changes in disease (e.g., progression, change in treatment plan), they may need to be sooner than 1 month. We would encourage flexibility around follow-up with PC patients with HM as their clinical situations can change quickly. Patients might also have input related to how often they are seen, some asking for more support and frequent visits, others preferring longer stretches between interactions.

## Goals-of-Care Conversations and Hospice Referrals

### Challenges with GOC Conversations in Patients with HM

As we conclude this chapter, we focus on end-of-life management of individuals with HM. Historically, PC referrals are often triggered by the need to discuss poor prognosis with patients with terminal cancer. PC clinicians are experts in difficult communication, specifically assessing the patient's understanding of their illness and goals of their treatment. In HM, there is more prognostic uncertainty, which understandably results in fewer PC referrals, as oncologists may be more focused on disease-directed treatment for potential cure. In comparison to solid tumor patients, HM may be more amenable to treatment. In fact, "a small proportion of these patients are indeed cured with aggressive therapy, though many do also die in pursuit of a cure" [18]. Oftentimes patients do not have a clear understanding that while the goal of their treatment may be curative, their hematologic cancer is in fact terminal. LeBlanc and El-Jawahri identified that patients with significant misperceptions about their illness trajectory and overall prognosis can benefit from PC involvement to help clarify their treatment goals and overall disease understanding [11].

Through ongoing conversations with outpatient PC clinicians, patients have the opportunity to build rapport and forge a relationship with a member of their team who can enhance the patient's overall understanding. PC clinicians can delve deeper into the patient's thoughts and emotions following their hematology/oncology clinic visits, providing more structure to supportive care. By reviewing what is important to the patient, as well as addressing hopes and fears related to their illness, PC clinicians explore the patient's goals and values and ensure that they receive goal-concordant care. Studies have shown that "patients may engage in different conversations with different clinicians, focusing on cancer with the cancer specialist, and other issues like pain or psychosocial distress with the [PC] specialist" [11]. Discussions about improving symptom control and preserving QOL will ultimately lead to a better understanding of what is important to the patient as their health declines. In turn, this additional layer of support allows the hematology/oncology clinician to have a more in-depth understanding of their patient and can direct their care accordingly.

There have been several studies exploring communication skills between PC clinicians and patients, specifically discussing hope. Busolo and Woodgate [19] described that cultural backgrounds have a significant impact on patient communication of emotional symptoms, which ultimately affects decision-making. While some may worry that having such conversations could impact patient's hope negatively, patients receiving PC support are often "able to transition their hopes from a complete focus on cure to hoping for other important goals, such as good symptom control, prolonging life while preserving [QOL], and spending quality time with their loved ones" [4].

The landmark SUPPORT study [20] demonstrated that "poor communication about [end of life] issues resulted in many patients receiving life-sustaining care that they did not want" [21]. Knowing this, one can envision the importance of exploring patient goals in a realistic fashion, as patients with HM are "often hospitalized during the last month of life and frequently die in the hospital" [21]. In addition to informative and practical conversations regarding the end of life, PC clinicians can also facilitate completion of advance directives as a means of helping patients advocate for themselves at times of crisis and end of life.

## Hospice Referral Barriers (Transfusion Dependency, When to Stop Treatment)

In considering end-of-life care for people with HM, it is essential to explore why they are less likely to die with hospice support. "Only a minority of patients who die of hematologic cancers in the US enroll [in hospice]. Moreover, they have the lowest rates of hospice use among all oncology patients" [20]. One can surmise there are many barriers that lead to less hospice use in this population. LeBlanc et al. [15] explain that hospice referrals seem more clearly defined for patients with solid tumors who have exhausted treatment options or become too frail for further lines of treatment. For patients with relapsed or refractory HM, "the treatment goal may even remain cure in these refractory settings, if [HCT] is an option, yet the longer-term prognosis may remain statistically quite poor." Because many with HM remain dependent on transfusions at end of life, transitioning to hospice care becomes impossible as many hospice agencies cannot provide transfusions as these are considerd to be "active treatment". "Yet evidence suggests that home transfusion programs are feasible and may even be cost saving in comparison to hospitalizations, while allowing patients to spend more time at home with loved ones" [15].

The American Society of Hematology released a statement in 2019 imploring Medicare to cover platelet and blood transfusions for HM patients at end of life as "transfusions can address palliative needs related to breathlessness, bothersome bleeding, and profound fatigue. Relieving these symptoms should be arguably a goal similar to treatment of pain, constipation, or obstructive symptoms typical for patients with solid tumors."

Another barrier to hospice is cancer-directed treatments which can be quite costly for hospice agencies to absorb. "One typical example is the use of low-dose cytarabine or hypomethylating therapy in older patients with AML. While transient remissions are possible with these therapies, cure is not; rather, they can help patients achieve important goals by improving longevity, reducing transfusion needs or symptoms by improving blood counts" [15].

Finally, many patients with HM die of complications from infection at the end of life. Cheng [22] discusses that antibiotics are not routinely prescribed at end of life for patients on hospice. "The decision to use antibiotics in PC is difficult and often complicated by physician, patient, and family beliefs. The probability of symptom improvement must be weighed against the burdens imposed on patients as well as the public health concerns regarding antibiotic resistance" [22]. It is known that earlier involvement with hospice support is more beneficial to the patient and family, thus it is essential to find ways to work with local hospice agencies and regulatory agencies to accommodate hospice care earlier in the end-of-life process for patients with HM.

## Location of Death

As we consider the end-of-life needs for individuals with HM, one must consider the preferred location of care. As stated above, many patients prefer to die at home rather than in the hospital. That said, it is not always feasible for patients with HM. According to Cheng [22], "more than half of elderly individuals with AML (51.2%) spent the whole period of their last 30 days of life (final month) in hospital. The average number of days being hospitalized in their final month of life was 21.4 days" [22]. The trajectory for patients dying with HM is different from their solid tumor counterparts. Patients dying from AML tend to have acute exacerbations of their illness, requiring more intense medical treatment including blood transfusions, management of infections, and intense medical care which cannot always be delivered sufficiently in the home. "Studies show that in the last 30 days of life, patients with HM, when compared to patients with solid tumors, have a greater number of emergency room visits, hospital admissions, intensive care unit admissions, hospital deaths, and deaths in the ICU. These adverse events at the end of life are linked to lack of hospice care" [22].

## Conclusion

This chapter has provided an overall review of a typical outpatient PC clinic specifically as it relates to the needs of patients with HM. We have reviewed consultative versus co-management methods of patient care. We have defined early PC for patients with HM and delved into some of the barriers that have historically made PC underutilized in this patient population. There is much to learn about improving collaboration between PC and hematology clinicians. Finally, we have highlighted the importance of goals-of-care conversations and some common barriers to hospice access.

## References

1. Calton BA, Alvarez-Perez A, Portman DG, Ramchandran KJ, Sugalski J, Rabow MW. The current state of palliative care for patients care for at leading US Cancer Centers: the 2015 NCCN Palliative Care Survey. J Palliat Care. 2016;14:7.
2. Hui D, Kim S-H, Kwon JH, Tanco KC, Zhang T, et al. Access to palliative care among patients treated at a comprehensive cancer center. Oncologist. 2012;17:1574–80.
3. Porta-Sales J, Guerrero-Torrelles M, Moreno-Alonso D, Sarrà-Escarré J, Clapés-Puig V, et al. Is early palliative care feasible in patients with multiple myeloma? J Pain Symptom Manag. 2017;54(5):692–700.
4. World Health Organization. WHO definition of palliative care. 2015. http://www.who.int/cancer/palliative/definition/en/. Accessed 27 Jan 2016.
5. Desai AV, Klimek VM, Chow K, Epstein AS, Bernal C, Anderson K, Okpako M, Rawlins-Duell R, Kramer D, Romano D, Goldberg JI,

Nelson JE. 1-2-3 Project: A quality improvement initiative to normalize and systematize palliative care for all patients with cancer in the outpatient clinic setting. J Oncol Pract. 2018;14(12):e775–85.
6. Ruiz M, Reynolds P, Marranzini R, Khan A, Ketterer J, Brahim A. Role of early palliative care interventions in hematological malignancies and bone marrow transplant patients: barriers and potential solutions. Am J Hosp Palliat Care. 2018;35(11):1456–60.
7. Zhuang H, Ma Y, Wang L, Zhang H. Effect of early palliative care on quality of life in patients with non-small-cell lung cancer. Curr Oncol. 2018;25(1):e54–8. https://doi.org/10.3747/co.25.3639.
8. Temel JS, Greer JA, Muzikansky A, Gallagher ER, Admane S, Jackson VA, Dahlin CM, Blinderman CD, Jacobsen J, Pirl WF, Billings JA, Lynch TJ. Early palliative care for patients with metastatic non-small-cell lung cancer. N Engl J Med. 2010;363:733–42.
9. Mah K, Chow B, Swami N, Pope A, Rydall A, Earle C, Krzyzanowska M, Le L, Hales S, Rodin G, Hannon B, Zimmermann C. Early palliative care and quality of dying and death in patients with advanced cancer. BMJ Support Palliat Care. 2021;2021:002893. https://doi.org/10.1136/bmjspcare-2021-002893.
10. Porta-Sales J, Guerrero-Torrelles M, Moreno-Alonso D, et al. Is early palliative care feasible in patients with multiple myeloma? J Pain Symptom Manag. 2017;54(5):692–700.
11. LeBlanc TW, El-Jawahri A. When and why should patients with hematologic malignancies see a palliative care specialist? Hematology. 2015;2015:471–8.
12. Watanabe SM, et al. A multicenter study comparing two numerical versions of the Edmonton Symptom Assessment System in palliative care patients. J Pain Symptom Manag. 2011;41(2):456–68.
13. Nekolaichuk CL, Fainsinger RL, Lawlor PG. A validation study of a pain classification system for advanced cancer patients using content experts: the Edmonton Classification System for Cancer Pain. Palliat Med. 2005;19(6):466–76.
14. Anderson F, Downing GM, Hill J, Casorso L, Lerch N. Palliative Performance Scale (PPS): a new tool. J Palliat Care. 1996;12(1):5–11.
15. LeBlanc TW, Roeland EJ, El-Jawahri A. Early palliative care for patients with hematologic malignancies: is it really so difficult to achieve? Curr Hematol Malig Rep. 2017;12(4):300–8. https://doi.org/10.1007/s11899-017-0392-z.
16. El-Jawahri A, Nelson-Lowe M, VanDusen H, Traeger L, Abel GA, Greer JA, Fathi A, Steensma DP, LeBlanc TW, Li Z, DeAngelo D, Wadleigh M, Hobbs G, Foster J, Brunner A, Amrein P, Stone RM, Temel JS. Patient-clinician discordance in perceptions of treatment risks and benefits in older patients with acute myeloid leukemia. Oncologist. 2019;24(2):247–54. https://doi.org/10.1634/theoncologist.2018-0317.
17. El-Jawahri A, Nelson AM, Gray TF, Lee SJ, Leblanc TW. Palliative and end-of-life care for patients with hematologic malignancies. J Clin Oncol. 2019;38(9):944.
18. Fadul NA, El Osta B, Dalal S, Poulter VA, Bruera E. Comparison of symptom burden among patients referred to palliative care with hematologic malignancies versus those with solid tumors. J Palliat Med. 2008;11:422–7.
19. Busolo D, Woodgate R. Palliative care experiences of adult cancer patients from ethnocultural groups: a qualitative systematic review protocol. JBI Database Syst Rev Implement Rep. 2015;12(1):99–111.
20. Connors AF, Dawson NV, Desbiens NA, et al. A controlled trial to improve care for seriously III hospitalized patients: the study to understand prognoses and preferences for outcomes and risks of treatments (SUPPORT). JAMA. 1995;274(20):1591–8. https://doi.org/10.1001/jama.1995.03530200027032.
21. Adams JA, Bailey DE Jr, Anderson RA, Docherty SL. Nursing roles and strategies in end-of-life decision making in acute care: a systematic review of the literature. Nurs Res Pract. 2011;2011:527834. https://doi.org/10.1155/2011/527834.
22. Cheng HB, Li C, Chan K, et al. End-of-life characteristics and palliative care provision for elderly patients suffering from acute myeloid leukemia. Support Care Cancer. 2015;23:111–6. https://doi.org/10.1007/s00520-014-2333-x.

# Part III

# The Intersection of Palliative Care and Hematologic Malignancies and Serious Blood Disorders: Key Issues

# Communication Throughout the Illness Trajectory

9

Marc-Antoine Marquis, Monia Marzouki, and Lysanne Daoust

## Introduction

"What the scalpel is to the surgeon, words are to the clinician… the conversation between doctor and patient is the heart of the practice of medicine" [1].

Nowhere are the above words truer than in palliative care. (PC) The identification and alleviation of suffering, lying at the core of palliative care practice, involve being able to communicate information sensibly and precisely, support patients and caregivers in the setting of a life-threatening illness, identify and adjust goals of care, and engage in uncertainty. Communication must be precise enough to allow individuals to make informed decisions and feel supported, and flexible enough to adapt to each patient's unique characteristics and preferences. Excellent communication is pertinent throughout the trajectory of an illness: patients and caregivers' hopes and goals may evolve over time, as can information preferences and need for support.

## The Language of Palliative Care

Discussing advance care planning is linked to an increase in goal-concordant end-of-life care [2], improvement in caregiver satisfaction, without increasing stress, anxiety, and depression in patients and relatives [2, 3]. Furthermore, the terminology clinicians use has an impact on management preferences as well as psychological outcomes in patients with the same underlying condition [4].

### Patient and Caregiver-Centered Language

The way we speak frames how we approach a given situation. Patient or caregiver-centered care may and should be mirrored in the language clinicians use. A focus on the illness rather than the patient runs the risk of shifting our attention away from the patient herself, her priorities, and particular needs. A first step in this direction is to avoid labeling a patient with her or his disease. Doing so helps keep the patient and caregiver at the center of conversations, which in turn may be more conducive to building strong partnerships.

#### Non-abandonment

Non-abandonment is a crucial responsibility of palliative care practitioners [5–7]. Such commitment to walk alongside a patient no matter what can be strongly expressed in the language we use. Clearly stating one's intention to remain engaged is one way, but there are additional changes in the way we discuss medical interventions that can reduce the unnecessary worry of being abandoned.

Statements about "stopping" or "withdrawing" care inadvertently send the message that when disease-directed or life-sustaining treatments are discontinued, patients stop receiving care altogether. This overlooks the fact that comfort measures are often as active and intense as other, disease-oriented interventions. Reframing those statements by offering to "change the focus of care in favor of comfort measures," for instance, may be both more accurate and less frightening for patients and clinicians alike.

Similarly, declarations such as "there is nothing more that we can do" are often used as a shortcut to "there is no curative option available." While the former suggests that all pos-

M.-A. Marquis (✉)
Department of Pediatrics, Sainte-Justine Hospital, Montreal, QC, Canada

Department of Pediatric Palliative Care, Sainte-Justine Hospital, Montreal, QC, Canada
e-mail: marc-antoine.marquis@umontreal.ca

M. Marzouki
Department of Pediatrics, Sainte-Justine Hospital, Montreal, QC, Canada
e-mail: monia.marzouki.hsj@ssss.gouv.qc.ca

L. Daoust
Department of Pediatric Palliative Care, Sainte-Justine Hospital, Montreal, QC, Canada
e-mail: lysanne.daoust.hsj@ssss.gouv.qc.ca


C. K. Ullrich, E. J. Roeland (eds.), *Palliative Care in Hematologic Malignancies and Serious Blood Disorders*, https://doi.org/10.1007/978-3-031-38058-7_9

sibilities have been exhausted, the latter leaves the door open for considerations other than cure.

### Failure

Treatments or tests are seldom guaranteed to provide a benefit to a patient. In many instances, it is difficult to predict if an intervention will be successful. Attempts at resuscitation, extubation, or pharmacologic treatments as well as time-limited trials, all have the potential to fail. In some cases, the responsibility for the failure of an intervention is transferred involuntarily onto a patient, having "failed extubation" or "failed the treatment." In reality, interventions sometimes do not achieve the results clinicians and caregivers hope for: it is the treatment, or the resuscitation attempt, that fails, rather than the patient.

### Dignity, Quality of Life, and Suffering

Some words are deeply ingrained in a society or culture's collective vocabulary, while holding very different meaning from one individual to another. Such is the case with terms like "dignity," "quality of life," (QOL) and "suffering"—all of which may be relevant to goals-of-care conversations. Asking patients (and parents or surrogate when appropriate) to describe what "dignity" or "suffering" means to them as well as what represents an acceptable QOL, greatly increases the chance to have meaningful, productive conversations and leaving the patient feel understood and considered.

### Metaphors

In a similar fashion, using the vocabulary of a patient or caregiver allows a clinician to enter her patient's world more easily and convey information in a way that will resonate more comprehensively. Patients and caregivers bring up metaphors for various reasons. Some may attempt to better understand how an illness is developing or affecting one's body, while others use symbolic language to voice feelings or questions that are difficult to articulate. Clinicians attentive to the reasons a specific metaphor is brought up may use the same language to reframe a patient or caregiver's way of thinking, help them see their situation through different lenses, and foster new coping strategies [8]. Applied skillfully, it is also a helpful strategy in engaging young children and their siblings around abstract topics such as uncertainty, serious illness, and death.

In other circumstances, metaphors help introduce difficult news in a gentle manner, such as the idea of a serious health decline or death. Metaphors can help personalize conversations, promote advance care planning, and improve patients and caregivers' understanding [9, 10]. While euphemisms are at times used to communicate difficult news, clinicians must remember that clarity is key: to avoid causing more confusion, metaphors should be introduced when helpful for a patient's or caregiver's understanding or to provide support.

## Communication Between Professionals

Communication between clinicians should use the same framework as with patients. Although the use of medical jargon between practitioners is relevant for precise communication, some shortcuts, including those discussed above, may be the source of unnecessary misunderstandings. Clinicians who frequently engage in difficult conversations have an opportunity to model this language to colleagues.

### Resuscitation Status

Using "Do Not Attempt Resuscitation" (DNAR) as opposed to "Do Not Resuscitate" (DNR) emphasizes that resuscitation is not always successful when initiated—a more accurate reflection of the reality of such interventions. In addition, "the patient has a DNAR order" is more consistent with patient-centered language than "the patient is DNR."

### Appropriate

The use of the term may, at times, inadvertently allow clinicians to introduce values and judgment into clinical encounters [11]. It is often incorrect and unhelpful to label emotions as inappropriate; one cannot help but feel the way one feels. Similarly, while grieving individuals may have varying levels of adjustment to a loved one's death, there is rarely an appropriate way to grieve: it is a multifaceted experience encompassing cultural, spiritual, and individual dimensions.

### Chronic Patient

The term "chronic" is best suited to a disease, illness, or condition, rather than a patient. It is often the case that an individual with a chronic illness will have prolonged or recurrent hospitalizations, a protracted course, or unremitting symptoms. An individual may be chronically ill; however, "chronic patient" is a shortcut that risks substituting the ill person for the diseased state.

### Denial

Denial may impede a patient's ability to make informed decisions in the setting of a life-threatening or progressing illness [12]. More commonly, individuals oscillate between more and less realistic understandings of their illness and prognosis [13]. This adaptive mental process is often mistaken for denial. Contemplating one's death or the possibility of a loved one's death at every moment may be intolerable; allowing a patient and caregiver space to escape those thoughts temporarily may, at times, ease adaptation to the reality of a life-threatening illness. It may help caregivers acclimatize to serious news at their own pace.

In some cases, difficult news is met with few outward emotional expressions or stoicism. Clinicians may interpret such reactions as a sign that they have not been able to convey the severity of the illness or the seriousness of the news adequately. Careful attention to other signs of understanding may prevent unnecessary repetition of an already distressing information to a patient or loved ones [14].

## Discussing Difficult News

### Why Disclose Difficult News?

Clinicians tend to underestimate an individual's desire for information and overestimate their awareness and understanding of their prognosis [15]. Although clinicians believe that patients should know the truth, many provide partial information or avoid discussing the subject altogether [16].

People with serious illness and their surrogates want to receive realistic information and appropriate hope [17]. Increasing evidence shows that delivering difficult news does not bring about harm or break a patient's hope. In fact, advance care planning and end-of-life discussions do not increase anxiety or distress [2, 18] and do not lead to hopelessness [19, 20]. Such conversations improve clinical outcomes for patients with serious illness [12]. They are associated with better QOL, less intensive care near death, and earlier referral to hospice [3] along with improved mood [21] and higher rates of goal-concordant care at the end of life [2, 22].

While it is true that many patients who understand their prognosis often opt for fewer intensive measures at the end of their lives, discussing difficult news and prognosis should not be expected to yield this result every time [23]. Patients who have a clearer sense of their prognosis are more likely to receive care that is consistent with their own goals and values, be it comfort-focused, life-sustaining, or a blend of both [24].

### Who Should Discuss Difficult News?

Patients usually expect clinicians to initiate advance care planning conversations and would have appreciated discussing the subject earlier in the course of their illness [16]. There are a variety of reasons why clinicians are reluctant to engage in such conversations with patients: lack of training or time, fear of harming the patient or destroying hope, prognostic uncertainty or hopelessness related to lack of curative interventions, and requests from family members to withhold information [16]. Furthermore, many individuals with serious illness are followed by multiple specialists, resulting in confusion about who should be initiating conversations about goals of care, disclose prognosis, or discuss treatment options [12]. The fact that patients have different preferences about which clinician they prefer to have difficult conversations with adds another layer of complexity [25]. In most instances, particularly when multiple clinicians are involved, a clinician known and trusted by the patient and caregiver should be identified and responsible for leading difficult conversations [12, 26].

Caregivers of children with cancer can also benefit from conversations with a trusted clinician. In one study involving children with a diagnosis other than cancer, strength of the relationship and understanding of the family were deemed as two major elements in identifying the ideal interlocutor [27].

### When Should Difficult News Be Discussed?

Clinicians commonly express a worry that patients or caregivers are not ready to engage in conversations around goals of care, disease progression, or end-of-life care. When asked about the timing of conversations about prognosis, adult patients often express that they would have liked to know earlier; at least some of the information could be discussed at the diagnosis of a life-threatening illness, or shortly after [26]. In pediatrics, many parents think about the possibility of their child dying before the subject is raised for the first time in a clinical encounter [28, 29]. It is common for parents to wait for clinicians to initiate such conversations [30].

While some opportunities to discuss prognosis or end-of-life care may appear throughout a patient's life, waiting for the ideal moment runs the risk of rushing conversations in the future, when a patient is experiencing a serious decline or progression of symptoms. Conversely, the multiplication of treatment options in oncology (e.g., experimental treatments and immunotherapies) further complicates prognostication. Combined with easier access to information by patients and caregivers, having many possible trajectories makes the determination of an adequate moment to discuss prognosis even more difficult.

Initiating conversations when a patient is stable, but is likely to decline, gives time to address difficult topics calmly without the pressure of making decisions [31]. Another opportunity, including in the pediatric setting, is to reflect on a recent episode of clinical deterioration (be it an aggravation of symptoms, a prolonged hospitalization, or an admission to the intensive care unit): discussing what the patient's experience was and how this impacts her or his way of thinking about similar episodes in the future. These conversations often can take place in the outpatient setting.

Ultimately, there is no right timing to discuss prognosis. When a patient is ambivalent about receiving information, such disclosure should be preceded by an assessment of whether the information would make a difference at the time [13, 32].

## Effective Communication Techniques

Communication in hematology/oncology and palliative care settings require that clinicians address two types of patient needs, often simultaneously: the need to know and the need to feel known [33, 34]. The first involves asking questions and providing information. The second includes accepting emotions and showing empathy through verbal and nonverbal means.

### Cognitive Needs—The Need to Know

All patients require information to make sense of their illness and navigate through it. Cognitive needs may be addressed by disclosing test results or a diagnosis, clarifying treatment options, answering questions about side effects or the expected impact of a given intervention, as well as explaining a prognosis or the expected course of a disease. In a social context where information of varying levels of quality is readily available, providing timely and precise information is even more important to help individuals and caregivers make informed decisions.

Clinicians caring for individuals with serious, chronic, or life-threatening illness inevitably need to disclose difficult news to their patients. The SPIKES model (see Table 9.1) is a well-recognized six-step tool for sharing difficult news to a patient and caregiver [35].

Although delivering factual information may seem relatively straightforward, informational preferences vary from one individual to another. When discussing difficult news with a patient or caregiver, two initial steps are important: determining *how much* and *what kind* of information a patient wants to receive [32, 36].

First, patients and caregivers have varying preferences about the amount of information they wish to receive. Open-ended questions are a useful way to explore those preferences such as "How much do you want to know about what to expect from your illness?" Some patients appreciate discussing detailed information with their clinician; others find the "big picture" more useful; others, still, defer to family members. Any one of those options are permissible, as long as they truly reflect a patient's preference.

In pediatrics, asking a child or adolescent what she prefers to know and what she prefers to defer to her parents is a useful strategy. Many parents of younger children choose to have conversations alone with the clinician and disclose the news afterwards to their child, with or without help. Another strategy is to allow a young patient to be present during discussions with her parents, while clearly leaving open the possibility for her to stop being part of the conversation at any time (e.g., leaving the room, listening to music, or using some other form of distraction).

Second, clinicians should clarify what kind of information a patient wants to receive. When discussing prognosis, for instance, individuals may prefer orienting the conversation around time (how much time a patient has), function (what is the expected trajectory of an illness is and what is the likely impact on QOL, physical autonomy, and cogni-

**Table 9.1** Adapted SPIKES model for sharing difficult news [35]

| | |
|---|---|
| S—Setup | Ensure the physical setting is conducive to serious conversations<br>Mentally prepare and rehearse delivering the news |
| P—Perception | Assess how the patient perceives her medical situation<br>– "What have you been told about your illness so far?"<br>– "Can you tell me what is your understanding of your illness?"<br>– "Based on what you know, what do you expect are the next steps (or next decisions) with regard to your health?"<br>Correct any misconceptions or misunderstandings<br>Be attentive to denial, wishful thinking, and unrealistic expectations |
| I—Invitation | Solicit the patient's invitation (or permission) to disclose information<br>– "Would it be okay if we talked about what lies ahead with your illness?"<br>Ask how much and what kind of information a patient prefers to receive<br>– "Some individuals want to receive detailed information about test results, others prefer to focus of the big picture and spend more time discussing a treatment plan. Where would you say your preference falls?" |
| K—Knowledge | Give knowledge and information to the patient<br>Giving a warning shot may be helpful ("I have difficult news to tell you")<br>Use patient's vocabulary and avoid jargon whenever possible<br>Give the patient time to understand the new information |
| E—Emotions | Give the patient space to express what she or he feels<br>Give empathic statements or gestures<br>– "I was also hoping for better news"<br>– "I wish things were different for you"<br>Resist the urge to minimize or discuss care options immediately<br>Avoid telling the patient how to feel or what not to feel<br>Refer to the NURSE model (Table 9.2) as needed |
| S—Strategy and summary | Ask the patient if she or he is ready to discuss next steps<br>– If so, summarize the information and discuss treatment or care options<br>– If not, reassure the patient, summarize the information and plan for a follow-up meeting |

tion), or symptom burden. In addition, there are many ways to approach any of these elements. Some patients appreciate information provided in the form of numbers (e.g., statistics); others have a better grasp when discussing best, worse, and most likely scenarios. Others, still, might prefer putting the prognosis in context, for example, thinking about specific upcoming events (holidays, graduations, anniversaries, etc.) [36].

Although patients or caregivers sometimes inquire directly about prognosis, they may be uncertain about the kind of information they wish to receive. In these circumstances, as well as with patients who know what kind of information they want, using the "Ask-Tell-Ask" model to delineate how to disclose prognosis is useful [37–39]. Following this model, the clinician might say to a patient who asks about her prognosis: "There are many ways to answer your question and I want to make sure to give you this information the right way. Can you tell me more about what you would like to know?" In some cases, offering specific ways in which the answer may be given (time, function, specific events in the future, symptom burden, etc.) can help the patient determine what is best suited to her needs.

As mentioned earlier, some patients may resist or feel ambivalent about receiving difficult news; inquiring about their informational preferences is a good starting point in preparing for such conversations. It may also help build partnership between a patient and her providers. In addition, clinicians can help a patient prepare for or anticipate difficult conversations. A fruitful approach is to "talk about talking about it": exploring with a patient what such conversations would look like, who it would be important to include and what the right moment would be, as well as what the advantages and disadvantages of having the conversation may be. For some patients, those discussions may occur using a metaphorical box that is opened and closed at selected moments, then put away until the clinician and her patient agree to open it again.

## Emotional Needs—The Need to Feel Known

While patients' desire for information is generally acknowledged by clinicians, emotional needs are less commonly recognized and addressed [40]. Receiving a serious disease diagnosis, enduring intense treatment with at times heavy symptom burden, grappling with uncertainty about the future, and adjusting to a new life are all potential sources of emotional suffering. In the clinical encounter, clinicians often miss opportunities to provide empathic statements [40, 41]. Furthermore, emotions are rarely expressed the same way facts are emphasizing the importance of clinician attunement to indirect manifestations of emotions from patients.

Even when they notice manifestations of emotions in a patient, clinicians are not always comfortable responding or may feel ill-equipped to do so. Some may shift the subject or worry about initiating a discussion about what the patient is feeling will take more time than is available. Yet, brief empathic statements, taking even less than a minute, may be sufficient to acknowledge a patient's feelings and strengthen the therapeutic relationship [42]. In addition, empathic responses by clinicians increase patient satisfaction and make them more likely to adhere to treatment plans [41].

**Table 9.2** Adapted NURSE model for responding to emotion [39, 41]

| | |
|---|---|
| N—Naming | Name the patient's emotion<br>– "It sounds like this is a surprise for you"<br>– "I wonder if you might be feeling angry"<br>– "Am I hearing disappointment in your voice?" |
| U—Understanding | Legitimize the patient's feelings and let her know she is heard<br>– "Many people would feel frustrated in this situation"<br>– "I cannot imagine how difficult this must be for you"<br>– "There is no right or wrong way to feel after receiving this kind of news" |
| R—Respecting | Acknowledge the patient's coping efforts and strengths<br>– "I am impressed by your ability to approach your illness in a way that remains true to who you are"<br>– "You care for your son beautifully and I'm thankful for being able to witness what a loving family you have"<br>– "I am grateful for being part of your care team" |
| S—Supporting | Formulate the desire to remain involved and to help<br>– "I plan to be at your side no matter what lies ahead"<br>– "I want to be helpful in any way I can" |
| E—Exploring | Show concern and curiosity about a patient's statements<br>– "What do you mean when you say you can't live like this?"<br>– "What I'm hearing is that you feel guilty about considering stopping chemotherapy. Can you tell me more about this?" |

While clinicians do not need to agree with the way their patients feel about their medical condition, treatment plan, or hopes, it is important for them to recognize that patients' feelings are legitimate. Accepting a patient's emotions, acknowledging their lived experience, and respecting their need to be heard are crucial for maintaining an effective therapeutic bond. There are many strategies to respond to direct or indirect patient emotions. A useful method is the NURSE model summarized in Table 9.2 [39, 41].

Often, emotional cues are nonverbal. Facial expressions, avoidance of eye contact, fidgeting, posture, tears are all potential manifestations of a patient's distress, feeling, or concern. Being attentive to nonverbal signs of emotion is another way for clinicians to respect a patient's feelings, respond accordingly, and make the patient feel heard. In the same way, a clinician does not always have to respond to emotions using words: a hand gesture, an open posture, eye contact, the use of silence, or simply being present may be as powerful as a well-formulated empathic statement.

## Putting It All Together

When delivering difficult news, both cognitive and emotional needs must be addressed, often concurrently [33]. Providing information alone, without attending to feelings or emotional distress, may negatively affect information recall, and leave the patient feeling misunderstood or isolated [43, 44]. Conversely, responding solely to emotion may be insufficient to move the conversation forward [45]. The result is that, in a given conversation, clinicians will often find themselves oscillating between giving information and responding to emotion. Moving back-and-forth requires practice in order to keep the conversation moving while making sure the patient receives enough support.

Other elements are worth considering when delivering difficult news. First, asking permission to open a conversation about what lies ahead is a good way to gently prepare the patient; by giving permission, the patient is agreeing to engage, even if it may be frightening or uncertain. Sometimes a patient will not give permission to broach a difficult subject right away—in these instances, suggesting this conversation should be held later on, or discussing "what ifs" may be useful (e.g., "If your illness were to progress despite the chemotherapy, what would you be most important to you?").

Second, patient and caregiver-centered care, coupled with medical practices that emphasize patient autonomy, may put the responsibility of decision-making in the hands of the patient or their loved ones. In many cases, this aligns with the way an individual or a family wishes to make decisions. Sometimes, patients clearly state that they prefer to defer to their loved ones or the medical team. Others will ask a clinician what she or he would do. Often, the opinion of trusted care providers is sought. In all these circumstances, making a recommendation has the potential to help move the conversation forward, correspond better to a patient's decision-making preferences, and remove an unwanted burden on the patient and the family [46].

Third, difficult conversations require that nuanced information be conveyed in a precise and sensible manner. Words matter, as do cultural and social backgrounds. The expertise of interpreters in clinical encounters is important and should be sought out.

## Family Meetings

Family meetings are often proposed, prepared, and led by clinicians caring for individuals with serious illness or approaching the end of life [47, 48]. Reasons to hold family meetings include delivering difficult news to a family when a patient is critically ill and establishing goals of care when a patient's status changes. In addition, family meetings are a regular occurrence in pediatric palliative care, as parents usually hold the responsibility to decide for their child's care. Family meetings should take place on an as needed basis, with clearly stated goals [49]. When done appropriately, family meetings have the potential to increase communication quality, and patient and caregiver-centeredness of care [50–52]. Care conferences are also associated with a reduction in critical care length of stay [50, 53].

A family meeting is a process requiring expertise, adaptability, and good preparation in order to achieve its goals effectively. It requires coordination between clinicians, attention to a patient and family's dynamic and information preferences, the ability to provide clear information in a transparent way, and to attend to the emotional needs of mul-

**Table 9.3** Family meeting checklist

| | |
|---|---|
| Before the meeting | 1. Determine the goal of the meeting<br>2. Determine who will attend (medical clinicians, psychosocial clinicians, chaplaincy, trusted clinician, important family members, surrogate(s), individuals the patient would like to have present)<br>3. Identify and prepare an adequate setting for the meeting (rounded seating, quiet room with minimal interruptions) |
| During the meeting | **Pre-meeting between clinicians**<br>4. Review the goal of the meeting and allow everyone to give updates about the patient's status<br>5. Determine who will be leading the conversation with the patient and/or caregiver<br>**Meeting with the patient and her or his family**<br>6. Introduce every member present (clinicians and loved ones)<br>7. Review meeting goals<br>8. Determine what the patient and her caregiver already know about her medical condition<br>9. Disclose relevant information (current medical status, trajectory, or prognosis)<br>10. Attend to emotional reactions of loved ones; respect silence<br>11. Present and discuss care options moving forward, allowing all members to voice their thoughts, and keeping the patient at the center of the conversation<br>**Wrapping up**<br>12. Summarize the plan and next steps; name the disagreements<br>13. Plan for a follow-up meeting if necessary |
| After the meeting | 14. Notify relevant clinicians of the conclusions of the meeting and next steps<br>15. Document the meeting: members present, content of the conversation, decisions made and follow-up plan |

tiple family members simultaneously [47, 54, 55]. A summary of the steps involved is presented in Table 9.3.

## Before the Meeting

When preparing for a family meeting, an important first step is to clarify the goals of the meeting, whether it is delivering new or important information about a patient's health, establishing goals of care, or addressing specific decisions or plans of care (e.g., resuscitation status, next steps when the status of a patient has changed, etc.). This helps set an agenda and determine who is best suited to join the meeting.

The individuals present at the meeting should include the patient if she or he is capable of participating, the surrogate decision maker (if pertinent), and any loved ones to assist with decision-making, hear information, or provide support. Key clinicians may include medical specialists, psychosocial clinicians, and pastoral care. Having a high number of clinicians present during a family meeting may be overwhelming or intimidating to a patient or family; if so, seeking the opinion of specific clinicians is sufficient if the information can be relayed by another during the meeting. Often patients and parents will appreciate the presence of a trusted clinician (sometimes a primary care provider or a long-time treating physician). For instance, the family of a child admitted to the intensive care unit may wish to have a long-time clinician at their side when considering important decisions.

Attention to the setting where the meeting takes place is also important. A circular seating avoids separation between clinicians and family members and may be more conducive to collaboration. The selected room should also allow privacy with minimal interruptions.

## During the Meeting

Clinicians often benefit from a pre-meeting where they can discuss the current status of the patient, review treatment options, determine if a preferred treatment path is possible, and identify who will lead the meeting. By doing so, clinicians have a better chance of delivering information in a cohesive manner.

Ideally, individuals present at the meeting should have met with the patient or family beforehand. This is not always possible, however. In such circumstances, taking time to build a therapeutic bond by asking questions about the patient as a person and what is important to her or him is helpful both for the clinicians, the patient, and family.

Once the participants of the meeting are assembled, introductions are completed, and the goals of the conference are clarified. Starting with what the patient and his family's understanding of his current condition and his illness trajectory is an effective way to start, allowing clinicians to clarify questions and provide additional information, as needed. An update on the medical status, prognosis, and treatment options may then be provided in fuller detail, if necessary.

Throughout the meeting, clinicians should be alert to the emotional reactions of the patient and caregivers. Responding to emotions (using NURSE, for instance), using pauses and silence, and gently inviting the members present to express how they feel is important to show the patient is heard, and to let the information sink in before any decision is made.

If a decision regarding which treatment path is to be made, the patient or surrogate should be asked directly what options she is considering; the caregivers may also have further questions or worries that must be addressed. In every case, it is crucial to keep the patient at the center of the conversation. Even when the patient is unable to participate to the meeting, asking *"What would she want to do in this circumstance"* rather than *"What should we do,"* serves as a reminder that the patient must remain central to the decision.

It is common for patients or caregivers to be unsure about the best path forward. Some may ask clinicians directly about their opinion; others may openly voice their preference to defer medical decisions to healthcare providers. In many instances, clinicians can use their expertise and offer to recommend a treatment path based on a patient's hopes, goals, and values. This approach helps to relieve the burden of decision-making for some patients and caregivers who are hesitant.

At times, participants reach a decision on a treatment plan or resuscitation status that can be implemented immediately. Commonly, individuals will have differing opinions on how to move forward. It is important to take the time to clarify what values underpin the opinion of disagreeing members. In some circumstances, family members wish to have some time to ponder the different options available, in which case the team may offer to leave the room and come back at a later time or schedule a follow-up meeting.

## After the Meeting

Once the options, decisions, or next steps are summarized and a follow-up meeting is planned (if needed), it is important to document the content of the conversation in the patient's chart, and inform other key clinicians about the decisions and clarify the plan moving forward.

## Conclusion

Excellent communication is central to efficient and quality care for patients with cancer and their caregivers throughout the illness trajectory. Attending to cognitive and emotional needs requires skill and practice as much as any other aspect of clinical practice. Effective, compassionate communication by clinicians will enable patients and caregivers to make informed decisions and feel supported and empowered, while remaining true to their values.

## References


1. Tumulty PA. What is a clinician and what does he do? N Engl J Med. 1970;283(1):20–4.
2. Detering KM, Hancock AD, Reade MC, Silvester W. The impact of advance care planning on end of life care in elderly patients: randomised controlled trial. BMJ. 2010;340:c1345.
3. Wright AA, Zhang B, Ray A, Mack JW, Trice E, Balboni T, et al. Associations between end-of-life discussions, patient mental health, medical care near death, and caregiver bereavement adjustment. JAMA. 2008;300(14):1665–73.
4. Nickel B, Barratt A, Copp T, Moynihan R, McCaffery K. Words do matter: a systematic review on how different terminology for the same condition influences management preferences. BMJ Open. 2017;7(7):e014129.
5. Quill TE, Cassel CK. Nonabandonment: a central obligation for physicians. Ann Intern Med. 1995;122(5):368–74.
6. van Vliet LM, van der Wall E, Plum NM, Bensing JM. Explicit prognostic information and reassurance about nonabandonment when entering palliative breast cancer care: findings from a scripted video-vignette study. J Clin Oncol. 2013;31(26):3242–9.
7. West HF, Engelberg RA, Wenrich MD, Curtis JR. Expressions of nonabandonment during the intensive care unit family conference. J Palliat Med. 2005;8(4):797–807.
8. Southall D. The patient's use of metaphor within a palliative care setting: theory, function and efficacy. A narrative literature review. Palliat Med. 2013;27(4):304–13.
9. Gustafsson AW, Hommerberg C, Sandgren A. Coping by metaphors: the versatile function of metaphors in blogs about living with advanced cancer. Med Humanit. 2019;46:267.
10. Hui D, Zhukovsky DS, Bruera E. Serious illness conversations: paving the road with metaphors. Oncologist. 2018;23(6):730–3.
11. MacDonald ME, Murray MA. The appropriateness of appropriate: smuggling values into clinical practice. Can J Nurs Res. 2007;39(4):59–73.
12. Bernacki RE, Block SD, American College of Physicians High Value Care Task F. Communication about serious illness care goals: a review and synthesis of best practices. JAMA Intern Med. 2014;174(12):1994–2003.
13. Jackson VA, Jacobsen J, Greer JA, Pirl WF, Temel JS, Back AL. The cultivation of prognostic awareness through the provision of early palliative care in the ambulatory setting: a communication guide. J Palliat Med. 2013;16(8):894–900.
14. Caruso Brown AE. Porous boundaries. JAMA. 2017;317(24):2487–8.
15. Hancock K, Clayton JM, Parker SM, Walder S, Butow PN, Carrick S, et al. Discrepant perceptions about end-of-life communication: a systematic review. J Pain Symptom Manag. 2007;34(2):190–200.
16. Hancock K, Clayton JM, Parker SM, Wal der S, Butow PN, Carrick S, et al. Truth-telling in discussing prognosis in advanced life-limiting illnesses: a systematic review. Palliat Med. 2007;21(6):507–17.
17. Apatira L, Boyd EA, Malvar G, Evans LR, Luce JM, Lo B, et al. Hope, truth, and preparing for death: perspectives of surrogate decision makers. Ann Intern Med. 2008;149(12):861–8.
18. Mack JW, Cronin A, Taback N, Huskamp HA, Keating NL, Malin JL, et al. End-of-life care discussions among patients with advanced cancer: a cohort study. Ann Intern Med. 2012;156(3):204–10.
19. Clayton JM, Hancock K, Parker S, Butow PN, Walder S, Carrick S, et al. Sustaining hope when communicating with terminally ill patients and their families: a systematic review. Psychooncology. 2008;17(7):641–59.
20. Emanuel EJ, Fairclough DL, Wolfe P, Emanuel LL. Talking with terminally ill patients and their caregivers about death, dying, and bereavement: is it stressful? Is it helpful? Arch Intern Med. 2004;164(18):1999–2004.
21. Temel JS, Greer JA, Muzikansky A, Gallagher ER, Admane S, Jackson VA, et al. Early palliative care for patients with metastatic non-small-cell lung cancer. N Engl J Med. 2010;363(8):733–42.
22. Silveira MJ, Kim SY, Langa KM. Advance directives and outcomes of surrogate decision making before death. N Engl J Med. 2010;362(13):1211–8.
23. Mack JW, Joffe S. Communicating about prognosis: ethical responsibilities of pediatricians and parents. Pediatrics. 2014;133(Suppl 1):S24–30.
24. Mack JW, Weeks JC, Wright AA, Block SD, Prigerson HG. End-of-life discussions, goal attainment, and distress at the end of life: predictors and outcomes of receipt of care consistent with preferences. J Clin Oncol. 2010;28(7):1203–8.
25. Dow LA, Matsuyama RK, Ramakrishnan V, Kuhn L, Lamont EB, Lyckholm L, et al. Paradoxes in advance care planning: the complex relationship of oncology patients, their physicians, and advance medical directives. J Clin Oncol. 2010;28(2):299–304.
26. Parker SM, Clayton JM, Hancock K, Walder S, Butow PN, Carrick S, et al. A systematic review of prognostic/end-of-life communication with adults in the advanced stages of a life-limiting illness: patient/caregiver preferences for the content, style, and timing of information. J Pain Symptom Manag. 2007;34(1):81–93.
27. Orkin J, Beaune L, Moore C, Weiser N, Arje D, Rapoport A, et al. Toward an understanding of advance care planning in children with medical complexity. Pediatrics. 2020;145(3):e20192241.
28. Hinds PS, Kelly KP. Helping parents make and survive end of life decisions for their seriously ill child. Nurs Clin N Am. 2010;45(3):465–74.
29. Mack JW, Wolfe J, Cook EF, Grier HE, Cleary PD, Weeks JC. Hope and prognostic disclosure. J Clin Oncol. 2007;25(35):5636–42.
30. Meyer EC, Burns JP, Griffith JL, Truog RD. Parental perspectives on end-of-life care in the pediatric intensive care unit. Crit Care Med. 2002;30(1):226–31.
31. Quill TE. Perspectives on care at the close of life. Initiating end-of-life discussions with seriously ill patients: addressing the "elephant in the room". JAMA. 2000;284(19):2502–7.
32. Back AL, Arnold RM. Discussing prognosis: "how much do you want to know?" talking to patients who do not want information or who are ambivalent. J Clin Oncol. 2006;24(25):4214–7.
33. van Vliet LM, Epstein AS. Current state of the art and science of patient-clinician communication in progressive disease: patients' need to know and need to feel known. J Clin Oncol. 2014;32(31):3474–8.
34. Levetown M, American Academy of Pediatrics Committee on B. Communicating with children and families: from everyday interactions to skill in conveying distressing information. Pediatrics. 2008;121(5):e1441–60.

35. Baile WF, Buckman R, Lenzi R, Glober G, Beale EA, Kudelka AP. SPIKES-A six-step protocol for delivering bad news: application to the patient with cancer. Oncologist. 2000;5(4):302–11.
36. Back AL, Arnold RM. Discussing prognosis: "how much do you want to know?" talking to patients who are prepared for explicit information. J Clin Oncol. 2006;24(25):4209–13.
37. Campbell TC, Carey EC, Jackson VA, Saraiya B, Yang HB, Back AL, et al. Discussing prognosis: balancing hope and realism. Cancer J. 2010;16(5):461–6.
38. Svarovsky T. Having difficult conversations: the advanced practitioner's role. J Adv Pract Oncol. 2013;4(1):47–52.
39. Back AL, Arnold RM, Baile WF, Tulsky JA, Fryer-Edwards K. Approaching difficult communication tasks in oncology. CA Cancer J Clin. 2005;55(3):164–77.
40. Butow PN, Brown RF, Cogar S, Tattersall MH, Dunn SM. Oncologists' reactions to cancer patients' verbal cues. Psychooncology. 2002;11(1):47–58.
41. Pollak KI, Arnold RM, Jeffreys AS, Alexander SC, Olsen MK, Abernethy AP, et al. Oncologist communication about emotion during visits with patients with advanced cancer. J Clin Oncol. 2007;25(36):5748–52.
42. Fogarty LA, Curbow BA, Wingard JR, McDonnell K, Somerfield MR. Can 40 s of compassion reduce patient anxiety? J Clin Oncol. 1999;17(1):371–9.
43. Sep MS, van Osch M, van Vliet LM, Smets EM, Bensing JM. The power of clinicians' affective communication: how reassurance about non-abandonment can reduce patients' physiological arousal and increase information recall in bad news consultations. An experimental study using analogue patients. Patient Educ Couns. 2014;95(1):45–52.
44. Jansen J, van Weert JC, de Groot J, van Dulmen S, Heeren TJ, Bensing JM. Emotional and informational patient cues: the impact of nurses' responses on recall. Patient Educ Couns. 2010;79(2):218–24.
45. Back AL, Arnold RM. "Yes it's sad, but what should I do?" moving from empathy to action in discussing goals of care. J Palliat Med. 2014;17(2):141–4.
46. Jacobsen J, Blinderman C, Alexander Cole C, Jackson V. "I'd Recommend ..." How to incorporate your recommendation into shared decision making for patients with serious illness. J Pain Symptom Manag. 2018;55(4):1224–30.
47. Michelson KN, Emanuel L, Carter A, Brinkman P, Clayman ML, Frader J. Pediatric intensive care unit family conferences: one mode of communication for discussing end-of-life care decisions. Pediatr Crit Care Med. 2011;12(6):e336–43.
48. Cahill PJ, Lobb EA, Sanderson C, Phillips JL. What is the evidence for conducting palliative care family meetings? A systematic review. Palliat Med. 2017;31(3):197–211.
49. Carson SS, Cox CE, Wallenstein S, Hanson LC, Danis M, Tulsky JA, et al. Effect of palliative care-led meetings for families of patients with chronic critical illness: a randomized clinical trial. JAMA. 2016;316(1):51–62.
50. White DB, Angus DC, Shields AM, Buddadhumaruk P, Pidro C, Paner C, et al. A randomized trial of a family-support intervention in intensive care units. N Engl J Med. 2018;378(25):2365–75.
51. Hudson P, Thomas T, Quinn K, Aranda S. Family meetings in palliative care: are they effective? Palliat Med. 2009;23(2):150–7.
52. Curtis JR, White DB. Practical guidance for evidence-based ICU family conferences. Chest. 2008;134(4):835–43.
53. Lilly CM, De Meo DL, Sonna LA, Haley KJ, Massaro AF, Wallace RF, et al. An intensive communication intervention for the critically ill. Am J Med. 2000;109(6):469–75.
54. Lautrette A, Ciroldi M, Ksibi H, Azoulay E. End-of-life family conferences: rooted in the evidence. Crit Care Med. 2006;34(11 Suppl):S364–72.
55. October TW, Dizon ZB, Arnold RM, Rosenberg AR. Characteristics of physician empathetic statements during pediatric intensive care conferences with family members: a qualitative study. JAMA Netw Open. 2018;1(3):e180351.

# Decision-Making Involvement Throughout the Illness Trajectory

# 10

Maura A. Miglioretti, Emily M. Fredericks, and Melissa K. Cousino

## Introduction

In recent decades, there has been a strong movement toward including children and adolescents in decisions about their health. In 1995, the American Academy of Pediatrics (AAP) [1] updated their policy on informed consent to state that pediatric patients should participate in decision-making at a level commensurate with their development. Various terms have been used to describe this shift in practice to involve youth in healthcare decision-making, including "shared decision making," "collaborative decision making," and "decision-making involvement." For the purposes of this text, the term decision-making involvement will be used to describe the practice of including pediatric patients in decisions about their health care. Decision-making involvement is a relational approach that focuses on strategies that adults, including caregivers and health care clinicians, can use to support a pediatric patient's involvement in decision-making throughout their developmental and illness trajectories [2]. Policy statements and practice guidelines released by the AAP acknowledge that pediatric patient perspectives and experiences are critical to enhancing health outcomes and improving trust in the healthcare system [3, 4].

The extent to which clinicians should solicit the involvement of pediatric patients in decision-making throughout their illness course is dependent on an array of factors, including (a) individual patient factors such as developmental level, (b) family-systems factors, and (c) disease-specific factors. As pediatric clinicians, we focus here on outlining the various factors to consider when including pediatric patients in care decisions and provides suggestions for soliciting appropriate levels of involvement for individual patients. However, we also believe that many of the assessments and approaches in the care of pediatric patients also have direct implications in the care of adult patients. Therefore, we also discuss what can be learned from our experience in decision-making involvement with children with hematologic malignancies (HM) and how this approach can be applied to the care of adults with HM.

## Role of the Pediatric Patient in Decision-Making

Decision-making involvement encompasses a wide range of behaviors, from very low-stakes decisions (e.g., which arm to use for blood draw) to high-stakes decisions (e.g., DNR wishes) [5–7]. Decision-making involvement also includes passive participation in care, such as adult solicitation of the child's preferences, questions, or concerns, and adult provision of information [5]. Critical to decision-making involvement is the heavy emphasis on collaboration between all parties (i.e., children, caregivers, and clinicians) to come to a joint decision. This process is one which appreciates the developmental nature of decision-making, and emphasizes that while children seek to be involved in their care, they tend to feel that making decisions independently of their caregivers and clinicians is somewhat burdensome [8, 9].

### Factors Influencing Patient Decision-Making

Cognitive development and psychosocial development can influence decision-making and communication skills. As it pertains to healthcare decision-making for children and adolescents, developmental level is particularly important to consider when aiming to promote individual autonomy while simultaneously reducing risk of harm. Bluebond-Langner

M. A. Miglioretti · M. K. Cousino (✉)
Department of Pediatrics, C.S. Mott Children's Hospital, Ann Arbor, MI, USA
e-mail: melcousi@med.umich.edu

E. M. Fredericks
Department of Pediatrics, C.S. Mott Children's Hospital, University of Michigan Medical School, Ann Arbor, MI, USA
e-mail: emfred@med.umich.edu


C. K. Ullrich, E. J. Roeland (eds.), *Palliative Care in Hematologic Malignancies and Serious Blood Disorders*,
https://doi.org/10.1007/978-3-031-38058-7_10

**Table 10.1** Key components of stages of development

| Age | Key components of developmental stage |
|---|---|
| Baby | • Based in trust<br>• Reliance on caregiver as source of comfort<br>• Reliance on routine |
| Toddler and preschool | • Forming symbolic relationships<br>• Developing sense of personal control<br>• Uses literal language<br>• Reliance on routine |
| School-age | • More logical, less egocentric<br>• Concrete thinking<br>• Beginning to make decisions and assert themselves<br>• Asks many questions<br>• Struggles to make inferences<br>• Developing problem solving skills and abstraction |
| Adolescent | • Have fully developed abstract thinking ability<br>• Can problem solve, make sense of information and draw inferences<br>• Engages in risk taking behavior<br>• Seeks control |
| Emerging adult | • Capable of abstract thinking and problem solving<br>• View themselves as autonomous<br>• Continuing to develop a sense of identity<br>• Engages in risk taking behavior<br>• Self-management skills are highly dependent on social context |

Modified from Refs. [11, 12]

and colleagues [10] explain that age and stage of development should be considered when involving children in care decisions, though not exclusively. Cognitive development follows a predictable trajectory for most individuals (Table 10.1). Chronological age can be used as a starting point for determining the appropriate level of involvement in healthcare decisions, however, individual differences in neurodevelopment, personal preferences, experience, health status, and family values are also likely to play an important role in determining appropriate decision-making involvement. Research suggests that involving youth in decision-making can facilitate self-efficacy, promote adherence, enhance coping, and provide the necessary foundational skills to eventually shift responsibility for health-management tasks to the individual patient as they approach adulthood [13–15]. Some recommendations for including pediatric patients in decision-making based on developmental level are outlined in Table 10.2.

Children's decision-making abilities are likewise dependent on the opinions and attitudes of others due to their susceptibility to social influence [21]. Susceptibility to social influence, particularly that of caregivers, is developmentally appropriate for children and should also be a consideration for adults when assessing decision-making skills. The AAP [3] acknowledges this susceptibility in stating that it would be inappropriate to expect children and adolescents to make decisions autonomously, nor would it be appropriate to

**Table 10.2** Decision-making by age and developmental level

| Age | Decision-making abilities | Suggestions for decision-making Involvement |
|---|---|---|
| Baby | • Expresses likes, dislikes, wants through eye contact and movement | • Verbally respond to child's indicators of like/dislike<br>• Be attentive to eye gaze and movements toward/away from stimuli |
| Toddler and preschool | • Can express likes and dislikes<br>• Can express desires, wants, needs to some extent | • Use forced-choice questions<br>• Be sure to only offer choice when choice can be honored<br>• Ask questions directly to child about symptoms |
| School-age | • Can engage in problem solving, though may not be logical<br>• Can express desires, wants, needs, concerns<br>• Likely to have questions and fears that influence their decisions | • Same as above<br>• Talk directly to the child using age-appropriate language<br>• Assess preferences for information and involvement<br>• Permit choice in low-stakes care decisions |
| Adolescent | • Difficulty making decisions in emotionally charged situations<br>• Decisions may be more focused on short-term outcomes | • Talk directly to child<br>• Assess preferences for information and involvement<br>• Ensure child has opportunity talk with clinicians independently<br>• Continue use of forced-choice for non-negotiable aspects of care<br>• If able, can involve adolescents in more high-stakes decisions if this is in line with family and patient values |
| Emerging adult | • Legally capable of making decisions independently<br>• Financially and socially independent individuals are likely most autonomous<br>• Benefit from older adult involvement | • Individual patient preferences, values, and wishes must be respected (assuming competence)<br>• Involvement of older adults in decision-making should be encouraged<br>• Care should be taken to not inadvertently suggest that the patient is child-like |

Modified from Refs. [2, 5, 10, 11, 16–20]

require patients to participate voluntarily in all aspects of care. Parental involvement is the norm for younger patients, but for older adolescents who seek more control or who are preparing for transition to adult care, increasing levels of independence are desired. It is important to note that while adolescents may have the cognitive skills necessary to make decisions, in general they consider the balance of cost and benefit to a lesser degree than adults do, and may not fully consider the risks associated with a particular decision [22]. Parental influence is appropriate, to some extent, throughout all of childhood and adolescence.

## Capacity, Competence, and Assent

In pediatrics, consent for medical treatment must be given by the guardian because of the notion that those under the age of 18 are not capable of understanding and making medical decisions; in other words, they lack the *capacity* to make such decisions [23]. Despite this lack of legal capacity, children and adolescents are able to *assent* to treatment and make decisions about their care in a way that reflects their development. Previous research has shown that children as young as 9 years of age can meaningfully participate in health-related decision-making [24]. Determining an appropriate level of involvement requires an assessment of individual patient competence, either formally or informally, with consideration of both social and cognitive factors such as those outlined above. For adults, clinicians should carefully consider the social and developmental skills of their patients when determining how to best facilitate understanding of medical information to build the skills necessary for competent decision-making. When in doubt, we recommend that providers consult with colleagues in specialties such as psychology and ethics when there are concerns for a patients ability to make informed choices.

Clinicians are encouraged to obtain assent from patients when the patient has the skills necessary to do so. When seeking to obtain assent, the AAP [3] recommends that the following be considered: (a) the patient should be helped to acquire a developmentally appropriate understanding of their condition, (b) the patient should know what to expect with tests and treatment, (c) the clinician should assess for the patient's understanding and be mindful of factors influencing assent, such as pressure from others, and (d) and the patient's expressed desire to accept the care plan should be solicited. Even when children lack decision-making skills to assent to treatment, they can make decisions about how to receive treatment in the most comfortable way.

There is a lack of consensus on the assessment of capacity and competence in youth. There is a need for institutional-level guidelines for determining individual decision-making capacity in pediatrics. We and other research recommend assessing individual patient competence using interview style questions, standardized measures, or vignettes [25]. When assessing competence of either children or adults informally in an interview format, we recommend taking 4 pillars of competence into consideration. These include (a) understanding of information, (b) ability to appreciate the potential outcomes of the given situation based on the information received, (c) the ability to reason (consider costs and benefits), and (d) the ability to express or communicate a choice [26]. Recommendations for clinical application of these pillars of competence in decision-making involvement are provided in Table 10.3. Decision-making involvement is more a question of *how* children can participate in their care,

**Table 10.3** Application of the 4 pillars of competency decision-making involvement in pediatrics

| | Understanding | Appreciation | Reasoning | Expression of choice |
|---|---|---|---|---|
| Ask | • What part of your body is affected?<br>• What are your doctors doing to help?<br>• What will happen when you get (surgery, chemotherapy, etc.)? | • What might happen to you because of (disease)?<br>• Why do you need to (take this medicine, get this surgery etc.)?<br>• What could happen if you do not do what the doctors ask? | • What things do you want the adults taking care of you to know?<br>• Is there anyone else you think we should include in this conversation?<br>• What led you to make this decision? | • Do you want your medicine now or in 5 min?<br>• How much do you want to know about what is happening?<br>• How do you want to be involved in this decision?<br>• What do you think is the best decision for you? |
| Assess | • General intellectual abilities<br>• Language skills<br>• Health literacy | • Ability to understand options<br>• Ability to recognize potential outcomes | • Outside influence<br>• Mental health concerns<br>Patient and family values | • Preferences for involvement<br>• Patient and family values |
| Measures/ tools | • Refer to neuro-psychological or psycho-educational testing<br>• Health literacy measures (REALM-SF, REALM-TeenS) [27]<br>• Utilize ask-tell-ask and teach-back | • Motivational interviewing<br>• Refer back to measures<br>• Tools used to assess knowledge | • Motivational interviewing<br>• Ottawa personal decision-making tool [28]<br>• Psychology<br>• Psychiatry evaluation<br>• Social work evaluation | • MyCHATT [29]<br>• Voicing my Choices [30]<br>• My Wishes [31] |

Inclusive of Refs. [26–34]

rather than *if* they can participate in their care [35]. Even when a child is not competent to make a treatment decision, there are a variety of ways in which children can be passively involved in their care.

### Guardianship and Surrogate Decision-Making

Neurodevelopmental differences can require increased levels of caregiver involvement beyond what is expected given chronological age for both children and adults. Patients with differences in cognitive abilities, expressive/receptive language skills, social-emotional skills, and/or executive functioning skills may require more oversight than others their age. Specifically for emerging adult patients, neurodevelopmental differences may require that parents or caregivers obtain legal guardianship granting them the ability to act as the surrogate decision maker on the patient's behalf. Typically, the guardianship process involves the caregiver petitioning the court, an evaluation of the individual patient's capacity (typically completed by a psychologist or psychiatrist, depending on state law), and a hearing in a local court. Guardianship can be temporary/time limited and pertaining to a specific decision, or permanent encompassing all decisions to be made now and in the future. When the medical team has questions about the need for guardianship, they should seek consultation from psychosocial clinicians and legal experts for guidance.

### Disease Characteristics

As experience often helps to develop competence in decision-making, children with chronic illness or other personal experience with illness may have better developed insight and understanding than others their age in terms of their medical decision-making skills [10]. When newly diagnosed, children generally have limited understanding of their condition and treatment options, as information is entirely new to them, and they likely have had no prior experience with acute or chronic illness. Skills in medical decision-making are developed in most individuals over time following exposure to hospitals, medical staff, procedures, and treatments. They are strengthened after patients have gained experience in receiving information about their condition, asking questions, and being permitted to make choices [36]. As children become more accustomed to accessing healthcare, they gain experience in navigating their condition, health-management tasks, and the healthcare system as a whole. Some become well-informed and eventual "experts" in their own care [37].

## Patient Decision-Making Preferences

In addition to developmental level, a young person's preferences for decision-making involvement are important to understand. It is highly recommended that the level of individual participation in health care decisions be based on the individual child's situation and preferences [7, 38]. It may be helpful to obtain information from patients and families/caregivers about how they prefer difficult information to be shared and how involved a patient and family feels that the child should be in their own care. Information can be gathered in an interview with the patient and caregiver, or through published measures of communication preferences such as MyCHATT [29] and the SDM-Q-9 [39].

Overall, research suggest that children want to be informed about their care, even when there is difficult news to share [40, 41]. Children and adolescents have reported that they feel more valued when involved in discussions with clinicians [42] and that they are able to report their feelings than their caregivers [43]. Pediatric patients tend to feel better prepared for procedures and feel less scared when they are able to understand what is going on [43]. Adolescents tend to prefer that physicians use a direct communication style and communicate with them directly instead of with their caregivers [44]. Many adolescents want to be able to voice their preferences and choose how they receive their treatments [45]. Even when discussing end of life (EOL) and advance care planning (ACP), pediatric patients have a preference for involvement [46, 47].

While research shows that children and adolescents are capable of understanding complex decisions and the potential impacts on themselves and others [48], many children acknowledge that they cannot make health care choices completely independently and still value the input of their caregivers [49]. In a recent study [41], patients and their caregivers alike reported that patients often sought information and advice from their caregivers. Likewise, adolescents reported having a strong preference for family involvement at the EOL [41]; when decision-making involvement at the EOL is facilitated, there is a higher degree of concordance between patients and their caregivers [50]. Other research on decision-making involvement shows that patients generally report a preference for their physicians leading decision-making or for the decisions to be shared between the patient and the clinician [51, 52]. This information can be used to soothe families who believe that their children are unable to make decisions on their own, or those who believe that pediatric patients will unwisely make care decisions independently of adults.

## Role of the Caregiver in Decision-Making

Historically, caregivers have been the primary focus during interactions with pediatric clinicians [53]. Caregivers are often the primary source of information, particularly for infants and toddlers who are unable to contribute to discussions with clinicians in the same way as older children and adults. As a child ages and is able to participate meaningfully with clinicians during appointments, the shift toward including children in decisions may feel uncomfortable for families [49]. Thus, part of the decision-making involvement process is addressing these concerns and helping caregivers to understand the collaborative nature of the process as well as the benefits of decision-making involvement for the patient. Caregiver preferences and concerns about decision-making involvement are outlined below.

## Caregiver Decision-Making Preferences

Parents or caregivers are ideally situated to help children, adolescents, and young adults navigate decision-making while taking into consideration the individual child's preferences, goals, and values. For adults, the value placed in the opinions of loved ones when making decisions is variable and should be considered on a case-by-case basis. With children, caregivers have reported that they feel they are best situated to determine when and how a child should be involved in decision-making [49]. Caregivers tend toward desiring that their child's physician talk first with the family about medical information, which permits the family to screen information that the child should receive [43, 54]. This tendency toward protectiveness seems to decrease with prolonged illness or severe illness, with caregivers of chronically or severely ill children becoming stronger advocates for their child's needs, rights, and wishes over time [43, 48, 55]. Caregivers may prefer to exclude children from conversations at the EOL in an attempt to protect their children from harm despite the fact that communicating with children about death and dying can actually reduce psychological harm to the child [56]. When caregivers do talk to their children about the EOL, they do not tend to regret it [57]. On the whole, most caregivers want their children to be involved to some degree, with caregivers placing increased value on their child's opinion and role as illness or disease progresses toward the EOL [49].

## Caregiver Interference and Discordant Beliefs

As children age, young people and their caregivers may have different values and beliefs about care decisions. Clinicians should be mindful of caregiver interference, which is cited frequently within the medical decision-making literature and is a known barrier to decision-making involvement [53, 58–60]. Caregivers may restrict communication between the clinician and the child because of a desire to protect the child from experiencing distress and to retain hope [49]. The desire to reduce distress may also impact caregiver understanding or medical information and alter willingness to ask questions of clinicians [54].

Careful consideration of individual patient/family values and beliefs is warranted in these situations. By understanding individual factors contributing to discordance, clinicians can work to find common ground with patients and families/caregivers and can them move forward together toward a mutually agreed upon goal. Sometimes, simple communication between children and their caregivers about health care decision-making can be effective. Likewise, the benefits of shared decision-making can be discussed with hesitant families. Decision-making involvement can lead to increased self-efficacy [15], perceptions of control and competence on behalf of the patient [61], improved rates of adherence [13, 62, 63], improved coping [64], increased visit satisfaction [65], and can lead to pediatric patients feeling more valued [42]. Families can likewise be reassured that children will only be permitted to make developmentally appropriate decisions; providing families with examples of developmentally appropriate decisions may aid in a transition toward a more inclusive decision-making process.

However, there are times when communicating openly with a family and focusing on relationship building does not help to resolve discordance. Consultation with psychosocial clinicians such as psychologists, social workers, and ethicists is highly recommended in these cases, particularly when decisions made by families to exclude their children from decision-making could potentially cause harm to the patient. For adolescent patients in particular, sometimes caregivers are unable to recognize their child's capacity to understand and participate in their care. While children under the legal age of consent are generally considered unable to make decisions on their own behalf, in certain instances, adolescent patients may be deemed legally competent to make individual decisions by a court of law.

## Role of the Clinician

Clinicians should also be mindful of their own beliefs regarding decision-making involvement, as these beliefs can influence the ways in which they communicate with children and adolescents. Some clinicians may believe that youth lack the capacity to make decisions [55]. Some may expect that pediatric patients simply prefer not to be involved and thereby limit their attempts to engage the patient in conversations about their care [53]. Additional barriers to including children in their health care decisions have long been cited in the literature to include time constraints, fear of having their opinions challenged, lack of consistent methods for which to include children, difficulty in assessing capacity, challenges with developmentally appropriate language, and conflict with caregivers related to their protective tendencies [41, 43, 66–68]. Regardless of personal opinions and beliefs, it is the role of the clinician to facilitate decision-making involvement in order to promote optimal social, emotional, and health outcomes for children and families.

## Facilitating Pediatric Patient Involvement in Decision-Making

During the course of any medical encounter, clinicians can facilitate involvement by asking children questions directly and soliciting the child's own questions and concerns; communication can be as simple as greeting the child first during the encounter, and asking them who is accompanying them to their appointment. Simple gestures like this can set a precedent in medical visits that children are encouraged to participate in their care, and that they are the focus of the medical visit. Research shows that involvement early in developmental and disease trajectory sets the expectation that children are stakeholders in their medical care, and prepares the stage for increased participation over time [69].

Once a precedent is set with a family that children will be involved in some capacity, formal conversations about decision-making involvement can proceed. It can be helpful to first ask the child about their preferences for involvement in the presence of their caregivers so that caregivers are made aware of the child's feelings. Oftentimes, this conversation between caregiver, child, and clinician can help all parties to be on the same page. If the caregiver and child have different preferences for decision-making involvement, the clinician can privately discuss options with the caregiver for how to include children in decision-making in a way that aligns with the family's values.

When facilitating pediatric involvement in decision-making, use of structured clinical tools such as The Ottawa Personal Decision Guide [28] or the Shared Decision Making Questionnaire (SDM-Q-9) [39] could be useful. The AAP [4] recommends the following, based on the SDM-Q-9 [39]: acknowledge that there is a decision to be made, identify stakeholders and form partnerships, present all treatment options without bias with attention to the risk and benefit of each, inquire about the patient and family's understanding of the situation, inquire about preferences and priorities of all stakeholders, facilitate negotiation between parties, come to a decision upon which to act (review this decision again at later date). Similar styled interview questions and considerations apply to adult populations as well and could be a useful clinical tool. Strategies to aid in holding discussions with families, such as the "Ask-Tell-Ask" method [32] and the "Teach Back" [33] method are also recommended by the AAP [4].

## Treatment-Related Decision-Making and the Appropriate Use of Choice

Providing patients with choice can occur across a continuum, taking individual factors into account. Age and stage of development is a starting point for consideration, yet as noted previously, should not be the only factors considered when determining the appropriate use of choice in health care decisions. In line with AAP [4] guidelines, children should always be told when they have a choice in doing something, and when offered a choice, their choice should always be respected. Considering this, choice should not be offered if the child's decision cannot or will not be honored. For example, do not ask a child or patient, "Can I give you your medicine now?" if a "no" answer is unacceptable. Instead, ask a child or patient, "Do you want your medication now or in 5 minutes?" Adolescents with higher-level decision-making skills may be able to participate in some higher stakes decisions with the input of their caregivers and clinicians, such as whether to participate in a clinical trial. The AAP outlines methods for having conversations such as the "options talk," "choice talk," and "decision talk" with patients in detail in their clinical report *Shared-Decision Making and Children with Disabilities: Pathways to Consensus* [4].

The onus remains on caregivers and clinicians alike to create an environment in which the pediatric patient is able to make use of their developing decision-making skills and to use these skills appropriately over time [70]. Clinicians should be mindful of what tasks and decisions are appropriate for a patient based on their individual capacity, noting that adverse outcomes, such as declines in adherence [71–74], can occur if a child is expected to take on too much, too soon.

## End-of-Life Decision-Making Involvement

Decision-making at the EOL and ACP in pediatrics has been identified as having a critical need for improvement [75]. Pediatric patients have a preference for involvement in EOL discussions, yet these discussions occur rather infrequently [41, 47]. This lack of decision-making involvement is likely related to barriers such as clinician discomfort, caregiver preferences to withhold information in an effort to protect their child, and concerns about reducing hope [41, 46].

It is the responsibility of the clinician to engage patients and their families/caregivers about discussions surrounding communication preferences and goals of care as noted previously in this chapter. When communicating with patients and families about diagnoses, prognoses, and goals of care, clinicians should specifically ask the patients and caregivers what they already understand and what they want to know about their or their child's illness [76, 77]. This recommendation extends tangentially to communication with children and adolescents; pediatric patients often know or understand more than their caregivers believe [78]. Without knowing what children know and understand about their illness, caregivers and clinicians may be unable to appropriately answer questions, correct misconceptions, and soothe worries. Likewise, clinicians should offer information and check for understanding once information has been provided, taking care to also respond to expressed emotions regarding diagnosis and prognosis. Some children may need time to process the information they have received and may appear disinterested or distracted during conversation; clinicians are cautioned against assuming that this indicates a lack of desire for involvement. Preferences should frequently be revisited, particularly as changes in care occur. Doing so protects children and families/caregivers from having unexpected conversations about decision-making during high-stress times [16, 46].

Conversations with patients and families about EOL decisions should be honest and direct, yet compassionate with particular attention to the developmental appropriateness of the material [46]. Various guidelines for discussing EOL decision-making have been put forth elsewhere and should be referenced [16, 46, 79–81]. There are also semi-structured interview tools designed to help facilitate these conversations, such as *This is My World* [82], *Voicing My Choices* [30], *My Wishes* [31], and *My CHATT* [29]. Further guidance for facilitating EOL conversations with pediatric patients is offered elsewhere [11, 80].

## Conclusions

### Caring for Patients with Hematologic Malignancies

While the literature reviewed in this chapter spans various pediatric and adult chronic illness groups, caring for patients with pediatric hematologic malignancies offers many opportunities to foster decision-making involvement throughout the illness trajectory. At diagnosis, even when treatment is heavily protocolized, decision-making involvement can include inclusion of pediatric patients in diagnostic, prognositic, and treatment planning conversations to the extent that is appropriate for the child's level of development and preferences, which often includes psychosoical experts such as child life specialists and psychologists. Involvement at the initiation of treatment can include education about how treatment is administered and soliciting the child's input on how they can be comforted during difficult aspects of care. Decisions related to various oncologic research studies at diagnosis and throughout the illness course can be approached with the skills and strategies outlined in above sections. At relapse or when complications arise, decisions specific to end of life are likely to become more relevant, yet, many patients and families may also welcome these decision-making discussions during earlier periods of good health or positive prognostic outlook. From which finger to have a pulse oximeter placed, whether to allow hair to fall out gradually or get a haircut, or to the placement of DNR orders a thoughtful approach to decision-making involvement is of utmost important throughout the pediatric hematologic malignancy course.

## Summary

Despite literature recommending involving children in their health care decisions, decision-making involvement remains challenging for patients, caregivers, and clinicians alike. Much of the difficulty in decision-making involvement for caregivers and clinicians seems to pertain to fears of burdening children with information and decisions that they are not developmentally ready for. Largely this fear is unfounded, as decision-making involvement can occur along a continuum where patient developmental level, decision-making experience, preferences, and values can be taken into consideration along with the preferences and values of the patient's primary caregivers. Pediatric patients themselves have a desire for involvement [40, 42, 44–47, 50], and this involvement is supported by the AAP [1, 3, 4].

In order for pediatric decision-making involvement to occur, clinicians must be well-educated about barriers to decision-making involvement, methods for facilitating decision-making involvement, and equipped to trouble shoot when discordance between patient, caregiver, and clinician inevitably surface. Patient and caregiver preferences should be solicited early in the diagnostic and treatment process and should continue to be revisited periodically throughout the illness course. Pediatric patients of all ages can be involved in health care communication and decision-making to some degree, and mutual goals of communication or care can be established between patients, caregivers, and clinicians in an effort to form an alliance between all stakeholders. Developmentally appropriate language, consideration of individual contextual factors, and the appropriate use of choice, and assent are critical to this process. A multitude of clinical tools are available to guide clinicians in this process, and it is highly recommended that clinicians rely on or consult these tools in guiding their practice.

## References


1. Committee on Bioethics AA of P. Informed consent, parental permission, and assent in pediatric practice. Pediatrics. 1995;95(2):314.
2. Miller VA. Involving youth with a chronic illness in decision-making: highlighting the role of providers. Pediatrics. 2018;142(Supplement 3):S142–8. https://doi.org/10.1542/peds.2018-0516D.
3. Katz AL, Webb SA. Informed consent in decision-making in pediatric practice. Pediatrics. 2016;138(2):e20161485. https://doi.org/10.1542/peds.2016-1485.
4. Adams RC, Levy SE. Shared decision-making and children with disabilities: pathways to consensus. Pediatrics. 2017;139(6):e20170956. https://doi.org/10.1542/peds.2017-0956.
5. Miller VA, Harris D. Measuring children's decision-making involvement regarding chronic illness management. J Pediatr Psychol. 2012;37(3):292–306. https://doi.org/10.1093/jpepsy/jsr097.
6. Alderson P. Competent children? Minors' consent to health care treatment and research. Soc Sci Med. 2007;65(11):2272–83.
7. Treseder P. Empowering children and young people: training manual: promoting involvement in decision making. London: Save the Children; 1997.
8. Lipstein EA, Muething KA, Dodds CM, Britto MT. "I'm the one taking it": adolescent participation in chronic disease treatment decisions. J Adolesc Health. 2013;53(2):253–9.
9. Miller VA. Parent–child collaborative decision making for the management of chronic illness: a qualitative analysis. Fam Syst Health. 2009;27(3):249–66. https://doi.org/10.1037/a0017308.
10. Bluebond-Langner M, Belasco JB, DeMesquita WM. "I want to live, until I don't want to live anymore": involving children with life-threatening and life-shortening illnesses in decision making about care and treatment. Nurs Clin N Am. 2010;45(3):329–43.
11. Hammes B, Briggs L. Building a systems approach to advance care planning. La Crosse: Gundersen Lutheran Medical Foundation, Inc.; 2011.
12. Erikson E. Identity: youth and crisis. New York: Norton & Co.; 1968.
13. Miller VA, Jawad AF. Relationship of youth involvement in diabetes-related decisions to treatment adherence. J Clin Psychol Med Settings. 2014;21(2):183–9. https://doi.org/10.1007/s10880-014-9388-1.
14. Monaghan M, Hilliard M, Sweenie R, Riekert K. Transition readiness in adolescents and emerging adults with diabetes: the role of patient-provider communication. Curr Diabetes Rep. 2013;13(6):900–8. https://doi.org/10.1007/s11892-013-0420-x.
15. White FA. Parent-adolescent communication and adolescent decision-making*. J Fam Stud. 1996;2(1):41–56. https://doi.org/10.5172/jfs.2.1.41.
16. Wiener L, Zadeh S, Wexler LH, Pao M. When silence is not golden: engaging adolescents and young adults in discussions around end-of-life care choices. Pediatr Blood Cancer. 2013;60(5):715–8. https://doi.org/10.1002/pbc.24490.
17. Arnett JJ. Emerging adulthood: a theory of development from the late teens through the twenties. Am Psychol. 2000;55(5):469–80. https://doi.org/10.1037/0003-066X.55.5.469.
18. Miller VA, Cousino MK. The role of children and adolescents in decision making about life-threatening illness. Oxford: Oxford University Press; 2021.
19. Rosenblum KL, Dayton CJ, Muzik M. Infant social and emotional development: emerging competence in a relational context. In: Zeannah Jr CH, editor. Handbook of infant mental health. 3rd ed. New York: The Guilford Press; 2009. p. 80–103.
20. Vern-Gross T. Establishing communication within the field of pediatric oncology: a palliative care approach. Curr Probl Cancer. 2011;35(6):337–50.
21. Mårtenson EK, Fägerskiöld AM. A review of children's decision-making competence in health care. J Clin Nurs. 2008;17(23):3131–41. https://doi.org/10.1111/j.1365-2702.2006.01920.x.
22. Halpern-Felsher BL, Millstein SG, Ellen JM, Adler NE, Tschann JM, Biehl M. The role of behavioral experience in judging risks. Health Psychol. 2001;20(2):120–6. https://doi.org/10.1037/0278-6133.20.2.120.
23. Melton G. Decision making by children: psychological risks and benefits. In: Melton GB, Koocher GP, Saks MJ, editors. Children's competence to consent. New York: Plenum Press; 1983. p. 21–40.
24. Weithorn LA, Campbell SB. The competency of children and adolescents to make informed treatment decisions. Child Dev. 1982;53(6):1589.
25. Miller VA, Drotar D, Kodish E. Children's competence for assent and consent: a review of empirical findings. Ethics Behav. 2004;14(3):255–95. https://doi.org/10.1207/s15327019eb1403_3.
26. Grisso T, Appelbaum PS. Assessing competence to consent to treatment: a guide for physicians and other health professionals. New York: Oxford University Press; 1998.
27. Manganello JA, Colvin KF, Chisolm DJ, Arnold C, Hancock J, Davis T. Validation of the rapid estimate for adolescent literacy in medicine short form (REALM-TeenS). Pediatrics. 2017;139(5):e20163286. https://doi.org/10.1542/peds.2016-3286.
28. Ottawa Health Research Institute. Ottawa Personal Decision Guide. 2015. https://decisionaid.ohri.ca/docs/das/OPDG.pdf.
29. Cousino MK, Rea KE, Mednick LM. Understanding the healthcare communication needs of pediatric patients through the my CHATT tool: a pilot study. J Commun Healthc. 2017;10(1):16–21. https://doi.org/10.1080/17538068.2017.1278637.
30. Aging With Dignity. Voicing my choices. Tallahassee: Aging With Dignity; 2012.
31. Aging With Dignity. My wishes. Tallahassee: Aging With Dignity; 2015.
32. Institute for Healthcare Improvement. What Is "Ask, Tell, Ask"? http://www.ihi.org/education/IHIOpenSchool/resources/Pages/AudioandVideo/ConnieDavis-WhatIsAskTellAsk.aspx.
33. Always Use Teach-back! [Training toolkit]. http://www.teachback-training.org. Accessed 24 Apr 2020.
34. Arozullah AM, Yarnold PR, Bennett CL, Soltysik RC, Wolf MS, Ferreira RM, et al. Development and validation of a short-form, rapid estimate of adult literacy in medicine. Med Care. 2007;45(11):1026–33.
35. Ruhe KM, Wangmo T, Badarau DO, Elger BS, Niggli F. Decision-making capacity of children and adolescents—suggestions for advancing the concept's implementation in pediatric healthcare. Eur J Pediatr. 2015;174(6):775–82. https://doi.org/10.1007/s00431-014-2462-8.
36. Holaday B, Lamontagne L, Marciel J. Vygotsky's zone of proximal development: implications for nurse assistance of children's learning. Issues Compr Pediatr Nurs. 1994;17(1):15–27. https://doi.org/10.3109/01460869409078285.
37. Alderson P, Sutcliffe K, Curtis K. Children's competence to consent to medical treatment. Hast Cent Rep. 2006;36(6):25–34. http://muse.jhu.edu/content/crossref/journals/hastings_center_report/v036/36.6alderson.pdf
38. Coyne I, Gallagher P. Participation in communication and decision-making: children and young people's experiences in a hospital setting. J Clin Nurs. 2011;20(15–16):2334–43. https://doi.org/10.1111/j.1365-2702.2010.03582.x.
39. Kriston L, Scholl I, Hölzel L, Simon D, Loh A, Härter M. The 9-item shared decision making questionnaire (SDM-Q-9). Development and psychometric properties in a primary care sample. Patient Educ Couns. 2010;80(1):94–9.
40. Dunsmore J, Quine S. Information, support, and decision-making needs and preferences of adolescents with cancer. J

Psychosoc Oncol. 1996;13(4):39–56. https://doi.org/10.1300/J077V13N04_03.

41. Cousino MK, Schumacher KR, Magee JC, Wolfe J, Yu S, Eder SJ, et al. Communication about prognosis and end-of-life in pediatric organ failure and transplantation. Pediatr Transplant. 2019;23(3):13373. https://doi.org/10.1111/petr.13373.
42. Angst DB, Deatrick JA. Involvement in health care decisions: parents and children with chronic illness. J Fam Nurs. 1996;2(2):174–94. https://doi.org/10.1177/107484079600200205.
43. Kilkelly U, Donnelly M. The child's right to be heard in the healthcare setting: perspectives of children. Dublin: Parents and Health Professionals; 2006.
44. Britto MT, Slap GB, DeVellis RF, Hornung RW, Atherton HD, Knopf JM, et al. Specialists understanding of the health care preferences of chronically ill adolescents. J Adolesc Health. 2007;40(4):334–41.
45. Coyne I, Amory A, Kiernan G, Gibson F. Children's participation in shared decision-making: children, adolescents, parents and healthcare professionals' perspectives and experiences. Eur J Oncol Nurs. 2014;18(3):273–80.
46. Rosenberg AR, Wolfe J, Wiener L, Lyon M, Feudtner C. Ethics, emotions, and the skills of talking about progressing disease with terminally ill adolescents. JAMA Pediatr. 2016;170(12):1216. https://doi.org/10.1001/jamapediatrics.2016.2142.
47. Cousino MK, Miller VA, Smith C, Uzark K, Lowery R, Rottach N, et al. Medical and end-of-life decision making in adolescents' pre-heart transplant: a descriptive pilot study. Palliat Med. 2020;34(3):272–80. https://doi.org/10.1177/0269216319874689.
48. Hinds PS, Schum L, Baker JN, Wolfe J. Key factors affecting dying children and their families. J Palliat Med. 2005;8(supplement 1):s-70–8. https://doi.org/10.1089/jpm.2005.8.s-70.
49. Wangmo T, De Clercq E, Ruhe KM, Beck-Popovic M, Rischewski J, Angst R, et al. Better to know than to imagine: including children in their health care. AJOB Empir Bioeth. 2017;8(1):11–20. https://doi.org/10.1080/23294515.2016.1207724.
50. Jacobs S, Perez J, Cheng YI, Sill A, Wang J, Lyon ME. Adolescent end of life preferences and congruence with their parents' preferences: results of a survey of adolescents with cancer. Pediatr Blood Cancer. 2015;62(4):710–4. https://doi.org/10.1002/pbc.25358.
51. Britto M, Cote M, Horning R, Slap G. Do adolescents with chronic illness want to make decisions about their treatment. J Adolesc Health. 2004;34(2):120.
52. Knopf JM, Hornung RW, Slap GB, DeVellis RF, Britto MT. Views of treatment decision making from adolescents with chronic illnesses and their parents: a pilot study. Health Expect. 2008;11(4):343–54. https://doi.org/10.1111/j.1369-7625.2008.00508.x.
53. van Staa A. Unraveling triadic communication in hospital consultations with adolescents with chronic conditions: the added value of mixed methods research. Patient Educ Couns. 2011;82(3):455–64.
54. Young B, Ward J, Salmon P, Gravenhorst K, Hill J, Eden T. Parents' experiences of their children's presence in discussions with physicians about leukemia. Pediatrics. 2011;127(5):e1230–8. https://doi.org/10.1542/peds.2010-2402.
55. de Vries MC, Bresters D, Kaspers GJL, Houtlosser M, Wit JM, Engberts DP, et al. What constitutes the best interest of a child? Views of parents, children, and physicians in a pediatric oncology setting. AJOB Prim Res. 2013;4(2):1–10. https://doi.org/10.1080/21507716.2012.757254.
56. Hilden JM, Watterson J, Chrastek J, Anderson PM. Tell the children. J Clin Oncol. 2000;18(17):3193–5. https://doi.org/10.1200/JCO.2000.18.17.3193.
57. Kreicbergs U, Valdimarsdóttir U, Onelöv E, Henter J-I, Steineck G. Talking about death with children who have severe malignant disease. N Engl J Med. 2004;351(12):1175–86. https://doi.org/10.1056/NEJMoa040366.
58. Beresford BA, Sloper P. Chronically ill adolescents' experiences of communicating with doctors: a qualitative study. J Adolesc Health. 2003;33(3):172–9.
59. Tates K, Meeuwesen L, Elbers E, Bensing J. "I've come for his throat": roles and identities in doctor-parent-child communication. Child Care Health Dev. 2002;28(1):109–16. https://doi.org/10.1046/j.1365-2214.2002.00248.x.
60. Savage E, Callery P. Clinic consultations with children and parents on the dietary management of cystic fibrosis. Soc Sci Med. 2007;64(2):363–74.
61. Croom A, Wiebe DJ, Berg CA, Lindsay R, Donaldson D, Foster C, et al. Adolescent and parent perceptions of patient-centered communication while managing type 1 diabetes. J Pediatr Psychol. 2011;36(2):206–15. https://doi.org/10.1093/jpepsy/jsq072.
62. Kyngäs H, Hentinen M, Barlow JH. Adolescents' perceptions of physicians, nurses, parents and friends: help or hindrance in compliance with diabetes self-care? J Adv Nurs. 1998;27(4):760–9. https://doi.org/10.1046/j.1365-2648.1998.00608.x.
63. Kyngas H, Rissanen M. Support as a crucial predictor of good compliance of adolescents with a chronic disease. J Clin Nurs. 2001;10(6):767–74. https://doi.org/10.1046/j.1365-2702.2001.00538.x.
64. Drotar D, Crawford P, Bonner M. Collaborative decision-making and promoting treatment adherence in pediatric chronic illness. In: Patient intelligence. Taylor & Francis; 2010. http://www.dovepress.com/collaborative-decision-making-and-promoting-treatment-adherence-in-ped-peer-reviewed-article-PI.
65. Freed LH, Ellen JM, Irwin CE, Millstein SG. Determinants of adolescents' satisfaction with health care providers and intentions to keep follow-up appointments. J Adolesc Health. 1998;22(6):475–9.
66. Coyne I. Children's participation in consultations and decision-making at health service level: a review of the literature. Int J Nurs Stud. 2008;45(11):1682–9.
67. Runeson I, Enskar K, Elander G, Hermeren G. Professionals' perceptions of children's participation in decision making in healthcare. J Clin Nurs. 2001;10(1):70–8. https://doi.org/10.1046/j.1365-2702.2001.00433.x.
68. Never MJ. Too young: how young children can take responsibility and make decisions: a handbook for early years workers. National Early Years Network; 1997.
69. Edwards A, Elwyn G. Inside the black box of shared decision making: distinguishing between the process of involvement and who makes the decision. Health Expect. 2006;9(4):307–20. https://doi.org/10.1111/j.1369-7625.2006.00401.x.
70. Ruhe KM, De Clercq E, Wangmo T, Elger BS. Relational capacity: broadening the notion of decision-making capacity in paediatric healthcare. J Bioeth Inq. 2016;13(4):515–24. https://doi.org/10.1007/s11673-016-9735-z.
71. Bender B, Milgrom H, Rand C, Ackerson L. Psychological factors associated with medication nonadherence in asthmatic children. J Asthma. 1998;35(4):347–53. https://doi.org/10.3109/02770909809075667.
72. Kovacs M, Obrosky DS, Goldston D, Drash A. Major depressive disorder in youths with IDDM: a controlled prospective study of course and outcome. Diabetes Care. 1997;20(1):45–51. https://doi.org/10.2337/diacare.20.1.45.
73. Ricker JH, Delamater AM, Hsu J. Correlates of regimen adherence in cystic fibrosis. J Clin Psychol Med Settings. 1998;5(2):159–72.
74. Silva K, Miller VA. The role of cognitive and psychosocial maturity in type 1 diabetes management. J Adolesc Health. 2019;64(5):622–30.
75. Institute of Medicine. Dying in America. Washington, DC: National Academic Press; 2015. http://www.nap.edu/catalog/18748

76. Masera G, Chesler MA, Jankovic M, Ablin AR, Ben Arush MW, Breatnach F, et al. SIOP working committee on psychosocial issues in pediatric oncology: guidelines for communication of the diagnosis. Med Pediatr Oncol. 1997;28(5):382–5. https://doi.org/10.1002/(sici)1096-911x(199705)28:5<382::aid-mpo12>3.0.co;2-d.
77. Baile WF, Buckman R, Lenzi R, Glober G, Beale EA, Kudelka AP. SPIKES—A six-step protocol for delivering bad news: application to the patient with cancer. Oncologist. 2000;5(4):302–11. https://doi.org/10.1634/theoncologist.5-4-302.
78. Bluebond-Langner M. The private words of dying children. Princeton: Princeton University Press; 1980.
79. Blazin L, Cecchini C, Habashy C, Kaye E, Baker J. Communicating effectively in pediatric cancer care: translating evidence into practice. Children. 2018;5(3):40.
80. Zadeh S, Pao M, Wiener L. Opening end-of-life discussions: how to introduce voicing my CHOiCESTM, an advance care planning guide for adolescents and young adults. Palliat Support Care. 2015;13(3):591–9.
81. Sisk BA, Bluebond-Langner M, Wiener L, Mack J, Wolfe J. Prognostic disclosures to children: a historical perspective. Pediatrics. 2016;138(3):e20161278. https://doi.org/10.1542/peds.2016-1278.
82. Zadeh S, Wiener L. This is my world. 2nd ed. Bethesda: National Institute of Health; 2011.

# Advance Care Planning in Hematologic Malignancies and Other Serious Blood Disorders

# 11

Vinay Rao and Dana Guyer

**Case**

Ms. W is a 42-year-old woman with a remote history of post-partum depression who presented to her primary care physician with progressive fatigue over 2 months and a 1-week history of shortness of breath. Her primary care physician did a thorough history and physical examination and noted pallor and a few ecchymoses. The physician ordered blood work that revealed leukocytosis (white blood cell count 88,000), anemia (hemoglobin 7.2 g/dL), and thrombocytopenia (platelets 55,000). The physician called Ms. W with the results, and she presented urgently to the tertiary care hospital. She was admitted to the hematology service, and after a thorough work-up, she was diagnosed with acute myeloid leukemia (AML). Ms. W was treated with induction chemotherapy and tolerated the treatment thus far. What is the role of advance care planning with Ms. W?

## Definitions of Advance Care Planning

Advance care planning (ACP) is the process of exploring a person's goals and values for future medical care and communicating these goals and values to caregivers and clinicians. ACP is a process, not an isolated event, and can occur before diagnosis and throughout an illness. Despite its importance, most healthy people have done little to no ACP. Moreover, many healthy young people have a sense of invincibility, and without exposure to serious illness, they spend little time considering what future problems may occur. Some people will have designated a surrogate decision-maker or completed a durable power of attorney for health care (dPOA-h), but most healthy individuals have not engaged in any meaningful ACP beyond designating a proxy. There has been a nationwide effort to engage people in ACP with The Conversation Project and other similar organizations. Yet, the percentage of those with any ACP at diagnosis remains low [1]. Therefore, when a serious illness is diagnosed, having ACP conversations is critical.

ACP encompasses many different types of planning, but there are four important aspects to all ACP: (1) considering goals and values, (2) learning about the illness and associated prognosis, (3) making medical decisions, and (4) communicating those decisions. The first critical part of ACP is for a patient to consider personal values and what matters most during the course of the illness. Certain people value life prolongation above all other things, whereas other people care more about the quality of life (QOL), maintaining independence, and/or not becoming burdensome to family members. Patients want and deserve autonomy in healthcare, and the physician's paternalistic role has become less prominent. However, there is a balance between what a person desires and what is medically reasonable. ACP affords an opportunity to align an individual's goals and desire for autonomy with medical reality.

When a person receives a diagnosis of serious illness, the second and third components of ACP become important and available. The second component includes learning about the specific care related to the illness and what potential decisions may be required. Every disease has unique characteristics that may inform what kind of planning is needed. For example, when a person is diagnosed with chronic kidney disease, a nuanced discussion regarding dialysis should

V. Rao (✉)
Division of Palliative Medicine, Yale University School of Medicine, New Haven, CT, USA
e-mail: vinay.rao@yale.edu

D. Guyer
Division of Palliative Medicine, Warren Alpert Medical School of Brown University, Providence, RI, USA
e-mail: dguyer@hopehealthco.org


C. K. Ullrich, E. J. Roeland (eds.), *Palliative Care in Hematologic Malignancies and Serious Blood Disorders*,
https://doi.org/10.1007/978-3-031-38058-7_11

occur. However, that discussion would be less important for someone with esophageal cancer, with whom discussing feeding tubes and artificial nutrition is much more salient. When a person is diagnosed with a high-risk hematologic malignancy (HM), the person should work with the health-care team to learn about the disease and prognosis, the expected course, and what decisions may lie ahead.

The third component of ACP involves making decisions about the type of care a person would choose in certain situations. When faced with similar situations, every person reacts differently because every person has different values. The third component integrates the first two components. When people know what matters most to them and know about their disease and the decisions they may face, they can formulate their own opinions about the care they would choose in certain medical situations. Consider the example of Ms. W from the case. Suppose Ms. W cares most about her teenage son's development and future when cardiopulmonary arrest is discussed as a potential complication during transplant and cellular therapies. In that case, she may decide to undergo cardiopulmonary resuscitation (CPR) and intubation so that she has every remote possibility to see him graduate from high school. ACP allows individuals to express how they would react and how they want their caregivers and clinicians to react when faced with certain medical situations.

The fourth aspect of ACP is communicating the goals, values, and decisions a person has made to an individual's caregiver network, including family, friends, and clinicians. This aspect is most critical because, if not completed, it has the potential to negate all the other important work that a person has done. Consider a scenario in which a person has made extensive decisions about the kind of care she prefers but has not told anyone about it or completed a document with those wishes. If that person becomes unable to make her own decisions, the surrogate decision-maker will not know what decisions to make, and the person may not be treated in the way she envisioned. The communication of one's wishes can be done orally or in writing and will be discussed in further detail below.

ACP should not be an isolated event, and the previously described four steps of meaningful ACP—considering goals and values, learning about the illness, making medical decisions, and communicating those decisions—can and should be repeated as often as needed when changes occur in the patient's disease or frame of mind.

## Benefits of Advance Care Planning

ACP promotes patient autonomy by giving patients control over the type of care they hope to receive in the future and under certain circumstances. Being proactive rather than reactive can prevent needless suffering or unwanted care. These conversations are crucial for the patient and the selected proxy. When a person is no longer able to make his own medical decisions, proxies must decide whether life-sustaining treatments make sense for that person. These proxies can face significant emotional, psychological, and social burdens during this process. There are times when proxies experience guilt when deciding to forgo certain treatments for the patient. Proxies may experience disagreement with other family members or other caregivers, leading to distress for everyone involved. When people discuss their EOL care preferences with their selected proxies ahead of time, the proxy's role becomes communicating those decisions rather than making them and effectively unburdens them of decisional guilt.

HMs add a significant layer of complexity to ACP, given the unpredictable nature of these diseases. Prognosis within each disease varies widely based on tumor genetics, and an individual patient's outcome can simultaneously range from cure to death. Compared to solid tumors, HMs tend to involve younger patients who may not have previously considered future care preferences. These factors make ACP both more challenging and more crucial. This is especially true in patients undergoing high-risk treatments, such as hemopoietic cell transplantation (HCT) or chimeric antigen receptor T-cell (CAR T-cell) therapy, resulting in loss of decisional capacity at some point during treatment. The distinction between solid tumors and HMs is important to highlight. A person with advanced pancreatic cancer at diagnosis has never been offered the possibility of cure. This situation may lead the person to be more conscious of the stepwise decline in health, have a better understanding of prognosis, and the possibility of being more prepared to share EOL care preferences with the healthcare team and his proxy. In contrast, a person with a high-risk HM, such as Ms. W in the case above, may be focused on getting better with the possibility of cure and thus less likely to consider and share her EOL care preferences. Unfortunately, Ms. W could become sick very quickly at any point in her illness and may not have enough time to consider and share her EOL care preferences thoughtfully. The moments to engage in meaningful ACP after a patient with a HM becomes seriously ill are often fleeting. Consequently, ACP in HMs is as crucial as in solid tumor malignancies, even when treatment intent is curative.

Studies on ACP benefits in patients with HMs often use completion of ADs and resuscitation status documentation as surrogate markers for ACP because the frequency, quality, and depth of ACP conversations are difficult to measure. These studies have shown that the frequency of AD completion in patients with HMs in different settings was approximately 50% [2–6].

Research also suggests that ACP reduces the use of intensive and unwanted interventions at the EOL. In patients undergoing allogeneic HCT at a single center institution, patients with completed ADs had less intensive care unit (ICU) and mechanical ventilation utilization [2]. These results suggest that ACP conversations lead to better disease understanding and decreased desire for intensive and invasive measures in critically ill patients.

## Barriers to Advance Care Planning

While the benefits of ACP are well recognized, there are many barriers to these conversations and the completion of ADs. Talking about EOL care, dying, and death can be hard for numerous reasons related to the individual patient, the individual clinician, and the practical challenges of the situation.

Common patient factors that serve as barriers to ACP include age, race, culture/ethnicity, religion, and socioeconomic status. Younger patients are less likely to have considered future health outcomes and EOL care preferences; they may believe they will remain healthy and do not need to worry about getting sick or dying [7]. Race and ethnicity also play a role in ACP; black and Hispanic older Americans are less likely to have completed ADs than white Americans [8]. These populations are more likely to receive life-sustaining treatments despite poor prognoses. There are many known and unknown reasons why minority populations receive more intensive EOL care. Religion and personal faith also influence ACP for a variety of reasons. Some people believe that a miracle can prevent death, and that negativity, which they may equate with ACP, could interfere with that miracle. Low socioeconomic status also affects access to care and healthcare outcomes, such as the use of intensive life-sustaining treatments [9]. Lack of education and health literacy can serve as barriers to an accurate understanding of prognosis and treatment options, leading to misalignment with goals and care received.

Clinicians have a wide variety of opinions on ACP as patients. A clinician's difficulty with prognostic uncertainty and desire to protect patients' psychological well-being can serve as barriers to ACP [10]. Prognostication is always challenging; usually, clinicians overestimate prognosis and believe their patients are healthier than they are [11–13]. This overestimation can give clinicians the false impression that they can wait until their patients show signs of health deterioration before having ACP conversations. Clinicians' fear of taking away hope and/or causing psychological and emotional distress to patients is another barrier to ACP, despite limited evidence to support such concerns [3, 5, 7, 10, 14]. A clinician's comfort level and experience in having these conversations can also impede ACP. Communication skills for ACP are seldom taught in formal medical training, and improving these skills takes time and practice. Health system barriers include the limited time available to spend with each patient and language barriers to effective ACP communication.

Personal experience, beliefs, and values affect a clinician's views on mortality and influence her or his ability and desire to engage in ACP conversations. The following factors influence clinician engagement in these conversations: identification with the patient, personal loss, fear of death and disability, personal mental health, and difficulty tolerating uncertainty [15]. Clinicians should have self-awareness of their own emotions and risk factors for excessive emotional engagement or disengagement with their patients' experiences. They should make time for personal reflection and consider discussing how they feel with other colleagues, their interdisciplinary team, and personal support systems. Recognizing these individual barriers is the first step to overcoming them.

Logistical barriers prevent many people from engaging in ACP and completing AD forms. Access to appropriate forms can be limited; patients and clinicians may not know how to access these forms, and the forms may not be available in their preferred language. Clinicians may not be able to provide an adequate explanation about how to complete these forms. Patients may not know what the purpose of each form is. They may not understand the language/wording used in the document and/or may not know how to translate their preferences from a conversation to the form. Additionally, patients may have limited access to a public notary or two non-medical witnesses. They also may have difficulty distributing these forms to the appropriate places (e.g., hospital electronic medical records, other clinician clinics, and/or other family members' homes). There are also financial and logistical barriers to ACP. Access to the necessary resources used to complete ADs and engage in meaningful ACP discussions may be limited.

HMs present unique challenges to ACP. Differences in patient populations, attitudes/beliefs of patients and clinicians, and prognostic uncertainty are a few of the barriers to these conversations [16]. In general, high-risk HMs affect younger patients with fewer medical comorbidities than solid tumors. Many young patients struggle to accept and adapt to a cancer diagnosis more so than older patients who have had more time and life experience to accept their current health condition. These patients are more likely to have children and young families who depend on them financially, emotionally, and logistically. Considering death and dying is so foreign to most 30-year-olds that it may feel impossible.

Like the general population, some patients with HMs believe they are not sick enough to engage in ACP. In the case of Ms. W, although she presented in a critical condition, because she is now tolerating treatment and has the potential for cure, she may be less inclined to consider rapid health deterioration at this moment. She may not be aware that future treatment toxicity or disease relapse could significantly limit her life expectancy. She may also think that since she has only had the diagnosis for a few weeks, ACP does not apply to her. This lack of awareness could prevent her from engaging in ACP.

Another patient barrier is the belief that health outcomes occur due to chance or accidental happenings and that people have little control over their situation [3]. For example, when a clinician tries to engage a patient in ACP but also states that prognosis is difficult to predict, the patient may say, "I could also get struck by lightning or get run over by a bus," as a reason for avoiding the conversation. Unfortunately, this type of thinking assumes that death is instantaneous, and until the moment of death, most people live well. In contrast, patients with HMs can experience significant physical and psychological symptom burden at the EOL and are more likely to spend their last days in the hospital [17]. ACP can give patients more control over their situation as their EOL draws near.

The chance for cure in HMs is higher compared to advanced solid tumor malignancies. As a result, hematologists/oncologists may recommend more intensive disease-directed treatments compared to solid tumor oncologists. They may also assume that patients have the same goal of cure and may not recommend ACP. Clinicians may believe that ACP conversations decrease patient hope and raise doubt about the healthcare team's commitment to doing "everything" possible to provide a cure. Data from patients undergoing HCT show that discussing mortality risk did not decrease hope or perceptions of clinician commitment [7]. Some clinicians believe their role is to "fight" for their patients rather than prepare them for all potential poor outcomes, including death [10]. Reassuring their patients, providing motivation, staying positive, and re-inspiring confidence after disease recurrence takes precedence over ACP. Some clinicians even believe that these roles are not compatible with ACP. They fear that discussing death and dying will harm their patient's psychological well-being and result in worse survival outcomes, although empirical data to support these claims are limited.

Prognosis in HMs is challenging to predict due to fluctuations in deterioration and recovery of functional status. Sometimes, clinicians wait to initiate ACP conversations until a patient shows signs of clinical deterioration or a poor prognosis. Unfortunately, clinical deterioration in HMs could occur rapidly and without warning, and a patient's prognosis may not be obvious until the final hours and days of a patient's life. Conversely, the concept of "super-responders" can be an additional barrier to initiating these conversations. When clinicians, patients, and caregivers witness exceptionally positive patient cases, known as "super-responders," this anecdotal experience can skew expected outcomes and delay ACP conversations for all patients. Although ACP is appropriate for all individuals with HMs, the timing, frequency, and content of these conversations need to be tailored to each patient.

## Recommended Approach to ACP Discussions

When to have an ACP discussion with a patient is complex and can be a challenge to navigate. While having a resuscitation status discussion makes sense when a person is nearing EOL, the timing of other conversations may be less obvious. There are numerous opportunities throughout the trajectory of a person's illness with an HM to discuss ACP. One helpful way to consider when to encourage a patient and caregiver to engage in ACP is to recommend it during times of change. Any change in the disease process, any change in the treatment, any change in a patient's location, and any change in the patient's function should prompt clinicians to talk to patients about ACP.

The initial diagnosis of a high-risk HM is ideal for starting ACP conversations with patients and caregivers. This conversation can also serve as an anchor for future discussions and give the clinician a picture of the patient as a person with goals, values, and hopes surrounding life and the disease. A main topic for early conversations with patients is surrogate decision-makers and asking a patient, "who will best represent your voice if you become unable to speak for yourself?" Other important topics at or near diagnosis include initial conversations about prognosis and introduction of the concept of a time-limited trial. A time-limited trial depicts every treatment as something that is tried for a certain period before the efficacy of the treatment is re-evaluated. For example, six cycles of chemotherapy before a CT scan is a "time-limited trial" of chemotherapy. Preparing patients early on for this concept, that no medical treatment is indefinite, serves clinicians well in future conversations.

Hospitalization is an excellent time to have a significant conversation with patients and caregivers about one's goals and preferences for care. In addition to having more time to talk with their patients, clinicians can also evaluate how functional a person is during a hospitalization. Many hospitals have a standard protocol to discuss resuscitation status with every patient. While the resuscitation status of "full code" (the preference to receive CPR and mechanical ventilation) may be the appropriate code status for many patients with a potentially curable HM, there are also many patients who either would not choose CPR or mechanical ventilation or to whom these medical interventions would not be beneficial. Engaging in ACP at every admission allows patients to make these wishes known.

Another prime opportunity for an ACP discussion is at the start of a new treatment. When a patient's current treatment is not working, or there are unacceptable side effects to the treatment, she or he may switch to a different chemotherapy regimen or consider advanced therapies if eligible. In these situations, it is appropriate for a clinician to ask difficult questions about the future. The clinician can align with the patient to hope for a successful outcome, while reinforcing the possibility that treatment may be ineffective. Suppose a clinician feels that the next line of treatment has an incredibly low likelihood of meeting a patient's previously stated goals or is more likely to be burdensome than beneficial. In that case, she or he may choose not to offer treatment or make a recommendation against further disease-directed treatment. When a recommendation against certain treatments or procedures comes from the clinician, it alleviates some of the decisional burden on patients and caregivers. Unlike paternalism, this approach respects a patient's autonomy by aligning treatment decisions with the patient's goals and values.

The final opportunity for ACP is when a patient's clinical status worsens and death draws near. This deterioration is when a clinician should clearly explain to the patient and caregivers about the very limited prognosis. It is an opportunity to delineate a person's EOL care preferences and make recommendations about hospice care when it aligns with these preferences.

Figure 11.1 illustrates the appropriate times to initiate ACP conversations for an incurable illness such as an advanced solid tumor malignancy. In contrast, Fig. 11.2 shows when to initiate ACP conversations in HMs even when cure is a possibility. Discussing the concept of "hoping for the best-case scenario (cure) while preparing for other possibilities (when a person's disease progresses and/or when functional status decreases)" is crucial before and at the time of changing treatment. If cure is achieved, ACP should still be continued as some disease types may relapse. Figure 11.3 summarizes topics discussed at each stage of illness, and Fig. 11.4 gives examples of words and phrases that can be used for certain topics. Lastly, Table 11.1 provides a list of additional ACP resources.

In addition to HMs, ACP is imperative for patients with other blood disorders such as sickle cell disease (SCD). Compared to the general population, patients with SCD have lower life expectancies and encounter many disease-related challenges [18]. ACP discussions should happen early for these patients, even childhood, and throughout a patient's disease trajectory. Although parents of children with SCD often serve as surrogate decision-makers and make medical decisions based on the children's best interest, engaging children in the decision-making process and encouraging them to assent to medical interventions can promote disease and prognostic understanding and prepare them to make their own decisions when they become adults. Please refer to Chap. 9 for more details regarding decision-making involvement.

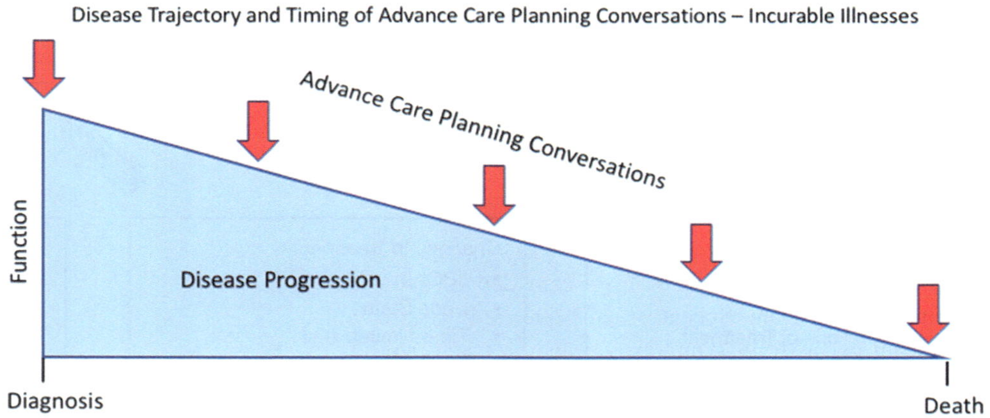


**Fig. 11.1** Disease trajectory and timing of ACP conversations in incurable illnesses. ACP conversations should occur at the time of diagnosis, at times of disease progression, and before the EOL

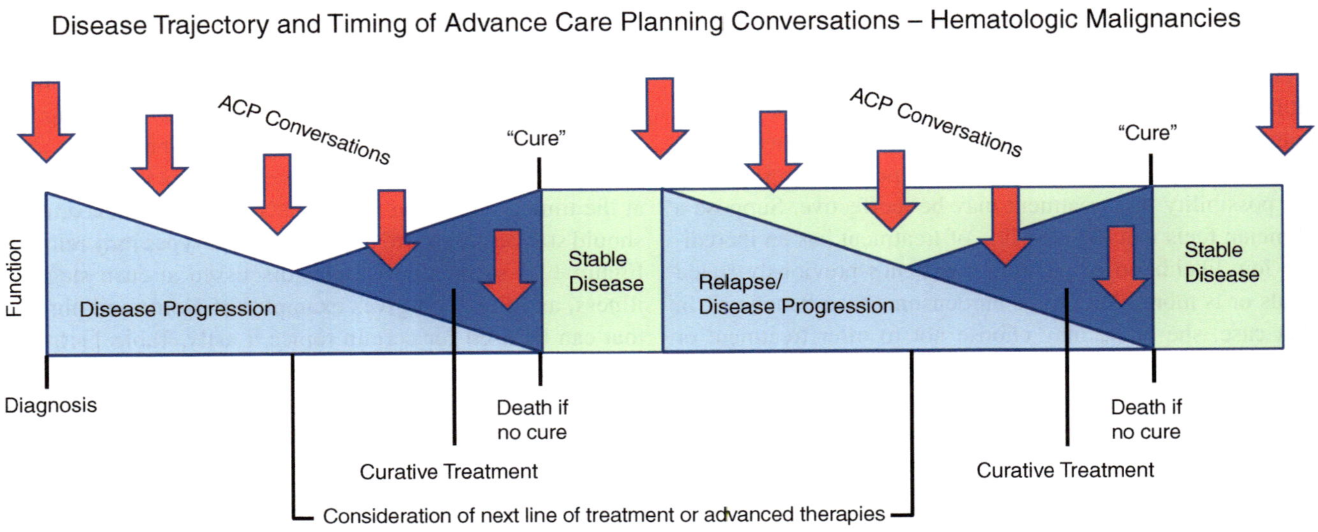


**Fig. 11.2** Disease trajectory and time of ACP conversations in high-risk HMs. Even with potentially curable diseases, ACP conversations should occur at the following time points: diagnosis, disease progression/functional decline, changes in treatments or consideration of advanced therapies, and near the EOL. Even if cure is achieved, ACP should continue as relapse may occur at any point for certain disease types

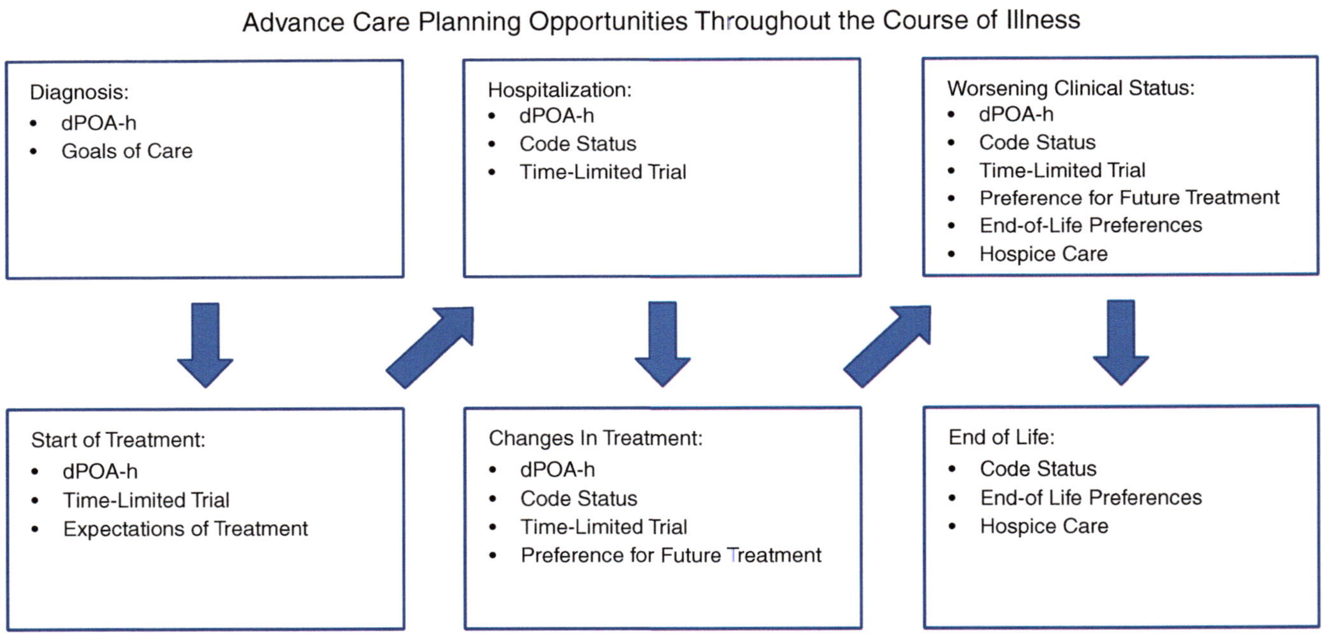


**Fig. 11.3** Opportunities for ACP along the illness continuum. At each stage of illness, certain topics can be discussed

**Fig. 11.4** Words that work when identifying a surrogate decision-maker, discussing code status, and discussing hospice

## Words that work for advance care planning conversations

### Identifying a surrogate decision maker

- If there comes a time when you can't make your own medical decisions, who would be the person you want to make them for you?
- Who do you lean on to help you make your medical decisions?
- If for some reason you can't speak or communicate with your doctors, who would the doctors speak with on your behalf?
- Is there someone who helps you make big decisions now?

### Code status discussion

- When your heart stops and you die, how do you want the doctors to treat you?
- Have you ever had thoughts about being on life support?
- What matters most to you at the end of life?
- How might we know when God thinks it's your time?

### Hospice discussion

- When it becomes clear that there are no more treatments that will help you live longer, what kind of medical care do you see for yourself?
- This is a difficult topic to discuss, but I am wondering if you have thought about where you would want to die.
- What are the things that matter most to you?
- My job is to make you comfortable so that God can decide what is next for you. Can we talk about what that might look like?

**Table 11.1** Advance care planning resources with websites and descriptions

| ACP resources | Website | Description |
|---|---|---|
| Five wishes | fivewishes.org | Living will that provides an approach to discussing and documenting care choices |
| Voicing my choices | fivewishes.org/Voicing-my-choices | Living will for adolescents and children to give them a voice in their own care and legacies |
| Serious illness conversation guide | https://www.ariadnelabs.org/areas-of-work/serious-illness-care/resources | A program for clinicians to give language and strategies to discuss goals, values and wishes |
| The conversation project | theconversationproject.org | A public engagement initiative to promote widespread discussion about expressing and respecting end-of-life care wishes |
| VitalTalk | vitaltalk.org | Training for clinicians to improve communication skills surrounding serious illnesses |
| Dying matters | dyingmatters.org | A card game that aims to increase discussion about end-of-life care preferences in an easy manner |
| Prepare for your care | prepareforyourcare.org | Website that is a step-by-step program with video stories to help patients understand and voice care choices |

## Communication About ACP

Discussing death and dying with patients can be uncomfortable. Clinicians have many worries about ACP conversations: the patient reaction, its impact on the patient's mood and spirits, the effect on the patient–clinician relationship, and the personal reaction of the clinician to the patient's emotions. This discomfort is normal; it shows the humanity of the clinician. Becoming comfortable with one's emotional discomfort is important; when a clinician can sit with her own emotions, she becomes better at sitting with the patient's emotions. Once a patient and clinician have overcome the barriers and recognize the benefits of ACP, they must find ways to communicate effectively. Having an ACP conversation can be difficult, and getting started is one of the most complex parts for many clinicians, but excellent communication strategies can make it easier.

A good starting place for a conversation is to ensure that the appropriate people are present and that the patient agrees to discuss planning for the future. This framework gives patients some control in a situation in which they may have very little control. In addition, it is helpful for the clinician to ask what the patient wants to know and not give too much or unwanted information. The clinician may introduce an ACP conversation this way: "Ms. W, is it an okay time to talk? I hope to talk with you about your leukemia and how we can help you plan. But before I begin, I want to get a sense of how you prefer to receive medical information. Do you want to know all the details, or do you prefer just the big picture?" This type of introduction elicits permission to start the conversation, lays out an agenda, and gets information on how patients want to receive information. Although many patients want to know medical and prognostic information, some patients prefer that their caregivers receive this information instead, especially within certain cultures. It is important to explore and document this. It is also important to consider approaching a patient who is reluctant to talk about her or his medical status and prognosis. A clinician should delve into the patient's particular worries about these topics. The responses to this question can give the clinician insight into the patient's knowledge and perceptions about her or his illness and can better guide effective communication.

After receiving permission to talk, asking patients what they know is a good next step. Patients hear things differently from what the clinicians say, and knowing a patient's true understanding at each ACP discussion is valuable and saves time. Simply asking, "Ms. W, tell me what you know about your leukemia," can provide a wealth of information, including disease understanding, health literacy, decisional capacity, and trust in the medical system.

Once a clinician has heard about the patient's understanding, another challenging part of an ACP conversation comes—the discussion of prognosis. Even a clinician who is comfortable answering the question, "How much time have I got, Doc?" may not be comfortable offering prognostic information if a patient does not ask. The desire for prognostic information varies among patients with HMs [11]. Many patients want to ask their clinicians about life expectancy, while others do not. Avoiding the topic of dying can worsen fear and anxiety. Exploring the best-case and worst-case scenarios gives patients a better understanding and some semblance of control in what a patient wants these outcomes to look like [19]. Even when exploring a limited life expectancy and death, patients provide valuable information about what is meaningful to them and what may bring them joy in times of sadness and uncertainty. For example, a clinician could say: "We've been talking about doing everything we can to cure you of this cancer. We are all hoping for you to get better, and this would certainly be the best-case scenario. At the same time, it is also my job to explore the worst-case scenario. If we find that your cancer is getting worse despite all treatments and you are reaching the EOL, what things would you find most important to you?"

When patients want to know their prognosis, being honest and upfront about prognostic uncertainty is essential [16]. Clinicians do not know everything, and that does not lessen their skill or expertise. Being honest and realistic about one's medical knowledge and its limitations can build trust in the patient–clinician relationship. It can also prevent patients from thinking that their healthcare team is withholding prognostic information from them or using an ACP conversation as a surrogate to sharing bad news. Here is one example of what could be said: "Ms. W, with this type of cancer, it is very difficult to know what your prognosis truly is. Some people improve with treatments, but others do not. Those who do well may see their cancer go away completely. Others may see a rapid decline in their health from either cancer or treatment toxicity." Not knowing what to expect can be difficult for patients and clinicians, but uncertainty should not be used as a reason to avoid the discussion. Acknowledging the uncertainty and the anxiety it causes allows clinicians to align with the patient: "This is scary. Most of us want to know what to expect. What you are feeling is normal. I would be feeling the same way right now."

A common reason clinicians cite for not engaging in ACP is that they do not want to take away a patient's hope or dampen the spirit of the patient and family [12]. Yet hope is dynamic and multidimensional. Over time, a patient's hope for cure and longevity may transition to hoping for other things such as spending time with family, having relief of symptoms, being at home, etc. This change is reflected in the concept of "regoaling," which suggests that when patients are confronted with changes in their condition, they may choose to disengage in their initial goals and reengage in a new set of goals that are more achievable and/or desirable [20]. Patients can simultaneously engage in ACP and still have hope; they are not mutually exclusive. Here is one way to communicate this concept to patients and families: "When our health declines and we reach the end of our lives, whether this is from cancer or something else, we can still have hope. Although we may no longer be hoping for a cure or trying to prolong time, we can still hope for different things. For example, we can hope for spending as much time with family, not being in pain, and being at home for as long as possible." It is always appropriate, helpful, and caring to ask a person, "what are you hoping for?" Acknowledge the response and then, regardless of the answer, the next appropriate question may be "what else are you hoping for?"

Some patients cope well with an EOL conversation, while others may find it challenging. Positive reframing is a technique that helps shift a person's perspective on a situation to a more positive perspective [21]. After allowing for patients to reflect and share their emotions, the clinician can positively reframe the conversation away from what the patient cannot control and toward what they still can control. One example of this is when poor prognostic information can help patients prioritize important things in life. Maybe this means spending more time with grandchildren, going to the beach, or doing things on one's "bucket list." This information can also help patients specify which medical interventions they would choose in the context of their life expectancy. Some may say, "If I only have 3 months to live, I don't want to undergo further disease-directed therapies." Here is an example of how to introduce positive reframing into a conversation: "Although we are not able to change how much time you have left in life, you may still have some say in what that time could look like. Our focus should be on how to help you live as well as possible for whatever time you have left."

Normalizing the ACP conversation can reduce patient anxiety and mistrust while allowing patients to open up during the discussion. These conversations should be standardized to all patients with high-risk HMs and ideally as part of the pre-transplant preparation process. If the conversation is not normalized, patients may worry that they are being singled out for having an exceptionally poor prognosis. Patients may ask, "Why are they having this conversation with *me*? Things must be really bad." Normalizing the conversation can also prevent patients from asking whether clinicians are withholding information. "Are my doctors hiding something from me? Why has no one talked to me about this before?" Instead, patients should know that these conversations are common and are being held with many other patients similar to themselves. This routine approach can be explained to patients as follows: "Any time a patient has a high-risk blood cancer like the one you have, we try to sit down and help you plan for possible future outcomes, both good and bad. We try to do this with all of our patients regardless of their life expectancy." When developing a plan of care, it is also important not to put the onus on the patient, but rather, the clinician should partner with the patient to develop this plan together. "We want to come up with a plan together so that we know how to best care for you if things don't turn out the way we hope." Likewise, clinicians should focus the plan of care on what will be done to promote the patient's goals as opposed to what will not be done. Both of these strategies can help the patient feel supported and seen.

Early referral to specialty palliative care (PC) at the time of diagnosis is important for patients who could potentially have a prognosis of less than 1 year, even when cure is still a possibility. Any clinician can conduct an ACP conversation. However, some patients may not want to discuss possibilities other than cure with their hematologist/oncologist. Having a different healthcare team member, such as a PC specialist, can provide more time and space to facilitate these conversations [22]. In fact, evidence shows that patients referred to specialized PC teams are more likely to receive direct communication about EOL care [23]. In such cases, the hematologist/oncologist can still provide hope for clinical improvement while the specialty PC clinician can help them prepare for the other possibilities. Communication between specialty PC and the hematology/oncology team is crucial to building trust between patients and the entire healthcare team. Topics such as estimated disease trajectory and prognosis, as well as roles and expectations for each clinician, should be discussed and agreed upon by all team members.

## Resuscitation Status Discussion

A cardiopulmonary arrest is a terminal event. Although there are instances where CPR and intubation may bring someone back to life to receive curative therapies, this is usually the exception to the rule. In general, patients with high-risk HMs do not survive cardiopulmonary arrest to return to a prior functional level. A population-level study of hospitalized patients who received HCT showed that CPR was associated with very high in-hospital mortality and low survival rates to discharge [24]. These statistics parallel the general population of hospitalized patients with all disease types. In addition to low survival rates, it is also important to consider a patient's functional status and QOL after surviving a cardiopulmonary arrest, which rarely recovers to what a patient was like prior to the arrest and may be much worse.

When a clinician presents options for resuscitation status, it is essential that the chances of surviving CPR and the chances of surviving successfully to hospital discharge are considered. When the chances of both are high, presenting CPR and intubation (full code) versus allowing a natural death (do not resuscitate and do not intubate, DNR/DNI) as two potential options is most appropriate. In contrast, when the chances of a meaningful recovery are low, clinicians need to make balanced recommendations based on the patient's clinical situation and her or his preferences for EOL care.

Resuscitation status should be discussed within a comprehensive ACP discussion that includes disease trajectory, prognosis, and the chances for a meaningful recovery after resuscitation, as well as exploration of a patient's goals and preferences for EOL care. This information will help the clinician formulate recommendations about resuscitation that are meaningful to the patient. In contrast, if resuscitation status is being discussed outside of the comprehensive ACP conversation, such as when admitting a patient to the hospital, patients may perceive full code and DNR/DNI as two items on a menu, each with similar value and consequences, which may not be the case as stated above. In such circumstances, patients may be forced to decide without being properly informed and without proper guidance (i.e., uninformed patient autonomy). This lack of guidance may lead to severe consequences such as receiving care inconsistent with their goals and values.

During a resuscitatgion status discussion, the words clinicians use should be clear and reflect the severity of cardiopulmonary arrest. Rather than saying "if your heart stops," one should say "when your heart stops and you die." A way to impart the difference in effect for CPR in someone who was electrocuted versus someone with a high-risk cancer is as follows: "When a person is young and healthy and has an accidental death, doing things like chest compressions, electric shocks, and putting people on breathing machines, may make sense if we can fix the underlying cause of the cardiopulmonary arrest. But when someone dies from a high-risk leukemia, the chances of dying are extremely high even despite these aggressive measures, because CPR does not fix the underlying cancer." CPR and advanced cardiac life support (ACLS) is not a solution if a high-risk cancer causes a patient's death.

The resuscitation status discussion should be documented directly in the electronic medical record. This documentation should include the date of the conversation, the people present, what was discussed, and the patient's preferences. If there is a question of a patient's decisional capacity, this should be documented prior to the documentation of the conversation with the proxy. If a patient or proxy chooses DNR/DNI, then a portable order for life-sustaining treatment (POLST) form or an inpatient DNR order form should also be completed (see below).

Discussing resuscitation status is a delicate process that should occur within a comprehensive ACP conversation. If the recommendation to a patient is to forgo CPR and intubation, this should be based on the patient's preferences for EOL care in the context of what is medically feasible, not based on the clinician's preferences alone.

## Written Advance Directives

ADs are documents that outline a patient's ACP. This is a general term that can apply to any document that provides information on a patient's plans for future medical care [25]. Patients who are healthy or ill can complete ADs with no standard requirement about what must be included. ADs are intended to help patients and caregivers plan for future health problems and provide an opportunity to be proactive about health care decisions rather than reactive during a medical crisis. There are different types of ADs that a patient can complete.

The first kind of AD is a healthcare power of attorney, sometimes called a Durable Power of Attorney for healthcare (dPOA-h) or healthcare proxy (HCP). This document legally designates a surrogate decision-maker who will help a patient make medical decisions or make decisions in the patient's stead if the patient becomes too ill to do so [26]. The dPOA-h is unrelated to the financial power of attorney, although the designated person can be the same for both documents. The dPOA-h only identifies the surrogate decision-maker. It does not specify a patient's health care preferences. Each state has different specifications for these documents, but most require either two witnesses, a notary, or both to make the document legal. Most states prohibit the designated health care agent from being a witness to the document, and many states prohibit members of the health-care team from witnessing the document to avoid any coercion or conflicts of interest [27]. Most dPOA-h forms have no expiration date but revisiting the document yearly is important in case a patient changes her or his mind about who she or he trusts to be her or his voice or if there are changes in the health of the assigned health care agent. The Department of Health website for each state has downloadable forms and specific requirements for completing dPOA-h documents.

The next type of AD is a living will. This type of document is broader than a dPOA-h and can also delineate a patient's wishes. Topics usually included in generic living wills are CPR, life support, intubation, and feeding tubes. Hemodialysis is sometimes discussed as well. Patients can create a living will with a lawyer or use a form document. Individually created living wills often have vague wording such as "if there is no reasonable chance of recovery…" and "life-sustaining measures" that provide only very general guidance. Form living wills often have a more detailed approach, outlining specific treatments and a patient's opinion about each one. There are many branded and state-specific combined documents that serve as both a dPOA-h and a living will. Table 11.1 provides more information about two specific living wills, Five Wishes and Voicing My Choices.

The final type of AD is a POLST. The POLST form is appropriate for patients who have a terminal illness and limit medical interventions at the EOL. In a medical emergency such as cardiopulmonary arrest, emergency medical service (EMS) clinicians need to respond quickly. Unlike other AD forms, the POLST form is a legally binding medical order that must be followed by all clinicians, including EMS. Each state has its state-specific document that often does not cross state lines. The POLST form is often printed on hot pink or bright green paper (state-specific) so that emergency medical service clinicians can easily locate it. Figure 11.5 is an example of a POLST form used by EMS clinicians when a patient undergoes cardiopulmonary arrest. This example form was derived from the National POLST Form [28].

When a patient desires full treatment, a POLST form is not necessary; the default is that EMS clinicians provide all interventions indicated to support cardiopulmonary function. In fact, there are instances when completing a POLST form and indicating full treatment could be detrimental to the patient and proxy. Take, for example, a patient who completes a POLST form and chooses full treatment when he has a low-risk disease. If his condition worsens in a way that makes full treatment medically inappropriate and the patient loses the capacity to change his decision, this leaves her proxy in a difficult situation. The proxy may have difficulty deciding between what is recommended by the clinicians and what was previously indicated by the patient on the form.

Some states have an electronic database for POLST forms, and many more are moving toward such a database. A POLST is intended to protect someone who does not want intensive medical interventions from receiving CPR and intubation. If a patient has a POLST form, but the document is not physically present during a crisis, the patient may receive such treatment instead of the desired comfort-focused care. For example, a patient may have a signed POLST indicating DNR/DNI hanging on the refrigerator at home. If she is at a restaurant and has a cardiopulmonary arrest, EMS clinicians will attempt resuscitation by default. If there were an electronic database, the EMS team could quickly check a patient's identification in the database and then provide the appropriate care based on the most up-to-date order.

Completing a POLST form with a patient should not be the start of a conversation but should occur as part of a conversation about EOL care preferences. After discussing CPR and intubation, the clinician can say, "based on our conversation, let's complete this document that will help us ensure that when you die, you can die naturally without CPR or being placed on a breathing machine." This approach is a more natural approach to the conversation. Patients are often leery of completing the POLST form without a clear understanding of why they are filling out the form and what each choice represents. Of note, while a living will or dPOA-h form can be completed by a patient on her or his own or with family, the clinician must be part of the conversation when completing a POLST form.

As a medical order, most state-specific documents require a signature of a physician or advance practice provider and a signature from the patient or surrogate decision-maker. However, in response to the COVID-19 pandemic, many states have allowed for flexibility as family members and caregivers have had limited physical access to the patient. New recommendations may allow for witnessed telephone conversations to serve in place of a surrogate decision-maker's physical signature.

Many clinicians have had this conversation with a patient: "Do you have an AD?" and the patient replies, "Yes, it's at my lawyer's office." "What does it say?" asks the clinician, and the patient replies, "I'm not sure." A document filed away in a lockbox or a lawyer's office is of little utility for a patient with active cancer. Patients should be encouraged to know what their documents outline. These documents are

## Example POLST Form

**Patient information.**

**A. Cardiopulmonary Resuscitation Orders** (If patient has no pulse and is not breathing).

| | |
|---|---|
| ☐ **YES CPR: Attempt Resuscitation, including mechanical ventilation, defibrillation and cardioversion** | ☐ **NO CPR: Do Not Attempt Resuscitation (allow natural death)** |

**B. Initial Treatment Orders** (if patient has a pulse and/or is breathing).

☐ **Full Treatments.** Goal: Attempt to sustain life by all medically effective means. Provide appropriate medical and surgical treatments as indicated to attempt to prolong life, including intensive care.

☐ **Selective Treatments.** Goal: Attempt to restore function while avoiding intensive care and resuscitation efforts (ventilator, defibrillation and cardioversion). May use non-invasive positive airway pressure, antibiotics and IV fluids as indicated. Avoid intensive care. Transfer to hospital if treatment needs cannot be met in current location.

☐ **Comfort-focused Treatments.** Goal: Maximize comfort through symptom management; allow natural death. Use oxygen, suction and manual treatment of airway obstruction as needed for comfort. Avoid treatments listed in full or select treatments unless consistent with comfort goal. Transfer to hospital **only** if comfort cannot be achieved in current setting.

**C. SIGNITURE: Patient or Patient Representative**

**D. SIGNATURE: Health Care Provider**

**Fig. 11.5** Example of a POLST form that emergency medical service clinicians could use for a person who undergoes cardiopulmonary arrest. This form was derived from the National POLST Form: Portable Medical Order [18]

meant to be available to the patient and clinician so that they can be easily accessed and understood in the event of an emergency or crisis.

Despite a person's best efforts to document her or his wishes, clinicians often find themselves in situations not covered by an AD. In these circumstances, clinicians should work with a patient's proxy to interpret the information from the AD and apply it to the situation at hand. This interpretation can be a challenge and is why serial conversations between patients, caregivers, and clinicians are so valuable.

## Practical Considerations

"Oh yeah, I should do that," is one of the most common phrases a clinician hears when she or he asks about ADs. Therefore, it is important to have the tools and skills to help patients move the process of completing ADs forward. One of the simplest things for clinicians to do is ask patients if they have an AD and then request a copy for the electronic medical record. As mentioned earlier, an important follow-up question to the answer "yes, I have a living will" is "what does it say?" If the answer is "I don't know," then the patient and proxy will need to revisit that document to determine if the choices still make sense for the current medical situation.

If the patient responds that she or he does not have an AD or completed it so long ago that she or he does not recall what it says, the clinician's job is to encourage the patient to complete a new one. The timing of ACP discussions in terms of illness trajectory was previously addressed, and certain documents can be completed at specific times during a patient's disease course. The dPOA-h form is appropriate to complete at any point in time, and clinicians can keep state-specific dPOA-h forms in their office to give to patients. Some clinicians may be able to provide state-specific or branded ADs in addition to the dPOA-h form.

When a patient decides to complete a dPOA-h form, a few steps must take place. The first is to decide on the proxy and up to two alternates. The next step is to complete the document, and, in most states, this must be witnessed, notarized, or occasionally both. This step does not require any lawyer involvement, and therefore there should be no costs associated with completing a dPOA-h form. Once the patient has selected the proxy, the patient must inform this decision-maker about her or his preferences for care, including EOL care.

Any skilled member of the healthcare team can help patients understand and complete a dPOA-h and an AD, including physicians, nurse practitioners, physician assistants, social workers, nurses, and oncology navigators. These conversations can occur during routine office visits either in person or during telehealth video/telephone visits. ACP conversations and completion of ADs are also appropriate for hospitalized patients, especially if they have not previously had these conversations or if their medical condition has changed.

The length of time required to have an ACP discussion varies based on the setting, topics discussed, illness, and individuals involved in the conversation. On average, a conversation may last between 15 and 30 min but could be much quicker if a patient has relatively clear goals. Completing a POLST form with a patient usually takes less than 10 min.

While picking a surrogate decision-maker may seem straightforward, some aspects of ACP conversations are much more nuanced and can take time. Therefore, physicians and advanced practice providers (nurse practitioners, physician assistants, and clinical nurse specialists) can bill for these services [29, 30]. Billing for ACP requires a face-to-face encounter between a physician or other qualified healthcare professional and a patient, family member, or surrogate. Billing codes for these conversations are 99497 for 16–45 min and 99498 for 46 min or more. If a conversation is greater than 46 min, a clinician should bill for both the 99497 and 99498 codes [29, 30]. Reimbursement for these billing codes is specific to one's region and insurance company policies. There are no specific guidelines for what a clinician must document when billing for ACP, but a recommended template is as follows:

"I met with [people present] [in person or over video conferencing/telephone], and we discussed the patient's illness and goals. The patient shared [key details of patient's story, values, and goals of care]. We reviewed [POLST] form [and completed the document together]. [Please see scanned document]. Time spent in care planning: [time in minutes]."

## Conclusion

In conclusion, ACP is a process in which patients, caregivers, and clinicians work together throughout the disease trajectory to plan for future care. ACP allows patients to proactively guide their care based on their goals and values rather than reactively making forced decisions when there is a clinical change. ACP also supports caregivers and clinicians to feel they are providing care that makes sense for the patient and everyone involved. Early ACP removes the stigma about EOL discussions and makes it easier for patients to know in detail what they want for their future. ACP is the best way for patients to hope for the best while preparing for all other possibilities.

## References


1. The conversation project. Who will speak for you? How to choose and be a health care proxy. Institute for Healthcare Improvement. 2017. https://theconversationproject.org/wp-content/uploads/2017/03/ConversationProject-ProxyKit-English.pdf.
2. Cappell K, Sundaram V, Park A, Shiraz P, Gupta R, Jenkins P, et al. Advance directive utilization is associated with less aggressive end-of-life care in patients undergoing allogeneic hematopoietic cell transplantation. Biol Blood Marrow Transplant. 2018;24(5):1035–40.
3. Duckworth KE, Forti AM, Russell GB, Naik S, Hurd D, McQuellon RP. The process of advance care planning in HCT candidates and proxies: self-efficacy, locus of control, and anxiety levels. Am J Hosp Palliat Care. 2014;31(7):710–6.
4. Ganti AK, Lee SJ, Vose JM, Devetten MP, Bociek RG, Armitage JO, et al. Outcomes after hematopoietic stem-cell transplantation for hematologic malignancies in patients with or without advance care planning. J Clin Oncol. 2007;25(35):5643–8.
5. Loberiza FR Jr, Swore-Fletcher BA, Block SD, Back AL, Goldman RE, Tulsky JA, et al. Coping styles, health status and advance care planning in patients with hematologic malignancies. Leuk Lymphoma. 2011;52(12):2342–8.
6. Wang WS, Ma JD, Nelson SH, Revta C, Buckholz GT, Mulroney CM, et al. Advance care planning and palliative care integration for patients undergoing hematopoietic stem-cell transplantation. J Oncol Pract. 2017;13(9):e721–e8.
7. Loggers ET, Lee S, Chilson K, Back AL, Block S, Loberiza FR. Advance care planning among hematopoietic cell transplant patients and bereaved caregivers. Bone Marrow Transplant. 2014;49(10):1317–22.
8. Huang IA, Neuhaus JM, Chiong W. Racial and ethnic differences in advance directive possession: role of demographic factors, religious affiliation, and personal health values in a National Survey of older adults. J Palliat Med. 2016;19(2):149–56.
9. Barwise A, Wilson M. Socioeconomic status and advance care planning in the ICU. Soc Crit Care Med. 2017;44(12):212. https://www.sccm.org/Communications/Critical-Connections/Archives/2017/Socioeconomic-Status-and-Advance-Care-Planning-in
10. Prod'homme C, Jacquemin D, Touzet L, Aubry R, Daneault S, Knoops L. Barriers to end-of-life discussions among hematologists: a qualitative study. Palliat Med. 2018;32(5):1021–9.
11. Gray TF, Temel JS, El-Jawahri A. Illness and prognostic understanding in patients with hematologic malignancies. Blood Rev. 2020;45:100692.
12. LeBlanc TW, El-Jawahri A. When and why should patients with hematologic malignancies see a palliative care specialist? Hematology Am Soc Hematol Educ Program. 2015;2015:471–8.
13. Perez-Cruz PE, Dos Santos R, Silva TB, Crovador CS, Nascimento MS, Hall S, et al. Longitudinal temporal and probabilistic prediction of survival in a cohort of patients with advanced cancer. J Pain Symptom Manag. 2014;48(5):875–82.
14. Mack JW, Wolfe J, Cook EF, Grier HE, Cleary PD, Weeks JC. Hope and prognostic disclosure. J Clin Oncol. 2007;25(35):5636–42.
15. Meier DE, Back AL, Morrison RS. The inner life of physicians and care of the seriously ill. JAMA. 2001;286(23):3007–14.
16. Temel JS, Shaw AT, Greer JA. Challenge of prognostic uncertainty in the modern era of cancer therapeutics. J Clin Oncol. 2016;34(30):3605–8.
17. El-Jawahri A, Nelson AM, Gray TF, Lee SJ, LeBlanc TW. Palliative and end-of-life care for patients with hematologic malignancies. J Clin Oncol. 2020;38(9):944–53.
18. Wilkie DJ, Johnson B, Mack AK, Labotka R, Molokie RE. Sickle cell disease: an opportunity for palliative care across the life span. Nurs Clin N Am. 2010;45(3):375–97.
19. Kruser JM, Nabozny MJ, Steffens NM, Brasel KJ, Campbell TC, Gaines ME, et al. "Best Case/Worst Case": qualitative evaluation of a novel communication tool for difficult in-the-moment surgical decisions. J Am Geriatr Soc. 2015;63(9):1805–11.
20. Hill DL, Miller V, Walter JK, Carroll KW, Morrison WE, Munson DA, et al. Regoaling: a conceptual model of how parents of children with serious illness change medical care goals. BMC Palliat Care. 2014;13(1):9.
21. Lambert NM, Fincham FD, Stillman TF. Gratitude and depressive symptoms: the role of positive reframing and positive emotion. Cogn Emot. 2012;26(4):615–33.
22. Leblanc TW. Advance care planning and palliative care specialists in malignant hematology and stem-cell transplantation: on why it takes a village. J Oncol Pract. 2018;14(1):3–4.
23. Kassam A, Skiadaresis J, Alexander S, Wolfe J. Differences in end-of-life communication for children with advanced cancer who were referred to a palliative care team. Pediatr Blood Cancer. 2015;62(8):1409–13.
24. Martinez-Schlurmann NI, Rampa S, Speicher DG, Allareddy V, Rotta AT, Allareddy V. Prevalence, predictors and outcomes of cardiopulmonary resuscitation in hospitalized adult stem cell transplant recipients in the United States: not just opening the black box but exploring an opportunity to optimize! Bone Marrow Transplant. 2015;50(12):1578–81.
25. National Cancer Institute—Advance Directives. https://www.cancer.gov/about-cancer/managing-care/advance-directives. Accessed 2015.
26. The Conversation Project—who will speak for you? https://theconversationproject.org/wp-content/uploads/2017/03/ConversationProject-ProxyKit-English.pdf.
27. American Bar Association—State health care power of attorney statutes. https://www.americanbar.org/content/dam/aba/administrative/law_aging/state-health-care-power-of-attorney-statutes.authcheckdam.pdf.
28. National POLST Form: Portable Medical Order. https://polst.org/wp-content/uploads/2019/10/2019.09.02-National-POLST-Form-with-Instructions.pdf.
29. Centers for Medicare and Medicaid Services—Advance Care Planning Services Fact Sheet. https://www.cms.gov/outreach-and-education/medicare-learning-network-mln/mlnproducts/downloads/advancecareplanning.pdf.
30. Jones CA, Acevedo J, Bull J, Kamal AH. Top 10 tips for using advance care planning codes in palliative medicine and beyond. J Palliat Med. 2016;19(12):1249–53.

# Measuring Quality of Life and Health-Related Quality of Life

# 12

Susan Parsons, Nadine Linendoll, and Courtney Schroeder

## Introduction

Quality of life (QOL) is a seminal concept integral to the understanding and practical delivery of palliative care (PC). Pointing to its significance, the World Health Organization (WHO) included QOL as an outcome in its definition of PC stating, "[PC] will enhance QOL and may also positively influence the course of illness" [1]. If a significant goal of PC is to improve the patient's overall QOL, then it is important for clinicians and clinical researchers to have a clear understanding of QOL and how it can be effectively measured and evaluated; however, although QOL is a concept that is widely used in healthcare settings, it is not always clearly defined. The first section of this chapter will explore the conceptual work that has been over the last four decades to define QOL and integrate it into mainstream medicine—recognizing that since QOL is both highly personal and constantly evolving over time, this work has historically been challenging and complex.

In addition to the development of a conceptual framework of QOL, clinicians and researchers have also worked diligently to develop tools, which can accurately measure QOL in real-world settings. These instruments can be helpful in eliciting diverse information and range in both their depth and specificity. For example, summary scales, such as the Patient-Reported Outcomes Measurement Information System (PROMIS)™ Global Scale, developed by the National Institutes of Health (NIH) can be completed by the patient within 1–2 min, requiring a low burden of time and effort for both the staff/patient [2]. In contrast, more in-depth instruments can take upwards of 30–40 min to complete, necessitating a higher burden of time and effort for the staff/patient, but ultimately generate richer information, which can lead to more specific and tailored interventions. Since the current scope of QOL instruments is so vast, choosing the best option can feel strategically overwhelming. The second section of this chapter will provide a landscape overview of QOL instruments, while also sharing practical advice on how to match specific clinical questions with optimal QOL measures.

Building upon the extensive foundational work done to develop the conceptual framework and instrumentation of QOL, experts in the field have branched out to address specific patient populations. The third section of this chapter will present applications of QOL assessment in clinical trials and clinical care, including innovative PC research, strategies to enhance inclusion of QOL assessment in clinical trials, and ongoing research on the QOL impact of chronic conditions, such as sickle cell disease (SCD). This final section will also discuss specific recommendations for further QOL research such as exploring the interrelatedness of symptom burden and QOL and considering standardized measurement batteries across the development of clinical trials.

## Defining Quality of Life

QOL is a latent construct—something that cannot be directly measured—but rather, approximated through validated and reliable instruments. Because human beings live rich and

S. Parsons (✉) · N. Linendoll
Tufts University School of Medicine, Boston, MA, USA

Division of Hematology/Oncology, Department of Medicine, Institute for Clinical Research and Health Policy Studies, Tufts Medical Center, Boston, MA, USA
e-mail: sparsons@tuftsmedicalcenter.org; nlinendoll@tuftsmedicalcenter.org

C. Schroeder
Division of Hematology/Oncology, Department of Medicine, Tufts Medical Center, Boston, MA, USA
e-mail: cschroeder@tuftsmedicalcenter.org


C. K. Ullrich, E. J. Roeland (eds.), *Palliative Care in Hematologic Malignancies and Serious Blood Disorders*,
https://doi.org/10.1007/978-3-031-38058-7_12

complex lives, the concept of QOL is inevitably complex and multi-faceted. While QOL can incorporate objective data such as the patient's diagnosis and their treatment regimen, QOL is essentially a subjective concept, a constantly evolving perspective or a personal point of view.

As a multidimensional construct, QOL reflects the World Health Organization's holistic definition of health presented at an international health conference in 1946 as incorporating the physical, mental, and social health [3] of the individual. Taking this one step further, in 1995 the WHO published a position paper on QOL which recognized that QOL does not exist in a state of homeostasis, but rather it is dynamic and embedded within the individual's culture and value systems stating, "The individual's perception of their position in life is in the context of the culture and value systems in which they live in relation to their goals, expectations, standards and concerns" [4]. In this position paper, the WHO identified six broad domains that are pertinent when assessing QOL including: physical, psychological, level of independence, social relationships, environment and spirituality/religion/personal beliefs. Each of these constructs contain two additional components, the individual's ability to function and their sense of well-being within that domain.

Clinicians have a natural inclination to foster a positive outlook with their patients. Similarly, patients want to present favorably to their care team, risking underreporting of problems or impact of the disease/treatment. To avoid this, the WHO recommends not conflating assessments with an overly optimistic representation. In other words, when assessing QOL, it is important to balance both the positive and the negative. For example, when asking a patient about their level of independence, it would be important to address both the possibility of positive components (contentment, mobility) with negative components (fatigue, pain) to obtain a true panoramic perspective of their experience [4].

## Health-Related Quality of Life (HRQL)

When QOL is considered in the context of health and disease, it is commonly referred to as health-related quality of life (HRQL). One of the pioneers of HRQL research, Dr. David Osoba, reminds us that HRQL is really the grounding foundation of all that the healthcare system strives for—with the purpose of health care being to maintain, preserve, or restore the individual's health and thereby their HRQL.

In 1995, Wilson and Cleary created one of the first conceptual models of HRQL which linked clinical variables and subjective health constructs, thus combining the disciplines of biomedicine and social science [5]. Their model (Fig. 12.1) presents the complex and dynamic interplay between five main concepts including: biologic/physiologic, symptoms, functional status, general health perception, and overall QOL. Each concept is anchored within the characteristics of the individual and the characteristics of the environment, reinforcing the highly personal nature of QOL. Concise and applicable to diverse health care settings, this model has been widely used and is one of the most cited HRQL models in research literature [7].

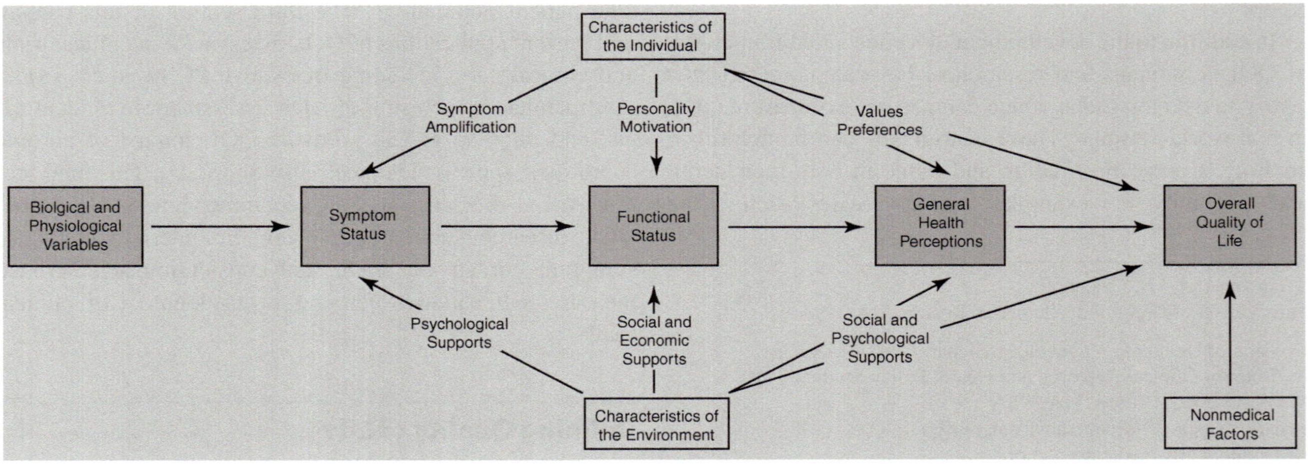


**Fig. 12.1** Wilson and Cleary QOL conceptual model, 1995 [6]. (Reproduced with permission from JAMA. 1995. 273(1). Copyright 1995 American Medical Association. All rights reserved)

## HRQL Instrument Development: Applications to PC Clinical Practice

Over the last three decades, extensive work has been done to develop well-validated, easy-to-administer instruments within both adult and pediatric settings. HRQL instruments can help to assess where people are in their illness trajectory and where they would like to be. Clinicians can use HRQL data to assess the patient's strengths and weaknesses and then to develop a care plan with tailored interventions to help them to reach their goals. When choosing an HRQL measures, it is important to assess both the type of instrument and the level of technology available to leverage as much information as possible with the lowest burden to the patient, caregiver, and staff.

Historically, HRQL instruments began to be included in clinical research trials beginning in the 1980s in adults. In 1986, Croog and colleagues conducted one of the first studies which included HRQL as an outcome [8]. This multicenter, randomized, double-blind clinical trial evaluated the effect of three antihypertensive drugs on blood pressure control and HRQL. In this study, the HRQL assessment addressed five categories including physical state, emotional state, intellectual function, ability to perform social roles, degree of satisfaction from those roles, sense of well-being, and satisfaction with life. Ultimately, the researchers found that although the drug effects did not differ, their impact on participants' HRQL did, thus linking the relationship between medication selection and HRQL.

Original HRQL measure performance relied on principles of classic test theory with measurement performance based on psychometric properties, including reliability, validity, responsiveness to change. Early inventories, such as the Sickness Impact Profile [9], contained many items (e.g., 136 items) in an attempt to broadly and inclusively cover the constructs being measures. Subsequently, these extensive inventories gave rise to "short forms," in which a fixed number of items was selected per domain to minimize burden and enhance acceptability. While initially completed on paper and pencil, further advances in technology and demonstrable comparability by mode of administration have led increasingly to electronic data capture.

Over the past 15 years, instrument development has been based on item response theory, which focus on the performance of individual items, rather than the overall test or scale. Items are characterized by their difficulty or usefulness in differentiating levels of functioning. Item response theory has been successfully used in educational testing for some time. One of the innovations is the use of dynamic testing in which the set of items an individual receives is directly informed by previous responses. For example, if a respondent said he could walk a mile without difficulty, he would not then be asked if he could stand unsupported. We and others have capitalized on this approach, particularly with populations at the lower end of functioning [10] due to disease or decline. Not only does this limit the number of questions a respondent is asked to complete, it ensures that those items are more relevant to the current condition.

Instrument length, modes of administration, and use of "smart" short forms or dynamic testing are all designed to ensure optimal completeness of assessments—both in terms of minimizing missing items within a measure or missing assessments completely. Missing data are values that are not available, but would be meaningful for the analysis if they were observed. Individual items can be missed or skipped, particularly if they are seen as not relevant to the health condition or perhaps are too difficult for the respondent to answer. Scoring rules unique to each measure allow for some degree of missingness at the item level without complete loss of information (e.g., 50% rule). Missing entire assessments, particularly due to respondent's health condition, can lead to biased results. This is referred to as missing not at random [11]. For example, if a respondent was too sick to complete an assessment, their HRQL and level of functioning would likely to be lower than those of the remaining respondents. This is especially important to consider in PC, given the anticipated decline in the patient's health and thus, HRQL. To avoid missing data at the assessment level, consideration should be given to the brevity of the assessment, including targeted toxicities, rather than comprehensive coverage. If missing data cannot be avoided, it needs to be addressed analytically. In our research in the hematopoietic stem cell population, we collected the reason(s) for missingness (e.g., related to the child's health or a non-health/logistical issue). We then developed pattern mixture models, stratified by reason for missingness [12, 13]. Other options include multiple imputation, which assumes data are missing at random [14]. Strategies such as last observation carried forward or analysis of completed cases only should be avoided due to bias.

## Instrument Selection

There are many considerations in selecting a measure or measures for either research or clinical care, including the purpose of measurement, any desire to compare within or across populations, and the capacity of the rater to respond. Additionally, measures can yield summary scores overall or by domain (so-called profile measures) or can be used to generate utility weights, particularly if the purpose of the measurement is to assess cost effectiveness or compare outcomes, such as quality-adjusted life expectancy. Measures can also be generic—across diseases or conditions—or can be condition-specific. Further, within oncology, there are generic cancer measures, such as the European Organization for Research and Treatment of Cancer Quality of Life Questionnaire-Core 30 (EORTC-QLQ-C30) [15], introduced below, or disease-specific modules, such as the Functional Assessment of Cancer Therapy-Lymphoma (FACT-Lymphoma) [16], which are designed to be used within a particular diagnosis.

Beyond the multidimensional measures, there are also single-domain measures and symptom assessments. Within the FACT family of instruments, for example, there is a specific scale about chemotherapy-induced peripheral neuropathy (FACT-GOG-Ntx), an 11-item symptom scale. Driven by the purpose of measurement, a battery of instruments can be compiled that include one or more of these types of instruments [17]. The majority of these instruments were developed in research settings as a way to compare QOL across different studies, populations, diseases, and/or treatments and were later adapted for use in the clinical setting. Examples of different types of instruments follow.

## Short Form-36 (SF-36) and Short Form-12 (SF-12)

The SF-36 is a 36 item multi-purpose health profile measure. Originally developed in the 1980s as part of the Medical Outcomes Study, the SF-36 was designed to evaluate health status across multiple chronic conditions, including cancer. Rigorously evaluated psychometrically, the SF-36 and its derivative versions have been used for more than 30 years in both research and clinical practice [18]. The SF-36 is a generic multidimensional scale, which assesses eight health concepts including physical functioning, physical role, bodily pain, general health, vitality, social functioning, emotional role, and mental health. These eight health concepts are scored individually and also categorized under physical or mental health to provide two summary scores. The survey was constructed for self-administration for those 14 years or older and can be also completed by interview [18]. The SF-36 has been validated and used for assessment of health status in patients with cancer and can detect deleterious effects in both physical and mental health in this population [19]. The SF-36 was later shortened to 12 questions in the SF-12, to provide a shorter, yet valid alternative to the SF-36. The 12 questions were selected from the SF-36 and combined and weighted to create two subscales that provide information on mental health, physical functioning, and overall HRQL [20]. Additionally, Brazier and colleagues developed algorithms to transform data from the SF-36 to the SF-6D, as a utility measure to be used in health economics and policy studies [21].

## European Organization for Research and Treatment of Cancer Quality of Life Questionnaire-Core 30 (EORTC QLQ-C30)

Like the SF-36, the EORTC-QLC-C30 was initially developed in the research setting and is now used in the clinical setting. EORTC-QLQ-C30 was initially created as an integrative, modular approach to evaluate the HRQL of cancer patients participating in international clinical trials [22]. The EORTC-QLC-C30 is a core questionnaire that comprises 30 questions to evaluate five functional scales (physical, role, cognitive, emotional, and social), three symptom scales (fatigue, pain, and nausea and vomiting), and a global health and HRQL scale [23]. The EORTC-QLQ-C30 is one of the most widely used global HRQL scales used in oncology, and pretreatment QLQ-C30 scores have been shown to provide strong prognostic value for overall survival in both research and clinical settings [24–26]. An adaptive version of the EORTC QLQ-C30 is also available to maximize measurement precision and minimize response burden on patients with cancer. Using computerized adaptive testing, this version also has the added benefit of reducing floor and ceiling effects [27]. The EORTC QLC-C30 was later shortened to 15 questions (EORTC QLQ-C15-PAL) to be used in the PC setting [28].

## EuroQOL-Five Dimensions (EQ-5D)

Widely used as a source of utility weights, the EQ-5D is a set of three questionnaires (EQ-5D-3L, EQ-5D-5L, EQ-5D-Y) developed by the EuroQOL research group and is used in clinical trials, population studies, and real-world settings [29]. It is a short survey that measures 5 dimensions of health including mobility, self-care, usual activities, pain and discomfort, and anxiety and depression. This is a generic questionnaire that can be used across patients, disease states, and treatments. It is available in 200 languages and is available in both electronic and paper versions and can be completed by the patient, proxy, or interviewer. The original EQ-5D-3L uses 3 response levels, whereas the EQ-5D-5L has 5 response levels to pick up more subtle differences in health. Studies have shown that the 5L version has similar to improved measurement properties, distributional parameters, and informativity compared to the 3L version. The third questionnaire, EQ-5D-Y, is a youth-friendly version that is designed for children and adolescents [30]. Like the SF-6D, the EQ-5D is an indirect measure of estimating utilities, although the two instruments rely on different methods to estimate the utilities. The EQ-5D using a time trade-off approach, whereas the SF-6D employs a standard gamble. The utility weights generated by these indirect approaches, using HRQL measures, are generally lower ("worse") than those obtained through direct measurement. From a policy perspective, the indirect measures may represent a lower bound of health effect [31].

## The Functional Assessment of Chronic Illness Therapy (FACIT) Measurement System

The FACIT Measurement System is a collection of HRQL questionnaires intended to assess the overall management of chronic illness [32]. The FACIT questionnaires can be administered by self-report (paper or computer) or through interview (face-to-face or telephone). The FACIT system was initially developed in collaboration with 845 cancer patients and 15 oncology specialists, who tested a battery of 370 overlapping items for breast, lung, and colorectal cancer [33]. Through factor and scale analysis, these items were condensed into the FACT-General (FACT-G). The FACT-G, now in its fourth version, is 27 item instrument with four domains of HRQL, physical, social, emotional, and functional well-being, which has been translated into many different languages and used worldwide. The FACT-G takes about 5–10 min to complete can be administered to individuals with any types of cancer. It has also been used and validated in other chronic illnesses such as HIV/AIDS; multiple sclerosis and rheumatoid arthritis [34].

## Health Utilities Index (HUI)

The HUI is a prominent preference-based measure that was initially developed to create a standardized system to measure comprehensive health status and HRQL across a broad age range and clinical scenarios. It has been applied clinically in pediatric and adult oncology, as well as in benign hematology settings including hemophilia and von Willebrand disease [35].

HUI currently uses two independent, but complementary health status classifications known as HUI2 and HUI3, which measure ability or disability within different categories [35]. The HUI2 classification assesses seven attributes including sensation, mobility, emotion, cognition, self-care, pain, and fertility across 3–5 levels. The HUI3 classification evaluates 8 attributes including vision, hearing, speech, ambulation, dexterity, emotion, cognition, and pain and evaluates each over 5–6 levels of ability/disability. In addition, providing descriptive measures of the specific attributes, each HUI provides a composite description of overall health status. There are several different versions of the surveys to allow for self-assessment versus proxy assessment, self-completion versus interview administered, different recall periods (1, 2, or 4 week time periods) [35]. Each survey is available in both a 15-item (15Q) and 40-item (40Q) questionnaire. The 15Q is designed for self-completion and takes approximately 5–10 min to complete [36]. The 40Q is for interviewer administration with a built-in skip pattern based on item response and takes approximately 3 min to complete [37]. The HUI has been used for clinical trials, cost effectiveness analyses, general population health, and in routine clinical practice.

The HUI is also an indirect method of utility elicitation. In contrast to the other measures described above, such as the SF-6D and EQ-5D, the HUI uses a visual analogue scale transformed into a standard gamble.

## Adult Instruments: Single Domain

When assessing patients, clinicians may desire a more in-depth assessment of a particular HRQL domain, rather than assessing HRQL from a global perspective or its multidimensionality. For instance, a systematic review of HRQL in Hodgkin Lymphoma found that the two most common single domains explored within this patient population included the psychological domain and the sexual health domain [38]. Within the psychological domain, the Brief Symptom Inventory (BSI) was reported as of the most commonly used scale. The BSI is a screening tool for psychological distress among individuals 18 years and older and has been frequently used for adults with cancer [39] and cancer survivors [40]. This measure takes approximately 5 min to complete and contains 18 questions. It assesses three symptom scales: anxiety, depression, and somatization. An overall summary score known as the Global Severity Index (GSI) is also obtained. Within the sexual health domain, the systematic review found that the Brief Sexual Function Inventory Test (BSFI) was a commonly used instrument. This BSFI includes 11 questions that are evaluated on a series of 5-item Likert scales. Scores are calculated for each of the 5 functional domains (Sexual Dive, Erection, Ejaculation, Sexual Problems, Overall Sexual Satisfaction Score) along with a total BSFI score [41, 42]. The use of single domain scales depends on the population under investigation and the study goals.

## Adult Instruments: Symptom Assessments

Symptom assessment is a fundamental component of HRQL evaluation in PC. The presence and burden of symptoms in serious illnesses, such as hematologic malignancies (HM) and serious blood disorders, are known to directly influence patient distress and HRQL [43]. The number of symptoms reported by patients correlates with perception of HRQL and higher symptom burden results in decreased HRQL [44, 45]. For this reason, comprehensive symptom assessments are another important tool to utilize when assessing HRQL. We will review three of the available comprehensive symptom assessment tools in this section.

## MD Anderson Symptom Inventory (MDASI)

The MDASI is multi-symptom measure for patients with cancer to assess both symptom severity and the interference of these symptoms on daily life [46]. The MDASI evaluates 13 core symptoms that were chosen due to their high frequency and severity in the cancer population and these core symptoms make up the majority of symptom distress that patients with cancer report during both active treatment and post-treatment follow-up. This instrument was designed to be used in symptom surveys, clinical trials, and for clinical patient monitoring [47]. The core MDASI applies broadly across different cancer types and treatments and can also be adapted to specific cancer types by use of MDASI modules (e.g., acute myeloid leukemia, multiple myeloma) [46]. This instrument takes less than 5 min and specifically evaluates symptoms and their impact on daily life over the past 24 h, suggesting its utility in the follow-up setting [43]. It is available in written, electronic, and telephone-based interactive voice response formats which allows for possibility of remote symptom monitoring for both research and clinical care purposes [46].

## Memorial Symptom Assessment Scale (MSAS) and Memorial Symptom Assessment Scale Short Form (MSAS-SF)

The MSAS is a multidimensional symptom assessment instrument that was initially validated in the cancer population. It evaluates 32 highly prevalent symptoms within physical and psychological domains to determine symptom severity, frequency, and associated distress related to those symptoms. It was initially developed to evaluate QOL in clinical trials and studies of symptom epidemiology. The MSAS physical distress dimension and frequency of psychologic symptoms correlated most with QOL measures [33]. The MSAS physical symptom subscale score has been shown to predict survival independent of disease extent and provides additional prognostic information in patients with cancer [48]. Due to the comprehensive and, therefore, time-consuming nature of the MSAS instrument, it has been suggested to be best suited for initial clinical assessment and research purposes [43].

The MSAS was later abbreviated to the MSAS-short form (MSAS-SF) and validated in adults with cancer which includes a physical subscale, psychological subscale, and global distress index. The MSAS-SF takes less than 5 min to administer and allows for rapid, comprehensive assessment of symptoms. For this reason, the MSAS-SF may be ideal for evaluation of symptoms in patients with limited stamina [49] such as patients with HM and serious blood disorders in the PC setting.

The MSAS was also adapted for use in children with cancer. Initially when studied within a pediatric population, the MSAS was administered to children aged 10–18. Researchers found that children could complete the scale easily within a mean of 11 min. When the child's report was compared to the parent's perspective and information from the medical chart, statistical analysis showed reliability and validity within the domains of physical, mental, and global symptom distress [50]. The MSAS was further validated for use in younger pediatric populations. Researchers found that children as young as 7 years old, who were receiving cancer treatment, could consistently report their own symptom experience [51].

## Patient-Reported Outcome Common Terminology Criteria for Adverse Events (PRO-CTCAE)

Clinician reporting of adverse events via CTCAE has been essential in the characterization of safety in clinical trials, principally severe adverse events that can lead to dose modification or treatment discontinuation. To more fully characterize the patients' experience with and burden of treatment, the PRO-CTCAE measurement system was developed to characterize the frequency, severity, interference, and presence or absence of symptomatic toxicities over the past 7 days through patient self-report [52]. The instrument can be built or tailored to a particular study or situation by selecting from among the 78 symptomatic toxicities in the library and from among 25 available languages. The PRO-CTCAE is publicly available in paper, electronic, and interactive voice response system forms; completion times vary based on the number of symptoms probed, typically in the 8–17 range. In one study, the 20-item inventory took less than 5 min, regardless of mode of administration [53]. Research is underway to enhance the interpretation and display of results from the PRO-CTCAE to allow for comparisons in clinical trials between study arms and highlight the impact of symptom severity, as well as persistence over time [54].

Overall the goal of the PRO-CTCAE measurement system is to enhance the precision and reproducibility of adverse event reporting in cancer clinical trials, to provide data that complement and extend the information provided by clinician reporting using CTCAE, and to represent the patient perspective of the experience of symptomatic adverse events [52]. Currently, the PRO-CTCAE is not designed to lead directly to protocol-directed action, such as dose modification.

The pediatric versions (PED-PRO-CTCAE) were developed with a 64-item library and both a self-report tool for youth ages 7–17 and a caregiver tool for ages less than 7 [55]. Although originally developed in English, translation is underway to ensure broader participation.

## Pediatric HRQL and Instrument Development

Although HRQL began to be integrated into clinical trials beginning in the 1980s in adults, related work in pediatrics lagged behind. Historically through the 1980s and 1990s, very few instruments were available to children for self-report with most relying heavily on their parents as proxy reporter [56]. In 1995, Bradlyn and colleagues published a retrospective review of 70 Phase III clinical trials from the Pediatric Oncology Group and Children's Cancer Group assessing for HRQL and/or toxicity data. They found that only about 3% of the studies included any data on QOL data, whereas toxicity data were collected in over 75% of the studies [57]. The authors recommended further education to the medical community on the value of including QOL measures in clinical trials as well as addressing potential barriers such as the burden and cost of increased data collection.

In 1996, the American Cancer Society convened the first summit on QOL in pediatric oncology. Bradlyn and colleagues made specific recommendations about how to conduct QOL research in pediatric oncology. They proposed that pediatric QOL should include several of its own age-specific themes [58]. First, there should be focus on the biology, treatment, and outcomes of childhood cancer. Providing the example of acute lymphoblastic leukemia, they explained that variables such as the age at diagnosis, disease stage, and range of treatments can all affect QOL outcomes. They also recognized that since treatment protocols are like "moving targets" and constantly changing—QOL instruments should also be flexible and able to adapt. Second, pediatric QOL should incorporate a fundamental understanding of childhood and adolescent development, recognizing that no single measure can capture the scope of changes that occur from elementary school through the older teenage years. Third, and most importantly, concepts of pediatric QOL should seek to understand the child within the context of her or his family, since the impact of serious disease on QOL extends beyond the patient to her or his siblings and extended family systems.

Over the past 25 years, there has been a steady growth in the development of psychometrically robust instruments to measure children's QOL, including the creation of age-based pediatric measures for child self-report, as well as parent proxy reports with a growing appreciation that, where possible, the voice of the child is preferred [59]. Modeled after prominent behavioral scales, such as the Child Behavior Checklist, completed by parents, and its Youth Self-Report [60], completed by adolescents, several early pediatric instruments, such as the PedsQL™ [61] and the Child Health Ratings Inventories (CHRIs) [62], created separate versions of the instruments for younger children and for teens with parent proxy measure including parallel content to the youth measures [63]. To assist school-aged children, Parsons et al. supplemented the text-based response scales with pictorial representations, allowing children "to pick the kid most like them" (Fig. 12.2). They also used animation, which included narration to circumvent literacy issues [64]. Both the PedsQL™ and the CHRIs are generic profile measures, designed to be used across disease and conditions. The PedsQL™ contains a cancer-specific module [63], whereas the CHRIs has a hematopoietic cell transplantation (HCT) module—each to be used with the generic core.

More recently, developers have created measures to be used across the broader age range of childhood and adolescence (e.g., 8–18 years) with the continued appreciation that younger children (under 8 years) may be more reliably represented by their parent proxies. In addition to the CHRIs, some measures, such as the KIDSCREEN [65] family of instruments, have developed a global index.

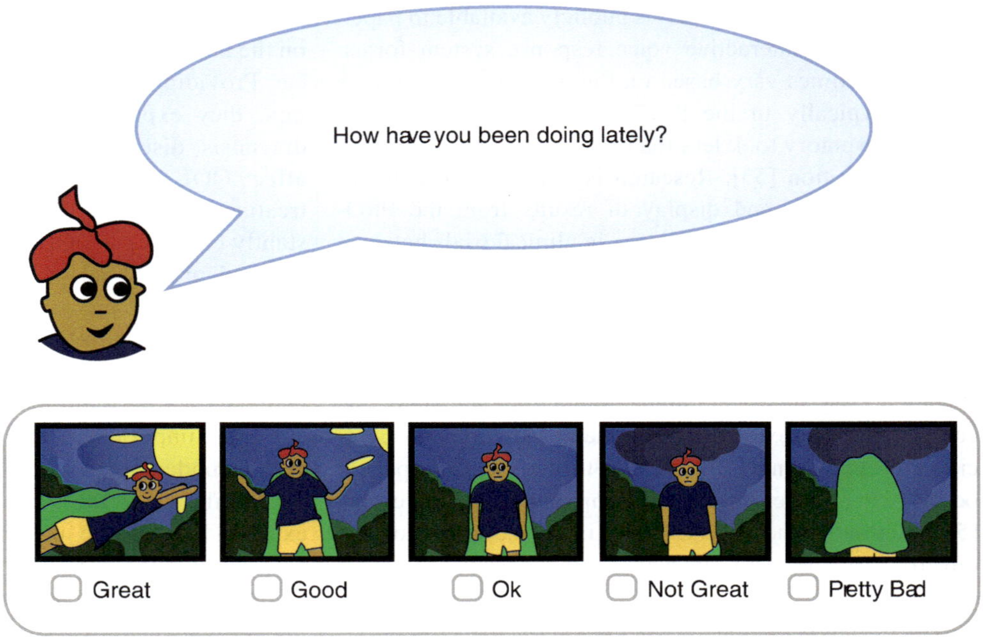


**Fig. 12.2** CHRIs (Child Health Rating Inventories): Sample question in which illustrations at each response level provide additional input to text-based response scale

## Patient-Reported Measurement Information System (PROMIS)

One of the major breakthroughs in HRQL measurement over the past 15 years has been the PROMIS, a trans-NIH roadmap initiative, designed to create a widely available, mutually understood language for studying and reporting universally relevant patient-reported outcome measures that would revolutionize patient-reported outcomes use in both research and clinical settings [66].

Beginning in 2004, item banks have been created for use with children and PROMIS includes over 300 measures that can evaluate global, physical, mental, and social health and specific domains within those categories (i.e., fatigue, pain intensity, anxiety, ability to participate in social activities). These measures are available as "smart" short forms of varying lengths, as well as in computer adaptive tests [67]. Computer adaptive tests use dynamically selected questions from an item bank, based on the respondents' previous answers. The questions are tailored to be relevant to the respondent and allow for precise measurements with use of fewer questions and reduced respondent burden. Each PROMIS measure is scored on common metrics and is centered on general population data, where a T-score is transformed to a mean of 50 represents the mean in the general US population and a standard deviation of 10. This allows for comparison across different populations and diseases [2]. In addition, custom questionnaires can be developed from the rich item bank. Rodday and coworkers leveraged the item bank for physical functioning to create a custom short form for patients with severe impairment in physical functioning, demonstrating ability to differentiate among participants even at the lower end of the scale [10].

As it applies to clinical care, PROMIS determines precise results across both broad health categories and specific symptoms, with as little burden on the patient as possible. As it pertains to PC, PROMIS measures have been shown to reliably estimate where patients are on the trajectory of declining health status leading towards end of life (EOL) in oncology patients including those with HM. PROMIS have also been successful in detecting worsening symptoms that warrant more aggressive palliative symptom management [68].

In addition to the strength of the measurement properties, the PROMIS instrument is available within the public domain and has been translated and tested for cross-language fidelity, allowing for broad-based use [69, 70]. Further, several studies have shown that the constructs are comparable across the age continuum, which greatly enhances the conduct of clinical studies across diverse age-groups. As an illustration, the Southwest Oncology Group (SWOG) is currently leading a trans-National Clinical Trials Network clinical trial of adolescents, young adults, and older adults with advanced stage Hodgkin Lymphoma (NCT03907488) [71]. To accommodate both adolescent and adult participants, age-specific generic scales (PROMIS Global) and targeted single domain (e.g., fatigue) and symptom scales (e.g., neuropathy) are being used to compare outcomes by treatment arm.

Historically, and in contrast to adult clinical trials, few pediatric trials have incorporated longitudinal HRQL assessment, based on concerns about site and participant burden. This trend is slowly changing. For example, Parsons and colleagues recently completed an embedded QOL study within a Phase III clinical trial for newly diagnosed Hodgkin lymphoma through the Children's Oncology Group (COG) (NCT02166463) [72, 73]. Baseline completion rates across exceeded 97% with on-treatment follow-up rates greater than 92%. These data suggest that patients (and parents) are very willing to provide this information. To alleviate site burden, the study relied on externally funded research staff to supplement infrastructure support from the cooperative group.

Gaps still exist in selected diseases and populations. Within COG, ~20% of clinical trials for adolescents and young adults (AYA) included patient-reported outcomes and/or HRQL endpoints [74]. To address this deficit and funded through the National Cancer Institute's Childhood Cancer Data Initiative, AYA investigators and HRQL topic experts are currently collaborating to identify a consensus-based instrument battery, enhanced infrastructure support, and statistical expertise in the design and analysis of this type of study.

## Real-Life Clinical Examples

Beyond clinical trials, HRQL is gradually making its way into clinical practice. As part of routine practice in the Reid R Sacco AYA Survivorship Clinic patients complete a 10-item PROMIS™ Global Health Measure at every visit [75]. This instrument was implemented to provide clinicians with a quick snapshot of the patient's subjective rating of their own physical and mental health. Having this information, particularly when seeing new patients, can help clinicians "break the ice" with a "jumping off point" to initiate more sensitive discussions. Secondly, distributing the PROMIS to all patients, who is able to independently complete it before the visit, normalizes the discussion so that patients do not feel that they are being singled out. Rather, the PROMIS assessment has become part of the clinic's overall approach to care.

Previous clinical research demonstrated that the PROMIS global instrument was feasible and straight-forward to implement within an AYA oncology clinical setting at the point of care [76]. The 10-item PROMIS global measure asks patients to rate their physical and mental health, using a five-point Likert scale [77]. Prior to the clinicians' initiation of the clinical visit, the patients' responses to the PROMIS™ global are scored in real-time, using established algorithms, yielding summary subscale scores for Global Physical Health and Global Mental Health, again, with a standardized mean score of 50 (standard deviation of 10). When reviewing the results of the PROMIS, clinicians can explain to patients how their scores compare with the general population and in subsequent visits, how current scores compare to previous scores.

To implement the PROMIS global in the AYA clinic, it was imperative to identify which staff member could consistently meet each patient prior to their visit and ask them to complete the instrument. Additionally, understanding when to administer the measure within the context of the clinical flow was essential. Once these two issues were addressed, the completion of the PROMIS global became a routine part of clinical practice and neither the staff nor the patients reported that completing the PROMIS was burdensome. The AYA clinic's successful administration of the PROMIS global echoed previous research which suggests that the instrument's high completion rate is likely due to its brevity and ease to which it can become part of the clinical routine when it is universally distributed versus targeting specific patients [76]. After the PROMIS™—global is scored, results are shared with the clinicians prior to the visit. In additional to subscale scores, the scores are also plotted on a graph to visually compare the current scores with scores from the previous visits (Fig. 12.3). Having this information readily available prior to seeing the patient has been very valuable in caring for patients within the AYA demographic, who may be less forthright with clinicians about how they are feeling [78]. A low score provides an immediate alert for the provider, who can then ask more specific questions to understand why the patient rated their mental or physical health low.

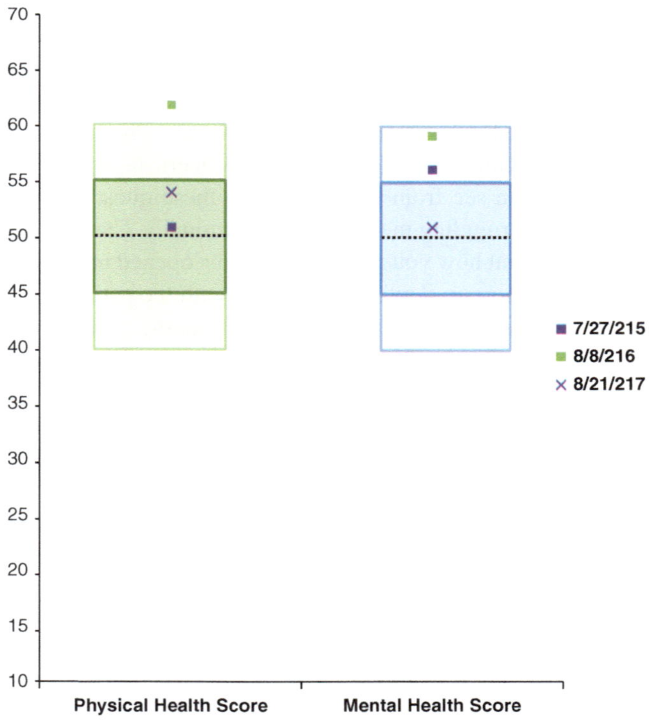


**Fig. 12.3** Sample scoring of several PROMIS global measure by subscale

Discussions related to the PROMIS™—global scores have uncovered serious physical and mental health concerns, which may not have been identified if the patients had not provided a subjective rating of their HRQL. In one example, a young woman presented with a low PROMIS™ global physical health subscale score. A young mother, she explained that her daily activity had become impaired by lower extremity sensory discomfort with recurrent trips and falls. Because her symptoms were subtle, she had been reluctant to mention them at previous doctors' appointments. After further discussion and a physical exam, the AYA care team was able to diagnosis her with persistent peripheral neuropathy related to her previous chemotherapy treatment. They made a referral to physiatrist in rehabilitation medicine who prescribed a tailored physical therapy regimen to improve her overall gait and balance. With this newfound knowledge regarding her deficits and clearly prescribed interventions for improvement, them this young woman's PROMIS™ global physical health scores improved at subsequent visits.

The PROMIS™ Global Mental Health subscale has also helped to uncover serious psychological distress within the AYA Survivorship Clinic. Data collected in the clinic found that 40% of AYA survivors present to the clinic with a preexisting psychological conditions ranging from anxiety and depression to post-traumatic stress disorder [75]. Reviewing the patient's PROMIS™ global mental health subscale scores prior to the visit can help clinicians prepare to address these sensitive psychological concerns. For example, one young man presented to his initial visit with a negative review of systems, but a PROMIS™ global mental health score well below the mean. Per clinic protocol, patients who score two standard deviations below the mean are immediately referred for psychological services. The clinician opened the conversation voicing her concern regarding his scores, "I can see from the answers to these questions you seem to be struggling mentally and emotionally. Can you tell me more about how you are feeling?" This opened up a much longer and more in-depth conversation with the patient, who disclosed that he was struggling with ongoing anxiety and depression related to his cancer diagnosis and long-term effects. He was also self-medicating with a mixture of drugs and alcohol. An immediate referral was made for him to establish care with both a therapist and psychiatrist. With structured psychological care in place and ongoing support through the AYA clinic, this young man's PROMIS™ global mental health scores steadily improved at subsequent visits.

## Innovations in the Incorporation of QOL and Symptom Assessment in PC

Within the area of pediatric PC, the Pediatric Quality of Life and Evaluation of Symptoms Technology (PediQUEST) is a highly innovative system to capture and report HRQL and symptoms assessment about children with advanced cancer [79]. The assessment incorporates validated HRQL measures (PedsQL) [61], the PediQUEST-MSAS [79], and measures of parental well-being. Previous studies have demonstrated the feasibility of this approach. In an ongoing randomized controlled trial at four pediatric oncology centers, children are randomly assigned to an enhanced response system with feedback reports to clinicians versus usual care (NCT03408314). The goal of the study is to ascertain if the standardization of family reports and clinicians' response results in less parental distress and enhanced child HRQL. The richness of this approach is that it examines the interconnectedness between HRQL and symptom burden for the child, as well as the intimate relationship between the child's and the parents' illness experience. If the current trial is successful, the field will benefit from broader dissemination of this powerful tool.

Recent research in the sickle cell population in both the adult and the pediatric age groups has demonstrated that, despite the level of disease acuity, patients hospitalized for management or treatment of sickle cell disease (SCD) are willing and able to complete reports of HRQL. In a recent study by Esham and coworkers, serial HRQL and SCD-specific patient-reported outcomes were obtained from young adult SCD patients who are admitted for vaso-occlusive crisis (VOC) [80, 81]. Understanding the multidimensional pain experience and its impact on those with SCD is critical for disease management and improvement of HRQL for patients with SCD [82]. Patient-reported outcome measures provide a standardized way to assess the impact of multidimensional pain and VOC on HRQL in SCD patients [82, 83].

The Esham study demonstrated that although pain intensity scores improved during the hospitalization, many other factors that contribute to the pain experience remained low after discharge, such as global mental health, emotional impact, social functioning, stiffness impact, and sleep impact. These findings suggest that SCD patients endure substantial suffering that cannot be assessed with numeric pain scores alone and incorporating patient-reported outcomes to fully evaluate HRQL in the adult SCD population is critical [84].

HRQL was also evaluated in children with SCD and thalassemia who underwent HCT. One study evaluated and compared HRQL of 13 patients with hemoglobinopathies that underwent HCT to patients with acquired conditions who underwent HCT (i.e., malignancy, aplastic anemia) by collecting serial HRQL separately from the children and parents [85]. Patients with hemoglobinopathies had a higher data completion rate (85%) than the acquired condition comparison group (64%). This study showed that children with hemoglobinopathies had higher physical and emotional functioning scores prior to HCT but experienced a similar pattern of recovery to baseline functioning when compared to children who received HCT for acquired conditions. Child emotional functioning ratings and parent ratings of all domains showed a nadir at 45 days with recovery to baseline at 3 months. This emphasized the importance of measuring HRQL in the initial weeks following HCT to capture decline in functional outcomes in the acute post-HCT period for patients with SCD and thalassemia. In the hemoglobinopathy group, it was also found that child HRQL ratings were higher than the parent ratings across physical, emotional, and role functioning domains. Overall, this study showed that completing HRQL scores was acceptable for pediatric hemoglobinopathy HCT patients and highlighted the importance of incorporating information from both the child and parent with an emphasis on the early post-HCT period [85].

The serial assessment of HRQL in the PC setting for patients with cancer or other debilitating conditions, such as chronic pain disorders, can only enhance communication between the patient, family, and clinicians. To ensure that participation is optimized across racial, ethnic, and cultural groups, validated measures need to be available in multiple languages with demonstrated fidelity. The current NCI-led Moonshot initiative is addressing this critical issue. Innovative platforms for data collection and integration of results, such as PediQUEST [79], ensure that the patient/family voice is heard and responded to in a timely manner.

Despite these inroads, gaps still persist in selected populations. Inclusion of HRQL assessment in cancer clinical trials is still low among AYAs, whose care often sits on the age-based care divide of pediatric and adult medicine. Ongoing initiatives through the National Community Oncology Research Program (NCORP) are addressing this issue within COG and across the NCTN research bases with consideration to developing standardized measurement batteries across trials and enhancing infrastructure support to assist patient participation. Finally, through the NCI Moonshot Patient Tolerability investigator teams are working on methods to enhance interpretation of patient-reported symptoms and toxicity. All of these efforts, taken together, will advance our understanding of the impact of illness, treatment, and symptoms on the patient, allowing us to intervene and support the patients across the continuum of care.

## References


1. World Health Organization. WHO definition of palliative care. https://www.who.int/cancer/palliative/definition/en/. Accessed 5 Feb 2020.
2. HealthMeasures. Intro to PROMIS. https://www.healthmeasures.net/explore-measurement-systems/promis/intro-to-promis. Accessed 20 Mar 2020.
3. International Health Conference. Constitution of the World Health Organization. 1946. Bull World Health Organ. 2002;80(12):983–4.
4. Whoqol Group. The World Health Organization Quality of Life assessment (WHOQOL): position paper from the World Health Organization. Soc Sci Med. 1995;41(10):1403–9.
5. Ojelabi AO, Graham Y, Haighton C, Ling J. A systematic review of the application of Wilson and Cleary health-related quality of life model in chronic diseases. Health Qual Life Outcomes. 2017;15(1):241.
6. Wilson IB, Cleary PD. Linking clinical variables with health-related quality of life. A conceptual model of patient outcomes. JAMA. 1995;273(1):59–65.
7. Bakas T, McLennon SM, Carpenter JS, Buelow JM, Otte JL, Hanna KM, et al. Systematic review of health-related quality of life models. Health Qual Life Outcomes. 2012;10:134.
8. Croog SH, Levine S, Testa MA, Brown B, Bulpitt CJ, Jenkins CD, et al. The effects of antihypertensive therapy on the quality of life. N Engl J Med. 1986;314(26):1657–64.
9. Bergner M, Bobbitt RA, Carter WB, Gilson BS. The sickness impact profile: development and final revision of a health status measure. Med Care. 1981;19(8):787–805.
10. Rodday AM, Graham RJ, Weidner RA, Rothrock NE, Dewalt DA, Parsons SK. Leveraging pediatric PROMIS item banks to assess physical functioning in children at risk for severe functional loss. J Patient Rep Outcomes. 2017;1(1):10.
11. Little RJ, D'Agostino R, Cohen ML, Dickersin K, Emerson SS, Farrar JT, et al. The prevention and treatment of missing data in clinical trials. N Engl J Med. 2012;367(14):1355–60.
12. Rodday AM, Terrin N, Parsons SK, Journeys to Recovery Study; HSCT-CHESS™ Study. Measuring global health-related quality of life in children undergoing hematopoietic stem cell transplant: a longitudinal study. Health Qual Life Outcomes. 2013;11:26.
13. Son H, Friedmann E, Thomas SA. Application of pattern mixture models to address missing data in longitudinal data analysis using SPSS. Nurs Res. 2012;61(3):195–203.
14. Barnard J, Meng XL. Applications of multiple imputation in medical studies: from AIDS to NHANES. Stat Methods Med Res. 1999;8(1):17–36.
15. EORTC. Quality of life of cancer patients: EORTC Quality of Life Group. 1995. https://qol.eortc.org/questionnaire/eortc-qlq-c30/.
16. Hlubocky FJ, Webster K, Cashy J, Beaumont J, Cella D. The Development and Validation of a Measure of Health-Related Quality of Life for Non-Hodgkin's Lymphoma: The Functional Assessment of Cancer Therapy—Lymphoma (FACT-Lym). Lymphoma. 2013;2013:147176.
17. Calhoun EA, Welshman EE, Chang CH, Lurain JR, Fishman DA, Hunt TL, et al. Psychometric evaluation of the functional assessment of cancer therapy/gynecologic oncology group-neurotoxicity (Fact/GOG-Ntx) questionnaire for patients receiving systemic chemotherapy. Int J Gynecol Cancer. 2003;13(6):741–8.
18. Ware JE Jr, Sherbourne CD. The MOS 36-item short-form health survey (SF-36). I. Conceptual framework and item selection. Med Care. 1992;30(6):473–83.
19. Reeve BB, Potosky AL, Smith AW, Han PK, Hays RD, Davis WW, et al. Impact of cancer on health-related quality of life of older Americans. J Natl Cancer Inst. 2009;101(12):860–8.
20. Ware J Jr, Kosinski M, Keller SD. A 12-Item Short-Form Health Survey: construction of scales and preliminary tests of reliability and validity. Med Care. 1996;34(3):220–33.
21. Brazier J, Roberts J, Deverill M. The estimation of a preference-based measure of health from the SF-36. J Health Econ. 2002;21(2):271–92.
22. Mystakidou K, Tsilika E, Parpa E, Kalaidopoulou O, Smyrniotis V, Vlahos L. The EORTC core quality of life questionnaire (QLQ-C30, version 3.0) in terminally ill cancer patients under palliative care: Validity and reliability in a Hellenic sample. Int J Cancer. 2001;94(1):135–9.
23. Aaronson NK, Ahmedzai S, Bergman B, Bullinger M, Cull A, Duez NJ, et al. The European Organization for Research and Treatment of Cancer QLQ-C30: a quality-of-life instrument for use

in international clinical trials in oncology. JNCI J Natl Cancer Inst. 1993;85(5):365–76.
24. Montazeri A. Quality of life data as prognostic indicators of survival in cancer patients: an overview of the literature from 1982 to 2008. Health Qual Life Outcomes. 2009;7:102.
25. Gotay CC, Kawamoto CT, Bottomley A, Efficace F. The prognostic significance of patient-reported outcomes in cancer clinical trials. J Clin Oncol. 2008;26(8):1355–63.
26. Husson O, de Rooij BH, Kieffer J, Oerlemans S, Mols F, Aaronson NK, et al. The EORTC QLQ-C30 summary score as prognostic factor for survival of patients with cancer in the "real-world": results from the population-based PROFILES registry. Oncologist. 2020;25(4):e722–e32.
27. EORTC. Quality of Life Group website. https://qol.eortc.org/.
28. Groenvold M, Petersen MA, Aaronson NK, Arraras JI, Blazeby JM, Bottomley A, et al. The development of the EORTC QLQ-C15-PAL: a shortened questionnaire for cancer patients in palliative care. Eur J Cancer. 2006;42(1):55–64.
29. Szende A, Janssen B, Cabases J, editors. Self-reported population health: an international perspective based on EQ-5D. Dordrecht, NL: Springer; 2014.
30. Euroqol. EQ-5D. https://euroqol.org/. Accessed 19 Oct 2020.
31. Arnold D, Girling A, Stevens A, Lilford R. Comparison of direct and indirect methods of estimating health state utilities for resource allocation: review and empirical analysis. BMJ. 2009;339:b2688.
32. Webster K, Cella D, Yost K. The functional assessment of chronic illness therapy (FACIT) measurement system: properties, applications, and interpretation. Health Qual Life Outcomes. 2003;1:79.
33. Cella DF, Tulsky DS, Gray G, Sarafian B, Linn E, Bonomi A, et al. The functional assessment of cancer therapy scale: development and validation of the general measure. J Clin Oncol. 1993;11(3):570–9.
34. FACIT.org. FACIT Measures and Searchable Library: FACIT Group. https://www.facit.org/facit-measures-searchable-library.
35. Horsman J, Furlong W, Feeny D, Torrance G. The Health Utilities Index (HUI): concepts, measurement properties and applications. Health Qual Life Outcomes. 2003;1:54.
36. Hawthorne G, Richardson J, Day NA. A comparison of the Assessment of Quality of Life (AQoL) with four other generic utility instruments. Ann Med. 2001;33(5):358–70.
37. Houle C, Berthelot J-M. A head-to-head comparison of the Health Utilities Index Mark 3 and the EQ-5D for the population living in private households in Canada. Qual Life Newslett. 2000;24:5–6.
38. Linendoll N, Saunders T, Burns R, Nyce JD, Wendell KB, Evens AM, et al. Health-related quality of life in Hodgkin lymphoma: a systematic review. Health Qual Life Outcomes. 2016;14(1):114.
39. Zabora J, BrintzenhofeSzoc K, Jacobsen P, Curbow B, Piantadosi S, Hooker C, et al. A new psychosocial screening instrument for use with cancer patients. Psychosomatics. 2001;42(3):241–6.
40. Recklitis CJ, Parsons SK, Shih MC, Mertens A, Robison LL, Zeltzer L. Factor structure of the brief symptom inventory--18 in adult survivors of childhood cancer: results from the childhood cancer survivor study. Psychol Assess. 2006;18(1):22–32.
41. Nedea D. Brief Sexual Function Inventory (BSFI) Test: 2020. Accessed 20 May 2017.
42. O'Leary MP, Fowler FJ, Lenderking WR, Barber B, Sagnier PP, Guess HA, et al. A brief male sexual function inventory for urology. Urology. 1995;46(5):697–706.
43. Kirkova J, Davis MP, Walsh D, Tiernan E, O'Leary N, LeGrand SB, et al. Cancer symptom assessment instruments: a systematic review. J Clin Oncol. 2006;24(9):1459–73.
44. Portenoy RK, Thaler HT, Kornblith AB, Lepore JM, Friedlander-Klar H, Kiyasu E, et al. The Memorial Symptom Assessment Scale: an instrument for the evaluation of symptom prevalence, characteristics and distress. Eur J Cancer. 1994;30A(9):1326–36.
45. Chang VT, Hwang SS, Feuerman M, Kasimis BS. Symptom and quality of life survey of medical oncology patients at a veterans affairs medical center: a role for symptom assessment. Cancer. 2000;88(5):1175–83.
46. Center MAC. The MD Anderson Symptom Inventory. https://www.mdanderson.org/research/departments-labs-institutes/departments-divisions/symptom-research/symptom-assessment-tools/md-anderson-symptom-inventory.html. Accessed 18 May 2020.
47. Cleeland CS, Mendoza TR, Wang XS, Chou C, Harle MT, Morrissey M, et al. Assessing symptom distress in cancer patients: the M.D. Anderson Symptom Inventory. Cancer. 2000;89(7):1634–46.
48. Chang VT, Thaler HT, Polyak TA, Kornblith AB, Lepore JM, Portenoy RK. Quality of life and survival: the role of multidimensional symptom assessment. Cancer. 1998;83(1):173–9.
49. Chang VT, Hwang SS, Feuerman M, Kasimis BS, Thaler HT. The memorial symptom assessment scale short form (MSAS-SF). Cancer. 2000;89(5):1162–71.
50. Collins JJ, Byrnes ME, Dunkel IJ, Lapin J, Nadel T, Thaler HT, et al. The measurement of symptoms in children with cancer. J Pain Symptom Manage. 2000;19(5):363–77.
51. Collins JJ, Devine TD, Dick GS, Johnson EA, Kilham HA, Pinkerton CR, et al. The measurement of symptoms in young children with cancer: the validation of the Memorial Symptom Assessment Scale in children aged 7-12. J Pain Symptom Manage. 2002;23(1):10–6.
52. National Cancer Institute. Patient-reported outcomes version of the common terminology criteria for adverse events (PRO-CTCAE™). 2020. https://healthcaredelivery.cancer.gov/pro-ctcae/. Accessed 19 May 2020.
53. Bennett AV, Dueck AC, Mitchell SA, Mendoza TR, Reeve BB, Atkinson TM, et al. Mode equivalence and acceptability of tablet computer-, interactive voice response system-, and paper-based administration of the U.S. National Cancer Institute's patient-reported outcomes version of the common terminology criteria for adverse events (PRO-CTCAE). Health Qual Life Outcomes. 2016;14:24.
54. Thanarajasingam G, Atherton PJ, Novotny PJ, Loprinzi CL, Sloan JA, Grothey A. Longitudinal adverse event assessment in oncology clinical trials: the toxicity over time (ToxT) analysis of alliance trials NCCTG N9741 and 979254. Lancet Oncol. 2016;17(5):663–70.
55. Reeve BB, McFatrich M, Mack JW, Maurer SH, Jacobs SS, Freyer DR, et al. Validity and reliability of the pediatric patient-reported outcomes - common terminology criteria for adverse events. J Natl Cancer Inst. 2020;112:1143.
56. Parsons SK, Barlow SE, Levy SL, Supran SE, Kaplan SH. Health-related quality of life in pediatric bone marrow transplant survivors: according to whom? Int J Cancer Suppl. 1999;12:46–51.
57. Bradlyn AS, Harris CV, Spieth LE. Quality of life assessment in pediatric oncology: a retrospective review of phase III reports. Soc Sci Med. 1995;41(10):1463–5.
58. Bradlyn AS, Ritchey AK, Harris CV, Moore IM, O'Brien RT, Parsons SK, et al. Quality of life research in pediatric oncology. Research methods and barriers. Cancer. 1996;78(6):1333–9.
59. Parsons SK, Tighiouart H, Terrin N. Assessment of health-related quality of life in pediatric hematopoietic stem cell transplant recipients: progress, challenges and future directions. Expert Rev Pharmacoecon Outcomes Res. 2013;13(2):217–25.
60. Achenbach TM, Rescorla LA. Manual for the ASEBA School-Age Forms & Profiles. Burlington, VT: University of Vermont, Research Center for Children, Youth, & Families; 2001.
61. Varni JW. The PedsQL™ measurement model for the Pediatric Quality of Life Inventory™. https://www.pedsql.org/.
62. Parsons SK, Shih MC, Mayer DK, Barlow SE, Supran SE, Levy SL, et al. Preliminary psychometric evaluation of the Child Health Ratings Inventory (CHRIs) and Disease-Specific Impairment Inventory-Hematopoietic Stem Cell Transplantation (DSII-HSCT) in parents and children. Qual Life Res. 2005;14(6):1613–25.

63. Varni JW, Burwinkle TM, Katz ER, Meeske K, Dickinson P. The PedsQL in pediatric cancer: reliability and validity of the Pediatric Quality of Life Inventory Generic Core Scales, Multidimensional Fatigue Scale, and Cancer Module. Cancer. 2002;94(7):2090–106.
64. Morone JF, Mayer DK, Parsons SK. Computer animation in health related quality of life (HRQL) assessment using the Child Health Rating Inventories (CHRIs©). PRONewsletter. 2006;37:5–8.
65. Ravens-Sieberer U, Gosch A, Abel T, Auquier P, Bellach BM, Bruil J, et al. Quality of life in children and adolescents: a European public health perspective. Soz Praventivmed. 2001;46(5):294–302.
66. Cella D, Riley W, Stone A, Rothrock N, Reeve B, Yount S, et al. The Patient-Reported Outcomes Measurement Information System (PROMIS) developed and tested its first wave of adult self-reported health outcome item banks: 2005-2008. J Clin Epidemiol. 2010;63(11):1179–94.
67. HealthMeasures. PROMIS®. https://www.healthmeasures.net/explore-measurement-systems/promis.
68. Stukenborg GJ, Blackhall LJ, Harrison JH, Dillon PM, Read PW. Longitudinal patterns of cancer patient reported outcomes in end of life care predict survival. Support Care Cancer. 2016;24(5):2217–24.
69. Chapman CH. How patients lose their own voices: disparities in patient-reported outcome capture in clinical trials. 2020. https://www.cancertherapyadvisor.com/home/cancer-topics/general-oncology/healthcare-disparities-how-patients-lose-their-voice-racism-clinical-trials/. Accessed 18 Oct 2020.
70. Pugh SL, Rodgers JP, Yeager KA, Chen RC, Movsas B, Bonanni R, et al. Characteristics of Participation in Patient-Reported Outcomes and Electronic Data Capture Components of NRG Oncology Clinical Trials. Int J Radiat Oncol Biol Phys. 2020;108(4):950–9.
71. National Cancer Institute. Immunotherapy (Nivolumab or Brentuximab Vedotin) plus combination chemotherapy in treating patients with newly diagnosed stage III-IV Classic Hodgkin lymphoma. 2019. https://clinicaltrials.gov/ct2/show/NCT03907488.
72. Castellino SM, Rodday AM, Pei Q, Bush R, Keller FG, Henderson TO, et al. Performance of FACT-GOG-Ntx to assess chemotherapy-induced peripheral neuropathy (CIPN) in pediatric Hodgkin lymphoma (HL) patients. J Clin Oncol. 2019;37(15_suppl):10064.
73. National Cancer Institute. Brentuximab Vedotin and combination chemotherapy in treating children and young adults with stage IIB or stage IIIB-IVB Hodgkin lymphoma. 2014. https://clinicaltrials.gov/ct2/show/NCT02166463.
74. Berkman AM, Murphy KM, Siembida EJ, Lau N, Geng Y, Parsons SK, et al. Inclusion of patient-reported outcomes in adolescent and young adult phase III therapeutic trials: an analysis of cancer clinical trials registered on clinicaltrials.gov. Value Health. 2021;24(12):1820–7.
75. Linendoll N, Murphy-Banks R, Barthel E, Bartucca L, Boehm L, Welch M, et al. The Creation of a Comprehensive Adolescent and Young Adult Cancer Survivorship Program: "Lost in Transition" No More. J Adolesc Young Adult Oncol. 2021;10(4):397–403.
76. Henderson JR, Kiernan E, McNeer JL, Rodday AM, Spencer K, Henderson TO, et al. Patient-reported health-related quality-of-life assessment at the point-of-care with adolescents and young adults with cancer. J Adolesc Young Adult Oncol. 2018;7(1):97–102.
77. PROMIS Health Organization (PHO). PROMIS® Scale v1.2 – Global Health. 2018. https://www.healthmeasures.net/index.php?option=com_instruments&view=measure&id=778&Itemid=992. Accessed 19 Oct 2020.
78. Zebrack B, Isaacson S. Psychosocial care of adolescent and young adult patients with cancer and survivors. J Clin Oncol. 2012;30(11):1221–6.
79. Wolfe J, Orellana L, Ullrich C, Cook EF, Kang TI, Rosenberg A, et al. Symptoms and distress in children with advanced cancer: prospective patient-reported outcomes from the PediQUEST study. J Clin Oncol. 2015;33(17):1928–35.
80. Brousseau DC, Panepinto JA, Nimmer M, Hoffmann RG. The number of people with sickle-cell disease in the United States: national and state estimates. Am J Hematol. 2010;85(1):77–8.
81. Dampier CD, Smith WR, Wager CG, Kim HY, Bell MC, Miller ST, et al. IMPROVE trial: a randomized controlled trial of patient-controlled analgesia for sickle cell painful episodes: rationale, design challenges, initial experience, and recommendations for future studies. Clin Trials. 2013;10(2):319–31.
82. Dampier C, Palermo TM, Darbari DS, Hassell K, Smith W, Zempsky W. AAPT Diagnostic Criteria for Chronic Sickle Cell Disease Pain. J Pain. 2017;18(5):490–8.
83. Rotenstein LS, Huckman RS, Wagle NW. Making patients and doctors happier - the potential of patient-reported outcomes. N Engl J Med. 2017;377(14):1309–12.
84. Esham KS, Rodday AM, Smith HP, Noubary F, Weidner RA, Buchsbaum RJ, et al. Assessment of health-related quality of life among adults hospitalized with sickle cell disease vaso-occlusive crisis. Blood Adv. 2020;4(1):19–27.
85. Kelly MJ, Pennarola BW, Rodday AM, Parsons SK, Journeys to Recovery Study H-CS. Health-related quality of life (HRQL) in children with sickle cell disease and thalassemia following hematopoietic stem cell transplant (HSCT). Pediatr Blood Cancer. 2012;59(4):725–31.

# Pain Syndromes of Hematologic Malignancies

# 13

Judith A. Paice and Jonathan Moreira

## Introduction

Pain is a frequent, yet unwanted, companion of those experiencing hematologic malignancies (HM). In the past 50 years, survival rates have improved for most cancers and have doubled for multiple myeloma (MM), non-Hodgkin lymphoma, and chronic myeloid leukemia [1]. Unfortunately, pain due to the disease or its treatment is also increasing. In a large study of patients recruited from a cancer registry, 55% experienced pain in the past week and 44% of those patients reported the pain to be moderate to severe. One of the predictors for the prevalence of pain was having a HM [2]. A meta-analyses of 122 cancer studies found pain prevalence rates at 39.3% after curative treatment, 55% during treatment, and 66.4% in advanced or terminal disease [3]. In a large cohort study of older adults undergoing hematopoietic cell transplantation (HCT) for HM, 39.4% reported severe pain that impaired performance [4]. The consequences of unrelieved pain include decreased function and diminished quality of life (QOL) [5, 6].

This chapter begins by detailing the unique pain syndromes experienced as a result of HM or their treatment. Pain associated with serious blood orders is addressed in Chap. 5. Treatment of these and other HM contributes significantly to the acute and chronic pain experience, including mucositis, avascular necrosis due to corticosteroid use, and pain as a result of granulocyte colony stimulating factor administration. Graft-versus-host disease (GVHD) is a multi-organ syndrome that develops after hematopoietic cell transplantation (HCT), leading to numerous serious painful complications. To best address these many syndromes, hematologists/oncologists and other clinicians providing care for these patients, must be aware of the painful sequelae of hematologic disorders and their treatment (Table 13.1). In addition, although there are no published studies suggesting the risk of substance use disorder is different in this population when compared to others with cancer, mitigation measures must be employed to reduce the risk of misuse [7] and manage pain when patients present with opioid use disorder [8].

J. A. Paice
Division, Hematology-Oncology, Northwestern University, Feinberg School of Medicine, Chicago, IL, USA
e-mail: j-paice@northwestern.edu

J. Moreira (✉)
Division of Hematology/Oncology, Department of Medicine, Robert H. Lurie Comprehensive Cancer Center, Northwestern University Feinberg School of Medicine, Chicago, IL, USA
e-mail: Jonathan.moreira@northwestern.edu



C. K. Ullrich, E. J. Roeland (eds.), *Palliative Care in Hematologic Malignancies and Serious Blood Disorders*,
https://doi.org/10.1007/978-3-031-38058-7_13

**Table 13.1** Pain syndromes associated with hematologic malignancies

| Disease/Condition | Pain syndrome | Etiology | Treatment(s) |
|---|---|---|---|
| Multiple myeloma | Lytic bone lesions<br>– Bone pain<br>– Bone fractures | Enhanced osteoclast activity, suppressed osteoblast activity | – Osteoclast inhibitors (i.e., bisphosphonate therapy)<br>– Vertebroplasty, kyphoplasty<br>– Radiation therapy<br>– Opioids |
| Waldenstrom Macroglobulinemia | Peripheral neuropathy<br>– Paresthesias<br>– Weakness | Possibly due to anti-MAG antibodies, anti-GM1 ganglioside antibodies | – Rituximab<br>– IVIG<br>– Fludarabine |
| Essential thrombocythemia/ polycythemia Vera | Secondary erythromelalgia<br>– Painful, erythematous extremities | – Changes to arterioles related to platelet activation<br>– Proliferation of intimal cells and smooth muscle of blood vessels<br>– Thrombotic occlusions from platelet aggregation | – Aspirin<br>– Gabapentin<br>– Pregabalin<br>– Venlafaxine<br>– Misoprostol<br>– Amitriptyline |
| Myeloproliferative neoplasms (e.g., essential thrombocythemia, polycythemia vera) | Aquagenic pruritus<br>– Pain, erythema and heat of the extremities, precipitated by exercise, warm/hot water and/or physical dependency | – Possible mast cell degranulation<br>– Histamine release, fibrinolytic factors, prostaglandins may also play a role | – Aspirin<br>– Paroxetine<br>– JAK inhibitors |
| Treatment-related (i.e., in various HMs, HCT candidates) | G-CSF associated bone pain | – Possibly due to marrow expansion leading to release of pro-inflammatory cytokines peripheral nerve remodeling<br>– Histamine production edema | – Opioids<br>– Loratadine<br>+/– famotidine |
| Treatment-related (i.e., various HMs, HCT candidates) | Mucositis | Cytotoxic chemotherapy mediated breakdown of the mucosal barrier of the alimentary tract | – Parenteral analgesic therapy<br>– Oral mucosal barrier gel |

*IVIG* intravenous immunoglobulin, *HM* Hematologic malignancies, *HCT* hematopoietic cell transplant

## Disease-Related Pain Syndromes

### Plasma Cell Dyscrasias

Plasma cell dyscrasias constitute a spectrum of diseases that involve malignant proliferation of plasma cells and/or the immunoglobulins they produce. With an incidence of 7 per 100,000 men and women per year [9], multiple myeloma (MM) is among the most frequently diagnosed plasma cell neoplasms.

#### Lytic Bone Disease

In addition to the multitude of hematologic, metabolic, nephrologic, and infectious complications, skeletal fractures are among the most significant morbidities attributed to MM. Osteolytic bone lesions that occur in MM are thought to be due to the compromised bone density and integrity that results from enhanced osteoclastic activity and suppressed osteoblastic activity. As a result, 60% of all individuals with MM present with skeletal lytic lesions at the time of diagnosis, and 20% may have osteopenia at the time of diagnosis as well [10]. Although the usage of osteoclast inhibitors (i.e., bisphosphonate therapy) is essential to the prevention of skeletal lytic lesions and fractures, the management of skeletal lytic fractures requires pharmacologic and nonpharmacologic methods to ensure appropriate pain control as well as improve functionality and QOL.

Radiation therapy, used in up to 40% of patients with MM at some point of their disease course [11], is an important therapeutic modality for cord compression, plasmacytomas, and adjunct therapy for pain control when systemic analgesic therapy is insufficient [12]. Other nonpharmacologic interventions play an important role in pain management and functional restoration due to vertebral body fracture and collapse. Vertebroplasty is a procedure that involves the injection of methyl methacrylate into a collapsed vertebral body to restore its height. Kyphoplasty is a procedure wherein an inflatable bone tamp is inserted into the vertebral body. Upon inflation, the bone tamp restores the height of the vertebral body, thus creating a cavity that can be filled with methyl methacrylate. Prospective trials demonstrated improved pain control, physical and/or social functioning with these interventions [13, 14], although their efficacy has not been evaluated in a blinded, randomized clinical trial for MM. Given the fact that bone cement injected into a vertebral body with lytic lesions may lead to altered spinal biomechanics, there is a concern for paradoxically increased risk of vertebral fractures following the procedure [15].

A retrospective study among patients with MM suggests that the number of previous fractures, the number of treated vertebrae, cement volume, pedicular disease, and disc leakage are important risk factors for the development of post-vertebroplasty fractures [16]. Thus, careful consideration must be given to optimal candidates for these procedures. Systemic analgesic therapy is an important component of pain control for patients with lytic fractures related to MM.

## Waldenstrom Macroglobulinemia

### Peripheral Neuropathy

Waldenstrom macroglobulinemia (WM) is a rare HM characterized by the presence of lymphoplasmacytic lymphoma in the bone marrow and an IgM monoclonal gammopathy in the blood. With an incidence of 3 per million people, only 1400 cases are diagnosed in the US each year [17, 18]. Symptoms associated with WM are related to the infiltration of hematopoietic tissues and/or the effects of monoclonal IgM accumulation in the bloodstream. Neuropathy is present in approximately 20% of patients at the time of diagnosis of WM, and 50% of patients will develop it during the course of their disease [19]. As the median age at diagnosis is 70 years, many individuals have other chronic conditions that may also drive neuropathy, thus compounding the severity of this manifestation. The most frequent neurologic abnormality is a distal, symmetric, and slowly progressive sensorimotor peripheral neuropathy causing paresthesias and weakness [19–21]. Anti-myelin associated glycoprotein (MAG) activity is found in about half of these patients [20] and other autoantibodies, including those directed against GM1 ganglioside or asialo-GM1 ganglioside, have also been identified. Although this is believed to be an autoantibody mediated process, there is no correlation between MAG antibodies and the severity of these symptoms, and the presence of other autoantibodies is of uncertain pathogenetic significance [22].

Treatment of the underlying disease remains the mainstay of therapy for management of peripheral neuropathy associated with WM [23]. Fludarabine, an agent that has been extensively used in the management of WM, has demonstrated some efficacy in reducing WM-associated peripheral neuropathy refractory to other therapies [24]. Rituximab, a CD20 monoclonal antibody that targets the clonal population responsible for WM, has limited demonstrated efficacy in the management of WM-associated peripheral neuropathy. Small studies have demonstrated significant median reduction in anti-myelin associated glycoprotein antibody titers by 93% at 12 months, 80% at 24 months, and 60% at 36 months after rituximab. And subjective and objective increases in strength at 3 and 6 months after completion of rituximab therapy [25]. A randomized trial of rituximab also demonstrated improvement in objective measurements of disability in patients with anti-myelin associated glycoprotein /sulfated glucoronyl paragloboside antibodies and IgM monoclonal gammopathy [26]. Data demonstrating efficacy of intravenous immunoglobulin (IVIG) is limited [27]. Efficacy of IVIG may related to neutralization of anti-myelin associated glycoprotein antibodies or to an antibody response to the anti-myelin associated glycoprotein producing CD5+ cells [28].

## Myeloproliferative Neoplasms

Myeloproliferative neoplasms (MPNs) constitute a constellation of malignancies characterized by the uncontrolled proliferation of terminal myeloid cells with expansion in the peripheral blood, resulting in various combinations of erythrocytosis, leukocytosis, thrombocytosis, bone marrow hypercellularity/fibrosis, and/or splenomegaly. The vast majority of MPNs are also characterized by mutations in either the JAK2, CALR, or MPL genes [29]. MPNs include polycythemia vera (PV), essential thrombocythemia (ET), chronic myelogenous leukemia (CML), primary myelofibrosis (PMF), chronic neutrophilic leukemia, and chronic eosinophilic leukemia. The resulting excessive proliferation of myeloid cells leads to a variety of painful clinical manifestations and symptoms.

### Secondary Erythromelalgia

Secondary erythromelalgia is characterized by painful and erythematous extremities and is seen in many myeloproliferative neoplasms. The pathogenesis of secondary erythromelalgia is thought to be due to changes to arterioles related to platelet activation, proliferation of their intimal cells and smooth muscle, as well as with thrombotic occlusions secondary to platelet aggregation [30]. Additionally, prostaglandin production from the above activation leads to coagulation pathways initiation, likely causing the inflammatory nature of the condition [31, 32]. Patients with secondary erythromelalgia often present with pain, erythema, swelling, and heat of the extremities, which is often precipitated by heat, exercise, and physical dependency [30]. As with many symptoms associated with HM, treatment of the underlying disease is the primary mode of therapy.

Case reports indicate that aspiring may be efficacious in the management of secondary erythromelalgia caused by MPNs [33]. Aspirin alleviates vasomotor (microvascular) disturbances associated with ET or PV [34, 35]. Additional therapies with demonstrated benefit include gabapentin, pregabalin, venlafaxine, oral amitriptyline, and oral misoprostol [30, 36–42]. Sertraline, carbamazepine, mexiletine, diltiazem, and oral nitroprusside also reduce erythromelalgia symptoms in small numbers of patients [36, 43–47].

### Pruritus

Aquagenic pruritus (pruritus following a warm bath or shower) is a common symptom in patients with PV, presenting in as many as 68% of patients. In a sizeable minority of patients, it can be debilitating, with 15% of patients presenting with this symptom describing it as "unbearable" [48]. Although the etiology of aquagenic pruritus is unclear, it has been suggested that mast cell degranulation, as well as histamine release, fibrinolytic factors, prostaglandins, or interleukin-31 may play a role [49–52]. Alternatively, the release of adenosine diphosphate from red blood cells or catecholamines from adrenergic vasoconstrictor nerves when the skin cools might also cause platelet aggregation in skin vessels, resulting in local production of pruritogenic factors, such as prostaglandins [49]. Aspirin is therefore often used to treat aquagenic pruritus in patients with PV, although there are data demonstrating efficacy of paroxetine [53] and JAK inhibitors [54], which also play a leading role in the management of various MPNs.

## Treatment-Related Pain Syndromes

### Bone Pain Associated with Granulocyte-Stimulating Factor

Granulocyte colony stimulating factor (G-CSF) is a commonly used agent for stem cell mobilization from the bone marrow to the peripheral blood stream, particularly as HCT centers worldwide increasingly adopt this method of stem cell harvesting over harvesting directly from the bone marrow. Bone pain has been associated with use of this agent in both HCT donors and recipients of chemotherapy for a myriad of malignancies [55]. A meta-analysis demonstrated that 33–50% of patients receiving G-CSF experience any grade bone pain, with severe bone pain reported in 3–7% of patients [56]. Stem cell donors often times receive doses of G-CSF higher than those administered for neutrophil recovery following cytotoxic chemotherapy, and severity of bone pain may follow. The incidence of G-CSF-associated bone pain, particularly among healthy donors and young patients, ranges from 20 to 71% [57–59]. A retrospective analysis of 22 clinical trials using pegfilgrastim (a depot formulation of G-CSF) in 1949 patients undergoing myelosuppressive chemotherapy demonstrated moderate to severe bone pain in 28% of cases [60]. The most common sites of G-CSF associated bone pain include the back, sternum, hips, and legs [61].

The etiology of G-CSF associated bone pain remains unclear. Some literature suggests that G-CSF-associated bone pain is due to bone marrow expansion from progenitor and myeloid cell proliferation, resulting in the recruitment of monocytes and macrophages [62]. These cells are then thought to release pro-inflammatory cytokines (i.e., interleukins, tumor necrosis factor) that lead to peripheral nerve remodeling and subsequent bone pain [63]. Other potential mechanisms of G-CSF-associated bone pain include histamine production within the bone marrow and subsequent edema, increased bone resorption from osteoclast and osteoblast stimulation, and sensitization of peripheral nociceptors from afferent nerve stimulation [64, 65].

Few studies have demonstrated strong evidence for any particular agent for the effective management of G-CSF associated. A randomized, phase II study evaluated the prophylactic usage of loratadine, a long-acting tricyclic antihistamine with selective histamine $H_1$-receptor antagonistic properties, on pegfilgrastim-induced bone pain among patients receiving taxane chemotherapy [66]. In sum, 213 patients who developed significant back or leg bone pain were enrolled into the treatment stage, and randomized to either daily loratadine 10 mg or placebo for 7 days. No statistically significant decrease in the incidence of severe bone pain or improvement in QOL was seen. Despite the lack of data demonstrating efficacy, single agent loratadine is used in the management of G-CSF associated bone pain at many HCT and Cancer Centers, including our own. Preliminary data suggests a combination of loratadine and famotidine may improve G-CSF induced bone pain, but requires prospective validation [65, 67]. Naproxen (500 mg twice daily for 5–8 days) has been found to reduce the severity and incidence of G-CSF associated bone pain [68], but given the risk of platelet dysfunction, bleeding, and nephrotoxicity, its utility in HCT recipients is extremely limited, as are most NSAIDs. Although some animal models suggest that meloxicam may increase serum G-CSF [69], we do not use celecoxib or meloxicam for bone pain associated with G-CSF due to concern for the risk for platelet dysfunction and bleeding.

### Mucositis

Chemotherapy-induced mucositis is a common and well-recognized complication of cytotoxic chemotherapy. The condition is characterized by the breakdown of the mucosal barrier of the alimentary tract that leads to ulceration of the oral cavity and/or gastrointestinal (GI) tract. It is characterized histologically by increased apoptosis, villus atrophy, crypt hypoplasia and dilatation, loss of epithelium, necrosis, inflammation, and excessive mucous secretion [70, 71]. The breakdown of the mucosal barrier leads to a wide variety of symptoms and potential complications, depending on the site(s) of involvement of the alimentary tract, but may include mouth, throat and/or esophageal pain, bleeding, diarrhea, and/or infection, owing to the translocation of alimentary tract bacteria into the bloodstream. Due to likely under-reporting of this complication, it is difficult to ascertain the exact incidence of this potentially fatal and debilitating condition. Estimates as to the incidence of mucositis range from 50 to 100% [70, 72].

The currently accepted pathobiological model of mucositis, which is based on the dynamic biochemical interactions between chemotherapeutic agents and constituents of the mucosa and indirect biological signaling pathophysiologic model, developed by Sonis and colleagues, consists of five overlapping phases [70, 73]. These include (1) initiation, (2) upregulation, (3) signal amplification, (4) ulceration, and (5) healing [70, 73]. There are a myriad of genomic, microbiological, and immunological factors that likely impact the risk of individuals developing mucositis [74], but these factors have limited if any incorporation into clinical decision-making. Thus, management of mucositis is primarily focused on symptom control, with usage of antimicrobial agents only if warranted by the development of mucosal surface infection.

Topical, systemic oral or parenteral analgesic therapies, in concert with oral hygiene, may be used to achieve appropriate pain control in patients with chemotherapy-associated mucositis. Topical analgesics, such as lidocaine, are often combined with cleansing and/or coating agents for pain relief. Although there are some commercially available mixed-medication mouthwashes available, they are often compounded in individual pharmacies with varying ratios of ingredients. A systematic review of the usage of these mixed-medication mouthwashes did not demonstrate any evidence supporting the use of mixed-medication mouthwashes for the management of chemotherapy-associated mucositis [75]. The American Academy of Nursing, in conjunction with the Oncology Nursing Society, has recommended against their use, owing to this lack of efficacy and cost, in their Choosing Wisely statement [76]. Additionally, there is a concern for systemic absorption, limiting the usage of topical lidocaine. We also refrain from employing lidocaine containing oral rinses at our institution due to the concern for aspiration. Systemic oral therapies may provide an effective route for pain control, but this may be limited by severe odynophagia, often seen with mucositis. Thus, parenteral analgesic therapy, often times in the form of patient-controlled analgesia (PCA), is often required for effective pain control. PCA allows for individualized pain control and allows patients to time its use around activities that may exacerbate pain associated with mucositis, including eating, drinking, and/or swallowing medications. Morphine is recommended as the first-line PCA opioid in this situation [77], with consideration of alternative opioids, such as hydromorphone or fentanyl, for patients with renal and/or hepatic insufficiency or intolerable side effects from morphine. Additional therapies that have demonstrated efficacy in the management of mucositis include palifermin and photobiomodulation [70, 75, 78, 79].

## Avascular Necrosis

Osteonecrosis or avascular necrosis (AVN) of bone is a devastating consequence of impaired blood flow, generally due to trauma, corticosteroid use, blood dyscrasias, alcohol intake, and coagulation disorders [80]. This often affects the femoral head, leading to severe pain and in some circumstances, collapse of the femoral head. Other affected joints include the shoulder, knee, elbow, wrist, or ankle. The prevalence in children with acute lymphoblastic leukemia is 2–14%, increasing to 29% in teenagers, and 20% in young adults [81]. Risk factors appear to be higher cumulative corticosteroid dose, age over 10 years at diagnosis, and treatment with transplantation [82]. AVN had a strong negative effect on QOL in adult survivors.

A thorough history should include review of past cancer treatments, particularly corticosteroid use. Patients may report pain in the hip, with extension to the groin and/or buttock. Imaging can provide confirmation and rule out other treatable causes. Referral to an orthopedic surgeon is warranted to determine surgical options. For those patients where surgery is delayed due to immunosuppression or frailty, pain management may incorporate nonsteroidal anti-inflammatory drugs (if not contraindicated), opioid therapy, and adjuvant analgesics, such as duloxetine. Although the evidence is limited, bisphosphonates, statins, anticoagulants, and vasodilators have all been suggested to slow progression of the necrosis [80]. The use of assistive devices may reduce pain associated with weight-bearing and enhance safety due to improved stability. Smoking cessation and limiting alcohol use may prevent further damage.

## Graft-Versus-Host Disease

Graft-versus-host disease (GVHD) is a multi-organ inflammatory and/or fibrotic syndrome that develops after an allogeneic HCT. GVHD arises when immune cells from the stem cell donor (i.e., the "graft") develop alloreactivity against the host's tissues, thereby eliciting an immune-mediated reaction. GVHD is a major cause of morbidity and mortality among recipients of an allogeneic HCT. Although the incidence of GVHD depends upon the population, it often affects a significant portion of allogeneic HCT recipients. As many as 9–50% of allogeneic HCT recipients are thought to develop acute GVHD (aGVHD), and while chronic GVHD (cGVHD) occurs in approximately 40% of allogeneic HCT recipients, reported incidence rates can vary from 6 to 80%, depending on the presence of risk factors and diagnostic criteria utilized for its classification [83, 84].

## Pathophysiology of Acute Graft-Versus-Host Disease

Historically, aGvHD was classified as the onset of GVHD occurring within 100 days of allogeneic HCT. As additional data emerges regarding the pathophysiology and distinctions between aGVHD and cGVHD, the classification of the two conditions relies less on the timing of onset of symptoms and more on the pathologic characteristics along with the affected tissue. Pathologically, aGVHD is due to an inflammatory T-cell infiltrate which leads to associated tissue destruction and apoptosis. A series of factors, including the transplantation conditioning regimen, the innate immune system, and the gastrointestinal (GI) microbiome facilitate the development of an inflammatory milieu in which the donor's transplanted T cells mediate inflammation and apoptosis of the affected tissues and subsequent symptoms [85, 86]. The transplantation conditioning regimen damages the GI epithelium of the host, leading to the subsequent translocation of bacteria, which in turns precipitates inflammation mediated by the innate immune system in conjunction with T and B lymphocytes of the adaptive immune system [87]. The resulting pro-inflammatory milieu also activates antigen presenting cells that in turn prime naïve T cells to $T_h1$ and $T_h17$ differentiation, leading to expansion of T effector cells and target host tissues. Several other immune cells further enhance antigen presentation and drive differentiation into $T_h1$ and $T_h17$ effector lineages [87]. There are several other factors that are found to impact a pro-inflammatory state and subsequent tissue damage in aGVHD, including activation of JAK1, JAK2, and STAT pathways [87]. The resulting inflammation and tissue damage occur primarily in the skin, liver, and/or GI tract, manifesting as a maculopapular rash, weight loss, diarrhea, and/or hepatitis (Table 13.2).

## Pathophysiology of Chronic Graft-Versus-Host Disease

Chronic GVHD represents a complex pathophysiologic process that encompasses chronic tissue injury and inflammation (which typically occurs in acute GVHD) and the subsequent fibrotic changes that take place in the target organ (typically presenting as chronic GVHD [cGVHD]) [87]. Tissues affected by GVHD are varied; Acute GVHD (aGVHD) tends to involve the skin, liver, and the GI tract. cGVHD generally involves other tissues that are relatively acellular and fibroproliferative. Historically, cGVHD was believed to develop greater than 100 days after allogeneic H CT. While this temporal characteristic continues to be present in a substantial number of cGVHD cases, diagnosis is more reliant on the unique pathologic findings associated with chronic inflammation and the resultant fibroproliferative changes observed in affected tissues. As in aGVHD, early inflammation results from the transplant conditioning regimen and activation of donor T cells. Injury of vascular endothelial cells facilitates migration donor immune cells into a myriad of target organs. As a result, donor-derived effector T lymphocytes, B lymphocytes, and antigen presenting cells initiate an immune response against these host tissues. The depletion and functional suppression of regulatory T ($T_{reg}$) cells, coupled with thymic injury and dysfunction, lead to altered immune tolerance that fails to inhibit immune-mediated damage to host tissue(s). Aberrant repair mechanisms facilitate activation of fibroblasts, collagen deposition, and fibrosis, ultimately leading to irreversible end-organ injury and dysfunction.

Experimental studies support a three-phase model of cGVHD [87] marked by early inflammation injury, chronic inflammation and tissue injury, and aberrant tissue repair and fibrosis.

**Table 13.2** Approaches to symptomn relief for graft versus host disease

| Disease | Pain syndrome/symptom | Treatment(s) |
|---|---|---|
| Gastrointestinal GVHD | Diarrhea | Loperamide, octreotide, budesonide, beclomethasone, extracorporeal photopheresis |
| | Abdominal pain, cramping | Dicyclomine, budesonide, beclomethasone, opioids |
| | Esophageal strictures, stenosis | Budesonide, beclomethasone, endoscopic esophageal dilatation |
| Oral cavity GVHD | Oral ulcerations, xerostomia, sensitivity | Narrow band-UVB, topical corticosteroids, topical calcineurin inhibitors |
| Musculoskeletal GVHD | Decreased range of motion, joint contractures | Calcineurin inhibitors, opioids, physical medicine and rehabilitation, +/– physical therapy/occupational therapy, orthotic devices, splinting |
| | Myalgias, weakness | Opioids, systemic corticosteroids +/– calcineurin inhibitors, physical medicine and rehabilitation |
| | Decreased bone mineral density pain | Vitamin D, calcium, bisphosphonate therapy, opioids, vertebroplasty/kyphoplasty |
| | Avascular necrosis | Corticosteroid injection(s) |
| Ocular GVHD | Keratoconjunctivitis sicca, gritty foreign-body sensation, photophobia, eye redness | Lubrication artificial +/– serum tears, tetracycline antibiotics, topical cyclosporine A, punctal plugs, warm compresses +/– erythromycin ointment, contact lenses |
| Cutaneous GvHD | Maculopapular rash, loss of sweat glands, atrophy, skin tightening, joint contractures | Topical corticosteroids, topical calcineurin inhibitors, extracorporeal photopheresis, thermal physical modalities, physical medicine and rehabilitation, orthotic devices |

*GVHD* graft versus host disease

#### Early Inflammation Injury

Similar to aGVHD, early inflammation in cGVHD is initiated and sustained by the innate immune system (i.e., dendritic cells, B cells, and macrophages), signaling mechanisms, and mediators (cytokines). This early inflammation leads to activation and injury of endothelial cells, which function as a barrier between donor and recipient tissues. Host donor T cells infused with the graft also contribute to this injury/inflammation model.

#### Chronic Inflammation and Tissue Injury

Chronic inflammation and tissue injury: As donor and/or host derived immune regulatory responses are insufficient to control this early inflammation, chronic inflammation and dysregulated immunity may result. Suppressed and/or dysregulated Tregs contribute to sustained inflammation in cGvHD. The deleterious effects of early inflammation on the thymus, coupled with diminished immune regulatory functions of B cells and natural killer (NK) cells, may also contribute to a lack of immune tolerance [88] and subsequent chronic inflammation.

#### Aberrant Tissue Repair and Fibrosis

The aforementioned dysregulated immunity and aberrant tissue repair contribute to scarring and fibrosis in cGVHD [87]. Early extracellular matrix damage also activates coagulation pathways that release chemotactic factors, and macrophages are a source of transforming growth factor (TGF) beta (TGFb), TNFa, IL-1b, platelet derived growth factor (PDGF), and matric metalloproteinases, resulting in a fibrotic cascade [89]. Activated Th2 and Th17 cells promote fibrosis by secretion of IL-13 and IL-17, respectively [87]. Additionally, B-cell activation contributes auto and allo-antibody production which, in conjunction with colony stimulating factor 1 (CSF-1), further activate monocytes and macrophages to release TGFb, which in turn activates myofibroblasts and collagen production, leading to further fibrosis and scarring [90] (Fig. 13.1).

### Pharmacologic Approaches to GVHD

Pharmacologic management of both acute and chronic GVHD is focused on the immunosuppression of donor T cells. Additional information on the therapeutic options for management of aGVHD and cGVHD is included in Chap. 3. Corticosteroids usually play a leading role as a systemic therapy option. Depending on the timing of the onset of GVHD, treatment may also involve the continuation or resumption of calcineurin inhibitors, used for GVHD prophylaxis during the peri- and post-engraftment period. This next section focused on an overview of symptoms, pharmacologic and nonpharmacologic approaches to pain associated with cGVHD of select organ systems.

### Gastrointestinal GVHD

#### Symptoms

GI involvement of aGVHD may involve both the upper and lower GI tracts. Diarrhea, cramping, and/or abdominal pain are most commonly associated with lower GI GVHD, whereas nausea, vomiting, and anorexia may be more commonly associated with upper GI tract GVHD, although these symptoms may also occur together. Patients with cGVHD of the GI tract may also experience a similar constellation of symptoms, in addition to chronic diarrhea, malabsorption, weight loss, and subsequent failure to thrive. cGVHD may also result in exocrine pancreatic insufficiency, and involvement of the oral cavity, seen much more frequently with cGVHD versus aGVHD, may result in xerostomia, mouth ulcers, and dysgeusia. Additionally, cGVHD may result in esophageal webs, strictures, or stenosis, which are all pathognomonic of GI cGVHD. Radiographically, these fibrotic changes may manifest as webs, ring-like narrowing, and/or a tapering of the mid and upper esophagus. Endoscopy with tissue biopsy is required for confirmation of GI GVHD, particularly that of the lower GI tract.

#### Pharmacologic Approaches to Pain

Antidiarrheal agents play an important adjunct to therapies directed toward management of GI cGVHD, provided that a concurrent infectious process has been safely ruled out or appropriately treated. Loperamide and/or diphenoxylate/atropine (Lomotil) provide patients with important oral alternatives for diarrheal control. For those patients refractory to these antidiarrheal agents, octreotide, a somatostatin analogue, may provide additional benefit. A pilot study of 21 patients with GI aGVHD demonstrated resolution of diarrhea in 15 of 21 (71%) of participants [91]. Systemic opioids play a central role in pain associated with GI GVHD, and pancreatic enzyme replacement may be necessary in those patients with pancreatic exocrine insufficiency. Topical corticosteroids, including dexamethasone for the oral cavity, and beclomethasone, and/or budesonide, with or without systemic corticosteroids and calcineurin inhibitors, serve as important adjuncts for systemic therapy and symptom management of oral cavity and upper/lower GI tract GVHD [87, 92].

#### Nonpharmacologic Approaches

Extracorporeal photopheresis is a therapeutic modality that consists of the infusion of ultraviolet-A irradiated autologous peripheral lymphocytes that have been collected by apheresis and incubated with 8-methoxypsoralen. The mechanism of action of this therapeutic approach remains unclear, but may involve the downregulation of activated T-cell clones and possible increase of Treg cells, as has been observed in murine models [93, 94]. Although there are no randomized

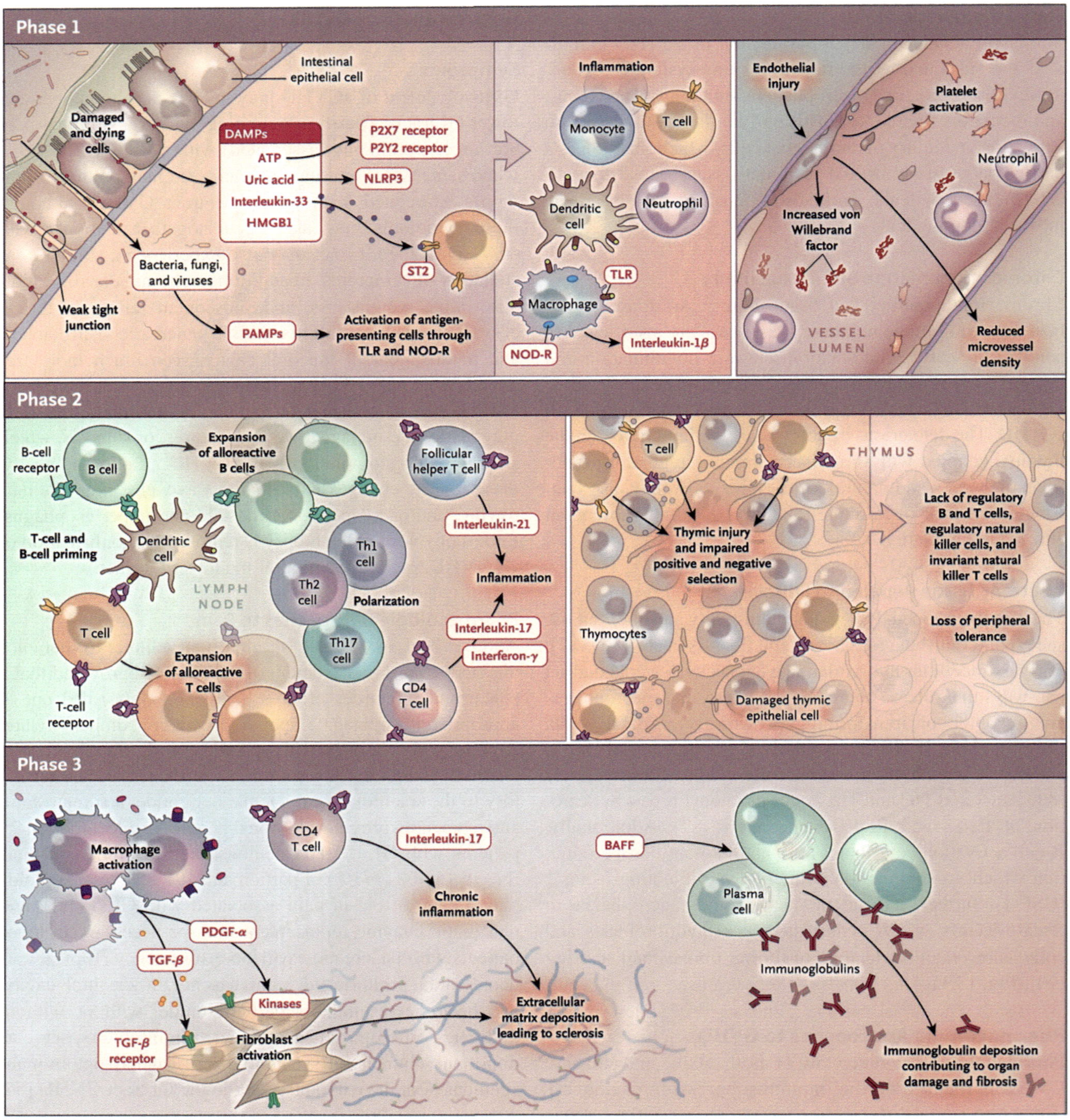


**Fig. 13.1** Chronic GVHD. (From The New England Journal of Medicine, Robert Zeiser and Bruce Blazar, Pathophysiology of Chronic Graft-versus-Host Disease and Therapeutic Targets, Vol 377, No. 26, 2020. Reprinted with permission from Massachusetts Medical Society)

clinical trials to date that have demonstrated efficacy, encouraging results have been obtained from retrospective analyses [95]. Narrow-band UV phototherapy has also been explored for the management of refractory oral cavity cGVHD. The mechanism of action appears to be a combination of factors, including interference with antigen presentation, diminished production of pro-inflammatory cytokines, and inactivation and/or suppression of T lymphocytes. A single institution, prospective study treated 11 patients with narrow-band-UVB treatments and noted at least partial improvement of xerostomia, sensitivity, and pain in 8 of 11 patients [96]. Esophageal dilatation and botulinum toxin injections can be useful adjuncts to systemic therapy for those patients with esophageal strictures, stenosis, and subsequent dysphagia and weight loss.

## Musculoskeletal GVHD

### Symptoms

Involvement of the musculoskeletal system is almost exclusively attributed to cGVHD. The hyperfibrotic changes classically associated with GVHD may have a disproportionate impact on mobility and range of motion when they impact the musculature or connective tissues. Muscles, joints, and other connective tissues may be impacted as a result. Symptoms associated with cGVHD of the joints may include decreased range of motion with resulting immobility, joint contractures, pain, and edema. This not only results in decreased mobility, but an impairment of the ability to perform activities of daily living [97]. Joints commonly involved include the wrists, shoulders, ankles, and hips, with distal joints affected first. cGVHD is an independent risk factor for joint destruction and associated pain and dysfunction [97]. Muscle mass loss and weakness are multifactorial in cGVHD, attributed to corticosteroid-induced myopathy, deconditioning from concomitant morbidities, and malnutrition. cGVHD may mimic an inflammatory myositis that is a direct, immune-mediated result of cGVHD [98]. This may often present with painful, symmetric proximal weakness with increased aldolase and creatine phosphokinase, as well as abnormal electromyography results in the proximal limbs and paraspinal muscles. As in GI GVHD, a tissue biopsy is essential for confirmation of the diagnosis [97].

Chronic corticosteroid use is well known to increase the risk of osteopenia and osteoporosis, and as many as 50% of patients who undergo an allogeneic HCT develop these conditions as a result [97, 99] . Calcineurin inhibitor usage, chemotherapy, and/or radiation therapy, gonadal dysfunction, and decreased weight-bearing activity further accentuate this risk. Bone density loss seen in HCT is typically seen more frequently in the femoral heads rather than the vertebrae, in contrast with menopausal osteoporosis [97]. These alterations in bone mineral density increase the risk of compression fractures, with subsequent immobility and pain as well as AVN of the femoral heads, which can be seen in 4–19% of allogeneic HCT recipients [97].

### Pharmacologic Approaches

Calcineurin inhibitors, in combination with systemic and/or topical corticosteroids, are the mainstays of management for musculoskeletal cGVHD. In addition to extracorporeal photopheresis, which also play an important role in the management of corticosteroid-refractory musculoskeletal GVHD (as it does in GI GVHD), there are a myriad of pharmacologic agents used in musculoskeletal cGVHD. However, an extensive review of their efficacy, risks, and benefits is beyond the scope of this chapter. Vitamin D, calcium, and bisphosphonate therapy are useful pharmacologic adjuncts for improvement of bone density and management and prevention of compression fractures. Opioid analgesics play a central role in the management of musculoskeletal GVHD. Additionally, a corticosteroid injection into a joint affected by AVN may help alleviate the inflammation and subsequent pain affecting the involved joint [97].

### Nonpharmacologic Approaches

Physical medicine and rehabilitation are central to any multidisciplinary effort to preserve and restore joint mobility, management painful joint contractures. The exact therapy is contingent on the joint(s) and/or muscle groups involved, the presence of absence of joint contractures, the presence or absence of compression fractures, and any subsequent loss of function. Passive stretching and resistance exercises may preserve muscle mass as well as prevent contractures [97]. Usage of splints and other orthotic devices, in conjunction with occupational therapy, has demonstrated efficacy in improving range of motion in patients with cGVHD and joint contractures [97]. Orthotic devices may also serve as useful adjuncts to kyphoplasty and/or vertebroplasty for management of vertebral compression fractures and require the intervention of skilled orthotists for appropriate usage of orthotic devices. Surgical intervention may be warranted when non-surgical modalities have been exhausted, including Y-V plasties, a technique in which incisions are cut and reattached in a manner to reduce tension on the resultant scar [100].

## Ocular GVHD

### Symptoms

Ocular GVHD is a term meant to encompass conjunctival disease, dry eye disease (keratoconjunctivitis sicca), and other ocular surface manifestations. Although ocular GVHD occurs primarily in the ocular surface, all parts of the eye may potentially be impacted by GVHD. Keratoconjunctivitis sicca is the most common presenting manifestation of chronic ocular GVHD. The lacrimal glands are affected and infiltrated by lymphocytes along with conjunctival inflammation, cicatricial scarring, and Meibomian gland dysfunction [101]. Researchers have also hypothesized that the conjunctiva may mimic systemic mucosal membranes, and thus serve as a target for inflammatory cell activity [102]. Although there are no distinctive symptoms that are unique to the presentation of ocular GVHD, symptoms most commonly attributed to it are analogous to typical dry eye symptoms, including dry, gritty feeling with foreign-body sensation, irritation, burning, or itching [103]. Patients may also present with eye redness, excessive tearing, blurred or fluctuating vision, photophobia, and pain along various stages of dry eye disease.

#### Pharmacologic Approaches

Treatment for ocular surface disease consists of multiple strategies, including lubrication of the ocular surface, tear preservation, prevention of tear evaporation, inflammation reduction, epithelial support, supportive care, and surgical intervention [103]. Phosphate-free and preservative-free artificial tears are the mainstays of eye lubrication. Systemic management of Meibomian gland dysfunction is addressed with oral tetracycline antibiotics such as doxycycline or minocycline, which aid in the reduction of inflammation of the Meibomian glands and subsequently improve meibum secretion and tear-film quality [103]. Azithromycin in either oral or topical form has also been demonstrated to statistically improve tear break-up time, Meibomian glad secretion, and symptoms in the treatment of posterior blepharitis [103]. Topical cyclosporine A inhibits T-cell activation, increases goblet-cell density, and downregulates release of pro-inflammatory cytokines in the conjunctiva and lacrimal gland [103, 104]. Topical corticosteroids also help alleviate conjunctival inflammation with cicatricial changes [105].

#### Nonpharmacologic Approaches

Punctal occlusion with collagen (temporary) or silicone (permanent) plugs helps preserve the tear film by inhibiting tear drainage, thus extending lubrication of the ocular surface [105]. Warm compresses twice daily, along with erythromycin ointment, may also augment Meibomian gland function. Contact lenses, frequently used in the management of several ocular surface diseases, are also used in ocular GvHD for the protection of the corneal surface and prevention of tear film evaporation [105]. Surgical intervention is often reserved for only the most severe cases of ocular GvHD where pharmacologic and other nonpharmacologic interventions have been insufficient to control complications and ophthalmologic damage from dry eye disease.

### Skin GvHD

#### Symptoms

Cutaneous involvement is the most common manifestation of cGVHD, affecting about 90–100% of patients and can result in significant impairment [106]. Cutaneous cGVHD can be further classified into two distinct anatomic subcategories, dermal and fascial, although many patients may have concurrent involvement [107]. Amongst patients with dermal cGVHD, the two typical manifestations are lichenoid and sclerodermatous. Lichenoid manifestations include a maculopapular rash that resembles lichen planus and can also affect the oral cavity and vaginal mucosa [97]. Sclerodermoid cGVHD mimics systemic sclerosis and can manifest as skin tightening, atrophy, blistering, ulceration, loss of sweat glands, and joint contracture [97]. Thus, sclerodermatous cGVHD, like musculoskeletal cGVHD, can lead to impaired mobility. This also further increases the risk of decubitus ulcers, resulting from immobility, inflammatory destruction of the skin, or the resulting shear forces of pressure, and subsequent risk for cellulitis and osteomyelitis [97]. As the presentation can range from mild to significant involvement, the severity of cGVHD is based on the extent to which skin and fascia are involved [97].

#### Pharmacologic Approaches

Topical corticosteroids, oral anti-histamines, and skin moisturizers may help alleviate pruritus and pain associated with inflammatory changes in the skin, although their efficacy may be limited to the outermost layers of skin [108]. Different corticosteroid potency formulations are considered based on the anatomic locations involved as well as severity of cGVHD. Topical calcineurin inhibitors may also be used for more severe cases. Systemic corticosteroids and calcineurin inhibitors are integral to the treatment of deeper dermal and/or fascial involvement and represent the mainstay for many advanced-stage cases of cGVHD. There are many systemic agents that are utilized or undergoing clinical trial assessment for corticosteroid-refractory cutaneous GVHD, but are beyond the scope of this chapter.

#### Nonpharmacologic Approaches

Extracorporeal photopheresis also plays an important role in the management of corticosteroid-refractory cutaneous cGVHD [108], much like other forms of GVHD. Physical medicine and rehabilitation, with usage of orthotic devices, also serve as an important adjunct to systemic and topical therapy in patients with cutaneous cGVHD, particularly those with fascial and/or sclerodermatous variants. As in musculoskeletal cGVHD, splinting and stretching have been shown to be effective in preventing skin contractures [109]. Thermal physical modalities, used to treat patients with systemic scleroderma, have not been validated in a randomized clinical trial setting among patients with cutaneous GVHD, but offer an intriguing and potentially beneficial pathway through which skin and joint contractures can be treated [97]. Intermittent ice application can alleviate pain and reduce inflammation, superficial heat can loosen bonds within collagen, and paraffin baths can heat tissues up to 1-cm deep, particularly in the hands and feet, thus allowing for the softening of collagen in deeper tissues [97]. These thermal modalities can be combined with physical/occupational therapy, stretching, orthotic devices, and systemic and topical therapies for a multimodality approach to pain and symptom control.

## Care of the Person with Substance Use Disorder

A particular challenge in caring for individuals with HM and serious blood disorders who also have persistent pain is the risk of misuse of opioids. Unfortunately, such individuals are not protected from the threat of substance misuse. And as alternate analgesics, such as nonsteroidal anti-inflammatory agents, are often contraindicated in this population, opioids may be necessary in selected circumstances. The challenge for clinicians is determining when chronic opioid therapy is warranted and safe [110].

### Pain Assessment

A thorough assessment of pain and risk factors for substance use disorder (SUD) is essential. Pain assessment, including a comprehensive history and physical exam, along with imaging and laboratory values, is directed at determining if the etiology of the pain warrants opioid use [111]. Generally, neuropathies are more effectively managed by gabapentinoids or serotonin-selective reuptake inhibitors, rather than opioids. Additionally, opioids are not indicated for pain that is, on average, mild intensity or when the pain does not interfere with function and activities of daily living. A thorough pain assessment will reveal the existence of comorbidities, such as deconditioning, that might be best approached with physical or occupational therapy [111].

### Risk Assessment

Risk assessment should be conducted during a comprehensive pain assessment and includes current or past use of substances (e.g., smoking, alcohol, cannabis, prescription opioids, illicit opioids, and other agents). Family history of substance use disorder may suggest genetic elements or environmental influences that increase risk [112]. Additionally, a history of abuse, trauma, or post-traumatic stress disorder has been shown to be a strong predictor of SUD [113].

Essential information can be obtained by review of prescription drug monitoring programs (PDMPs), which is mandatory in some states and institutions [114]. This information can reveal if there are controlled substances being prescribed by other providers [115]. Urine drug screening can confirm the intake of prescribed medications and rule out use of agents obtained illicitly [116]. Clinicians need to understand the limitations of the tests available in their setting and be aware of false positives and negatives that can occur with each type of test [117, 118].

### Mitigation

After collecting these data, the clinician stratifies risk of diversion and misuse, determines whether opioids are indicated and if it is safe to prescribe these agents [119]. Efforts to minimize risk include using multimodal pain therapies, such as optimizing adjuvant analgesics, referral to physical or occupational therapy, incorporating cognitive-behavioral approaches, and offering integrative treatments. Concomitant psychiatric illness, including anxiety, depression, and sleep disorders should be addressed. Rarely are these strategies all available within a typical oncology center. As a result, oncologists should identify professionals or programs within their institutions or communities that offer these services [120].

### Aberrant Behaviors

When aberrant behaviors occur, or when first prescribing opioids in people with risk of unsafe use, smaller supplies of medication can be provided to limit intake of unsafe amounts. Prescriptions can be written for 1 or 2 week increments and urine screening may be conducted with greater frequency. When these behaviors persist, referral to addiction providers is warranted [119].

## Conclusion

Pain associated with HM and their treatment is common and likely increasing with improved survival rates. Unrelieved pain leads to decreased function, impaired mood, diminished QOL, and in some cases, may affect the delivery of potentially curative therapies. Hematologists/oncologists caring for these patients must be aware of the unique pain syndromes experienced as a result of plasma cell dyscrasias and MPNs, as well as the treatment of these and other HM. Treatment-related painful syndromes, such as mucositis, AVN due to corticosteroid use, pain after G-CSF administration, and GVHD require careful assessment and management. Throughout this care, it is imperative to monitor for and attend to behaviors suggesting risk of opioid misuse. Knowledge of supportive pain services available in the area, including physical, cognitive-behavioral, integrative, interventional, and rehabilitative therapies, along with addiction specialists, will allow the provision of the multimodal care necessary to address these complex disorders.

## References


1. Siegel RL, Miller KD, Jemal A. Cancer statistics, 2019. CA Cancer J Clin. 2019;69:7–34.
2. Van den Beuken-Van Everdingen MH, De Rijke JM, Kessels AG, Schouten HC, Van Kleef M, Patijn J. High prevalence of pain in patients with cancer in a large population-based study in The Netherlands. Pain. 2007;132:312–20.
3. Van Den Beuken-Van Everdingen MH, Hochstenbach LM, Joosten EA, Tjan-Heijnen VC, Janssen DJ. Update on prevalence of pain in patients with cancer: systematic review and meta-analysis. J Pain Symptom Manag. 2016;51:1070–1090e9.
4. Farrukh N, Hageman L, Chen Y, Wu J, Ness E, Kung M, Francisco L, Parman M, Landier W, Arora M, Armenian S, Bhatia S, Williams GR. Pain in older survivors of hematologic malignancies after blood or marrow transplantation: a BMTSS report. Cancer. 2020;126:2003–12.
5. Boland E, Eiser C, Ezaydi Y, Greenfield DM, Ahmedzai SH, Snowden JA. Living with advanced but stable multiple myeloma: a study of the symptom burden and cumulative effects of disease and intensive (hematopoietic stem cell transplant-based) treatment on health-related quality of life. J Pain Symptom Manag. 2013;46:671–80.
6. Cohen MZ, Rozmus CL, Mendoza TR, Padhye NS, Neumann J, Gning I, Aleman A, Giralt S, Cleeland CS. Symptoms and quality of life in diverse patients undergoing hematopoietic stem cell transplantation. J Pain Symptom Manag. 2012;44:168–80.
7. Geyer HL, Gazelka H, Mesa R. How I treat pain in hematologic malignancies safely with opioid therapy. Blood. 2020;135:2354–64.
8. Loren AW. Harder to treat than leukemia—opioid use disorder in survivors of cancer. N Engl J Med. 2018;379:2485–7.
9. Kyle RA, Therneau TM, Rajkumar SV, Larson DR, Plevak MF, Melton LJ 3rd. Incidence of multiple myeloma in Olmsted County, Minnesota: trend over 6 decades. Cancer. 2004;101:2667–74.
10. Post TW, Rutgeerts P, Grover S, editors. Multiple myeloma: treatment of complications. Waltham: UpToDate; 2020.
11. Featherstone C, Delaney G, Jacob S, Barton M. Estimating the optimal utilization rates of radiotherapy for hematologic malignancies from a review of the evidence: part II-leukemia and myeloma. Cancer. 2005;103:393–401.
12. Mark D, Gilbo P, Meshrekey R, Ghaly M. Local radiation therapy for palliation in patients with multiple myeloma of the spine. Front Oncol. 2019;9:601.
13. Dudeney S, Lieberman IH, Reinhardt MK, Hussein M. Kyphoplasty in the treatment of osteolytic vertebral compression fractures as a result of multiple myeloma. J Clin Oncol. 2002;20:2382–7.
14. Fourney DR, Schomer DF, Nader R, Chlan-Fourney J, Suki D, Ahrar K, Rhines LD, Gokaslan ZL. Percutaneous vertebroplasty and kyphoplasty for painful vertebral body fractures in cancer patients. J Neurosurg. 2003;98:21–30.
15. Legroux-Gerot I, Lormeau C, Boutry N, Cotten A, Duquesnoy B, Cortet B. Long-term follow-up of vertebral osteoporotic fractures treated by percutaneous vertebroplasty. Clin Rheumatol. 2004;23:310–7.
16. Rocha Romero A, Hernandez-Porras BC, Plancarte-Sanchez R, Espinoza-Zamora JR, Carvajal G, Ramos Nataren RG, De Los Reyes Pacheco VA, Salazar Carrera IH. Risk of new fractures in vertebroplasty for multiple myeloma. A retrospective study, vol. 21. Pain Med; 2020. p. 3018.
17. Groves FD, Travis LB, Devesa SS, Ries LA, Fraumeni JF Jr. Waldenstrom's macroglobulinemia: incidence patterns in the United States, 1988–1994. Cancer. 1998;82:1078–81.
18. Fonseca R, Hayman S. Waldenstrom macroglobulinaemia. Br J Haematol. 2007;138:700–20.
19. Baehring JM, Hochberg EP, Raje N, Ulrickson M, Hochberg FH. Neurological manifestations of Waldenstrom macroglobulinemia. Nat Clin Pract Neurol. 2008;4:547–56.
20. Nobile-Orazio E, Marmiroli P, Baldini L, Spagnol G, Barbieri S, Moggio M, Polli N, Polli E, Scarlato G. Peripheral neuropathy in macroglobulinemia: incidence and antigen-specificity of M proteins. Neurology. 1987;37:1506–14.
21. Rudnicki SA, Harik SI, Dhodapkar M, Barlogie B, Eidelberg D. Nervous system dysfunction in Waldenstrom's macroglobulinemia: response to treatment. Neurology. 1998;51:1210–3.
22. Ansell SM. Epidemiology, pathogenesis, clinical manifestations, and diagnosis of Waldenstrom macroglobulinemia. Waltham: UpToDate; 2021.
23. Chaudhry HM, Mauermann ML, Rajkumar SV. Monoclonal gammopathy-associated peripheral neuropathy: diagnosis and management. Mayo Clin Proc. 2017;92:838–50.
24. Wilson HC, Lunn MP, Schey S, Hughes RA. Successful treatment of IgM paraproteinaemic neuropathy with fludarabine. J Neurol Neurosurg Psychiatry. 1999;66:575–80.
25. Levine TD, Pestronk A. IgM antibody-related polyneuropathies: B-cell depletion chemotherapy using rituximab. Neurology. 1999;52:1701–4.
26. Dalakas MC, Rakocevic G, Salajegheh M, Dambrosia JM, Hahn AF, Raju R, McElroy B. Placebo-controlled trial of rituximab in IgM anti-myelin-associated glycoprotein antibody demyelinating neuropathy. Ann Neurol. 2009;65:286–93.
27. Ellie E, Vital A, Steck A, Boiron JM, Vital C, Julien J. Neuropathy associated with "benign" anti-myelin-associated glycoprotein IgM gammopathy: clinical, immunological, neurophysiological pathological findings and response to treatment in 33 cases. J Neurol. 1996;243:34–43.
28. Gertz MA, Greipp PR. Hematologic malignancies: multiple myeloma and related plasma cell disorders. Berlin: Springer; 2003.
29. Dickstein JI, Vardiman JW. Hematopathologic findings in the myeloproliferative disorders. Semin Oncol. 1995;22:355–73.
30. Mann N, King T, Murphy R. Review of primary and secondary erythromelalgia. Clin Exp Dermatol. 2019;44:477–82.
31. Michiels JJ, Abels J, Steketee J, van Vliet HH, Vuzevski VD. Erythromelalgia caused by platelet-mediated arteriolar inflammation and thrombosis in thrombocythemia. Ann Intern Med. 1985;102:466–71.
32. Michiels JJ, Van Joost T. Erythromelalgia and thrombocythemia: a causal relation. J Am Acad Dermatol. 1990;22:107–11.
33. Krishnan SG, Yesudian DP, Jayaraman M, Janaki VR, Raj BJ. Erythromelalgia responding to aspirin. Indian J Dermatol Venereol Leprol. 1996;62:204–5.
34. Michiels JJ, Berneman Z, Schroyens W, Koudstaal PJ, Lindemans J, Neumann HM, Van Vliet HH. Platelet-mediated erythromelalgic, cerebral, ocular and coronary microvascular ischemic and thrombotic manifestations in patients with essential thrombocythemia and polycythemia vera: a distinct aspirin-responsive and coumadin-resistant arterial thrombophilia. Platelets. 2006;17:528–44.
35. Tefferi A, Barbui T. Polycythemia vera and essential thrombocythemia: 2019 update on diagnosis, risk-stratification and management. Am J Hematol. 2019;94:133–43.
36. Natkunarajah J, Atherton D, Elmslie F, Mansour S, Mortimer P. Treatment with carbamazepine and gabapentin of a patient with primary erythermalgia (erythromelalgia) identified to have a mutation in the SCN9A gene, encoding a voltage-gated sodium channel. Clin Exp Dermatol. 2009;34:e640–2.
37. Davis MD, Rooke T. Erythromelalgia. Curr Treat Options Cardiovasc Med. 2002;4:207–22.
38. Dicaudo DJ, Kelley LA. Alleviation of erythromelalgia with venlafaxine. Arch Dermatol. 2004;140:621–3.

39. Mork C, Salerud EG, Asker CL, Kvernebo K. The prostaglandin E1 analog misoprostol reduces symptoms and microvascular arteriovenous shunting in erythromelalgia—a double-blind, crossover, placebo-compared study. J Invest Dermatol. 2004;122:587–93.
40. Herskovitz S, Loh F, Berger AR, Kucherov M. Erythromelalgia: association with hereditary sensory neuropathy and response to amitriptyline. Neurology. 1993;43:621–2.
41. Kakizaki A, Fujimura T, Kambayashi Y, Watabe A, Aiba S. Successful treatment of adult-onset erythromelalgia with steroid pulse and pregabalin. Case Rep Dermatol. 2012;4:242–6.
42. Kalava K, Roberts C, Adair JD, Raman V. Response of primary erythromelalgia to pregabalin therapy. J Clin Rheumatol. 2013;19:284–5.
43. Rudikoff D, Jaffe IA. Erythromelalgia: response to serotonin reuptake inhibitors. J Am Acad Dermatol. 1997;37:281–3.
44. Kuhnert SM, Phillips WJ, Davis MD. Lidocaine and mexiletine therapy for erythromelalgia. Arch Dermatol. 1999;135:1447–9.
45. Nathan A, Rose JB, Guite JW, Hehir D, Milovcich K. Primary erythromelalgia in a child responding to intravenous lidocaine and oral mexiletine treatment. Pediatrics. 2005;115:e504–7.
46. Fischer TZ, Gilmore ES, Estacion M, Eastman E, Taylor S, Melanson M, Dib-Hajj SD, Waxman SG. A novel Nav1.7 mutation producing carbamazepine-responsive erythromelalgia. Ann Neurol. 2009;65:733–41.
47. Cregg R, Cox JJ, Bennett DL, Wood JN, Werdehausen R. Mexiletine as a treatment for primary erythromelalgia: normalization of biophysical properties of mutant L858F NaV 1.7 sodium channels. Br J Pharmacol. 2014;171:4455–63.
48. Siegel FP, Tauscher J, Petrides PE. Aquagenic pruritus in polycythemia vera: characteristics and influence on quality of life in 441 patients. Am J Hematol. 2013;88:665–9.
49. Fjellner B, Hagermark O. Pruritus in polycythemia vera: treatment with aspirin and possibility of platelet involvement. Acta Dermato Venereol. 1979;59:505–12.
50. Ishii T, Wang J, Zhang W, Mascarenhas J, Hoffman R, Dai Y, Wisch N, Xu M. Pivotal role of mast cells in pruritogenesis in patients with myeloproliferative disorders. Blood. 2009;113:5942–50.
51. Steinman HK, Kobza-Black A, Lotti TM, Brunetti L, Panconesi E, Greaves MW. Polycythaemia rubra vera and water-induced pruritus: blood histamine levels and cutaneous fibrinolytic activity before and after water challenge. Br J Dermatol. 1987;116:329–33.
52. Jackson N, Burt D, Crocker J, Boughton B. Skin mast cells in polycythaemia vera: relationship to the pathogenesis and treatment of pruritus. Br J Dermatol. 1987;116:21–9.
53. Tefferi A, Fonseca R. Selective serotonin reuptake inhibitors are effective in the treatment of polycythemia vera-associated pruritus. Blood. 2002;99:2627.
54. Pardanani A, Vannucchi AM, Passamonti F, Cervantes F, Barbui T, Tefferi A. JAK inhibitor therapy for myelofibrosis: critical assessment of value and limitations. Leukemia. 2011;25:218–25.
55. Lieschke GJ, Burgess AW. Granulocyte colony-stimulating factor and granulocyte-macrophage colony-stimulating factor. N Engl J Med. 1992;327:28–35.
56. Gregory SA. Evaluation of reported bone pain in cancer patients receiving chemotherapy in pegfilgrastim clinical trials: a retrospective analysis. Commun Oncol. 2010;7:297–308.
57. Crawford J, Ozer H, Stoller R, Johnson D, Lyman G, Tabbara I, Kris M, Grous J, Picozzi V, Rausch G, et al. Reduction by granulocyte colony-stimulating factor of fever and neutropenia induced by chemotherapy in patients with small-cell lung cancer. N Engl J Med. 1991;325:164–70.
58. Heil G, Hoelzer D, Sanz MA, Lechner K, Liu Yin JA, Papa G, Noens L, Szer J, Ganser A, O'Brien C, Matcham J, Barge A. A randomized, double-blind, placebo-controlled, phase III study of filgrastim in remission induction and consolidation therapy for adults with de novo acute myeloid leukemia. The International Acute Myeloid Leukemia Study Group. Blood. 1997;90:4710–8.
59. Vogel CL, Wojtukiewicz MZ, Carroll RR, Tjulandin SA, Barajas-Figueroa LJ, Wiens BL, Neumann TA, Schwartzberg LS. First and subsequent cycle use of pegfilgrastim prevents febrile neutropenia in patients with breast cancer: a multicenter, double-blind, placebo-controlled phase III study. J Clin Oncol. 2005;23:1178–84.
60. Xu H, Gong Q, Vogl FD, Reiner M, Page JH. Risk factors for bone pain among patients with cancer receiving myelosuppressive chemotherapy and pegfilgrastim. Support Care Cancer. 2016;24:723–30.
61. Karlsson L, Quinlan D, Guo D, Brown C, Selinger S, Klassen J, Russell JA. Mobilized blood cells vs bone marrow harvest: experience compared in 171 donors with particular reference to pain and fatigue. Bone Marrow Transplant. 2004;33:709–13.
62. Ma JD, El-Jawahri AR, TW LB, Roeland EJ. Pain syndromes and management in adult hematopoietic stem cell transplantation. Hematol Oncol Clin N Am. 2018;32:551–67.
63. Bennett A. The role of biochemical mediators in peripheral nociception and bone pain. Cancer Surv. 1988;7:55–67.
64. Lambertini M, del Mastro L, Bellodi A, Pronzato P. The five "Ws" for bone pain due to the administration of granulocyte-colony stimulating factors (G-CSFs). Crit Rev Oncol Hematol. 2014;89:112–28.
65. Moore DC, Pellegrino AE. Pegfilgrastim-induced bone pain: a review on incidence, risk factors, and evidence-based management. Ann Pharmacother. 2017;51:797–803.
66. Moukharskaya J, Abrams DM, Ashikaga T, Khan F, Schwartz J, Wilson K, Verschraegen C, Openshaw T, Valentine J, Eneman J, Unger P, Ades S. Randomized phase II study of loratadine for the prevention of bone pain caused by pegfilgrastim. Support Care Cancer. 2016;24:3085–93.
67. Gavioli E, Abrams M. Prevention of granulocyte-colony stimulating factor (G-CSF) induced bone pain using double histamine blockade. Support Care Cancer. 2017;25:817–22.
68. Kirshner JJ, Heckler CE, Janelsins MC, Dakhil SR, Hopkins JO, Coles C, Morrow GR. Prevention of pegfilgrastim-induced bone pain: a phase III double-blind placebo-controlled randomized clinical trial of the university of Rochester cancer center clinical community oncology program research base. J Clin Oncol. 2012;30:1974–9.
69. Hofer M, Pospíšil M, Znojil V, Holá J, Vacek A, Štreitová D. Meloxicam, an inhibitor of cyclooxygenase-2, increases the level of serum G-CSF and might be usable as an auxiliary means in G-CSF therapy. Physiol Res. 2008;57:307–10.
70. Van Sebille YZ, Stansborough R, Wardill HR, Bateman E, Gibson RJ, Keefe DM. Management of mucositis during chemotherapy: from pathophysiology to pragmatic therapeutics. Curr Oncol Rep. 2015;17:50.
71. Gibson RJ, Bowen JM, Inglis MR, Cummins AG, Keefe DM. Irinotecan causes severe small intestinal damage, as well as colonic damage, in the rat with implanted breast cancer. J Gastroenterol Hepatol. 2003;18:1095–100.
72. Benson AB III, Ajani JA, Catalano RB, Engelking C, Kornblau SM, Martenson JA Jr, McCallum R, Mitchell EP, O'Dorisio TM, Vokes EE, Wadler S. Recommended guidelines for the treatment of cancer treatment-induced diarrhea. J Clin Oncol. 2004;22:2918–26.
73. Sonis ST. The pathobiology of mucositis. Nat Rev Cancer. 2004;4:277–84.
74. Bachour PC, Sonis ST. Predicting mucositis risk associated with cytotoxic cancer treatment regimens: rationale, complexity, and challenges. Curr Opin Support Palliat Care. 2018;12:198–210.
75. McGuire DB, Fulton JS, Park J, Brown CG, Correa ME, Eilers J, Elad S, Gibson F, Oberle-Edwards LK, Bowen J, Lalla RV, Mucositis Study Group of the Multinational Association

of Supportive Care in Cancer/International Society of Oral, Oncology (MASCC/ISOO). Systematic review of basic oral care for the management of oral mucositis in cancer patients. Support Care Cancer. 2013;21:3165–77.
76. American Academy of Nursing. Twenty-five things nurses and patients should question. 2018. https://www.choosingwisely.org/societies/american-academy-of-nursing/. Accessed 31 Aug 2021.
77. Coda BA, O'Sullivan B, Donaldson G, Bohl S, Chapman CR, Shen DD. Comparative efficacy of patient-controlled administration of morphine, hydromorphone, or sufentanil for the treatment of oral mucositis pain following bone marrow transplantation. Pain. 1997;72:333–46.
78. Bensadoun RJ. Photobiomodulation or low-level laser therapy in the management of cancer therapy-induced mucositis, dermatitis and lymphedema. Curr Opin Oncol. 2018;30:226–32.
79. McDonnell AM, Lenz KL. Palifermin: role in the prevention of chemotherapy- and radiation-induced mucositis. Ann Pharmacother. 2007;41:86–94.
80. Cohen-Rosenblum A, Cui Q. Osteonecrosis of the femoral head. Orthop Clin N Am. 2019;50:139–49.
81. Patel B, Richards SM, Rowe JM, Goldstone AH, Fielding AK. High incidence of avascular necrosis in adolescents with acute lymphoblastic leukaemia: a UKALL XII analysis. Leukemia. 2008;22:308–12.
82. Girard P, Auquier P, Barlogis V, Contet A, Poiree M, Demeocq F, Berbis J, Herrmann I, Villes V, Sirvent N, Kanold J, Chastagner P, Chambost H, Plantaz D, Michel G. Symptomatic osteonecrosis in childhood leukemia survivors: prevalence, risk factors and impact on quality of life in adulthood. Haematologica. 2013;98:1089–97.
83. Carlens S, Ringden O, Remberger M, Lönnqvist B, Hägglund H, Klaesson S, Mattsson J, Svahn BM, Winiarski J, Ljungman P, Aschan J. Risk factors for chronic graft-versus-host disease after bone marrow transplantation: a retrospective single centre analysis. Bone Marrow Transplant. 1998;22:755–61.
84. Filipovich AH, Weisdorf D, Pavletic S, Socie G, Wingard JR, Lee SJ, Martin P, Chien J, Przepiorka D, Couriel D, Cowen EW, Dinndorf P, Farrell A, Hartzman R, Henslee-Downey J, Jacobsohn D, McDonald G, Mittleman B, Rizzo JD, Robinson M, Schubert M, Schultz K, Shulman H, Turner M, Vogelsang G, Flowers ME. National Institutes of Health consensus development project on criteria for clinical trials in chronic graft-versus-host disease: I. Diagnosis and staging working group report. Biol Blood Marrow Transplant. 2005;11:945–56.
85. Jenq RR, Ubeda C, Taur Y, Menezes CC, Khanin R, Dudakov JA, Liu C, West ML, Singer NV, Equinda MJ, Gobourne A, Lipuma L, Young LF, Smith OM, Ghosh A, Hanash AM, Goldberg JD, Aoyama K, Blazar BR, Pamer EG, van den Brink MR. Regulation of intestinal inflammation by microbiota following allogeneic bone marrow transplantation. J Exp Med. 2012;209:903–11.
86. Mathewson ND, Jenq R, Mathew AV, Koenigsknecht M, Hanash A, Toubai T, Oravecz-Wilson K, Wu SR, Sun Y, Rossi C, Fujiwara H, Byun J, Shono Y, Lindemans C, Calafiore M, Schmidt TM, Honda K, Young VB, Pennathur S, van den Brink M, Reddy P. Gut microbiome-derived metabolites modulate intestinal epithelial cell damage and mitigate graft-versus-host disease. Nat Immunol. 2016;17:505–13.
87. Cooke KR, Luznik L, Sarantopoulos S, Hakim FT, Jagasia M, Fowler DH, van den Brink MR, Hansen JA, Parkman R, Miklos DB, Martin PJ, Paczesny S, Vogelsang G, Pavletic S, Ritz J, Schultz KR, Blazar BR. The biology of chronic graft-versus-host disease: a task force report from the National Institutes of Health consensus development project on criteria for clinical trials in chronic graft-versus-host disease. Biol Blood Marrow Transplant. 2017;23:211–34.
88. Sakoda Y, Hashimoto D, Asakura S, Takeuchi K, Harada M, Tanimoto M, Teshima T. Donor-derived thymic-dependent T cells cause chronic graft-versus-host disease. Blood. 2007;109:1756–64.
89. Wynn TA, Ramalingam TR. Mechanisms of fibrosis: therapeutic translation for fibrotic disease. Nat Med. 2012;18:1028–40.
90. Alexander KA, Flynn R, Lineburg KE, Kuns RD, Teal BE, Olver SD, Lor M, Raffelt NC, Koyama M, Leveque L, Le Texier L, Melino M, Markey KA, Varelias A, Engwerda C, Serody JS, Janela B, Ginhoux F, Clouston AD, Blazar BR, Hill GR, MacDonald KP. CSF-1-dependant donor-derived macrophages mediate chronic graft-versus-host disease. J Clin Invest. 2014;124:4266–80.
91. Ippoliti C, Neumann J. Octreotide in the management of diarrhea induced by graft versus host disease. Oncol Nurs Forum. 1998;25:873–8.
92. Hockenbery DM, Cruickshank S, Rodell TC, Gooley T, Schuening F, Rowley S, David D, Brunvand M, Berryman B, Abhyankar S, Bouvier M, McDonald GB. A randomized, placebo-controlled trial of oral beclomethasone dipropionate as a prednisone-sparing therapy for gastrointestinal graft-versus-host disease. Blood. 2007;109:4557–63.
93. Gatza E, Rogers CE, Clouthier SG, Lowler KP, Tawara I, Liu C, Reddy P, Ferrara JL. Extracorporeal photopheresis reverses experimental graft-versus-host disease through regulatory T cells. Blood. 2008;112:1515–21.
94. Setterblad N, Garban F, Weigl R, Assier E, Drillat P, Charron D, Dickinson A, Greinix H, Mooney N. Extracorporeal photophoresis increases sensitivity of monocytes from patients with graft-versus-host disease to HLA-DR-mediated cell death. Transfusion. 2008;48:169–77.
95. Jagasia M, Greinix H, Robin M, Das-Gupta E, Jacobs R, Savani BN, Engelhardt BG, Kassim A, Worel N, Knobler R, Russell N, Socie G. Extracorporeal photopheresis versus anticytokine therapy as a second-line treatment for steroid-refractory acute GVHD: a multicenter comparative analysis. Biol Blood Marrow Transplant. 2013;19:1129–33.
96. Treister N, Li S, Lerman MA, Lee S, Soiffer R. Narrow-band UVB phototherapy for management of oral chronic graft-versus-host disease. Photodermatol Photoimmunol Photomed. 2015;31:75–82.
97. Smith SR, Haig AJ, Couriel DR. Musculoskeletal, neurologic, and cardiopulmonary aspects of physical rehabilitation in patients with chronic graft-versus-host disease. Biol Blood Marrow Transplant. 2015;21:799–808.
98. Stevens AM, Sullivan KM, Nelson JL. Polymyositis as a manifestation of chronic graft-versus-host disease. Rheumatology (Oxford). 2003;42:34–9.
99. McClune BL, Polgreen LE, Burmeister LA, Blaes AH, Mulrooney DA, Burns LJ, Majhail NS. Screening, prevention and management of osteoporosis and bone loss in adult and pediatric hematopoietic cell transplant recipients. Bone Marrow Transplant. 2011;46:1–9.
100. Kim JB, Liakopoulou E, Watson JS. Successful treatment of refractory joint contractures caused by sclerodermatous graft versus host disease. J Plast Reconstr Aesthet Surg. 2008;61:1235–8.
101. Munir SZ, Aylward J. A review of ocular graft-versus-host disease. Optometry Vis Sci. 2017;94:545–55.
102. Na KS, Yoo YS, Mok JW, Lee JW, Joo CK. Incidence and risk factors for ocular GVHD after allogeneic hematopoietic stem cell transplantation. Bone Marrow Transplant. 2015;50:1459–64.
103. Dietrich-Ntoukas T, Cursiefen C, Westekemper H, Eberwein P, Reinhard T, Bertz H, Nepp J, Lawitschka A, Heiligenhaus A, Seitz B, Messmer E, Meyer-Ter-Vehn T, Basara N, Greinix H, Datiles MB, Lee SJ, Pavletic SZ, Wolff D. Diagnosis and treatment of ocular chronic graft-versus-host disease: report from the German–Austrian–Swiss consensus conference on clinical practice in chronic GVHD. Cornea. 2012;31:299–310.
104. Hessen M, Akpek EK. Ocular graft-versus-host disease. Curr Opin Allergy Clin Immunol. 2012;12:540–7.

105. Townley JR, Dana R, Jacobs DS. Keratoconjunctivitis sicca manifestations in ocular graft versus host disease: pathogenesis, presentation, prevention, and treatment. Semin Ophthalmol. 2011;26:251–60.
106. Johnson ML, Farmer ER. Graft-versus-host reactions in dermatology. J Am Acad Dermatol. 1998;38:369–92.
107. Janin A, Socie G, Devergie A, Aractingi S, Esperou H, Verola O, Gluckman E. Fasciitis in chronic graft-versus-host disease. A clinicopathologic study of 14 cases. Ann Intern Med. 1994;120:993–8.
108. Strong Rodrigues K, Oliveira-Ribeiro C, de Abreu Fiuza Gomes S, Knobler R. Cutaneous graft-versus-host disease: diagnosis and treatment. Am J Clin Dermatol. 2018;19:33–50.
109. Choi IS, Jang IS, Han JY, Kim JH, Lee SG. Therapeutic experience on multiple contractures in sclerodermoid chronic graft versus host disease. Support Care Cancer. 2009;17:851–5.
110. Paice JA. Cancer pain management and the opioid crisis in America: how to preserve hard-earned gains in improving the quality of cancer pain management. Cancer. 2018a;124:2491.
111. Swarm RA, Paice JA, Anghelescu DL, Are M, Bruce JY, Buga S, Chwistek M, Cleeland C, Craig D, Gafford E, Greenlee H, Hansen E, Kamal AH, Kamdar MM, Legrand S, Mackey S, Mcdowell MR, Moryl N, Nabell LM, Nesbit S, BCPS, O'Connor N, Rabow MW, Rickerson E, Shatsky R, Sindt J, Urba SG, Youngwerth JM, Hammond LJ, Gurski LA. Adult cancer pain, version 3.2019, NCCN clinical practice guidelines in oncology. J Natl Compr Cancer Netw. 2019;17:977–1007.
112. Peck KR, Harman JL, Anghelescu DL. Family and peer-group substance abuse as a risk-factor for opioid misuse behaviors for a young adult with cancer-related pain—a case study. J Adolesc Young Adult Oncol. 2018;7:137–40.
113. Paice JA. Risk assessment and monitoring of patients with cancer receiving opioid therapy. Oncologist. 2019b;24:1294–8.
114. Paice JA. Navigating cancer pain management in the midst of the opioid epidemic. Oncology (Williston Park). 2018b;32:386–90.
115. Pardo B. Do more robust prescription drug monitoring programs reduce prescription opioid overdose? Addiction. 2017;112:1773–83.
116. Rauenzahn S, Sima A, Cassel B, Noreika D, Gomez TH, Ryan L, Wolf CE, Legakis L, Del Fabbro E. Urine drug screen findings among ambulatory oncology patients in a supportive care clinic. Support Care Cancer. 2017;25:1859–64.
117. Christo PJ, Manchikanti L, Ruan X, Bottros M, Hansen H, Solanki DR, Jordan AE, Colson J. Urine drug testing in chronic pain. Pain Physician. 2011;14:123–43.
118. Arthur JA. Urine drug testing in cancer pain management. Oncologist. 2020;25:99–104.
119. Paice JA, Portenoy R, Lacchetti C, Campbell T, Cheville A, Citron M, Constine LS, Cooper A, Glare P, Keefe F, Koyyalagunta L, Levy M, Miaskowski C, Otis-Green S, Sloan P, Bruera E. Management of chronic pain in survivors of adult cancers: American Society of Clinical Oncology clinical practice guideline. J Clin Oncol. 2016;34:3325–45.
120. Paice JA. Pain in cancer survivors: how to manage. Curr Treat Options Oncol. 2019;20:48.

# Symptoms in Advanced Hematologic Malignancies and Other Serious Hematologic Conditions

# 14

Mellar Davis, Carlos Fernandez, Nicki Vithalani, Lauren Elizabeth Nicholls, and Glen Digwood

## Introduction

Symptoms are more frequent than volunteered by patients with cancer. In a study of over 200 patients assessed with a 48-symptom question survey, the median number of volunteered symptoms was 1 (range of 0–6), but with assessment as many as 10 symptoms were present (range 0–25) [1]. Those symptoms that were not volunteered were often distressful to patients. For example, in this study, 69% of 522 severe symptoms and 79% of 1393 distressing symptoms detected by systematic assessment were not volunteered. Fatigue was the most common symptom that patients marked on the symptom checklist, but pain was the most volunteered symptom [1]. This study illustrates the importance of a systematic symptom assessment tool which should be used on a regular basis during a patient's cancer trajectory.

The Edmonton Symptom Assessment Scale (ESAS), which is the most common symptom assessment tool used internationally, assesses 9 symptoms and symptom burden. It has established psychometrics and minimally important clinical changes established within its 0 to 10 numerical rating for each symptom [2–8]. The ESAS can be easily completed by patients with a minimum of question burden. The Memorial Symptom Assessment-Short Form (MSAS-SF) [9] and Condensed Memorial Symptom Assessment Scale (CMSAS) questionnaires [9] scores correlate with prognosis and overall survival and can be used for planning palliative care (PC) services [10]. An abbreviated Pediatric Quality of Life and Evaluation of Symptoms Technology Memorial Symptom Assessment Scale was electronically administered in a cohort of children undergoing hematopoietic cellular transplants (HCT). Eliciting symptoms electronically improved nurses' understanding of symptoms and promoted timely assessment [11]. A patient-centered myeloma specific Myeloma Patient Outcome Scale (MyPOS) has been developed to assess and monitor symptoms and supportive care factors in routine care and has been translated into German allowing for international assessment of treatment responses [12]. A systematic review of randomized controlled trials with a patient-related outcome conducted in patients with leukemia and myelodysplastic syndromes has been published. Collecting patient-related outcomes was both feasible and provided unique information which facilitated decision-making [13]. The use of symptom tools by oncologists, therefore, should be intrinsic to their practice and is as relevant and important as measuring tumor by RECIST criteria, blood counts, light-chain levels in myeloma, and bone marrow and cytogenetic responses in leukemia.

This chapter will cover both common and uncommon non-pain symptoms associated with malignancies. Fatigue and cachexia are relatively common. Both can be caused by the underlying malignancy or the treatment of the cancer. Nausea and vomiting have usually been associated with the treatment of cancer, and there are well established protocol guidelines for managing chemotherapy-induced nausea and vomiting (CINV). CINV specific to patients with hematologic malignancies (HM) will be reviewed briefly, but the

M. Davis (✉)
Department of Palliative Care, Geisinger Medical Center, Danville, PA, USA
e-mail: mdavis2@geisinger.edu

C. Fernandez
Department of Palliative Medicine, Geisinger Medical Center, Danville, PA, USA
e-mail: cfernandez1@geisinger.edu

N. Vithalani
Department of Palliative Medicine, Geisinger Lewistown Hospital, Lewistown, PA, USA
e-mail: nvrao@geisinger.edu

L. E. Nicholls
Department of Palliative Care, Geisinger Community Medical Center, Scranton, PA, USA
e-mail: lnicholls@geisinger.edu

G. Digwood
Department of Palliative Medicine, Geisinger Community Medical Center, Scranton, PA, USA
e-mail: gdigwood@geisinger.edu


C. K. Ullrich, E. J. Roeland (eds.), *Palliative Care in Hematologic Malignancies and Serious Blood Disorders*,
https://doi.org/10.1007/978-3-031-38058-7_14

focus will be on nausea unrelated to treatment. Mucositis, hiccups, and pruritus do not appear on the ESAS but are important symptoms to address when they occur. Dyspnea, delirium, and depression are major symptoms which both impair a patient's quality of life (QOL) and have prognostic value [14–17].

## Fatigue

Fatigue is a multidimensional concept (i.e., physical, cognitive, affective, spiritual, psychosocial, and environmental) that needs better characterization. Clinically, cancer-related fatigue (CRF) is described as a subjective sensation of tiredness out of proportion to any change in activity and severe enough to affect function and QOL of patients with cancer. Between 70% and 100% of patients with cancer experience CRF regardless of the cancer type [18].

Studies of CRF have centered on patients with non-hematological malignancies, and CRF in patients with HM is poorly understood. At the same time, CRF in patients with HM is common and potentially more severe than in patients with advanced solid tumors [19]. CRF in HM is prevalent at the time of diagnosis, during and after cancer treatments, including hematopoietic cell transplant (HCT). The presence of CRF may limit the dose, frequency, and adherence to cancer treatments; therefore, it potentially affects survival rates [20, 21]. CRF impairs the ability of patients receiving treatment for HM as well as survivors to work. Despite CRF's high prevalence and significant impact on QOL, HM patients with CRF are less likely to be seen by PC [19].

CRF is associated with advanced cancer stage, surgery, chemotherapy, radiotherapy, biologic-response modifiers, hormone therapy, and symptoms such as pain, depression, and sleep disturbance [22]. Anemia correlates variably with fatigue and activity but does not correlate with muscle mass in patients with HM [23, 24]. The correlation is generally lost in terminally ill patients [25]. In advanced hematologic malignancies, multivariate analysis showed that low performance status, low platelet count, opioid based pain therapy, high LDH, and low albumin are associated with poor prognosis and not the degree of anemia [26]. In contrast, cachexia (described below) correlates with fatigue and decreased muscle strength [27]. In patients with myeloproliferative neoplasms (e.g., essential thrombocytopenia, polycythemia vera, and myelofibrosis) and those undergoing HCT, CRF is triggered by physical work, stress, exercise, sexual activity, and comorbidities such as depression [28, 29]. However, in patients undergoing therapy for a myeloproliferative disorder (myelofibrosis), the Functional Assessment of Cancer Therapy (FACT)-Anemia domains improved in anemia responders to therapy. These included the physical well-being, functional well-being, and trial outcome index scores [30].

### Mechanism

The molecular mechanism that causes CRF is unknown. Proposed mechanisms include proinflammatory cytokines, growth factors, circadian rhythm modulation, hypothalamic-pituitary-adrenal axis disruption, serotonin dysregulation, vagal-afferent activation, anemia, and abnormalities of generation of use of adenosine triphosphate [31]. The lack of consensus in the definition of fatigue and the reliance on scales that evaluate subjective fatigue limit our ability to understand fatigue and its etiology. Correlation of fatigue with objective measurements like tests of motor function, imaging, or biomarkers is necessary to identify phenotypes of CRF [32, 33].

It is likely that more than one mechanism affects an individual patient with CRF, and that the mechanisms underlying CRF vary depending on the circumstances. For example, radiotherapy promotes an inflammatory response and chemotherapy suppresses it [34]. Studies of solid cancers suggest that the origin of fatigue is predominantly in sustained and intermittent exercises [35, 36]. Peripheral fatigue arises from exhaustion of muscle force, velocity, or power, whereas central fatigue is a central activation failure related to the central nervous system or peripheral nervous system [37–39]. Within the hematologic malignancy population, it may be helpful to investigate fatigue in subgroups based on characteristics such as type of cancer and modality of cancer treatment. Unfortunately, such studies have not been published in patients with HM to determine whether specific factors such as anemia might play a more important role.

### Management

The management of CRF should be individualized depending on the patient's condition, treatment status, preferences, and goals. Factors that cause or contribute to fatigue should be assessed and treated when possible, such as deconditioning, pain, anemia, depression/anxiety, sleep disturbances, and cachexia. More research is needed to understand the effect of these interventions in improving CRF. The lack of mechanism-driven clinical trials exploring pharmacological therapies has hampered effective CRF management [22]. The evidence supporting pharmacological treatments for CRF is not conclusive, and there seems to be an important role for placebo that needs more investigation [40, 41]. The National Comprehensive Cancer Network (NCCN) additionally recommends education about the natural history of fatigue, counseling about physical activities, energy conservation, and distraction for coping with fatigue. But evidence supporting counseling and education is lacking [18].

Evidence suggests that exercise and psychological interventions help more in CRF than pharmacological interventions [42]. According to a meta-analysis of 113 studies of pharmacologic, psychological, and exercise interventions for CRF (11,525 patients), exercise, psychological interventions, and exercise plus psychological interventions improve CRF during and after cancer treatments [42]. There is not enough evidence to recommend a specific amount or intensity of exercise. Caution should be applied when recommending exercise to patients who have bone metastasis, thrombocytopenia, anemia, fever, active infection, limitations secondary to metastasis or other conditions, and risk of falls or accidents.

Unfortunately, most prior studies have involved participants with breast cancer, limiting application to HM. A pilot study of patients undergoing myeloablative HCT showed that a multimodal exercise training for 20 minutes, 5 days a week, compared to usual care improved physical performance and fatigue [43]. Another study revealed that a daily endurance-training program reduced the treatment-related loss of physical performance in patients with HM undergoing chemotherapy [44].

The use of integrative medicine for CRF is common among patients with cancer. According to a recent systematic review of randomized controlled trials [45], cognitive behavioral therapies plus hypnosis and American ginseng are "likely to be beneficial" in patients on active cancer treatments; while acupressure, mindfulness-based cognitive therapy, and qigong/tai chi are "likely to be beneficial" in patients after cancer treatments. However, due to the lack of rigorous trials and replication of the results, no therapies are recommended.

*Psychostimulants*: Mixed reports from a meta-analysis suggest the limited benefit of psychostimulants like methylphenidate to treat CRF [46]. No clear recommendation about the dose is given. Headache and nausea are some of the side effects reported [47]. Modafinil improves severe symptoms of fatigue, especially in patients with sleepiness and symptoms of depression. However, the results are inconsistent, not seen in mild to moderate fatigue, and its use is associated with increased toxicity from nausea and vomiting [48]. In general, modafinil is safe. However, for those with obstructive sleep apnea and a prior stroke, an adjusted hazard ratio of 1.96 (95% CI, 1.02 to 3.76) was observed for stroke among modafinil users [49].

*American ginseng*: Ginseng is an alternative superior to placebo after a consistent use of 2.000 mg for at least 8 weeks [50]. The advantage is that it is not associated with serious side effects. PT and INR monitoring is recommended for patients on warfarin.

*Erythropoiesis-stimulating agents*: The use of erythropoiesis-stimulating agents is associated with thromboembolism and increased mortality. These agents are recommended in patients with anemia secondary to chemotherapy and a hemoglobin level of less than 10 g/dL [51]. With the exception of myelodysplastic syndromes, erythropoietin should not be offered to most patients with nonchemotherapy-associated anemia [51]. In patients with myeloma, non-Hodgkin lymphoma, or chronic leukemia, clinicians should observe anemia response to cancer therapy before considering erythropoietin [51]. These American Society of Clinical Oncology/American Society of Hematology guidelines did not include the presence or degree of fatigue into the equation for using erythropoietin. The improvement of fatigue is likely modest and may not clinically significant as observed above in a previously cited study [52].

*Red blood cell transfusions*: Observational studies suggest that red blood cell transfusions improve symptoms of fatigue in patients with anemia and advanced cancer. However, the duration of the effects and the appropriate timing (i.e., at end of life) are unknown [53].

*Antidepressants*: The use of antidepressants does not improve fatigue in non-depressed patients with CRF [54].

*Corticosteroids*: Dexamethasone is better than placebo for CRF at day 8 and 15 of treatment [55]. Corticosteroids are an option when the benefits outweigh the well-known risks (e.g., osteopenia/osteoporosis, myopathy, and bleeding) like in those with expected survival of no more than a few weeks/months.

CRF is common and poorly understood in patients with HM. Psychological interventions and exercise and the combination of both are more effective as therapy than the pharmacological treatments available. It is necessary to better characterize CRF to improve the clinical assessment and the design of treatment trials to find more effective treatments.

## Cachexia

Cachexia (Greek "kakos" and "hexis" meaning "bad condition") is a multiorgan syndrome resulting from systemic inflammation. This complex metabolic syndrome is characterized primarily by weight loss (5% weight loss over 6 months) which is most often accompanied by of muscle, adipose tissue, anorexia, anemia, and reduced physical function [56]. The involuntary weight loss of greater than or equal to 5% over 6 months is based upon a body mass index (BMI) of greater than 20 kg per meter squared. If patients have a less than 20 kg per meter squared BMI, it is a 2% weight loss over 6 months [56]. The associated low muscle mass (sarcopenia), even in the setting of obesity, portends a poor survival and response to anticancer therapy [57]. The prevalence of cachexia ranges from 50% to 80% of individuals with cancer. It is estimated that 20% of patients die as a direct result of cachexia [58–61]. Cachexia is most common in patients with pancreatic and non-small cell lung cancer and occurs late in breast cancer and hematological malignancies [56, 62].

Anorexia often accompanies cachexia as a syndrome of hypogeusia, dysgeusia, diurnal variations in dietary intake, early satiety, smell changes, and loss of the rewarding experience of eating [63–65]. Cachexia can be differentiated from starvation by the presence of anorexia, dysgeusia, hypogeusia and early satiety, and the presence of inflammation and inflammatory markers such as the C-reactive protein or hypoalbuminemia [66, 67]. Cachexia must be differentiated from age-related muscle loss, primary depression, and hyperthyroidism. Additionally, malabsorption may mimic cachexia. Chemotherapy can cause anorexia, muscle loss, and fatigue which may be misdiagnosed as cancer cachexia [60].

Thirty-eight percent of 145 myeloma and lymphoma patients entered into a trial were found to be cachectic [68]. Patients undergoing allogeneic HCT develop significantly increased symptoms during the first 3 weeks, particularly appetite loss, nausea and vomiting, diarrhea, and fatigue. Patients with myeloablative transplants had worst QOL, anorexia, sleep disturbances, and pain. Graft-versus-host disease (GVHD) further worsened QOL and anorexia [69]. In regard to weight at the time of allogenic HCT, patients either underweight or obese at the time of transplant have an increased non-relapse mortality. In general, enteral nutrition is preferred in patients who are underweight, whether weight loss in the obese influences mortality is not known [70]. Nutritional support during the transplant improves oral intake but does not alter gastrointestinal graft-versus-host disease [71]. In pediatric patients, poor nutrition is a risk for acute graft-versus-host disease and mortality from transplant [72].

In regard to body composition during HCT, fat mass increases in both auto and allotransplants while muscle mass decreases in allotransplants [73]. This body composition change is likely to be missed by clinicians if weight alone is assessed during and after marrow transplants. Approximately half of patients undergoing allotransplant for Fanconi anemia have significant muscle loss [74]. There is a paucity of data which demonstrates the benefits of nutritional therapy and resistance exercises during transplantation on muscle mass, and some studies are several decades old [75, 76].

## Mechanisms

Cachexia is a complex metabolic syndrome which cannot be adequately discussed in a paragraph or two. Cytokines (interleukin [IL]1a, tumor necrosis factor [TNF], and IL6) are up-regulated by nuclear factor kappa-B as are prostaglandins in response to activated transcription factors induced by cancer [77]. Caspases, proteasomes, and associated E3 (ubiquitin ligases) cause breakdown of muscle proteins [78]. Caspases and calpains breakdown myofibrils before the myofibrils are ubiquitinated. Both enzymes are increased in cachexia A toxohormone L-polypeptide derived from tumor suppresses appetite [79]. The modulation of protein synthesis rates in patients with cancer is less clear. Increased resting energy expenditure in patients with cancer may depend on alterations in thermogenesis [80]. The tissues mainly involved in this process are the brown adipose tissue and the skeletal muscle. Both express high uncoupling proteins levels which have been shown to be further increased in tumor-bearing animals and patients with cancer. Muscle mitochondria in tumor-bearing animals with associated increased uncoupling proteins have reduced oxidative capacity and reduced biogenesis [80]. Cardiac muscle may also be involved with cachexia. Heart weight has been noted to be diminished in patients with cachexia and this may be the cause or at least a contributing factor to fatigue and dyspnea in advanced cancer [81]. The diaphragm is also adversely influenced by cancer cachexia. In an animal model, the atrophy of the diaphragm leads to the inability to increase breathing frequency, tidal volume, and minute ventilation under stress [82]. This may be the mechanism of dyspnea in patients with normal chest radiographs and the risk of respiratory failure in advanced cancer.

A recent review of cachexia after autologous stem cell transplant was published. Patients had myeloma and lymphoma. Assessment 30 days post-transplant patient revealed reduced aerobic capacity. Changes in weight and steroid exposure during and 30 days after transplant were significant factors for cachexia. There was no relationship to interleukin-1 beta, interleukin-6, or tumor necrosis factor alpha or bioavailable testosterone [83]. Inflammation may play a role in cachexia associated with hematologic cancers even though cytokines do not predict cachexia. C-reactive protein (CRP) > 54 mg/L is a risk factor of cachexia with an odds ratio 5.94 with wide confidence intervals (1.55–39.14) [68]. Interleukin levels and tumor necrosis factor blood levels may not reflect what is happening in tissues and vary widely during the day. There may not be an association between interleukin levels and C-reactive protein [84]. As mentioned in the previous paragraph, respiratory muscles may be influenced by weight loss. A recent study demonstrated that a peak expiratory flow rates and carbon monoxide diffusion capacity independently predicted survival in patients with myeloma. The loss of pulmonary function may reflect respiratory muscle loss over time with treatment. This also may reflect comorbid chronic obstructive lung disease [85].

## Management

The Subjective Global Assessment and Patient Generated Subjective Global Assessment (PG-SGA) tool are the most frequent nutritional assessment questionnaire in cancer. The

PG-SGA has a sensitivity, specificity and positive and negative predictive values of 98, 82, 95, and 93%, respectively [86]. The Glasgow Prognostic Index uses albumin and C-reactive protein as a 3-stage prognostic indicator and is an inflammatory index [87]. CT-derived measures of skeletal muscle at the third lumbar area [skeletal muscle index] and skeletal muscle density suggest that density (inversely related to myosteatosis) may be of equal or greater importance than skeletal muscle area in assessing cachexia [88]. Also, bioelectrical impedance measures phase angle reflecting both cellular health and muscle mass and provides an evaluation of nutritional and overall health status in patients with cancer. Measuring the phase angle is an easily measured noninvasive technique which is prognostic [89, 90].

The best treatment for cancer cachexia is cancer remission. There are no approved medications for the management of cachexia, and nutritional support alone is inadequate [91]. Combinations of exercise, nutritional support, medications to stimulate appetite (e.g., megestrol acetate, olanzapine), and anti-inflammatories (e.g., celecoxib, omega-3 fatty acids) in small randomized trials have been found to improve outcomes [92–97]. The ghrelin analogue, anamorelin, and the non-steroidal selective androgen receptor modulator, enobosarm, improved weight, lean body mass, and QOL but not physical function and hence were not approved for use in managing cancer cachexia by the Food and Drug Administration (FDA) in the United States (US) [98, 99]. The FDA requires both subjective, objective, and functional improvement as criteria for approval of anti-cachexia drugs in the US.

## Mucositis

The oral mucosa is normally exposed to a constant level of trauma which is thermal, mechanical, and chemical. The epithelium and saliva play a major role in protection. The mucosa consists of a stratified squamous epithelium with a basal layer from which new cells arise through cell division to replace the upper layer. This occurs over a 4–8-day period [100]. The layer between the stratified squamous epithelium—the lamina propria—consists largely of connective tissue. The mucosa is a source of anti-inflammatory cytokines and growth factors which counteract mucositis, promote regeneration and replacement of senescent cells [100].

Epithelial growth factor derived from the submandibular glands promotes cellular proliferation and maintenance of the stratified squamous epithelium. Loss of this growth factor promotes mucosal atrophy and mucositis [101–103]. Nerve growth factor (NGF) binds to tropomyosin receptor kinase A, prevents epithelial apoptosis, and promotes oral wound healing [104]. The precursor pro-NGF is found in salivary glands and mucosal epithelium. Fibroblast growth factor is also found in saliva and diminishes with age. This factor promotes maintenance of microvessels. Radiation to salivary glands reduces fibroblast growth factor and reduces microvessels, thus contributing to delayed wound healing and reducing mucosal health [105].

Saliva promotes food digestion, maintains oral pH for optimal health, and aids in food bolus formation to facilitate swallowing. Saliva lubrication prevents mechanical trauma to the underlying mucosa. Loss of saliva increases oral damage, promotes inflammation, delays wound healing, and increases tooth loss. Chemotherapy and radiation reduce saliva production and secretion leading to increased oral trauma and reduced dental health [100].

Mucositis from chemotherapy or radiation therapy is painful, interferes with nutritional intake, is associated with systemic infections and other complications, and increases the length of hospital stay and treatment costs [106–109]. Patients undergoing intensive chemotherapy for HM or high-dose chemotherapy with allogenic or autologous HCT are at a significant risk of mucositis. For example, 60–100% patients undergoing myeloablative hemopoietic stem cell transplants develop mucositis [110]. In a series of 20 patients who underwent bone marrow transplant who received either total body irradiation or busulfan in combination with cyclophosphamide and etoposide as pretransplant conditioning, mucosal changes began approximately 2 days before transplant and peaked approximately 8 days after transplant [109]. Mucositis from chemotherapy or radiation therapy is time limited. On the other hand, graft-versus-host disease, which may manifest itself with mucositis and oral pain, may be ongoing. The oral problems can be very debilitating and life-threatening.

## Mechanisms

Chemotherapy and radiation damage the basal cells causing the release of endogenous damage-associated molecular patterns molecules (DAMPs) which initiate an inflammatory response with up-regulation of inflammatory cytokines through activation of nuclear factor kappa-B [111–113]. Chemotherapy and radiation induce direct damage to the DNA, cause oxidative stress, and generate reactive oxygen species. Reactive oxygen species, innate immune response, and binding of DAMPS to receptors propagate further damage to mucosal cell membranes and activate several transcriptional pathways. Production of IL-1, TNF-α, IL-6, and cyclooxygenase-2 (COX-2), and cytokine modulators by fibroblasts and endothelial cells lead to cell apoptosis. Apoptotic pathways activated on submucosal and basal epithelial cells cause mucosal ulceration. Oral dysbiosis, an imbalance between the types of organism present in a person's natural microflora, occurs during this phase [114]. In the healing stage, epithelial proliferation, migration, and differentiation are stimulated by the extracellular matrix, and there is simultaneous restoration of the local microbial flora [115]. The stages of mucositis include initiation, primary damage response in signaling amplification, ulcer formation, and healing [116].

## Management

The World Health Organization oral toxicity scale is used to grade oral mucositis from 0 to 4. Grade 0 is no change. Grade 1 is soreness and erythema. Grade 2 is soreness, erythema, and ulceration but patients can take solid food. Grade 3 is soreness, erythema, and ulceration with intake limited to liquids. Lastly, grade 4 mucositis is soreness, erythema, and ulceration with no ability to take food or water by mouth [117]. Management should consist of preventive measures prior to initiation of radiation and/or chemotherapy. Professional dental care should be done 1–2 weeks prior to initiation of therapy and is recommended in conjunction with good oral hygiene. The evidence is largely expert opinion but is low risk [118]. Bland oral rinses with saline or sodium bicarbonate may help maintain oral hygiene and improve patient comfort during therapy. Chlorhexidine preventive mouthwash is not recommended [118]. Palifermin does not reduce mucositis from standard chemotherapy and of all modalities produces the greatest taste disturbances [119]. Guidelines for the prevention of mucositis during marrow transplants are scarce, but low-level laser therapy (photobiomodulation) and palifermin are recommended for prevention of oral mucositis [120].

The evidence for treating mucositis is sparse. Benzydamine, which is not available in the US, is the only anti-inflammatory drug that has some preventive and therapeutic benefit for patients undergoing head and neck cancer therapy [121]. Oral cryotherapy can reduce mucositis from 5-fluorouracil [122]. This has also been effective in patients undergoing HCT with high-dose melphalan conditioning [123].

With respect to analgesia, topical anesthetics reduce pain related to mucositis. Each institution has developed its own "magic mouthwash" which consists of diphenhydramine, lidocaine, and liquid antacid [124]. Bupivacaine lozenges or dyclonine produce longer lasting analgesia than lidocaine [125]. Gabapentin has been used to treat mucositis with mixed results [126–129]. Opioids are commonly used to treat the pain associated with mucositis. In a comparison of the safety and efficacy of two analgesic regimens for patients with head and neck cancer undergoing chemoradiation, high-dose prophylactic gabapentin increased the percentage of patients who did not require opioids during treatment. Methadone appeared to improve QOL compared with a regimen of short-acting opioids and fentanyl [130].

Integrative therapies have been used to treat mucositis. Aloe vera juice, curcumin mouthwashes, and chamomile have been reported to reduce mucositis pain [131, 132]. In one study, aloe vera mouthwash was as beneficial as benzydamine mouthwash in reducing the severity of radiation-induced mucositis with no side effects [133]. Honey has been used both prophylactically and therapeutically. A review of 19 randomized trials including 1276 patients found that honey mitigated mucositis prophylactically and was also an effective treatment. Intolerable mucositis was prevented with honey with a relative risk of 0.18 (95% confidence intervals 0.09–0.41) and decreased pain in the first month of treatment with a weighted mean difference of −3.25 (95% confidence intervals −4.41 to-2.09) [134].

Finally, there is evidence supporting the efficacy of low-level laser therapy and more recently termed photobiomodulation in the management of mucositis in patients undergoing radiotherapy for head and neck cancer [135, 136]. The Multinational Association of Supportive Care in cancer has included photobiomodulation (low-power laser) into its guidelines [137]. Recommendations are made for the prevention of mucositis and related pain with therapy in patients with cancer treated with one of the following modalities: HCT, head and neck radiotherapy (without chemotherapy), and radiotherapy with chemotherapy [138].

## Pruritus

Pruritus is a sensation that provokes the desire to scratch. The behavior associated with pruritus extends to the desire to rub or pinch damaged skin with devices. Scratching in a subset of patients may result in worse pruritus called urticaria factitia (pruritus induced secondarily by scratching). Chronic pruritus is daily pruritus lasting 6 weeks or longer, and the presence of chronic pruritus should trigger a diagnostic workup [139]. Chronic pruritus is divided into a dermatologic, systemic, neuropathic, somatoform or psychiatric, and mixed or other (idiopathic) [139]. Three groups of patients can be identified by skin examination. Patients may have pruritus occurring with disease or inflamed skin. Pruritus may occur with normal appearing skin, and pruritus may be associated with secondary skin lesions from chronic scratching (chronic nodular prurigo). Approximately 14% of the general population have chronic pruritus and 22% have a lifetime risk [140]. Associated features are eczema, dry skin, asthma, liver disease, increased BMI, and anxiety [140]. The origin of pruritus remains unknown in 20% of patients presenting to a primary care practice. Certain malignancies are associated with a significant frequency of pruritus. Pruritus occurs in greater than 30% of patients with Hodgkin disease and in 15–50% of non-Hodgkin lymphoma [141–143]. Cutaneous T-cell lymphomas are frequently associated with pruritus which has been reported to respond to mirtazapine and low-dose skin electron beam therapy [144–146]. Patients with biliary obstruction from perihepatic lymphadenopathy, intrahepatic biliary obstruction from malignancies involving the liver or tumors of the primary biliary tract will have pruritus in >50% of the time [140, 147–149]. Pruritus prevalence from chronic kidney disease which can frequently occur with myeloma or as an adverse effect from chemotherapy ranges between 25 and 75% [150].

Two clinical forms of cutaneous graft-versus-host disease are distinguished: Lichenoid cutaneous graft-versus-host disease develops within 3 or more months after transplantation and can be quite pruritic, and is characterized by violaceous, lichenoid papules usually starting at the extremities. The second is sclerodermoid cutaneous graft-versus-host disease and is distinguished by plaques of dermal sclerosis resembling morphea, and eventually by generalized scleroderma [151]. Checkpoint blockade is associated with vitiligo, pruritus, and morbilliform eruptions [152]. Paraneoplastic pruritus occurs in 6% of patients with cancer and is usually generalized and most frequently associated with gastrointestinal or HM [142, 153].

Among patients with non-malignant hematologic conditions, pruritus occurs in 15–40% of patients with polycythemia vera and usually occurs after a hot shower (aquagenic pruritus). Iron deficiency and overload have been associated with chronic pruritis, which is usually generalized. Certain endocrine disorders produce pruritus limited to the genitals such as hyperthyroidism or diabetes mellitus [141, 154–156].

Pruritus associated with psychiatric disease is particularly prevalent in depression, and depression is relatively common among patients with hematologic malignancies [157]. Nearly a third of patients with depression will have pruritus at some time during their illness. Characteristically, the scalp is often the site of pruritus and can be a precursor to psychosis. Pruritus is a major symptom for delusional parasitosis [158]. Medications account for 5% of pruritus with or without skin lesions. This can occur with liver injury and may be a presenting sign of cholestatic drug toxicity [159, 160].

## Mechanisms

The mechanism of pruritus in cancer is not understood. A subset will have neuropathic pruritus from compression neuropathy (brachioradialis pruritus, notalgia paresthetica). In HM, release of IL-31 has been described with T-cell lymphoma [161]. IL-31 may also be involved in morphine-related pruritus [162]. Histamine release from increased populations of basophils causes the pruritus of polycythemia vera [154, 163]. The mechanism of pruritus in cholestasis has been centered on elevated plasma levels of pruritogenic bile acids and accumulation in the skin. Lysophosphatidic acid has become the important mediator cholestatic itch. Although pain and itch are often thought of as independent sensory pathways, the two are interlinked. A series of inhibitory interneurons within the dorsal horn of the spinal cord connect the two sensory pathways. Pruritus varies depending on the activity of opioid receptor subtype. The activation of mu-opioid receptors causes pruritus, whereas kappa-opioid receptors inhibit itch [164].

## Management

The history of pruritus is important. One should determine if skin lesions, if present, predated or postdated the onset of pruritus. This is helpful in separating primary skin disorders from skin trauma secondary to pruritus. Localized (dermatomal) pruritus in non-inflamed skin is suggestive of neuropathic pruritus particularly if associated with numbness with burning or allodynia [165]. Individuals with chronic kidney disease frequently develop pruritus of the back and legs, whereas liver disease produces pruritus of the soles and palms. Localized vulvar pruritus can be a sign of iron deficiency. Generalized pruritus with normal skin, though suggestive of a systemic illness, can occur with neuropathic or psychogenic illnesses [165]. As a general rule, constant pruritus is more associated with systemic illnesses than in intermittent pruritis. Nocturnal pruritus associated with fever, night sweats, and weight loss suggests an underlying cancer [165].

The intensity of pruritus can be measured on a numerical or visual analog scale. The QOL can be assessed using the Itchy Quality of Life Scale [166]. Inspection of the skin for primary lesions versus secondary lesions from trauma such as excoriations, ulcers, crusts, papules, lichenified patches, papule-vesicles, and hyper or hypopigmented areas is important. Clinical examination should include inspection of the scalp, nails, oral cavity, and anogenital areas. Dermatological consultation can offer help in the differentiation, and a skin biopsy may be quite helpful. Radiologic and laboratory studies should be based on the history and physical examination.

Basic skin care is essential. Xerosis is quite common particularly among the elderly which will respond to basic care. Skin care measures include keeping room temperature low and applying skin emollients to improve the skin barrier and reduce pruritus. Colloidal oatmeal baths may restore the skin barrier. The use of urea (5–10% concentration), glycerol (20%), propylene glycol (20%), and lactic acid (1.5–5%) hydrates the skin. Application is best done after a bath or shower [165, 167]. Palmitoylethanolamide topical 0.3%, an acylethanolamine both improves the skin barrier and reduces pruritus [168].

Treatment of the underlying condition may also ameliorate pruritis. Lymphoma treatment quickly relieves pruritus related to Hodgkin disease and non-Hodgkin lymphoma. Stenting an obstructed common bile duct rapidly relieves pruritus and jaundice. Immunosuppressive therapy for skin GVHD may also relieve pruritis associated with it.

Selection of a symptomatic treatment is largely predicated on the cause. Second-generation non-sedating antihistaminic medications (e.g., loratadine, cetirizine) may be tried as the initial therapy and are excellent treatments for systemic mastocytosis. A short course of glucocorticoids (prednisone 30–40 mg per day or dexamethasone 4–8 mg per day) may relieve intractable paraneoplastic pruritus from lymphoma or cutaneous T-cell lymphomas prior to definitive therapy [169]. The mu-receptor antagonist naltrexone at doses of 50–100 mg daily may reduce cholestatic liver disease-related pruritus, pruritus from chronic kidney disease and from checkpoint inhibitors [170, 171]. Naltrexone has worked where ursodeoxycholic acid, various first- and second-generation antihistamines, and rifampin have failed to produce a response [172]. Naltrexone will reduce uremic pruritus as will the kappa-opioid-receptor-agonist, nalfurafine and nalbuphine [173, 174].

Gabapentin and pregabalin may relieve pruritus associated with uremia. Doses need to be attenuated since gabapentin is cleared by the kidneys [175, 176]. Doses are 100 to 300 mg of gabapentin three times a week or pregabalin 50 mg three times a week which should be given after dialysis if the patient is on hemodialysis [177]. Selective serotonin reuptake inhibitors (SSRIs) can reduce psychogenic pruritus, cholestatic pruritus, aquagenic pruritus from polycythemia vera, and paraneoplastic pruritus [178–181]. Mirtazapine is an alternative to an SSRI [178, 182–186]. Ondansetron reduces pruritus secondary to opioid therapy and liver disease [187–189].

Ultraviolet phototherapy reduces pruritus in many systemic illnesses including systemic mastocytosis, aquagenic pruritus, cholestatic liver disease, chronic kidney disease, and paraneoplastic pruritus [165, 190, 191]. Ultraviolet phototherapy should be considered in patients who have not responded to at least two different drug trials. An uncommon side effect to opioids is pruritus which may respond to opioid rotation. Low-dose nalbuphine, a kappa receptor agonist, added to morphine will also reduce pruritus [192–194].

## Hiccups

The first mention of hiccups "hickop" was described by Lupton in 1627 [195]. Hiccups were first thought to be related to diseases of the stomach and liver but it was Shortt in 1833 who first thought that hiccups involve the phrenic nerve [195]. The classification of hiccups is based on duration. Hiccups occur anywhere between four and 60 times a minute and can interfere with breathing, eating, and sleep, and can worsen pain, fatigue, weight loss, and dyspnea, dramatically reducing QOL [196]. Acute hiccups resolve within 48 h. Persistent hiccups last greater than 48 h but less than a month, whereas chronic hiccups last greater than a month. Persistent and chronic hiccups are commonly associated with diseases [196].

### Mechanism

Hiccups are caused by coordinated contractions of intercostal muscle and diaphragm followed by a few milliseconds with involuntary closure of the glottis producing the characteristic "hic" sound of hiccups. The reflex arc of hiccups involves an afferent signal from either the vagus, phrenic nerve, or sympathetic nerve fibers that ascend to the brainstem through T6-T12. The central component of the arc involves the medulla respiratory center, the nucleus tract solitarius, the nucleus ambiguous, the reticular formation, hypothalamus with modulating influences descending from the cerebral cortex [196, 197]. The efferent arc involves the phrenic nerve, the intercostal nerves, and recurrence laryngeal branch of the vagus [197]. Measures that stimulate the uvula or pharynx or disrupt diaphragmatic (respiratory) rhythm help to end otherwise benign, self-limited hiccups. Such maneuvers less frequently terminate persistent hiccups. Drug therapy becomes necessary for more intractable hiccups [195]. In utero, hiccups are common and appear to prepare the fetus for breathing and prevent aspiration of amniotic fluid [198]. There appears to be no purpose to hiccups after birth, or at least one that is known.

### Management

Peripheral causes of hiccups are divided into gastrointestinal or non-gastrointestinal. Gastrointestinal causes are the most common and include reflux, esophageal hernias, malignancies, peptic ulcers, and gastric paresis. Non-gastrointestinal causes include otitis media, myocardial infarction, pericarditis, pneumonia, pleural effusions, and bronchitis. Central causes include neurodegenerative diseases such as Parkinson disease, cerebral vascular accidents, brain trauma, intracranial tumors, and encephalitis [197, 199]. Hiccups occur with hyponatremia, hypocalcemia, hypokalemia, diabetes mellitus, progressive renal failure, hypocapnia, and alcohol withdrawal. Medications that are frequently associated with hiccups include alcohol, corticosteroids, benzodiazepines, dopamine agonists, and occasionally with chemotherapy such as cisplatin, paclitaxel, and docetaxel [200–202]. By case report persistent hiccups associated with the use of a fludarabine, cytarabine, and idarubicin [203]. The prevalence is rare as only 0.39% of chemotherapy patients on average (range = 0.08% to 6.03%) experience hiccups with treatment [204].

Evaluation of individuals with persistent hiccups starts with a history, assessing for fever or recent infections, preexisting illnesses, and recent gastrointestinal procedures or central nervous system events or diseases. A review of medications particularly over-the-counter medications should also be included. Red flag symptoms are anorexia, dysphagia, weight loss, and pain which may be concerning for an underlying intrathoracic cancer or lymphoma. The physical examination should focus on the respiratory tract, cardiovascular system, and gastrointestinal and nervous system. Basic laboratory tests include electrolytes and renal function as well as an electrocardiogram and or echocardiogram if the history and physical examination suggests a cardiac etiology. Brain imaging should be considered if the neurological examination is abnormal [197].

The initial treatment should focus on the underlying cause, though the underlying etiology is not frequently reversible. There are several "folk" remedies which have been used to break the hiccups cycle but have not been subject to randomized trials. The risks are low and so these maneuvers are often utilized initially for acute hiccups. These include breathing into a paper bag, taking a spoonful of sugar or drinking on the other side of a cup [199, 205]. Valsalva maneuvers or a knee-to-chest position can sometimes break the cycle of hiccups [199].

Pharmacologic management has centered on dopamine, GABA, and serotonin receptors [206]. Intravenous chlorpromazine at doses of 25–50 mg (equivalent to 100–200 mg by mouth) was originally approved based upon two single armed prospective studies. However, significant side effects led to the withdrawal of approval [200]. A randomized trial of metoclopramide compared to placebo in 34 patients with cancer, strokes, or cerebral tumors, demonstrated improvement (no hiccups for 1 week) in those who received metoclopramide 10 mg every 8 h [207]. In a randomized controlled trial of baclofen compared to placebo in 30 patients with strokes and persistent hiccups, 10 mg of baclofen every 8 h resulted in resolution of hiccups that lasted for 1 week in 14 of 15 patients treated, whereas placebo produced a response in only 2 of 15 [208]. It has been proposed that baclofen, a GABAb agonist, works through central mechanisms to palliate hiccups; however, baclofen reduces transient lower esophageal relaxation which is the cause of acid reflux and GERD and will improve hiccups failing to respond to proton pump inhibitors [209–211]. Baclofen causes muscle weakness, confusion, and sedation. Doses need to be reduced in renal failure to 2.5 mg every 8 h [197]. In contrast, gabapentin for the management of hiccups has been reported in multiple prospective studies and case series, at (relatively low) doses ranging from 200 to 1200 mg per day. Pregabalin 300–450 mg per day has also been evaluated. There are no randomized trials of gabapentin in the management of hiccups but multiple case reports [212–214]. The gabapentinoids have fewer side effects than baclofen [215]. Doses will need to be adjusted to renal function [197]. Other drugs have been used as second-line therapy including nifedipine, nimodipine, valproic acid, olanzapine, orphenadrine, and midazolam [197, 199, 216]. Drug combinations have been rarely reported. Baclofen has been added to gabapentin, and a triple combination of proton pump inhibitor, gabapentin, and baclofen has been used in refractory hiccups [197].

Given the above, metoclopramide or baclofen should be considered first-line therapy for persistent hiccups. If reflux symptoms are present, a proton pump inhibitor should be added. Though metoclopramide is assumed to work with peripheral causes and baclofen with central causes, both randomized trials involved patients with both central and peripheral causes for hiccups and both groups responded [197, 207]. Gastroenterologists will likely choose metoclopramide or neuroleptics while neurologists are more likely to use baclofen or gabapentin. Empiric use of either drug with rotation to the alternative drug seems to be the most reasonable approach. Gabapentin is a second-line agent while calcium channel blockers, valproic acid, olanzapine, or a benzodiazepine would be third-line drugs [199, 217, 218].

Interventional approaches should be considered if responses are not observed with at least two medication trials without benefit. Interventional approaches to managing hiccups include acupuncture, and radiofrequency ablation of the phrenic, cervical, or phrenic nerves. Electrostimulation of the phrenic nerve and vagus [197].

## Dyspnea

Dyspnea is a subjective experience of breathing discomfort that consists of qualitatively distinct sensations that vary in intensity [219]. Another definition is "awareness of breathing with difficulty."[217] Patients report several different descriptors such as "sense of air hunger," "ineffective breathing," inability to catch your breath," and "shortness of breath" [220]. Patients may state that they are "unable to get air in," or that they feel like they are "not getting enough air," or they state that they are "suffocating" [220]. Some are so frightened by the symptom that they feel like they are dying. Others use metaphors such as "an elephant on your chest" or "like I was running a race and when you stop suddenly and feel like you are going to collapse" [220]. Exertional dyspnea is seen in 6–10% of survivors of childhood cancer and in 50–70% of patients with advanced cancer. The symptom is often missed when assessed using the terms “dyspnea” because the patient does not have rest dyspnea. Dyspnea tends to be worst in the very advanced stages of cancer and end of life [221].

Breathlessness, a patient-centered term, is common among individuals with cancer. It may stem from a variety of causes, including pulmonary involvement of their underlying condition, lymphangitic metastases, pleural effusions, fluid overload, and infection will often report dyspnea. A progressive decline in lung function begins in childhood with patients who have sickle cell disease. Asthma, sleep-disordered breathing, and chronic hypoxemia are common and associated with increased morbidity. Pulmonary hypertension is more common in adults than in children with sickle cell disease. Although there is a growing attention toward respiratory care of patients with sickle cell disease, evidence regarding the prognostic meaning and optimal management of pulmonary issues in children with this condition is limited [222]. Forty-one percent of adults with sickle cell disease have mild dyspnea at rest which increases to 61% after a 6-minute walk test [223]. It is also a problem experienced by certain subpopulations, due to specific causes. Dyspnea during daily living activities, exercise capacity, and physical activity are considerably impaired in allogeneic-HCT recipients during post-engraftment period [224]. Treatment-related pulmonary vascular injury from radiation therapy and/or chemotherapy or checkpoint inhibitors will worsen dyspnea. Cancer complications such as pulmonary emboli may cause sudden worsening of dyspnea. Systemic chemotherapy causes muscle wasting and myopathy leading to reduced respiratory muscle function [60, 225–229]. Sepsis causes a rapid wasting of the diaphragm [230]. In activity, cancer-related fatigue with central activation failure of muscle, anorexia, and chest wall pain leads to skeletal respiratory muscle deconditioning and atrophy [231].

Individuals with cancer frequently have comorbid lung and cardiac diseases complicating the cause for their shortness of breath. For example, dyspnea is common with coronary artery disease and significantly improves after coronary artery bypass grafting [232]. Dyspnea frequency and severity marks the course of chronic lung disease and directly correlates with mortality [225, 233].

## Mechanisms

Physiologically, breathlessness is a mismatch between an increased inspiratory neural drive and a suboptimal mechanical response [233]. There are both central and peripheral contributors to dyspnea. The central contributing factors are not well studied. Both hypoxia and hypercapnia will increase central drive. In a group of patients with chronic obstructive lung disease subject to inspiratory occlusion and compared with healthy individuals, there was a greater unpleasantness and intensity of dyspnea in those with lung disease relative to healthy individuals. Electroencephalogram tracings demonstrated increased respiratory evoked potentials in emotion-related brain areas consistent with a central sensitization [234]. Individuals with chronic lung disease have greater perception and neural processing of respiratory sensations, reflecting a highly aversive, and attention-demanding character of dyspnea [234]. The perception of dyspnea shares characteristics with pain, and both sensations might be linked to affective states [235]. By multichannel functional near-infrared spectroscopy which measures oxygenated hemoglobin, the right medial prefrontal cortex activity in healthy individuals correlates with the magnitude of the dyspnea [236].

Peripheral causes of dyspnea in cancer are in part related to a weakened diaphragm from cachexia resulting in reduced inspiratory pressures [231]. Mice implanted with colon C-26 cancer developed diaphragmatic muscle atrophy which results in lower tidal volumes, and an inability to increase breathing frequency, tidal volume, and minute ventilation with respiratory challenge [82]. Individuals with chronic obstructive lung disease have increased lung compliance (“disappearing lung”), greater reserve volume, and reduced inspiratory volume with a plateauing of tidal volume with respiratory challenge [233]. The neuromechanical dissociation causes a sense of ineffective breathing. Increased respiratory rates further taxes already expanded and exhausted respiratory muscles as dynamic lung hyperinflation occurs. This leads to increased afferent feedback from type III and IV sensory fibers within muscle which ascend to the limbic and paralimbic system which worsens air hunger [235, 237]. The increased motor command from the respiratory control centers within the medulla, which monitor hypoxia and hypercapnia, and the limbic area which provides the emotional dimensions to dyspnea, are related to the somatosensory sensory cortex by way of central corollary discharge to produce the sense of dyspnea. Stimulation of the medullary pontine centers is in fact associated with a sense of dyspnea in the absence of respiratory muscle activity [238].

## Management

The correlation of chest radiographic findings and spirometry to dyspnea is quite poor [239]. The same is true for respiratory rate and pulse oximetry, hemoglobin levels, electrolytes, calcium, albumin, and magnesium blood levels, which do not correlate with dyspnea or its severity. There is a very weak correlation with anxiety (Pearson $r = 0.26$) [239]. Dyspnea correlates poorly with the presence of pain, fatigue, depression, anxiety, and drowsiness [240].

Patients should be asked about dyspnea at rest and with activity. Most manage their dyspnea by limiting activity. In those with chronic pulmonary disease, dyspnea is worse with morning activity and climbing up/down the stairs [241]. A visual analog scale or a numerical rating scale for severity can be used for dyspnea at rest and with activity [242, 243]. The Borg scale, a numerical scale, also measures dyspnea severity [244] The Intensive Care-Respiratory Distress Observation Scale (IC-RDOS) is designed for use in non-communicative ICU patients. The variables include supplemental oxygen, facial expression of fear, heart rate, accessory muscle use, and paradoxical motion of the abdomen during inspiration and correlate well with the visual analog scale [245]. There are several multidimensional scales that include dyspnea. The EORTC QLQ C-30 QOL scale, the Memorial Symptom Assessment-Short Form (MSAS-SF), and Condensed Memorial Symptom Assessment Scale (CMSAS) questionnaires include a dyspnea item [10, 246]. The Medical Research Council scale is commonly used in chronic obstructive pulmonary disease (COPD), and the Obstruction, Dyspnea, and Exercise capacity (BODE) index in patients with COPD is used to stage the severity of illness [247]. The New York Heart Association classification for congestive heart failure severity also includes dyspnea [242, 248].

The differential diagnosis of dyspnea is quite long, and patients usually have several causes for dyspnea as mentioned. The correct diagnosis by history and physical examination is only 50–66% accurate [249, 250]. A chest radiograph, digital oximetry, complete blood count, and electrolytes are used to screen for causes of dyspnea after physical examination [251]. The physical examination should focus on the heart and lungs. Stridor, egophony, lung dullness, crackles, elevated jugular venous pulse, distended chest veins (for severely or vena cava syndrome), a cardiac gallop, and murmur may be helpful findings. The use of accessory muscles and abdominal breathing provides clues to the severity of respiratory distress. There are limitations to the physical examination. In a systematic review, there was not a single symptom or sign sensitive enough to rule out heart failure, COPD, asthma, or pulmonary embolism. An elevated jugular venous, the presence of a S3 gallop and lung crepitus were useful in making a diagnosis of heart failure [252]. A normal pulse oximeter and respiratory rate should not be used to rule out life-threatening causes for dyspnea. Only a minority of patients with pulmonary emboli, COPD, or arrhythmia have oxygen saturations less than 90% and/or have a respiratory rate greater than 25 per minute [253].

Additional testing, when indicated, may be useful diagnostically. Natriuretic peptide, brain natriuretic peptide (BNP), and N-terminal pro hormone brain natriuretic peptide (NT-pro-BNP) are useful for excluding heart failure. Plasma NT-pro-BNP is elevated in patients with myocardial/pericardial cancer infiltrations [254]. A normal D-dimer rules out pulmonary emboli, though an elevated D-dimer is often a nonspecific finding. Additional tests that may be considered include a 12-lead ECG, a CT scan of the chest for pulmonary emboli and coronary calcifications, and echocardiogram and spirometry. Bedside sonography of the lung and heart has become a clinical reality and is likely to be used in the future as an initial evaluation [255–257].

Treatment of underlying causes of dyspnea depends upon the cause and goals of care. In those not imminently dying, angiotensin-converting enzyme inhibitors plus beta blockers, diuretics, and spironolactone will help systolic heart failure. Bronchodilators and corticosteroids will reduce air trapping and lung volumes and improve inspiratory reserve in those patients with obstructive lung disease. Diuretics may also be helpful even if patients are on comfort measures only. Anticoagulants for pulmonary emboli reduce the recurrence lung emboli and eventually improve dyspnea though this may be limited by thrombocytopenia. Superior vena cava stenting for the superior vena cava syndrome reduces dyspnea. Intrapleural catheterization and drainage relieve dyspnea related to a pleural effusion. Local radiation or stenting may be helpful if a bronchus is occluded. Antibiotic therapy may be beneficial when pneumonia is suspected.

Bronchiolitis obliterans organizing pneumonia is an inflammatory lung disease involving the distal bronchioles, respiratory bronchioles, bronchiolar ducts, and alveoli. Its cause is generally unknown, but there are several known causes and associated systemic diseases. It has been reported in individuals undergoing allogenic stem cell transplants [258]. High-resolution chest CT scan shows bilateral ground-glass opacities with air bronchograms and triangular, pleura-based opacities. Corticosteroid therapy is the best treatment option. Alternatively, azithromycin or erythromycin has been added to corticosteroids. Improvement has been noted in small case series [259–261].

Some patients with dyspnea and hypoxia will benefit from oxygen therapy and noninvasive ventilation. It is important to understand that dyspnea does not correlate with the degree of hypoxia. Oxygen therapy is no better than medical air or a fan in reducing dyspnea in patients with normal oxygen levels [262]. A fan directed at the trigeminal nerve will temporarily reduce dyspnea. High-flow oxygen (30–60 liters/minute) delivered either through nasal prongs or face mask reduces dyspnea where standard oxygen has failed to improve comfort, dyspnea, or oxygen levels. High-flow oxygen therapy is superior to conventional oxygen therapy in reducing dyspnea within an hour of starting therapy [263]. High-flow oxygen results in greater comfort, less mucosal dryness, and delivers a more reliable fraction of inspired oxygen. Physiologically high-flow oxygen reduces arterial pCO2, increases end-expiratory and tidal volumes, and decreases the respiratory rate and reduces dyspnea. High-flow oxygen is substituted for noninvasive ventilation in patients who are unable to tolerate noninvasive ventilation [264, 265]. High-flow oxygen therapy has a positive and-expiratory pressure (PEEP) benefit to patient [266]. High-flow oxygen does not increase mortality relative to noninvasive ventilation in patients who do not wish to be intubated. High-flow oxygen therapy reduces the intubation rate among individuals who would pursue intubation [267].

The use of opioids to treat dyspnea is controversial. Opioids have been used to reduce dyspnea and patients with an estimated survival of 2 weeks or less who have not responded to other measures [268]. In patients with longer prognosis, the risks and benefits of opioids to relieve dyspnea should be considered based on the patient's unique clinical condition, opioid tolerance, and goals of treatment [269]. In a systematic review of 48 randomized controlled trials and two retrospective cohort studies (n = 4029) of patients with solid tumor cancers [270], the baseline level of breathlessness varied in severity. Several nonpharmacological interventions were effective for breathlessness, including fans, bilevel ventilation, acupressure/reflexology, and multicomponent nonpharmacological interventions (behavioral/psychoeducational combined with activity/rehabilitation and integrative medicine). For pharmacological interventions, opioids were not more effective than placebo for improving breathlessness or exercise capacity; most studies were of exertional breathlessness. Different doses or routes of administration of opioids did not differ in effectiveness for breathlessness. Anxiolytics were not more effective than placebo for breathlessness. Evidence for other pharmacological interventions was limited.

The use of corticosteroids to reduce dyspnea in advanced cancer has mixed reviews. In a qualitative review, there was no evidence for improvement in dyspnea [271]. However, a recent randomized trial using dexamethasone 16 mg for 4 days and 8 mg for 3 days demonstrated improvement in dyspnea [272, 273]. Other symptom-relieving strategies include positioning, breathing retraining, relaxation and distraction techniques, pacing activities, and pulmonary rehabilitation.

Multiple integrative therapies are also useful in relieving dyspnea. Music therapy, acupressure, yoga and Tai Chi, relaxation, mindfulness, and guided imagery have been reported to be helpful [274–276]. L-menthol, a transient receptor potential M8 agonist, provided as a patch to stimulate the olfactory nerve reduces air hunger, effort, and unpleasantness of dyspnea in patients with COPD [277]. Dyspnea is often experienced at the end of life. Recommendations can be summarized as follows: 1. Start morphine at 1–2 mg IV every 15 min until dyspnea is reduced to mild (less than 4 on a 0–10 numerical rating scale). Higher doses may be needed in those who are opioid tolerant. 2. Monitor dyspnea, comfort, respiratory rate, and patients' response with sedation using the Richmond Agitation Sedation Scale. Patients who are nonverbal can be assessed by using the respiratory rate knowing that it is a poor correlate to dyspnea. In this case, morphine should be titrated to reduce the respiratory rate to less than 26 per minute. 3. Once dyspnea is controlled maintain the affective basal infusion rate. 4. If patients develop side effects such as nausea and vomiting, myoclonus or progressive confusion then treat symptomatically or rotate to hydromorphone using a conversion ratio of 5 mg of IV morphine to 1 mg of IV hydromorphone [268].

## Delirium

Delirium has several names including terms such as encephalopathy, acute brain failure, global brain failure, and critical care psychosis [278]. Delirium is the most common psychiatric syndrome diagnosed in hospitalized patients. On a general medicine ward, 11–42% will develop or be admitted with delirium, whereas 87% in the intensive care unit will develop delirium at some time during their critical care stay [279, 280]. Dementia increases the risk of in-hospital delirium five-fold [281]. Other risk factors include severe medical comorbidities, substance abuse and withdrawal, sensory deficits (visual and hearing), immobility, sleep disturbances, dehydration, electrolyte imbalances, and certain medications (e.g., anticholinergics, hypnotics, opioids, and benzodiazepines) [280]. Factors associated with delirium in a study which included it a significant number of patients with hematologic malignancies, older age, cognitive impairment, low albumin, bone metastases and the presence of a hematologic malignancy predisposed patients to delirium episodes [282]. Half of patients undergoing HCT experience delirium during therapy and the pre transplant risk factors are low cognitive functioning, lower physical functioning, higher creatinine, total body irradiation, older age and prior alcohol or drug abuse [283].

The core criteria for delirium comes from the DSM-IV and consists of disturbance of consciousness with loss of the ability to focus and shift attention. A change in cognition occurs which may include disorientation, memory deficits, and/or perception disturbances not related to a pre-existing condition. The disturbances develop over a short period of time, usually over days, and wax and wane during the day. There should be evidence from history, physical examination, and /or laboratory studies that the delirium is a consequence of the underlying medical condition [284, 285]. Delirium is often missed by clinicians. Forty percent of patients referred to psychiatry in the hospital for a presumed diagnosis of depression are delirious [286]. Within critical care, delirium is not recognized in as many as 66% of delirious patients [287]. There are several barriers and misconceptions to making a diagnosis of delirium (Table 14.1). Delirium symptoms fluctuate, making it difficult to conduct cognitive testing in the extremes of a psychomotor distur-

**Table 14.1** Misconceptions of delirium [289]

| |
|---|
| 1. Orientation does not rule out delirium and is not an effective screen |
| 2. Delirium is not always reversible particularly in the elderly and those with dementia |
| 3. Delirium will accelerate the course of dementia. Patients are unlikely to return to their baseline cognitive function |
| 4. Confusion in a frail elderly patient, even if only transient, should not be considered normal (even if on analgesics) |
| 5. Neuroleptics, particularly haloperidol, are effective drugs in reversing delirium |

bances. Hypoactive delirium is often overlooked or is assumed to be excessive sedation from medications or fatigue. Individuals with pre-existing dementia will have abnormal cognitive testing at baseline [288]. Unless there is an understanding of baseline cognitive function in those with cognitive failure or dementia diagnosing delirium in this population will be difficult.

Twenty percent of delirium is hyperactive and 80% is either hypoactive or mixed hypoactive-hyperactive. A subgroup particularly those with dementia will have persistent delirium. Diagnosis requires a minimum of assessing attention (such as spelling WORLD backwards or the months backwards or drawing a clock), orientation, memory, and thought processes. Ideally this is done per shift in the hospital to capture the fluctuating nature of delirium [289]. Patients may be oriented to person place and time yet be delirious. Some patients will have a "subsyndrome" phenotype which does not meet the diagnostic criteria for delirium. Patients with subsyndromal delirium may have personality changes, anxiety, irritability and are likely to have circadian rhythm changes during hospitalization manifested by sleep disturbances and sundowning [280].

New onset of psychiatric symptoms in late life is unlikely to be a psychotic disease but delirium. Non-auditory hallucinations (visual or tactile), hypnagogic (at sleep onset), and hypnopompic (upon awaking) hallucinations which occur at the boundaries of sleep are not psychotic but rather delirious symptoms. Strange or bizarre beliefs and misinterpretation of the environment or interpersonal cues should be considered a manifestation of delirium [289]. The hypoactive delirious patient is at risk for bedsores, pneumonia, and nutritional failure. Individuals do not become delirious just because they are hospitalized. In short, delirium should not be considered "a normal" experience [289].

## Mechanisms

There are several mechanisms causing delirium. Mechanisms include alterations in cerebral blood flow, cerebral hypoperfusion, degradation of the blood–brain barrier, loss of white matter integrity, endothelial dysfunction, and neuroinflammation. Neurotransmitters may be altered with delirium. Acetylcholine is diminished, and glutamate and dopamine are increased and have provided the rationale for psychotropic drug management and deprescribing anticholinergics [280, 287]. Functional connectivity is increased between the superchiasmatic nucleus, which governs circadian rhythms, and the anterior cingulate gyrus. There is decreased connectivity as determined by the functional MRI between superchiasmatic nucleus and the posterior cingulate gyrus, parahippocampal gyrus, cerebellum, and thalamus. This leads to loss of day/night orientation, loss of attention, changes in personality and affect. The posterior cingulate gyrus maintains consciousness to the external environment, the parahippocampal gyrus has governs memory and its retrieval, the cerebellum is involved with motor coordination and the thalamus is intrinsic to pain processing. There is also an increase connectivity between the dorsal lateral prefrontal cortex in the posterior cingulate gyrus [290].

## Management

A recent systematic review of delirium screening tools found that the Memorial Delirium Assessment scale, the Delirium Rating Scale including the DRS-R 98, and a Confusion Assessment Measurement-Short Form are the most commonly used tools to assess delirium [291]. Two scales, the Delirium-0-Meter and the Delirium Observation Scale are brief and can be completed in less than 5 min. Both tools facilitate continued assessment of delirium and require a minimum amount of training [291]. The 4 A's Test (4AT) consists of an assessment of alertness, an abbreviated mental test [4], a test of attention using the months backwards, and the presence of acute changes or fluctuating course. The scale takes 2 min to complete and does not require special training and has a sensitivity of 83–100% and a specificity of 70–99% [292, 293]. An EEG can be helpful in confirming the diagnosis of delirium. A single channel EEG over a very short period of time will demonstrate increased delta power (1–6 Hz) with a receiver operating characteristic of 0.78 (95% confidence interval 0.72 to 0.84) [294].

Prevention of delirium is more successful than treatment of delirium. Six factors are targeted in prevention: orientation, mobilization, medication reconciliation, sleep, sensory impairments, and dehydration [295]. This is the rationale behind the multicomponent intervention: Deprescribing psychotropics, resolving visual and hearing impairment, ambulation, sleep protocols, hydration, and nutrition that have been most successful in preventing delirium in the hospital [296]. The most successful treatment of delirium is to reverse the underlying cause. Reversible causes in the medical setting include medication toxicities which reverse delirium through deprescribing, electrolyte abnormalities, and infections [297]. Drug treatment of delirium is directed at the complications of delirium (such as agitation) but does not reverse delirium. When patients have a limited survival, the singular therapeutic goal is to control severe symptoms associated with delirium. There are no approved FDA medications for delirium [298]. Haloperidol, risperidone, ziprasidone, and olanzapine are ineffective in treating delirium [298–304]. Limiting anticholinergics including medications with anticholinergic activity, limiting benzodiazepines, and reducing corticosteroids and opioids if possible may help reduce or resolve delirium [305]. Opioid rotation may resolve delirium caused by opioids [306].

In intensive care unit (ICU), dexmedetomidine shortens the duration of delirium relative to placebo [304, 307, 308]. Melatonin has a very low risk for side effects or drug interactions. Melatonin for 48 h for patients in the intensive care unit reduces the frequency but not duration of delirium. In the elderly, 0.5 mg of melatonin nightly, reduced the frequency of delirium a relative to placebo (12% verses 31%). Ramelteon 8 mg at night also reduces the frequency of delirium in the elderly [309–313]. Inflammation is an important mechanism in the pathogenesis of delirium. Since delirium hence may be reduced by the anti-inflammatory effects of omega-3 fatty acids [314, 315]. Valproic acid 750–1500 mg a day has been shown to reduce agitation associated with hyperalert delirium in multiple prospective studies and case series and has been more effective than haloperidol in a randomized trial [316–321]. Conflicting results exist regarding bright light therapy. Bright light therapy (5000 lux) delivered between 9:00 a.m. and 11:00 a.m. in the ICU reduces the frequency of delirium though there is also a negative trial of bright light therapy in the ICU [322, 323].

## Depression and Anxiety

Psychological symptoms, including anxiety and depression, are common symptoms in oncology and can have a significant impact on QOL. Studies of prevalence have estimated a prevalence of depression ranging from 8 to 24% in patients with cancer and anxiety in at least 25%. Psychological symptoms are associated with a higher rate of pain, fatigue, shortness of breath. These symptoms can interfere with coping with the illness or its treatments and can worsen QOL as well as increase hospitalizations and suicide risk [324, 325]

Depression is often characterized with feelings of low mood, lack of interest in daily activities, hopelessness, guilt, or suicidal ideation [326]. Altered sleep or appetite commonly occurs in depression but may also occur in advanced malignancies independent of depression. Anhedonia is a helpful diagnostic characteristic of depression in cancer though in patients who underwent HCT anhedonia has been associated with fatigue [327]. Important, and potentially modifiable, risk factors include previous history of depression, lack of social support, advanced or progressive illness, unmet needs, and high symptom burden. A recommended screening tool from the US Preventative Services Task Force includes the Patient Health Questionnaire (PHQ)-2, asking "Over the past 2 weeks, have you ever felt down, depressed, or hopeless?" and "Over the past 2 weeks, have you ever felt little interest or pleasure in doing things?" If either question is positive, a more thorough assessment of depression should be completed. There is a wide spectrum of diagnoses for depression from adjustment disorder and normal grief to minor or mild depression in the middle, and major depressive disorder [328].

When considering treatment for depression, both pharmacotherapy and psychotherapy are effective, especially in combination. Psychotherapy is recommended at all stages of depression or anxiety. When pharmacotherapy is considered, prognosis should be evaluated as many medications may take about 4 weeks to reach an effect. For those with depressive symptoms and a prognosis less than 1-month, psychostimulant medications such as methylphenidate or dextroamphetamine could be considered in patients without delirium or cardiovascular disease after considering risks and benefits. Alternatively, ketamine at a dose of 0.5 mg/kg intravenously twice weekly can produce a very quick antidepressant effect. Side effects include depersonalization, hallucinations, and confusion [329–331].

For patients with a longer prognosis (1 month or more), there is no consensus on best antidepressant, so options should be considered on an individual patient level with side effect profiles of the medications in mind. Common classes of antidepressants include SSRIs or serotonin-norepinephrine reuptake inhibitors (SNRI). Prior to choosing an agent, it is important to consider any comorbid symptoms, such as anxiety, anorexia, insomnia, or neuropathic pain, because the side effect profile of some antidepressants can worsen these symptoms while others may treat more than one symptom. Of the SSRI class, sertraline (starting at 25 mg/day), citalopram (20 mg/day), and escitalopram (10 mg/day) have low side effect profiles and drug interactions and should be started at low doses and increased as tolerated. Other agents, such as mirtazapine, has histaminergic properties that can help patients with insomnia, anorexia, or frequent nausea; typical dose starts at 7.5-15 mg nightly. Bupropion is considered more energizing, with fewer sexual side effects, but may decrease seizure threshold; starting dose is typically 75-150 mg daily. SNRIs can be helpful with neuropathic pain, as well as anxiety-predominant depression and vasomotor instability. For prevention of chemotherapy-induced peripheral neuropathy (CIPN), venlafaxine is often used (starting at 37.5 mg/day). If there is concomitant CIPN, duloxetine is often a good choice (starting at 30 mg/day) [329, 332].

Anxiety is a common symptom and is often part of another diagnosis, including adjustment disorder, panic disorder, and depression, and could include hyperactivity, insomnia, restlessness, or agitation. Corticosteroids can commonly cause anxiety, as can withdrawal state from alcohol, benzodiazepines, or opioids. Common screening tools include the Hospital Anxiety and Depression Scale (HADS) and the Rotterdam Symptom Checklist [332, 333].

For acute anxiety, short-acting anxiolytics such as lorazepam, temazepam, or oxazepam are safer than their longer-acting counterparts, as they avoid toxic accumulation in the liver. If ineffective, neuroleptics such as haloperidol or chlorpromazine can be effective and may be safer in setting of respiratory compromise. SSRIs improve anxiety but may take 3–4 weeks to see improvement. For all patients with acute anxiety or other psychological symptoms, assessment should be made for suicidal ideation and referral to psychiatry, psychotherapy, or PC is warranted who screen positive.

Anxiety and depression can have notable significant impact on QOL, especially for patients with cancer. It is important to recognize symptoms early and provide treatment, whether with psychotherapy or pharmacotherapy, or both, and referral to psychiatry or palliative medicine if indicated.

## Nausea and Vomiting

Nausea and vomiting occur in about 60% of adults with advanced cancer [334] and 80% of patients actively receiving chemotherapy [335]. Newer agents for HM are also associated with an increased risk for nausea and vomiting. Brentuximab vedotin in lymphoma patients is associated with nausea (RR 1.51, 95% CI: 1.05–2.18), vomiting (RR 1.54, 95% CI: 1.08–2.19) relative to non-brentuximab vedotin regimens [336]. Patients undergoing HCT are at a high risk for nausea and vomiting and require prophylactic treatment similar to patients receiving highly emetogenic chemotherapy for solid tumors or HM [337, 338]. Fifty percent of patients undergoing induction therapy for acute leukemia have severe or moderate nausea [339]. Immunoglobulin light-chain amyloidosis (AL amyloidosis) is a rare and often fatal disease for which there is currently treated with drugs based on therapies for multiple myeloma. Half of patients experience nausea on treatment [340]. Despite improvements in prophylactic and treatment regimens, chemotherapy-induced nausea and vomiting (CINV) remains one of the most distressing side of effects of cancer-related treatment [341]. The consequences of poorly controlled nausea and vomiting are serious and can include metabolic derangements, nutritional deterioration, and impaired functional capacity and repeated hospitalizations. In treating nausea and vomiting, it is important to address the causes of nausea and the neurologic receptors activated to best treat the nausea.

### Mechanisms

Nausea and vomiting are multifactorial for most oncologic patients, but mainly mediated through the vomiting center, located in the medulla. The cerebral cortex, limbic system, vestibular system, gastrointestinal tract, and vagal or spinal sympathetic nerves respond to chemical and physical stimuli and transmit impulses to the vomiting center via the chemoreceptor trigger zone (Table 14.2).

The chemoreceptor trigger zone, also located in the medulla, responds to chemical stimuli in cerebrospinal fluid and blood. It is primarily activated by chemotherapeutic agents, toxins from food, and metabolic products, such as uremia. It contains multiple types of receptors: serotonin, dopamine, histamine, and neurokinin 1.

The cerebral cortex is stimulated by senses and learned associations. It is largely responsible for nausea and vomiting related to increased intracranial pressure, central nervous infection, and anticipatory nausea and vomiting. Anticipatory nausea and vomiting is also referred to as conditioned or learned nausea and vomiting. Roughly 25% of patients develop anticipatory nausea and vomiting by their fourth chemotherapy cycle. Risk factors for anticipatory nausea and vomiting include age less than 50 years, nausea, vomiting, or sweating after last chemotherapy session, expectation of posttreatment nausea, and anxiety [342].

The vestibular system includes the inner ear. Nausea and vomiting are triggered by nociceptors in the inner ear and visual system. Patients with motion-related nausea and vom-

**Table 14.2** Causes of nausea and vomiting and mechanisms [288]

| | Causes of nausea | Pathway activated | Receptors activated |
|---|---|---|---|
| A | Anxiety/ anticipatory | "Pavlovian conditioned reflex," cerebral cortex | Cholinergic, histaminic, NK1, 5HT-3 |
| V | Vestibular | Vestibular system, visual stimuli | Cholinergic, histaminic |
| O | Obstruction/ dysmotility | GI tract | Cholinergic, histaminic, 5HT-3 |
| M | Metabolic | Cerebral cortex | Cholinergic, histaminic, NK-1, 5HT-4 |
| M | Medications | CTZ | Dopamine-2, 5HT-3 |
| I | Infection/ inflammation | Cerebral cortex and gut / brain axis | Cholinergic, histaminic, NK-1, 5HT-3 |
| T | Toxins | CTZ | Dopamine-2, 5HT-3 |

*CTZ* chemoreceptor trigger zone, *5HT-3+* serotonin receptor-3, *5HT-4* serotonin receptor-4, *NK1* neurokinin1 receptor

iting have been noted in some studies to have higher rates of anticipatory nausea and vomiting, as discussed above [343]. This system can also be stimulated by medications such as opioids, chemotherapeutic agents, and aspirin.

The gastrointestinal tract has neurotransmitters and mechanoreceptors in the intestinal smooth muscle wall or peritoneum. These receptors stimulate nausea via the sympathetic nervous system or vagus nerve to the chemoreceptor trigger zone or vomiting center. Other inciting factors include gastric lining irritation by drugs, such as NSAIDS, antibiotics, iron supplementation, and obstruction or constipation.

Causes of nausea can be thought of using the "A VOMMIT" acronym, as in Table 14.1.

## Management

Assessment of nausea and vomiting should include a detailed history, including such topics as intensity, frequency, possible cyclical nature of the episodes, presence or absence of emesis, quality of emesis (bilious or stomach contents), association with mealtimes, associated movements, smells, tastes, or associations [344]. Assessment of nausea and vomiting should occur regularly during a patient's care. The revised Edmonton Symptom Assessment System (ESAS-r) is an assessment tool which is well validated across cultures, available readily in multiple languages, and easy for patients to understand [345]. Using tools such as the ESAS-r allows for temporal tracking of symptom management as well as tracking of symptom clusters.

As previously noted, there are a vast number of causative sources for nausea and vomiting. In the HM population, disease itself can be a primary etiology. One etiology may be a bowel obstruction caused by primary intestinal lymphoma or due to enlarged mesenteric lymph nodes [346–348]. Gastric amyloid may present with gastroparesis and intractable nausea and vomiting [349]. The same is true for cancer treatment, such as chemotherapy (discussed below) or radiation therapy. In the malignant hematology patient population, CINV remains an important focus point. The nature of nausea and vomiting can be subdivided into acute (within 24 h of chemotherapy) and delayed (2–5 days after treatment). Breakthrough CINV is that which occurs within 5 days of chemotherapy after the use of guideline-specified prophylactic medications.

Physical symptoms such as pain, anxiety, and constipation are known to be contributing factors. Pain is particularly prominent in patients with myeloma which is often difficult to manage with opioids due to incident bone pain and neuropathic pain from treatment [350]. Moreover, side effects of analgesics reduce the QOL in patients with myeloma [351]. Medications utilized for symptoms, such as opioids, can often result in nausea and vomiting. In patients treated for chronic cancer pain, point prevalence of 25% and 17% for nausea and vomiting, respectively, have been observed [352]. Most nausea will resolve over a period of days. However, strategies to mitigate this adverse effect may be necessary in a subset of patients which can include opioid switching, changing the route of administration, and the use of antiemetics [353].

It is important to tailor the antiemetic regimen to the suspected cause; however, clinicians should be mindful that most nausea is multifactorial and multiple receptors may be activated. Table 14.3 notes the locations of receptors along with agonists and antagonists to aid in identifying the cause of a patient's nausea and a treatment which may help with multiple etiologies. Notably omitted from Table 14.3 are corticosteroids (dexamethasone, prednisone, etc.). While they are a mainstay of many guidelines, and can be helpful in certain instances, such as postoperative nausea/vomiting, their specific mechanism of antiemetic action is poorly understood.

## Chemotherapy-Induced Nausea and Vomiting

Guidelines for specific regimens, dosing strategies, and durations provide guidance for different patient populations undergoing various treatment regimens [354]. Certain HM protocols prohibit corticosteroids. Given the heterogeneity of anticancer therapies, these agents have historically been divided into four categories to delineate their emetic risk and therefore the intensity of prophylaxis indicated [355]. Therapies are divided into categories of highly emetogenic chemotherapy (HEC), moderately emetogenic chemotherapy (MEC), low emetic risk, and minimal emetic risk. These categories are based solely on the incidence of acute chemotherapy-related vomiting, as opposed to delayed or overall CINV and thus may not accurately predict the burden on delayed phase CINV [356].

Acute CINV is predominantly mediated by 5-HT3 receptors in the intestine. Prophylactic 5-HT3 receptor antagonist use has resulted in improvement in acute CINV for most patients. These agents, however, have little efficacy with respect to delayed CINV [357]. The delayed phase of CINV is largely driven by the release of neurotransmitter substance P in response to chemotherapy. Substance P binds to neurokinin-1 (NK-1) receptors in the area postrema and nucleus tractus solitarius and can induce vomiting [358]. Efficacy of NK-1 receptor antagonists demonstrates the role of substance P in delayed CINV but is relatively ineffective in controlling nausea relative to vomiting. Olanzapine is the antiemetic of choice for delayed nausea which is also effective when used prophylactically [359].

Historically, CINV has been poorly studied in patients with HM receiving multiday chemotherapy regimens.

**Table 14.3** Receptors, their locations, and medications which target nausea and vomiting

| Types of receptor | Receptor location | Receptor agonists | Receptor antagonists |
|---|---|---|---|
| Dopamine 2 | Chemoreceptor trigger zone (CTZ)<br>Gastrointestinal tract | Gastric irritants, morphine, digoxin, hypercalcemia, and uremia | Chlorpromazine<br>Domperidone<br>Haloperidol<br>Levomepromazine<br>Metoclopramide<br>Prochlorperazine |
| Histamine 1 | Vestibular system, vomiting center, GI tract | Movement | Chlorpromazine<br>Cyclizine<br>Diphenhydramine<br>Hydroxyzine<br>Levomepromazine<br>Meclizine<br>Prochlorperazine |
| Acetylcholine | Vomiting center, GI tract | Movement | Cyclizine<br>Chlorpromazine<br>Hyoscine<br>Levomepromazine |
| 5HT2 | Vomiting center | Increased intracranial pressure, hyponatremia | Levomepromazine |
| 5HT3 | Intestinal wall, cerebral cortex | Abdominal distension, radiation, chemotherapy | Granisetron<br>Metoclopramide<br>Ondansetron<br>Palonosetron |
| 5HT4 | Gut wall, cerebral cortex | Tegaserod | Cisapride<br>Metoclopramide |
| Alpha 2 | Cerebral cortex, cerebellum, brain stem | Clonidine | Mirtazapine<br>Atypical antipsychotics |
| GABA | Limbic system | Fear, hyponatremia, increased intracranial pressure | Flumazenil |
| Neurokinin-1 | CTZ, area postrema, GI tract | | Aprepitant<br>Fosaprepitant<br>Rolapitant |
| Cannabinoid | Brainstem, basal ganglia, amygdala, and cortical regions | Dronabinol, nabilone | Rimonabant |

Therefore, the general approach to CINV prophylaxis in the multiday regimens has been to base antiemetic treatment on the highest emetic risk agent [360–362]. Recently, the 2016 Multinational Association of Supportive Care in Cancer (MASCC) and European Society of Medical Oncology (ESMO) CINV consensus guidelines include recommendations in the prevention and management of multiday chemotherapy regimens [363].

## Nausea and Vomiting Associated with Advanced Malignancies

Although etiology-based, guideline-directed therapies may offer quick benefit, a randomized trial of patients with advanced cancer and nausea not related to anticancer treatment did not show a significant difference between this strategy and a single-agent treatment with haloperidol at 72 h [364]. Other agents which are effective include metoclopramide and olanzapine [365, 366]. Although cannabinoids are popular, there are no good quality studies which demonstrate antiemetic activity in advanced cancer [367].

## Non-pharmacologic Approaches

Aromatherapy has been shown to reduce nausea in the postoperative and emergency room setting [368–373]. Nasal isopropyl alcohol reduces nausea within 10 min and is superior to placebo [374]. The antiemetic activity is equivalent or superior to ondansetron and is quicker in onset than oral antiemetics [368, 371–373]. In the limited trials available, there did not appear to be a benefit to combining isopropyl alcohol and a 5HT3 antagonist [372]. Behavioral interventions can be very effective, especially in anticipatory nausea and vomiting given it is a learned response and are recommended by the MASCC [375]. Hypnosis prevents anticipatory nausea and post treatment nausea in patients receiving chemotherapy, particularly in the pediatric population [376]. Acupuncture and acupressure have shown efficacy in decreasing chemotherapy-related nausea and post treatment vomiting [377]. It is important to keep in mind while discussing these with patients that they are not typically covered by insurance and may have a significant financial burden.

## References


1. Homsi J, Walsh D, Rivera N, Rybicki LA, Nelson KA, Legrand SB, et al. Symptom evaluation in palliative medicine: patient report vs systematic assessment. Support Care Cancer. 2006;14(5):444–53.
2. Palm RF, Jim HSL, Boulware D, Johnstone PAS, Naghavi AO. Using the revised Edmonton symptom assessment scale during neoadjuvant radiotherapy for retroperitoneal sarcoma. Clin Transl Radiat Oncol. 2020;22:22–8.
3. McGee SF, Zhang T, Jonker H, Laurie SA, Goss G, Nicholas G, et al. The impact of baseline Edmonton symptom assessment scale scores on treatment and survival in patients with advanced non-small-cell lung cancer. Clin Lung Cancer. 2018;19(1):e91–e9.
4. Hui D, Shamieh O, Paiva CE, Perez-Cruz PE, Kwon JH, Muckaden MA, et al. Minimal clinically important differences in the Edmonton symptom assessment scale in cancer patients: a prospective, multicenter study. Cancer. 2015;121(17):3027–35.
5. Selby D, Chakraborty A, Myers J, Saskin R, Mazzotta P, Gill A. High scores on the Edmonton symptom assessment scale identify patients with self-defined high symptom burden. J Palliat Med. 2011;14(12):1309–16.
6. Zeng L, Zhang L, Culleton S, Jon F, Holden L, Kwong J, et al. Edmonton symptom assessment scale as a prognosticative indicator in patients with advanced cancer. J Palliat Med. 2011;14(3):337–42.
7. Chang VT, Hwang SS, Feuerman M. Validation of the Edmonton symptom assessment scale. Cancer. 2000;88(9):2164–71.
8. Oldenmenger WH, de Raaf PJ, de Klerk C, van der Rijt CC. Cut points on 0-10 numeric rating scales for symptoms included in the Edmonton symptom assessment scale in cancer patients: a systematic review. J Pain Symptom Manag. 2013;45(6):1083–93.
9. Chang VT, Hwang SS, Kasimis B, Thaler HT. Shorter symptom assessment instruments: the condensed memorial symptom assessment scale (CMSAS). Cancer Investig. 2004;22(4):526–36.
10. Bircan HA, Yalcin GS, Fidanci S, Karaibrahimoglu A, Tuglu HC. The usefulness and prognostic value of memorial symptom assessment-short form and condensed memorial symptom assessment scale in assessment of lung cancer patients. Support Care Cancer. 2020;28(4):2005–14.
11. Ward JA, Balian C, Gilger E, Raybin JL, Li Z, Montgomery KE. Electronic symptom assessment in children and adolescents with advanced cancer undergoing hematopoietic stem cell transplantation. J Pediatr Oncol Nurs. 2020;37(4):255–64.
12. Gerlach C, Taylor K, Ferner M, Munder M, Weber M, Ramsenthaler C. Challenges in the cultural adaptation of the German myeloma patient outcome scale (MyPOS): an outcome measure to support routine symptom assessment in myeloma care. BMC Cancer. 2020;20(1):245.
13. Cannella L, Caocci G, Jacobs M, Vignetti M, Mandelli F, Efficace F. Health-related quality of life and symptom assessment in randomized controlled trials of patients with leukemia and myelodysplastic syndromes: what have we learned? Crit Rev Oncol Hematol. 2015;96(3):542–54.
14. Chow S, Wan BA, Pidduck W, Zhang L, DeAngelis C, Chan S, et al. Symptoms predictive of overall quality of life using the Edmonton symptom assessment scale in breast cancer patients receiving radiotherapy. Clin Breast Cancer. 2019;19(6):405–10.
15. McKenzie E, Zhang L, Chan S, Zaki P, Razvi Y, Tsao M, et al. Symptom correlates of dyspnea in advanced cancer patients using the Edmonton symptom assessment system. Support Care Cancer. 2020;28(1):87–98.
16. Merchant SJ, Brogly SB, Booth CM, Goldie C, Nanji S, Patel SV, et al. Palliative care and symptom burden in the last year of life: a population-based study of patients with gastrointestinal cancer. Ann Surg Oncol. 2019;26(8):2336–45.
17. Chen JJ, Huang SS, Li IF, Lin KP, Tsay SL. Prognostic association of demographic and clinical factors with the change rates of symptoms and depression among patients with hepatocellular carcinoma. Support Care Cancer. 2019;27(12):4665–74.
18. Berger A, et al. NCCN Guidelines Version 2.2019. Cancer-Related Fatigue 2019. https://www.nccn.org/store/login/login.aspx?ReturnURL=https://www.nccn.org/professionals/physician_gls/pdf/fatigue.pdf.
19. Manitta V, Zordan R, Cole-Sinclair M, Nandurkar H, Philip J. The symptom burden of patients with hematological malignancy: a cross-sectional observational study. J Pain Symptom Manag. 2011;42(3):432–42.
20. Hjermstad MJ, Knobel H, Brinch L, Fayers PM, Loge JH, Holte H, et al. A prospective study of health-related quality of life, fatigue, anxiety and depression 3-5 years after stem cell transplantation. Bone Marrow Transplant. 2004;34(3):257–66.
21. Horsboel TA, Bultmann U, Nielsen CV, Nielsen B, Andersen NT, de Thurah A. Are fatigue, depression and anxiety associated with labour market participation among patients diagnosed with haematological malignancies? A prospective study. Psychooncology. 2015;24(4):408–15.
22. Wang XS. Pathophysiology of cancer-related fatigue. Clin J Oncol Nurs. 2008;12(5 Suppl):11–20.
23. Fukushima T, Nakano J, Ishii S, Natsuzako A, Kawachi H, Sakamoto J, et al. Influence of hemoglobin level on muscle and physical functions, activities of daily living, and quality of life in patients with hematological malignancies. Integr Cancer Ther. 2019;18:1534735419842196.
24. Ben-Arye E, Dahan O, Shalom-Sharabi I, Samuels N. Inverse relationship between reduced fatigue and severity of anemia in oncology patients treated with integrative medicine: understanding the paradox. Support Care Cancer. 2018;26(12):4039–48.
25. Monti M, Castellani L, Berlusconi A, Cunietti E. Use of red blood cell transfusions in terminally ill cancer patients admitted to a palliative care unit. J Pain Symptom Manag. 1996;12(1):18–22.
26. Kripp M, Willer A, Schmidt C, Pilz LR, Gencer D, Buchheidt D, et al. Patients with malignant hematological disorders treated on a palliative care unit: prognostic impact of clinical factors. Ann Hematol. 2014;93(2):317–25.
27. Morishita S, Kaida K, Tanaka T, Itani Y, Ikegame K, Okada M, et al. Prevalence of sarcopenia and relevance of body composition, physiological function, fatigue, and health-related quality of life in patients before allogeneic hematopoietic stem cell transplantation. Support Care Cancer. 2012;20(12):3161–8.
28. Scherber RM, Kosiorek HE, Senyak Z, Dueck AC, Clark MM, Boxer MA, et al. Comprehensively understanding fatigue in patients with myeloproliferative neoplasms. Cancer. 2016;122(3):477–85.
29. Prieto JM, Blanch J, Atala J, Carreras E, Rovira M, Cirera E, et al. Clinical factors associated with fatigue in haematologic cancer patients receiving stem-cell transplantation. Eur J Cancer. 2006;42(12):1749–55.
30. Tefferi A, Hudgens S, Mesa R, Gale RP, Verstovsek S, Passamonti F, et al. Use of the Functional Assessment of Cancer Therapy--anemia in persons with myeloproliferative neoplasm-associated myelofibrosis and anemia. Clin Ther. 2014;36(4):560–6.
31. Yang S, Chu S, Gao Y, Ai Q, Liu Y, Li X, et al. A narrative review of cancer-related fatigue (CRF) and its possible pathogenesis. Cell. 2019;8(7):738.
32. Filler K, Saligan LN. Defining cancer-related fatigue for biomarker discovery. Support Care Cancer. 2016;24(1):5–7.

33. Fernandez C, Firdous S, Jehangir W, Behm B, Mehta Z, Berger A, et al. Cancer-related fatigue: perception of effort or task failure? Am J Hosp Palliat Care. 2019;37:1049909119849420.
34. Renner M, Saligan LN. Understanding cancer-related fatigue: advancing the science. Fatigue. 2016;4(4):189–92.
35. Cai B, Allexandre D, Rajagopalan V, Jiang Z, Siemionow V, Ranganathan VK, et al. Evidence of significant central fatigue in patients with cancer-related fatigue during repetitive elbow flexions till perceived exhaustion. PLoS One. 2014;9(12):e115370.
36. Kisiel-Sajewicz K, Siemionow V, Seyidova-Khoshknabi D, Davis MP, Wyant A, Ranganathan VK, et al. Myoelectrical manifestation of fatigue less prominent in patients with cancer related fatigue. PLoS One. 2013;8(12):e83636.
37. Taylor JL, Todd G, Gandevia SC. Evidence for a supraspinal contribution to human muscle fatigue. Clin Exp Pharmacol Physiol. 2006;33(4):400–5.
38. McComas AJ, Miller RG, Gandevia SC. Fatigue brought on by malfunction of the central and peripheral nervous systems. Adv Exp Med Biol. 1995;384:495–512.
39. Gandevia SC, Allen GM, McKenzie DK. Central fatigue. Critical issues, quantification and practical implications. Adv Exp Med Biol. 1995;384:281–94.
40. Zhou ES, Hall KT, Michaud AL, Blackmon JE, Partridge AH, Recklitis CJ. Open-label placebo reduces fatigue in cancer survivors: a randomized trial. Support Care Cancer. 2019;27(6):2179–87.
41. Berenson JR, Yellin O, Shamasunder HK, Chen CS, Charu V, Woliver TB, et al. A phase 3 trial of armodafinil for the treatment of cancer-related fatigue for patients with multiple myeloma. Support Care Cancer. 2015;23(6):1503–12.
42. Mustian KM, Alfano CM, Heckler C, Kleckner AS, Kleckner IR, Leach CR, et al. Comparison of pharmaceutical, psychological, and exercise treatments for cancer-related fatigue: a meta-analysis. JAMA Oncol. 2017;3(7):961–8.
43. Oechsle K, Aslan Z, Suesse Y, Jensen W, Bokemeyer C, de Wit M. Multimodal exercise training during myeloablative chemotherapy: a prospective randomized pilot trial. Support Care Cancer. 2014;22(1):63–9.
44. Dimeo F, Schwartz S, Fietz T, Wanjura T, Boning D, Thiel E. Effects of endurance training on the physical performance of patients with hematological malignancies during chemotherapy. Support Care Cancer. 2003;11(10):623–8.
45. Arring NM, Barton DL, Brooks T, Zick SM. Integrative therapies for cancer-related fatigue. Cancer J. 2019;25(5):349–56.
46. Yennurajalingam S, Bruera E. Review of clinical trials of pharmacologic interventions for cancer-related fatigue: focus on psychostimulants and steroids. Cancer J. 2014;20(5):319–24.
47. Qu D, Zhang Z, Yu X, Zhao J, Qiu F, Huang J. Psychotropic drugs for the management of cancer-related fatigue: a systematic review and meta-analysis. Eur J Cancer Care (Engl). 2016;25(6):970–9.
48. Jean-Pierre P, Morrow GR, Roscoe JA, Heckler C, Mohile S, Janelsins M, et al. A phase 3 randomized, placebo-controlled, double-blind, clinical trial of the effect of modafinil on cancer-related fatigue among 631 patients receiving chemotherapy: a University of Rochester Cancer Center Community Clinical Oncology Program Research base study. Cancer. 2010;116(14):3513–20.
49. Kaplan S, Goehring EL Jr, Melamed-Gal S, Nguyen-Khoa BA, Knebel H, Jones JK. Modafinil and the risk of cardiovascular events: findings from three US claims databases. Pharmacoepidemiol Drug Saf. 2018;27(11):1182–90.
50. Barton DL, Liu H, Dakhil SR, Linquist B, Sloan JA, Nichols CR, et al. Wisconsin ginseng (Panax quinquefolius) to improve cancer-related fatigue: a randomized, double-blind trial, N07C2. J Natl Cancer Inst. 2013;105(16):1230–8.
51. Bohlius J, Bohlke K, Castelli R, Djulbegovic B, Lustberg MB, Martino M, et al. Management of Cancer-associated anemia with erythropoiesis-stimulating agents: ASCO/ASH clinical practice guideline update. J Clin Oncol. 2019;37(15):1336–51.
52. Tonia T, Mettler A, Robert N, Schwarzer G, Seidenfeld J, Weingart O, et al. Erythropoietin or darbepoetin for patients with cancer. Cochrane Database Syst Rev. 2012;12:CD003407.
53. Preston NJ, Hurlow A, Brine J, Bennett MI. Blood transfusions for anaemia in patients with advanced cancer. Cochrane Database Syst Rev. 2012;2012(2):CD009007.
54. Minton O, Richardson A, Sharpe M, Hotopf M, Stone P. Drug therapy for the management of cancer-related fatigue. Cochrane Database Syst Rev. 2010;7:CD006704.
55. Yennurajalingam S, Frisbee-Hume S, Palmer JL, Delgado-Guay MO, Bull J, Phan AT, et al. Reduction of cancer-related fatigue with dexamethasone: a double-blind, randomized, placebo-controlled trial in patients with advanced cancer. J Clin Oncol. 2013;31(25):3076–82.
56. Fearon K, Strasser F, Anker SD, Bosaeus I, Bruera E, Fainsinger RL, et al. Definition and classification of cancer cachexia: an international consensus. Lancet Oncol. 2011;12(5):489–95.
57. Prado CM, Cushen SJ, Orsso CE, Ryan AM. Sarcopenia and cachexia in the era of obesity: clinical and nutritional impact. Proc Nutr Soc. 2016;75(2):188–98.
58. Ubachs J, Ziemons J, Minis-Rutten IJG, Kruitwagen R, Kleijnen J, Lambrechts S, et al. Sarcopenia and ovarian cancer survival: a systematic review and meta-analysis. J Cachexia Sarcopenia Muscle. 2019;10(6):1165–74.
59. Sasaki S, Oki E, Saeki H, Shimose T, Sakamoto S, Hu Q, et al. Skeletal muscle loss during systemic chemotherapy for colorectal cancer indicates treatment response: a pooled analysis of a multicenter clinical trial (KSCC 1605-a). Int J Clin Oncol. 2019;24(10):1204–13.
60. Davis MP, Panikkar R. Sarcopenia associated with chemotherapy and targeted agents for cancer therapy. Ann Palliat Med. 2019;8(1):86–101.
61. Tournadre A, Vial G, Capel F, Soubrier M, Boirie Y. Sarcopenia. Joint Bone Spine. 2019;86(3):309–14.
62. Fearon KC. Cancer cachexia and fat-muscle physiology. N Engl J Med. 2011;365(6):565–7.
63. Yavuzsen T, Walsh D, Davis MP, Kirkova J, Jin T, LeGrand S, et al. Components of the anorexia-cachexia syndrome: gastrointestinal symptom correlates of cancer anorexia. Support Care Cancer. 2009;17(12):1531–41.
64. Davis MP, Walsh D, Lagman R, Yavuzsen T. Early satiety in cancer patients: a common and important but underrecognized symptom. Support Care Cancer. 2006;14(7):693–8.
65. Davis MP, Dreicer R, Walsh D, Lagman R, LeGrand SB. Appetite and cancer-associated anorexia: a review. J Clin Oncol. 2004;22(8):1510–7.
66. Fearon KC, Barber MD, Falconer JS, McMillan DC, Ross JA, Preston T. Pancreatic cancer as a model: inflammatory mediators, acute-phase response, and cancer cachexia. World J Surg. 1999;23(6):584–8.
67. Fearon KC, Falconer JS, Slater C, McMillan DC, Ross JA, Preston T. Albumin synthesis rates are not decreased in hypoalbuminemic cachectic cancer patients with an ongoing acute-phase protein response. Ann Surg. 1998;227(2):249–54.
68. Mallard J, Gagez AL, Baudinet C, Herbinet A, Maury J, Bernard PL, et al. C-reactive protein level: a key predictive marker of cachexia in lymphoma and myeloma patients. J Hematol. 2019;8(2):55–9.
69. Frodin U, Lotfi K, Fomichov V, Juliusson G, Borjeson S. Frequent and long-term follow-up of health-related quality of life following allogeneic haematopoietic stem cell transplantation. Eur J Cancer Care (Engl). 2015;24(6):898–910.

70. Doney K, McMillen K, Buono L, Deeg HJ, Gooley T. Impact of body mass index on outcomes of hematopoietic stem cell transplantation in adults. Biol Blood Marrow Transplant. 2019;25(3):613–20.
71. Aoyama T, Yoshitsugu K, Fukaya M, Kume T, Kawashima M, Nakajima K, et al. Benefit of reducing body weight loss with a nutritional support pathway in patients undergoing allogeneic hematopoietic stem cell transplantation. Med Sci Monit Basic Res. 2019;25:187–98.
72. Kerby EH, Li Y, Getz KD, Smith EC, Smith LT, Bunin NJ, et al. Nutritional risk factors predict severe acute graft-versus-host disease and early mortality in pediatric allogeneic hematopoietic stem cell transplantation. Pediatr Blood Cancer. 2018;65(2):e26853.
73. DeFilipp Z, Troschel FM, Qualls DA, Li S, Kuklinski MW, Kempner ME, et al. Evolution of body composition following autologous and allogeneic hematopoietic cell transplantation: incidence of sarcopenia and association with clinical outcomes. Biol Blood Marrow Transplant. 2018;24(8):1741–7.
74. Silva P, Schmit D, Bonfim C, Campos DJ, Rabito EI, Vilela RM. Body composition of Fanconi anemia patients after hematopoietic stem cell transplantation. Rev Bras Hematol Hemoter. 2017;39(4):318–24.
75. Cheney CL, Abson KG, Aker SN, Lenssen P, Cunningham BA, Buergel NS, et al. Body composition changes in marrow transplant recipients receiving total parenteral nutrition. Cancer. 1987;59(8):1515–9.
76. Cunningham BA, Morris G, Cheney CL, Buergel N, Aker SN, Lenssen P. Effects of resistive exercise on skeletal muscle in marrow transplant recipients receiving total parenteral nutrition. JPEN J Parenter Enteral Nutr. 1986;10(6):558–63.
77. Argiles JM, Lopez-Soriano FJ, Busquets S. Mediators of cachexia in cancer patients. Nutrition. 2019;66:11–5.
78. Ebner N, Anker SD, von Haehling S. Recent developments in the field of cachexia, sarcopenia, and muscle wasting: highlights from the 11th cachexia conference. J Cachexia Sarcopenia Muscle. 2019;10(1):218–25.
79. Okabe Y, Sakata T, Kurokawa M, Fujimoto K, Ueda K, Masuno H, et al. Anorexia induced by toxohormone-L isolated from ascites fluid of patients with hepatoma. Physiol Behav. 1992;52(2):333–7.
80. Penna F, Ballaro R, Beltra M, De Lucia S, Garcia Castillo L, Costelli P. The skeletal muscle as an active player against cancer cachexia. Front Physiol. 2019;10:41.
81. Barkhudaryan A, Scherbakov N, Springer J, Doehner W. Cardiac muscle wasting in individuals with cancer cachexia. ESC heart Fail. 2017;4(4):458–67.
82. Roberts BM, Ahn B, Smuder AJ, Al-Rajhi M, Gill LC, Beharry AW, et al. Diaphragm and ventilatory dysfunction during cancer cachexia. FASEB J. 2013;27(7):2600–10.
83. Anderson LJ, Yin C, Burciaga R, Lee J, Crabtree S, Migula D, et al. Assessing cachexia acutely after autologous stem cell transplant. Cancers (Basel). 2019;11(9):1300.
84. Rief W, Mills PJ, Ancoli-Israel S, Ziegler MG, Pung MA, Dimsdale JE. Overnight changes of immune parameters and catecholamines are associated with mood and stress. Psychosom Med. 2010;72(8):755–62.
85. Trakada G, Kastritis E, Gavriatopoulou M, Velentza L, Fotiou D, Ziogas DC, et al. Pulmonary function abnormalities are common in patients with multiple myeloma and are independently associated with worse outcome. Ann Hematol. 2019;98(6):1427–34.
86. Mendes NP, Barros TA, Rosa COB, Franceschini S. Nutritional screening tools used and validated for cancer patients: a systematic review. Nutr Cancer. 2019;71(6):898–907.
87. Dolan RD, Daly L, Sim WMJ, Fallon M, Ryan A, McMillan DC, et al. Comparison of the prognostic value of ECOG-PS, mGPS and BMI/WL: implications for a clinically important framework in the assessment and treatment of advanced cancer. Clin Nutr. 2019;39:2889.
88. McDonald JJ, Fallon MT, Laird BJA. Meaningful measures in cancer cachexia: implications for practice and research. Curr Opinion Support Palliative care. 2019;13(4):323–7.
89. Grundmann O, Yoon SL, Williams JJ. The value of bioelectrical impedance analysis and phase angle in the evaluation of malnutrition and quality of life in cancer patients--a comprehensive review. Eur J Clin Nutr. 2015;69(12):1290–7.
90. Davis MP, Yavuzsen T, Khoshknabi D, Kirkova J, Walsh D, Lasheen W, et al. Bioelectrical impedance phase angle changes during hydration and prognosis in advanced cancer. Am J Hosp Palliat Care. 2009;26(3):180–7.
91. Roeland EJ, Bohlke K, Baracos VE, Bruera E, Del Fabbro E, Dixon S, et al. Management of cancer cachexia: ASCO guideline. J Clin Oncol. 2020;38:2438.
92. Miura S, Naito T, Mitsunaga S, Omae K, Mori K, Inano T, et al. A randomized phase II study of nutritional and exercise treatment for elderly patients with advanced non-small cell lung or pancreatic cancer: the NEXTAC-TWO study protocol. BMC Cancer. 2019;19(1):528.
93. Argiles JM, Lopez-Soriano FJ, Stemmler B, Busquets S. Therapeutic strategies against cancer cachexia. Eur J Transl Myol. 2019;29(1):7960.
94. Shirai Y, Okugawa Y, Hishida A, Ogawa A, Okamoto K, Shintani M, et al. Fish oil-enriched nutrition combined with systemic chemotherapy for gastrointestinal cancer patients with cancer cachexia. Sci Rep. 2017;7(1):4826.
95. Ravasco P. Nutrition in cancer patients. J Clin Med. 2019;8(8):1211.
96. Gorjao R, Dos Santos CMM, Serdan TDA, Diniz VLS, Alba-Loureiro TC, Cury-Boaventura MF, et al. New insights on the regulation of cancer cachexia by N-3 polyunsaturated fatty acids. Pharmacol Ther. 2019;196:117–34.
97. Okamoto H, Shono K, Nozaki-Taguchi N. Low-dose of olanzapine has ameliorating effects on cancer-related anorexia. Cancer Manag Res. 2019;11:2233–9.
98. Crawford J, Prado CM, Johnston MA, Gralla RJ, Taylor RP, Hancock ML, et al. Study design and rationale for the phase 3 clinical development program of enobosarm, a selective androgen receptor modulator, for the prevention and treatment of muscle wasting in cancer patients (POWER trials). Curr Oncol Rep. 2016;18(6):37.
99. Temel JS, Abernethy AP, Currow DC, Friend J, Duus EM, Yan Y, et al. Anamorelin in patients with non-small-cell lung cancer and cachexia (ROMANA 1 and ROMANA 2): results from two randomised, double-blind, phase 3 trials. Lancet Oncol. 2016;17(4):519–31.
100. Duncan M, Grant G. Oral and intestinal mucositis - causes and possible treatments. Aliment Pharmacol Ther. 2003;18(9):853–74.
101. Kasselberg AG, Orth DN, Gray ME, Stahlman MT. Immunocytochemical localization of human epidermal growth factor/urogastrone in several human tissues. J Histochem Cytochem. 1985;33(4):315–22.
102. Fujisawa K, Miyamoto Y, Nagayama M. Basic fibroblast growth factor and epidermal growth factor reverse impaired ulcer healing of the rabbit oral mucosa. J Oral Pathol Med. 2003;32(6):358–66.
103. Epstein JB, Gorsky M, Guglietta A, Le N, Sonis ST. The correlation between epidermal growth factor levels in saliva and the severity of oral mucositis during oropharyngeal radiation therapy. Cancer. 2000;89(11):2258–65.
104. Schenck K, Schreurs O, Hayashi K, Helgeland K. The role of nerve growth factor (ngf) and its precursor forms in oral wound healing. Int J Mol Sci. 2017;18(2):386.
105. van Setten GB. Basic fibroblast growth factor in human saliva: detection and physiological implications. Laryngoscope. 1995;105(6):610–2.

106. da Fonseca MA. Management of mucositis in bone marrow transplant patients. J Dent Hyg. 1999;73(1):17–21.
107. McGuire DB, Yeager KA, Dudley WN, Peterson DE, Owen DC, Lin LS, et al. Acute oral pain and mucositis in bone marrow transplant and leukemia patients: data from a pilot study. Cancer Nurs. 1998;21(6):385–93.
108. Woo SB, Sonis ST, Monopoli MM, Sonis AL. A longitudinal study of oral ulcerative mucositis in bone marrow transplant recipients. Cancer. 1993;72(5):1612–7.
109. Zerbe MB, Parkerson SG, Ortlieb ML, Spitzer T. Relationships between oral mucositis and treatment variables in bone marrow transplant patients. Cancer Nurs. 1992;15(3):196–205.
110. Rubenstein EB, Peterson DE, Schubert M, Keefe D, McGuire D, Epstein J, et al. Clinical practice guidelines for the prevention and treatment of cancer therapy-induced oral and gastrointestinal mucositis. Cancer. 2004;100(9 Suppl):2026–46.
111. Logan RM, Stringer AM, Bowen JM, Gibson RJ, Sonis ST, Keefe DM. Is the pathobiology of chemotherapy-induced alimentary tract mucositis influenced by the type of mucotoxic drug administered? Cancer Chemother Pharmacol. 2009;63(2):239–51.
112. Logan RM, Gibson RJ, Bowen JM, Stringer AM, Sonis ST, Keefe DM. Characterisation of mucosal changes in the alimentary tract following administration of irinotecan: implications for the pathobiology of mucositis. Cancer Chemother Pharmacol. 2008;62(1):33–41.
113. Lambros MP, Parsa C, Mulamalla H, Orlando R, Lau B, Huang Y, et al. Identifying cell and molecular stress after radiation in a three-dimensional (3-D) model of oral mucositis. Biochem Biophys Res Commun. 2011;405(1):102–6.
114. Hong BY, Sobue T, Choquette L, Dupuy AK, Thompson A, Burleson JA, et al. Chemotherapy-induced oral mucositis is associated with detrimental bacterial dysbiosis. Microbiome. 2019;7(1):66.
115. Basile D, Di Nardo P, Corvaja C, Garattini SK, Pelizzari G, Lisanti C, et al. Mucosal injury during anti-cancer treatment: from pathobiology to bedside. Cancer. 2019;11(6):857.
116. Sonis ST, Elting LS, Keefe D, Peterson DE, Schubert M, Hauer-Jensen M, et al. Perspectives on cancer therapy-induced mucosal injury: pathogenesis, measurement, epidemiology, and consequences for patients. Cancer. 2004;100(9 Suppl):1995–2025.
117. Maria OM, Eliopoulos N, Muanza T. Radiation-induced Oral mucositis. Front Oncol. 2017;7:89.
118. Hong CHL, Gueiros LA, Fulton JS, Cheng KKF, Kandwal A, Galiti D, et al. Systematic review of basic oral care for the management of oral mucositis in cancer patients and clinical practice guidelines. Support Care Cancer. 2019;27(10):3949–67.
119. Wilairat P, Kengkla K, Kaewpanan T, Kaewthong J, Ruankon S, Subthaweesin C, et al. Comparative efficacy and safety of interventions for preventing chemotherapy-induced oral mucositis in adult cancer patients: a systematic review and network meta-analysis. Eur J Hosp Pharm. 2020;27(2):103–10.
120. Bowen JM, Wardill HR. Advances in the understanding and management of mucositis during stem cell transplantation. Curr Opin Support Palliat Care. 2017;11(4):341–6.
121. Ariyawardana A, Cheng KKF, Kandwal A, Tilly V, Al-Azri AR, Galiti D, et al. Systematic review of anti-inflammatory agents for the management of oral mucositis in cancer patients and clinical practice guidelines. Support Care Cancer. 2019;27(10):3985–95.
122. Okamoto K, Ninomiya I, Yamaguchi T, Terai S, Nakanuma S, Kinoshita J, et al. Oral cryotherapy for prophylaxis of oral mucositis caused by docetaxel, cisplatin, and fluorouracil chemotherapy for esophageal cancer. Esophagus: official journal of the Japan esophageal. Society. 2019;16(2):207–13.
123. Correa MEP, Cheng KKF, Chiang K, Kandwal A, Loprinzi CL, Mori T, et al. Systematic review of oral cryotherapy for the management of oral mucositis in cancer patients and clinical practice guidelines. Support Care Cancer. 2020;28(5):2449–56.
124. Sherr DL. Finding the magic in magic mouthwash. JAMA Intern Med. 2019;179(5):723–4.
125. Carnel SB, Blakeslee DB, Oswald SG, Barnes M. Treatment of radiation- and chemotherapy-induced stomatitis. Otolaryngol Head Neck Surg. 1990;102(4):326–30.
126. Milazzo-Kiedaisch CA, Itano J, Dutta PR. Role of gabapentin in managing mucositis pain in patients undergoing radiation therapy to the head and neck. Clin J Oncol Nurs. 2016;20(6):623–8.
127. Kataoka T, Kiyota N, Shimada T, Funakoshi Y, Chayahara N, Toyoda M, et al. Randomized trial of standard pain control with or without gabapentin for pain related to radiation-induced mucositis in head and neck cancer. Auris Nasus Larynx. 2016;43(6):677–84.
128. Bar AV, Weinstein G, Dutta PR, Dosoretz A, Chalian A, Both S, et al. Gabapentin for the treatment of pain syndrome related to radiation-induced mucositis in patients with head and neck cancer treated with concurrent chemoradiotherapy. Cancer. 2010;116(17):4206–13.
129. Bar AV, Weinstein G, Dutta PR, Chalian A, Both S, Quon H. Gabapentin for the treatment of pain related to radiation-induced mucositis in patients with head and neck tumors treated with intensity-modulated radiation therapy. Head Neck. 2010;32(2):173–7.
130. Hermann GM, Iovoli AJ, Platek AJ, Wang C, Miller A, Attwood K, et al. A single-institution, randomized, pilot study evaluating the efficacy of gabapentin and methadone for patients undergoing chemoradiation for head and neck squamous cell cancer. Cancer. 2020;126(7):1480–91.
131. Elad S, Meidan I, Sellam G, Simaan S, Zeevi I, Waldman E, et al. Topical curcumin for the prevention of oral mucositis in pediatric patients: case series. Altern Ther Health Med. 2013;19(3):21–4.
132. Dos Reis PE, Ciol MA, de Melo NS, Figueiredo PT, Leite AF, Manzi NM. Chamomile infusion cryotherapy to prevent oral mucositis induced by chemotherapy: a pilot study. Support Care Cancer. 2016;24(10):4393–8.
133. Sahebjamee M, Mansourian A, Hajimirzamohammad M, Zadeh MT, Bekhradi R, Kazemian A, et al. Comparative efficacy of aloe vera and benzydamine mouthwashes on radiation-induced oral mucositis: a triple-blind, randomised, controlled clinical trial. Oral Health Prev Dent. 2015;13(4):309–15.
134. Liu TM, Luo YW, Tam KW, Lin CC, Huang TW. Prophylactic and therapeutic effects of honey on radiochemotherapy-induced mucositis: a meta-analysis of randomized controlled trials. Support Care Cancer. 2019;27(7):2361–70.
135. Zecha JA, Raber-Durlacher JE, Nair RG, Epstein JB, Sonis ST, Elad S, et al. Low level laser therapy/photobiomodulation in the management of side effects of chemoradiation therapy in head and neck cancer: part 1: mechanisms of action, dosimetric, and safety considerations. Support Care Cancer. 2016;24(6):2781–92.
136. Cronshaw M, Parker S, Anagnostaki E, Mylona V, Lynch E, Grootveld M. Photobiomodulation and oral mucositis: a systematic review. Dent J (Basel). 2020;8(3):87.
137. Elad S, Cheng KKF, Lalla RV, Yarom N, Hong C, Logan RM, et al. MASCC/ISOO clinical practice guidelines for the management of mucositis secondary to cancer therapy. Cancer. 2020;126:4423.
138. Zadik Y, Arany PR, Fregnani ER, Bossi P, Antunes HS, Bensadoun RJ, et al. Systematic review of photobiomodulation for the management of oral mucositis in cancer patients and clinical practice guidelines. Support Care Cancer. 2019;27(10):3969–83.
139. Stander S. Chronic pruritus: principals of diagnostics and therapy. Hautarzt. 2007;58(7):627–36. quiz 37
140. Matterne U, Apfelbacher CJ, Loerbroks A, Schwarzer T, Buttner M, Ofenloch R, et al. Prevalence, correlates and characteristics

of chronic pruritus: a population-based cross-sectional study. Acta Derm Venereol. 2011;91(6):674–9.
141. Alizadeh N, Mirpour SH, Golmohamadi R, Darjani A, Eftekhari H, Rafiei R, et al. Chronic generalized pruritus without primary skin lesions: a longitudinal prospective observational study. Int J Dermatol. 2019;58(3):273–8.
142. Larson VA, Tang O, Stander S, Kang S, Kwatra SG. Association between itch and cancer in 16,925 patients with pruritus: experience at a tertiary care center. J Am Acad Dermatol. 2019;80(4):931–7.
143. Beigi M, Haberle M, Gschwendtner A, Baum U, Weisshaar E. Generalized chronic itch as a first sign of malignancy resembling paraneoplastic sensomotoric neuropathy. Acta Derm Venereol. 2018;98(5):526–7.
144. Song A, Gochoco A, Zhan T, Sahu J, Alpdogan O, Porcu P, et al. A prospective cohort study of condensed low-dose total skin electron beam therapy for mycosis fungoides: reduction of disease burden and improvement in quality of life. J Am Acad Dermatol. 2020;83(1):78–85.
145. Bromberg H, Chang Y, Craig D. Pruritic manifestation of peripheral t cell lymphoma effectively managed with mirtazapine: a case report. J Pain Palliat Care Pharmacother. 2020;34(3):153–4.
146. Molloy K, Jonak C, Woei AJF, Guenova E, Busschots AM, Bervoets A, et al. Characteristics associated with significantly worse quality of life in mycosis fungoides/Sezary syndrome from the prospective cutaneous lymphoma international prognostic index (PROCLIPI) study. Br J Dermatol. 2020;182(3):770–9.
147. Luman W, Cull A, Palmer KR. Quality of life in patients stented for malignant biliary obstructions. Eur J Gastroenterol Hepatol. 1997;9(5):481–4.
148. Ballinger AB, McHugh M, Catnach SM, Alstead EM, Clark ML. Symptom relief and quality of life after stenting for malignant bile duct obstruction. Gut. 1994;35(4):467–70.
149. Elford AT, Dwyer JP, Fanning SB. Jaundice, hepatosplenomegaly, and portal lymphadenopathy in a middle-aged female: is it lymphoma? JGH Open. 2020;4(2):292–3.
150. Szepietowski JC, Salomon J. Uremic pruritus: still an important clinical problem. J Am Acad Dermatol. 2004;51(5):842–3.
151. Enk CD, Elad S, Vexler A, Kapelushnik J, Gorodetsky R, Kirschbaum M. Chronic graft-versus-host disease treated with UVB phototherapy. Bone Marrow Transplant. 1998;22(12):1179–83.
152. Mochel MC, Ming ME, Imadojemu S, Gangadhar TC, Schuchter LM, Elenitsas R, et al. Cutaneous autoimmune effects in the setting of therapeutic immune checkpoint inhibition for metastatic melanoma. J Cutan Pathol. 2016;43(9):787–91.
153. Kilic A, Gul U, Soylu S. Skin findings in internal malignant diseases. Int J Dermatol. 2007;46(10):1055–60.
154. Steinman HK, Greaves MW. Aquagenic pruritus. J Am Acad Dermatol. 1985;13(1):91–6.
155. Barnes HM, Sarkany I, Calnan CD. Pruritus and thyrotoxicosis. Trans St Johns Hosp Dermatol Soc. 1974;60(1):59–62.
156. Barrow MV, Bird ED. Pruritus in hyperthyroidism. Arch Dermatol. 1966;93(2):237–8.
157. Papathanasiou IV, Kelepouris K, Valari C, Papagiannis D, Tzavella F, Kourkouta L, et al. Depression, anxiety and stress among patients with hematological malignancies and the association with quality of life: a cross-sectional study. Med Pharm Rep. 2020;93(1):62–8.
158. Stander S, Weisshaar E, Mettang T, Szepietowski JC, Carstens E, Ikoma A, et al. Clinical classification of itch: a position paper of the international forum for the study of itch. Acta Derm Venereol. 2007;87(4):291–4.
159. Huang AH, Kaffenberger BH, Reich A, Szepietowski JC, Stander S, Kwatra SG. Pruritus associated with commonly prescribed medications in a tertiary care center. Medicine. 2019;6(3):84.
160. Peters J. Medication-related pruritis in older adults with long-term conditions. Br J Community Nurs. 2019;24(8):380–2.
161. Nocchi L, Roy N, D'Attilia M, Dhandapani R, Maffei M, Traista A, et al. Interleukin-31-mediated photoablation of pruritogenic epidermal neurons reduces itch-associated behaviours in mice. Nat Biomed Eng. 2019;3(2):114–25.
162. Tsuji M, Arai I, Miyagawa K, Miyagishi H, Saito A, Takeda K, et al. Involvement of interleukin-31 receptor a in morphine-induced itching and antinociception in mice. Eur J Pain. 2019;23(2):378–88.
163. Steinman HK, Kobza-Black A, Lotti TM, Brunetti L, Panconesi E, Greaves MW. Polycythaemia rubra vera and water-induced pruritus: blood histamine levels and cutaneous fibrinolytic activity before and after water challenge. Br J Dermatol. 1987;116(3):329–33.
164. Shah RA, Kowdley KV. Mechanisms and treatments of pruritus in primary biliary cholangitis. Semin Liver Dis. 2019;39(2):209–20.
165. Weisshaar E, Szepietowski JC, Dalgard FJ, Garcovich S, Gieler U, Gimenez-Arnau AM, et al. European S2k guideline on chronic pruritus. Acta Derm Venereol. 2019;99(5):469–506.
166. Krause K, Kessler B, Weller K, Veidt J, Chen SC, Martus P, et al. German version of ItchyQoL: validation and initial clinical findings. Acta Derm Venereol. 2013;93(5):562–8.
167. Lindh JD, Bradley M. Clinical effectiveness of moisturizers in atopic dermatitis and related disorders: a systematic review. Am J Clin Dermatol. 2015;16(5):341–59.
168. Rukwied R, Watkinson A, McGlone F, Dvorak M. Cannabinoid agonists attenuate capsaicin-induced responses in human skin. Pain. 2003;102(3):283–8.
169. Cedeno-Laurent F, Singer EM, Wysocka M, Benoit BM, Vittorio CC, Kim EJ, et al. Improved pruritus correlates with lower levels of IL-31 in CTCL patients under different therapeutic modalities. Clin Immunol. 2015;158(1):1–7.
170. Wolfhagen FH, Sternieri E, Hop WC, Vitale G, Bertolotti M, Van Buuren HR. Oral naltrexone treatment for cholestatic pruritus: a double-blind, placebo-controlled study. Gastroenterology. 1997;113(4):1264–9.
171. Kwatra SG, Stander S, Kang H. PD-1 blockade-induced pruritus treated with a mu-opioid receptor antagonist. N Engl J Med. 2018;379(16):1578–9.
172. Mozer-Glassberg Y, Hojsak I, Zevit N, Shapiro R, Shamir R. Pruritus responsive to naltrexone in a patient with cholestatic liver disease. Isr Medi Assoc J. 2011;13(2):111–2.
173. Mettang M, Weisshaar E. Pruritus: control of itch in patients undergoing dialysis. Skin Therapy Lett. 2010;15(2):1–5.
174. Reszke R, Szepietowski JC. End-stage renal disease chronic itch and its management. Dermatol Clin. 2018;36(3):277–92.
175. Razeghi E, Eskandari D, Ganji MR, Meysamie AP, Togha M, Khashayar P. Gabapentin and uremic pruritus in hemodialysis patients. Ren Fail. 2009;31(2):85–90.
176. Manenti L, Vaglio A, Costantino E, Danisi D, Oliva B, Pini S, et al. Gabapentin in the treatment of uremic itch: an index case and a pilot evaluation. J Nephrol. 2005;18(1):86–91.
177. Simonsen E, Komenda P, Lerner B, Askin N, Bohm C, Shaw J, et al. Treatment of uremic pruritus: a systematic review. Am J Kidney Dis. 2017;70(5):638–55.
178. Ataei S, Kord L, Larki A, Yasrebifar F, Mehrpooya M, Seyedtabib M, et al. Comparison of sertraline with rifampin in the treatment of cholestatic pruritus: a randomized clinical trial. Rev Recent Clin Trials. 2019;14(3):217–23.
179. Roulet T, Zdanowicz N. Delusional parasitosis treated by atypical antipsychotic and selective serotonin reuptake inhibitor: a case report. Psychiatr Danub. 2017;29(Suppl 3):219–21.
180. Greaves MW. Itch in systemic disease: therapeutic options. Dermatol Ther. 2005;18(4):323–7.

181. Gupta MA, Guptat AK. The use of antidepressant drugs in dermatology. J Eur Acad Dermatol Venereol. 2001;15(6):512–8.
182. Khanna R, Boozalis E, Belzberg M, Zampella JG, Kwatra SG. Mirtazapine for the treatment of chronic pruritus. Medicine. 2019;6(3):73.
183. Kaur R, Sinha VR. Antidepressants as antipruritic agents: a review. Eur Neuropsychopharmacol. 2018;28(3):341–52.
184. Kouwenhoven TA, van de Kerkhof PCM, Kamsteeg M. Use of oral antidepressants in patients with chronic pruritus: a systematic review. J Am Acad Dermatol. 2017;77(6):1068–73 e7.
185. Demierre MF, Taverna J. Mirtazapine and gabapentin for reducing pruritus in cutaneous T-cell lymphoma. J Am Acad Dermatol. 2006;55(3):543–4.
186. Davis MP, Frandsen JL, Walsh D, Andresen S, Taylor S. Mirtazapine for pruritus. J Pain Symptom Manag. 2003;25(3):288–91.
187. Rashid S, Trivedi DD, Al-Shathir M, Moulton M, Baumrucker SJ. Is there a role for 5-HT3 receptor antagonists in the treatment of opioid-induced pruritus? Am J Hosp Palliat Care. 2018;35(4):740–4.
188. Muller C, Pongratz S, Pidlich J, Penner E, Kaider A, Schemper M, et al. Treatment of pruritus in chronic liver disease with the 5-hydroxytryptamine receptor type 3 antagonist ondansetron: a randomized, placebo-controlled, double-blind cross-over trial. Eur J Gastroenterol Hepatol. 1998;10(10):865–70.
189. O'Donohue JW, Pereira SP, Ashdown AC, Haigh CG, Wilkinson JR, Williams R. A controlled trial of ondansetron in the pruritus of cholestasis. Aliment Pharmacol Ther. 2005;21(8):1041–5.
190. Swarna SS, Aziz K, Zubair T, Qadir N, Khan M. Pruritus associated with chronic kidney disease: a comprehensive literature review. Cureus. 2019;11(7):e5256.
191. Hussain AB, Samuel R, Hegade VS, Jones DE, Reynolds NJ. Pruritus secondary to primary biliary cholangitis: a review of the pathophysiology and management with phototherapy. Br J Dermatol. 2019;181(6):1138–45.
192. Inan S, Torres-Huerta A, Jensen LE, Dun NJ. Yy a kappa opioid receptor agonist and mu opioid receptor antagonist attenuates pruritus, decreases IL-31, and increases IL-10 in mice with contact dermatitis. Eur J Pharmacol. 2019;864:172702.
193. Mercadante S. Opioid analgesics adverse effects: the other side of the coin. Curr Pharm Des. 2019;25(30):3197–202.
194. Tubog TD, Harenberg JL, Buszta K, Hestand JD. Prophylactic Nalbuphine to prevent Neuraxial opioid-induced pruritus: a systematic review and meta-analysis of randomized controlled trials. J Perianesth Nurs. 2019;34(3):491–501 e8.
195. Lewis JH. Hiccups: causes and cures. J Clin Gastroenterol. 1985;7(6):539–52.
196. Steger M, Schneemann M, Fox M. Systemic review: the pathogenesis and pharmacological treatment of hiccups. Aliment Pharmacol Ther. 2015;42(9):1037–50.
197. Kohse EK, Hollmann MW, Bardenheuer HJ, Kessler J. Chronic hiccups: an underestimated problem. Anesth Analg. 2017;125(4):1169–83.
198. Chang FY, Lu CL. Hiccup: mystery, nature and treatment. J Neurogastroenterol Motil. 2012;18(2):123–30.
199. Jeon YS, Kearney AM, Baker PG. Management of hiccups in palliative care patients. BMJ Support Palliat Care. 2018;8(1):1–6.
200. Woelk CJ. Managing hiccups. Can Fam Physician. 2011;57(6):672–5. e198-201
201. Gilbar P, McPherson I. Severe hiccups during chemotherapy: corticosteroids the likely culprit. J Oncol Pharm Pract. 2009;15(4):233–6.
202. Zhou JN, Huang XE, Ye Z, Li C, Zhang Q, Lin Y, et al. Weekly paclitaxel/ docetaxel combined with a platinum in the treatment of advanced non-small cell lung cancer: a study on efficacy, safety and pre-medication. Asian Pac J Cancer Prev. 2009;10(6):1147–50.
203. Forghieri F, Maccaferri M, Morselli M, Potenza L, Volzone F, Bandieri E, et al. Persistent hiccups as an adverse event to FLAG-IDA regimen for leukemia. Acta Oncol. 2009;48(6):932–3.
204. Takiguchi Y, Watanabe R, Nagao K, Kuriyama T. Hiccups as an adverse reaction to cancer chemotherapy. J Natl Cancer Inst. 2002;94(10):772.
205. Engleman EG, Lankton J, Lankton B. Granulated sugar as treatment for hiccups in conscious patients. N Engl J Med. 1971;285(26):1489.
206. Nausheen F, Mohsin H, Lakhan SE. Neurotransmitters in hiccups. Springerplus. 2016;5(1):1357.
207. Wang T, Wang D. Metoclopramide for patients with intractable hiccups: a multicentre, randomised, controlled pilot study. Intern Med J. 2014;44(12a):1205–9.
208. Zhang C, Zhang R, Zhang S, Xu M, Zhang S. Baclofen for stroke patients with persistent hiccups: a randomized, double-blind, placebo-controlled trial. Trials. 2014;15:295.
209. Curcic J, Schwizer A, Kaufman E, Forras-Kaufman Z, Banerjee S, Roy S, et al. Effects of baclofen on the functional anatomy of the oesophago-gastric junction and proximal stomach in healthy volunteers and patients with GERD assessed by magnetic resonance imaging and high-resolution manometry: a randomised controlled double-blind study. Aliment Pharmacol Ther. 2014;40(10):1230–40.
210. Holloway RH, Boeckxstaens GE, Penagini R, Sifrim D, Smout AJ. Objective definition and detection of transient lower esophageal sphincter relaxation revisited: is there room for improvement? Neurogastroenterol Motil. 2012;24(1):54–60.
211. Lehmann A, Hansson-Branden L, Karrberg L. Effects of repeated administration of baclofen on transient lower esophageal sphincter relaxation in the dog. Eur J Pharmacol. 2000;403(1–2):163–7.
212. Ozturk O, Yavuz E, Yazicioglu B, Uzuner B. Treatment of resistant idiopathic hiccups with pulse radio frequency on phrenic nerve and gabapentin: a case report. Niger J Clin Pract. 2017;20(7):910–3.
213. Ong AM, Tan CS, Foo MW, Kee TY. Gabapentin for intractable hiccups in a patient undergoing peritoneal dialysis. Perit Dial Int. 2008;28(6):667–8.
214. Tegeler ML, Baumrucker SJ. Gabapentin for intractable hiccups in palliative care. Am J Hosp Palliat Care. 2008;25(1):52–4.
215. Dong R, Xu X, Yu L, Ding H, Pan J, Yu Y, et al. Randomised clinical trial: gabapentin vs baclofen in the treatment of suspected refractory gastro-oesophageal reflux-induced chronic cough. Aliment Pharmacol Ther. 2019;49(6):714–22.
216. Polito NB, Fellows SE. Pharmacologic interventions for intractable and persistent hiccups: a systematic review. J Emerg Med. 2017;53(4):540–9.
217. Adam E. A systematic review of the effectiveness of Oral baclofen in the Management of Hiccups in adult palliative care patients. J Pain Palliat Care Pharmacother. 2020;34(1):43–54.
218. Rouse S, Wodziak M. Intractable Hiccups. Curr Neurol Neurosci Rep. 2018;18(8):51.
219. Dyspnea. Mechanisms, assessment, and management: a consensus statement. American Thoracic Society. Am J Respir Crit Care Med. 1999;159(1):321–40.
220. Banzett RBB, Sheridan AR, Baker KM, Lansing RW, Stevens JP. Scared to death' dyspnoea from the hospitalised patient's perspective. BMJ Open Pespir Res. 2020;7(1):e000493.
221. Bruera E, Schmitz B, Pither J, Neumann CM, Hanson J. The frequency and correlates of dyspnea in patients with advanced cancer. J Pain Symptom Manag. 2000;19(5):357–62.
222. Arigliani M, Gupta A. Management of chronic respiratory complications in children and adolescents with sickle cell disease. Eur Respir Rev. 2020;29(157):200054.
223. Alameri HF, Aleem A, Kardas W, Jehangir A, Owais M, Al-Momen A. Dyspnea, pulmonary function and exercise capac-

ity in adult Saudi patients with sickle cell disease. Saudi Med J. 2008;29(5):707–13.
224. Bosnak Guclu M, Bargi G, Sucak GT. Impairments in dyspnea, exercise capacity, physical activity and quality of life of allogeneic hematopoietic stem cell transplantation survivors compared with healthy individuals: a cross sectional study. Physiother Theory Pract. 2019;37:1–12.
225. Roberts MH, Mapel DW, Bruse S, Petersen H, Nyunoya T. Development of a modified BODE index as a mortality risk measure among older adults with and without chronic obstructive pulmonary disease. Am J Epidemiol. 2013;178(7):1150–60.
226. Ueno R, Nemoto M, Uegami W, Fukuoka J, Misawa M. Pembrolizumab-induced pneumonitis with a perilymphatic nodular pattern in a lung cancer patient: a radio-pathologic correlation. Respir Med Case Rep. 2019;26:168–70.
227. Tateishi A, Nakashima K, Hoshi K, Oyama Y, Ebisudani T, Misawa M, et al. Pulmonary tumor thrombotic Microangiopathy mimicking inhalation lung injury. Intern Med. 2019;58(9):1311–4.
228. Kazemi-Bajestani SMR, Becher H, Butts C, Basappa NS, Smylie M, Joy AA, et al. Undiagnosed cardiac deficits in non-small cell carcinoma patients in the candidate population for anti-cachexia clinical trials. Support Care Cancer. 2019;27(4):1551–61.
229. Hecimovic A, Jakopovic M, Vukic Dugac A, Dzubur F, Samarzija M. Metastatic cancer mimics interstitial lung disease. Cases when we need fast diagnosis and treatment. Monaldi archives for chest disease. 2019;89(2)
230. Stana F, Vujovic M, Mayaki D, Leduc-Gaudet JP, Leblanc P, Huck L, et al. Differential regulation of the autophagy and proteasome pathways in skeletal muscles in sepsis. Crit Care Med. 2017;45(9):e971–e9.
231. Travers J, Dudgeon DJ, Amjadi K, McBride I, Dillon K, Laveneziana P, et al. Mechanisms of exertional dyspnea in patients with cancer. J Appl Physiol. 2008;104(1):57–66.
232. Sjoland H, Caidahl K, Karlsson BW, Karlsson T, Herlitz J. Limitation of physical activity, dyspnea and chest pain before and two years after coronary artery bypass grafting in relation to sex. Int J Cardiol. 1997;61(2):123–33.
233. O'Donnell DE, Milne KM, James MD, de Torres JP, Neder JA. Dyspnea in COPD: new mechanistic insights and management implications. Adv Ther. 2020;37(1):41–60.
234. Reijnders T, Troosters T, Janssens W, Gosselink R, Langer D, Davenport PW, et al. Brain activations to Dyspnea in patients with COPD. Front Physiol. 2020;11:7.
235. Schon D, Dahme B, von Leupoldt A. Associations between the perception of dyspnea, pain, and negative affect. Psychophysiology. 2008;45(6):1064–7.
236. Nakai H, Tsujimoto K, Fuchigami T, Ohmatsu S, Osumi M, Nakano H, et al. Effect of anticipation triggered by a prior dyspnea experience on brain activity. J Phys Ther Sci. 2015;27(3):635–9.
237. von Leupoldt A, Sommer T, Kegat S, Baumann HJ, Klose H, Dahme B, et al. The unpleasantness of perceived dyspnea is processed in the anterior insula and amygdala. Am J Respir Crit Care Med. 2008;177(9):1026–32.
238. Gandevia SC, Killian K, McKenzie DK, Crawford M, Allen GM, Gorman RB, et al. Respiratory sensations, cardiovascular control, kinaesthesia and transcranial stimulation during paralysis in humans. J Physiol. 1993;470:85–107.
239. Dudgeon DJ, Lertzman M, Askew GR. Physiological changes and clinical correlations of dyspnea in cancer outpatients. J Pain Symptom Manag. 2001;21(5):373–9.
240. Hui D, Morgado M, Vidal M, Withers L, Nguyen Q, Chisholm G, et al. Dyspnea in hospitalized advanced cancer patients: subjective and physiologic correlates. J Palliat Med. 2013;16(3):274–80.
241. Kuyucu T, Guclu SZ, Saylan B, Demir C, Senol T, Guner S, et al. A cross-sectional observational study to investigate daily symptom variability, effects of symptom on morning activities and therapeutic expectations of patients and physicians in COPD-SUNRISE study. Tuberkuloz ve toraks. 2011;59(4):328–39.
242. Berliner D, Schneider N, Welte T, Bauersachs J. The differential diagnosis of Dyspnea. Dtsch Arztebl Int. 2016;113(49):834–45.
243. Morris NR, Sabapathy S, Adams L, Kingsley RA, Schneider DA, Stulbarg MS. Verbal numerical scales are as reliable and sensitive as visual analog scales for rating dyspnea in young and older subjects. Respir Physiol Neurobiol. 2007;157(2–3):360–5.
244. Farncombe M. Dyspnea: assessment and treatment. Support Care Cancer. 1997;5(2):94–9.
245. Persichini R, Gay F, Schmidt M, Mayaux J, Demoule A, Morelot-Panzini C, et al. Diagnostic accuracy of respiratory distress observation scales as surrogates of Dyspnea self-report in intensive care unit patients. Anesthesiology. 2015;123(4):830–7.
246. Hechtner M, Eichler M, Wehler B, Buhl R, Sebastian M, Stratmann J, et al. Quality of life in NSCLC survivors - a multicenter cross-sectional study. J Thorac Oncol. 2019;14(3):420–35.
247. Camargo LA, Pereira CA. Dyspnea in COPD: beyond the modified Medical Research Council scale. J Bras Pneumol. 2010;36(5):571–8.
248. Blinderman CD, Homel P, Billings JA, Portenoy RK, Tennstedt SL. Symptom distress and quality of life in patients with advanced congestive heart failure. J Pain Symptom Manag. 2008;35(6):594–603.
249. Pratter MR, Curley FJ, Dubois J, Irwin RS. Cause and evaluation of chronic dyspnea in a pulmonary disease clinic. Arch Intern Med. 1989;149(10):2277–82.
250. Pratter MR, Abouzgheib W, Akers S, Kass J, Bartter T. An algorithmic approach to chronic dyspnea. Respir Med. 2011;105(7):1014–21.
251. Meriggi F. Dyspnea in cancer patients: a well-known and neglected symptom. Rev Recent Clin Trials. 2018;13(2):84–8.
252. Renier W, Winckelmann KH, Verbakel JY, Aertgeerts B, Buntinx F. Signs and symptoms in adult patients with acute dyspnea: a systematic review and meta-analysis. Eur J Emerg Med. 2018;25(1):3–11.
253. Hale ZE, Singhal A, Hsia RY. Causes of shortness of breath in the acute patient: a National Study. Acad Emerg Med. 2018;25(11):1227–34.
254. Masago K, Fujita S, Togashi Y, Irisa K, Sakamori Y, Hatachi Y, et al. Association between brain natriuretic peptide and distant metastases in advanced non-small cell lung cancer patients. Oncol Lett. 2011;2(2):253–6.
255. Wang XT, Liu DW, Zhang HM, Chai WZ. Integrated cardiopulmonary sonography: a useful tool for assessment of acute pulmonary edema in the intensive care unit. J Ultrasound Med. 2014;33(7):1231–9.
256. Volpicelli G, Silva F, Radeos M. Real-time lung ultrasound for the diagnosis of alveolar consolidation and interstitial syndrome in the emergency department. Eur J Emerg Med. 2010;17(2):63–72.
257. Frassi F, Gargani L, Tesorio P, Raciti M, Mottola G, Picano E. Prognostic value of extravascular lung water assessed with ultrasound lung comets by chest sonography in patients with dyspnea and/or chest pain. J Card Fail. 2007;13(10):830–5.
258. Uhlving HH, Buchvald F, Heilmann CJ, Nielsen KG, Gormsen M, Muller KG. Bronchiolitis obliterans after Allo-SCT: clinical criteria and treatment options. Bone Marrow Transplant. 2012;47(8):1020–9.
259. Wang X, Liu C, Wang M, Zhang YI, Li H, Liu G. Clinical features of post-infectious bronchiolitis obliterans in children undergoing long-term azithromycin treatment. Exp Ther Med. 2015;9(6):2379–83.
260. Ichikawa Y, Ninomiya H, Katsuki M, Hotta M, Tanaka M, Oizumi K. Low-dose/long-term erythromycin for treatment of bronchiolitis obliterans organizing pneumonia (BOOP). Kurume Med J. 1993;40(2):65–7.

261. Stover DE, Mangino D. Macrolides: a treatment alternative for bronchiolitis obliterans organizing pneumonia? Chest. 2005;128(5):3611–7.
262. Kako J, Kobayashi M, Oosono Y, Kajiwara K, Miyashita M. Immediate effect of fan therapy in terminal cancer with dyspnea at rest: a meta-analysis. Am J Hosp Palliat Care. 2020;37(4):294–9.
263. Ruangsomboon O, Dorongthom T, Chakorn T, Monsomboon A, Praphruetkit N, Limsuwat C, et al. High-flow nasal cannula versus conventional oxygen therapy in relieving dyspnea in emergency palliative patients with do-not-intubate status: a randomized crossover study. Ann Emerg Med. 2019;75:615.
264. Pisani L, Vega ML. Use of nasal high flow in stable COPD: rationale and physiology. COPD. 2017;14(3):346–50.
265. Pisani L, Fasano L, Corcione N, Comellini V, Musti MA, Brandao M, et al. Change in pulmonary mechanics and the effect on breathing pattern of high flow oxygen therapy in stable hypercapnic COPD. Thorax. 2017;72(4):373–5.
266. Nishimura M. High-flow nasal cannula oxygen therapy in adults: physiological benefits, indication, clinical benefits, and adverse effects. Respir Care. 2016;61(4):529–41.
267. Wilson ME, Mittal A, Dobler CC, Curtis JR, Majzoub AM, Soleimani J, et al. High-flow nasal cannula oxygen in patients with acute respiratory failure and do-not-intubate or do-not-resuscitate orders: a systematic review. J Hosp Med. 2020;15(2):101–6.
268. Pisani L, Hill NS, Pacilli AMG, Polastri M, Nava S. Management of dyspnea in the terminally ill. Chest. 2018;154(4):925–34.
269. Vozoris NT. Opioids, chronic obstructive pulmonary disease, and hyperbole. J Palliat Med. 2018;21(6):745.
270. Dy SM GA, Waldfogel JM, Sharma R, Zhang A, Feliciano JL, Sedhom R, Day J, Gersten RA, Davidson PM, Bass EB. Interventions for breathlessness in patients with advanced cancer. Comparative Effectiveness Review No. 232. (Prepared by the Johns Hopkins University Evidence-based Practice Center under Contract No 290–2015-00006-I for the Agency for Healthcare Research and Quality and the Patient-Centered Outcomes Research Institute) AHRQ Publication No 21-EHC024, PCORI Publication No 2020-SR-01. 2020.
271. Strieder M, Pecherstorfer M, Kreye G. Symptomatic treatment of dyspnea in advanced cancer patients : a narrative review of the current literature. Wien Med Wochenschr. 2018;168(13–14):333–43.
272. Haywood A, Duc J, Good P, Khan S, Rickett K, Vayne-Bossert P, et al. Systemic corticosteroids for the management of cancer-related breathlessness (dyspnoea) in adults. Cochrane Database Syst Rev. 2019;2:CD012704.
273. Hui D, Kilgore K, Frisbee-Hume S, Park M, Tsao A, Delgado Guay M, et al. Dexamethasone for dyspnea in cancer patients: a pilot double-blind, randomized, controlled trial. J Pain Symptom Manag. 2016;52(1):8–16 e1.
274. Dogan N, Tasci S. The effects of acupressure on quality of life and dyspnea in lung cancer: a randomized, controlled trial. Altern Ther Health Med. 2020;26(1):49–56.
275. Hernandez A, Bronas UG, Steffen AD, Marquez DX, Fritschi C, Quinn LT, et al. Rhythmic auditory stimulation increases 6-minute walk distance in individuals with COPD: a repeated measures study. Heart Lung. 2020;49:324.
276. Ratarasarn K, Kundu A. Yoga and tai chi: a mind-body approach in managing respiratory symptoms in obstructive lung diseases. Curr Opin Pulm Med. 2020;26(2):186–92.
277. Kanezaki M, Ebihara S. Effect of the cooling sensation induced by olfactory stimulation by L-menthol on dyspnoea: a pilot study. Eur Respir J. 2017;49(4):1601823.
278. Jackson P, Khan A. Delirium in critically ill patients. Crit Care Clin. 2015;31(3):589–603.
279. Siddiqi N, House AO, Holmes JD. Occurrence and outcome of delirium in medical in-patients: a systematic literature review. Age Ageing. 2006;35(4):350–64.
280. Maldonado JR. Acute brain failure: pathophysiology, diagnosis, management, and sequelae of delirium. Crit Care Clin. 2017;33(3):461–519.
281. Morandi A, Bellelli G. Delirium superimposed on dementia. Eur Geriatr Med. 2020;11(1):53–62.
282. Ljubisavljevic V, Kelly B. Risk factors for development of delirium among oncology patients. Gen Hosp Psychiatry. 2003;25(5):345–52.
283. Fann JR, Roth-Roemer S, Burington BE, Katon WJ, Syrjala KL. Delirium in patients undergoing hematopoietic stem cell transplantation. Cancer. 2002;95(9):1971–81.
284. Lawlor PG, Bush SH. Delirium diagnosis, screening and management. Curr Opin Support Palliat Care. 2014;8(3):286–95.
285. Leonard MM, Nekolaichuk C, Meagher DJ, Barnes C, Gaudreau JD, Watanabe S, et al. Practical assessment of delirium in palliative care. J Pain Symptom Manag. 2014;48(2):176–90.
286. Inouye SK, Foreman MD, Mion LC, Katz KH, Cooney LM Jr. Nurses' recognition of delirium and its symptoms: comparison of nurse and researcher ratings. Arch Intern Med. 2001;161(20):2467–73.
287. Maldonado JR. Delirium pathophysiology: an updated hypothesis of the etiology of acute brain failure. Int J Geriatr Psychiatry. 2018;33(11):1428–57.
288. Thom R, Silbersweig DA, Boland RJ. Major depressive disorder in medical illness: a review of assessment, prevalence, and treatment options. Psychosom Med. 2019;81(3):246–55.
289. Oldham MA, Flanagan NM, Khan A, Boukrina O, Marcantonio ER. Responding to ten common delirium misconceptions with best evidence: an educational review for clinicians. J Neuropsychiatr Clin Neurosci. 2018;30(1):51–7.
290. Choi SH, Lee H, Chung TS, Park KM, Jung YC, Kim SI, et al. Neural network functional connectivity during and after an episode of delirium. Am J Psychiatry. 2012;169(5):498–507.
291. Jones RN, Cizginer S, Pavlech L, Albuquerque A, Daiello LA, Dharmarajan K, et al. Assessment of instruments for measurement of delirium severity: a systematic review. JAMA Intern Med. 2019;179(2):231–9.
292. MacLullich AM, Shenkin SD, Goodacre S, Godfrey M, Hanley J, Stiobhairt A, et al. The 4 'A's test for detecting delirium in acute medical patients: a diagnostic accuracy study. Health Technol Assess. 2019;23(40):1–194.
293. Shenkin SD, Fox C, Godfrey M, Siddiqi N, Goodacre S, Young J, et al. Delirium detection in older acute medical inpatients: a multicentre prospective comparative diagnostic test accuracy study of the 4AT and the confusion assessment method. BMC Med. 2019;17(1):138.
294. Numan T, van den Boogaard M, Kamper AM, Rood PJT, Peelen LM, Slooter AJC, et al. Delirium detection using relative delta power based on 1-minute single-channel EEG: a multicentre study. Br J Anaesth. 2019;122(1):60–8.
295. Inouye SK, Bogardus ST Jr, Charpentier PA, Leo-Summers L, Acampora D, Holford TR, et al. A multicomponent intervention to prevent delirium in hospitalized older patients. N Engl J Med. 1999;340(9):669–76.
296. Hosie A, Phillips J, Lam L, Kochovska S, Noble B, Brassil M, et al. Multicomponent non-pharmacological intervention to prevent delirium for hospitalised people with advanced cancer: study protocol for a phase II cluster randomised controlled trial. BMJ Open. 2019;9(1):e026177.
297. Bush SH, Bruera E, Lawlor PG, Kanji S, Davis DH, Agar M, et al. Clinical practice guidelines for delirium management: potential application in palliative care. J Pain Symptom Manag. 2014;48(2):249–58.

298. Gaertner J, Eychmueller S, Leyhe T, Bueche D, Savaskan E, Schlogl M. Benzodiazepines and/or neuroleptics for the treatment of delirium in palliative care?-a critical appraisal of recent randomized controlled trials. Ann Palliat Med. 2019;8(4):504–15.
299. Shrikant KN. No reduction in delirium with the use of haloperidol or ziprasidone in critically ill patients. Am Fam Physician. 2019;99(7):460–1.
300. Riviere J, van der Mast RC, Vandenberghe J, Van Den Eede F. Efficacy and tolerability of atypical antipsychotics in the treatment of delirium: a systematic review of the literature. Psychosomatics. 2019;60(1):18–26.
301. Nikooie R, Neufeld KJ, Oh ES, Wilson LM, Zhang A, Robinson KA, et al. Antipsychotics for treating delirium in hospitalized adults: a systematic review. Ann Intern Med. 2019;171:485.
302. van der Vorst M, Neefjes ECW, Boddaert MSA, Verdegaal B, Beeker A, Teunissen SCC, et al. Olanzapine versus haloperidol for treatment of delirium in patients with advanced cancer: a phase III randomized clinical trial. Oncologist. 2019;25:e570.
303. Tenser RB. Haloperidol and ziprasidone for treatment of delirium in critical illness. N Engl J Med. 2019;380(18):1778.
304. Shen YZ, Peng K, Zhang J, Meng XW, Ji FH. Effects of haloperidol on delirium in adult patients: a systematic review and meta-analysis. Med Princ Pract. 2018;27(3):250–9.
305. Vondeling AM, Knol W, Egberts TCG, Slooter AJC. Anticholinergic drug exposure at intensive care unit admission affects the occurrence of delirium. A prospective cohort study. Eur J Intern Med. 2020;78:121–6.
306. Lawley H, Hewison A. An integrative literature review exploring the clinical management of delirium in patients with advanced cancer. J Clin Nurs. 2017;26(23–24):4172–83.
307. Sun R, Wang S, Li S, Yang C, Zhao Y, Luo A. Effects of dexmedetomidine on delirium and mortality during sedation in ICU patients: a systematic review and meta-analysis protocol. BMJ Open. 2019;9(4):e025850.
308. Maagaard M, Barbateskovic M, Perner A, Jakobsen JC, Wetterslev J. Dexmedetomidine for the management of delirium in critically ill patients-a protocol for a systematic review. Acta Anaesthesiol Scand. 2019;63(4):549–57.
309. Marra A, McGrane TJ, Henson CP, Pandharipande PP. Melatonin in critical care. Crit Care Clin. 2019;35(2):329–40.
310. Foster J, Burry LD, Thabane L, Choong K, Menon K, Duffett M, et al. Melatonin and melatonin agonists to prevent and treat delirium in critical illness: a systematic review protocol. Syst Rev. 2016;5(1):199.
311. Alagiakrishnan K. Melatonin based therapies for delirium and dementia. Discov Med. 2016;21(117):363–71.
312. Baumgartner L, Lam K, Lai J, Barnett M, Thompson A, Gross K, et al. Effectiveness of melatonin for the prevention of intensive care unit delirium. Pharmacotherapy. 2019;39(3):280–7.
313. Hatta K, Kishi Y, Wada K, Takeuchi T, Odawara T, Usui C, et al. Preventive effects of ramelteon on delirium: a randomized placebo-controlled trial. JAMA Psychiatry. 2014;71(4):397–403.
314. Sanford AM, Flaherty JH. Do nutrients play a role in delirium? Curr Opin Clin Nutr Metab Care. 2014;17(1):45–50.
315. Guo Y, Li Y, Zhang Y, Fang S, Xu X, Zhao A, et al. Post-operative delirium associated with metabolic alterations following hemi-arthroplasty in older patients. Age Ageing. 2019;49(1):88–95.
316. Crowley KE, Urben L, Hacobian G, Geiger KL. Valproic acid for the management of agitation and delirium in the intensive care setting: a retrospective analysis. Clin Ther. 2020;42:e65.
317. Yeo QM, Wiley TL, Smith MN, Hammond DA. Oral agents for the management of agitation and agitated delirium in critically ill patients. Crit Care Nurs Q. 2017;40(4):344–62.
318. Gagnon DJ, Fontaine GV, Riker RR, Fraser GL. Repurposing valproate, enteral clonidine, and phenobarbital for comfort in adult ICU patients: a literature review with practical considerations. Pharmacotherapy. 2017;37(10):1309–21.
319. Gagnon DJ, Fontaine GV, Smith KE, Riker RR, Miller RR 3rd, Lerwick PA, et al. Valproate for agitation in critically ill patients: a retrospective study. J Crit Care. 2017;37:119–25.
320. Sher Y, Miller Cramer AC, Ament A, Lolak S, Maldonado JR. Valproic acid for treatment of hyperactive or mixed delirium: rationale and literature review. Psychosomatics. 2015;56(6):615–25.
321. Asadollahi S, Heidari K, Hatamabadi H, Vafaee R, Yunesian S, Azadbakht A, et al. Efficacy and safety of valproic acid versus haloperidol in patients with acute agitation: results of a randomized, double-blind, parallel-group trial. Int Clin Psychopharmacol. 2015;30(3):142–50.
322. Potharajaroen S, Tangwongchai S, Tayjasanant T, Thawitsri T, Anderson G, Maes M. Bright light and oxygen therapies decrease delirium risk in critically ill surgical patients by targeting sleep and acid-base disturbances. Psychiatry Res. 2018;261:21–7.
323. Estrup S, Kjer CKW, Poulsen LM, Gogenur I, Mathiesen O. Delirium and effect of circadian light in the intensive care unit: a retrospective cohort study. Acta Anaesthesiol Scand. 2018;62(3):367–75.
324. Krebber AM, Buffart LM, Kleijn G, Riepma IC, de Bree R, Leemans CR, et al. Prevalence of depression in cancer patients: a meta-analysis of diagnostic interviews and self-report instruments. Psycho-Oncology. 2014;23(2):121–30.
325. Block SD. Psychological issues in end-of-life care. J Palliat Med. 2006;9(3):751–72.
326. Trivedi MH, Wisniewski SR, Morris DW, Fava M, Gollan JK, Warden D, et al. Concise health risk tracking scale: a brief self-report and clinician rating of suicidal risk. J Clin Psychiatry. 2011;72(6):757–64.
327. Amonoo HL, Fenech A, Greer JA, Temel JS, Huffman JC, El-Jawahri A. Does desire to pursue pleasurable activities matter? The impact of pretransplantation anhedonia on quality of life and fatigue in hematopoietic stem cell transplantation. Biol Blood Marrow Transplant. 2020;26(8):1477–81.
328. Fujisawa D. Depression in cancer care. Keio J Med. 2018;67(3):37–44.
329. Watanabe N, Omori IM, Nakagawa A, Cipriani A, Barbui C, Churchill R, et al. Mirtazapine versus other antidepressive agents for depression. Cochrane Database Syst Rev. 2011;12:CD006528.
330. Barbosa MG, Delfino RS, Sarin LM, Jackowski AP. Repeated subcutaneous esketamine administration for depressive symptoms and pain relief in a terminally ill cancer patient: a case report. Palliat Med. 2020;34(6):822–5.
331. Falk E, Schlieper D, van Caster P, Lutterbeck MJ, Schwartz J, Cordes J, et al. A rapid positive influence of S-ketamine on the anxiety of patients in palliative care: a retrospective pilot study. BMC Palliat Care. 2020;19(1):1.
332. Tremblay A, Breitbart W. Psychiatric dimensions of palliative care. Neurol Clin. 2001;19(4):949–67.
333. Lloyd-Williams M, Friedman T, Rudd N. An analysis of the validity of the hospital anxiety and depression scale as a screening tool in patients with advanced metastatic cancer. J Pain Symptom Manag. 2001;22(6):990–6.
334. Reuben DB, Mor V. Nausea and vomiting in terminal cancer patients. Arch Intern Med. 1986;146(10):2021–3.
335. Morran C, Smith DC, Anderson DA, McArdle CS. Incidence of nausea and vomiting with cytotoxic chemotherapy: a prospective randomised trial of antiemetics. Br Med J. 1979;1(6174):1323–4.
336. Gao S, Zhang M, Wu K, Zhu J, He Z, Li J, et al. Risk of adverse events in lymphoma patients treated with brentuximab vedotin: a systematic review and meta-analysis. Expert Opin Drug Saf. 2020;19(5):617–23.

337. Di Renzo N, Musso M, Scime R, Cupri A, Perrone T, De Risi C, et al. Efficacy and safety of multiple doses of NEPA without dexamethasone in preventing nausea and vomiting induced by multiple-day and high-dose chemotherapy in patients with non-Hodgkin's lymphoma undergoing autologous hematopoietic stem cell transplantation: a phase IIa, multicenter study. Bone Marrow Transplant. 2020;55:2114.
338. Tendas A, Marchesi F, Mengarelli A, Annibali O, Tomarchio V, Saltarelli D, et al. Prevention of chemotherapy-induced nausea and vomiting after high-dose melphalan and stem cell transplantation: review of the evidence and suggestions. Support Care Cancer. 2019;27(3):793–803.
339. Crossnohere NL, Richardson DR, Reinhart C, O'Donoghue B, Love SM, Smith BD, et al. Side effects from acute myeloid leukemia treatment: results from a national survey. Curr Med Res Opin. 2019;35(11):1965–70.
340. Rizio AA, White MK, McCausland KL, Quock TP, Guthrie SD, Yokota M, et al. Treatment tolerability in patients with immunoglobulin light-chain amyloidosis. Am Health Drug Benefits. 2018;11(8):430–7.
341. Kuchuk I, Bouganim N, Beusterien K, Grinspan J, Vandermeer L, Gertler S, et al. Preference weights for chemotherapy side effects from the perspective of women with breast cancer. Breast Cancer Res Treat. 2013;142(1):101–7.
342. Roscoe JA, Morrow GR, Aapro MS, Molassiotis A, Olver I. Anticipatory nausea and vomiting. Support Care Cancer. 2011;19(10):1533–8.
343. Morrow GR. Susceptibility to motion sickness and the development of anticipatory nausea and vomiting in cancer patients undergoing chemotherapy. Cancer Treat Rep. 1984;68(9):1177–8.
344. Stephenson J, Davies A. An assessment of aetiology-based guidelines for the management of nausea and vomiting in patients with advanced cancer. Support Care Cancer. 2006;14(4):348–53.
345. Hui D, Bruera E. The Edmonton symptom assessment system 25 years later: past, present, and future developments. J Pain Symptom Manag. 2017;53(3):630–43.
346. Cheng AW, Abdeljaber M, Lima NA, Shebrain S. Large bowel obstruction in the setting of small lymphocytic lymphoma. Cureus. 2020;12(8):e9640.
347. Kasparian S, Burns E, Shehabeldin A, Awar M, Pingali SR. Recurrent small bowel obstruction caused by Burkitt lymphoma in an elderly man: a case report and review of the literature. J Med Case Rep. 2020;14(1):127.
348. Shirwaikar Thomas A, Schwartz M, Quigley E. Gastrointestinal lymphoma: the new mimic. BMJ Open Gastroenterol. 2019;6(1):e000320.
349. Menke DM, Kyle RA, Fleming CR, Wolfe JT 3rd, Kurtin PJ, Oldenburg WA. Symptomatic gastric amyloidosis in patients with primary systemic amyloidosis. Mayo Clin Proc. 1993;68(8):763–7.
350. Coluzzi F, Rolke R, Mercadante S. Pain management in patients with multiple myeloma: an update. Cancers (Basel). 2019;11(12):2037.
351. Sloot S, Boland J, Snowden JA, Ezaydi Y, Foster A, Gethin A, et al. Side effects of analgesia may significantly reduce quality of life in symptomatic multiple myeloma: a cross-sectional prevalence study. Support Care Cancer. 2015;23(3):671–8.
352. Glare P, Walsh D, Sheehan D. The adverse effects of morphine: a prospective survey of common symptoms during repeated dosing for chronic cancer pain. Am J Hosp Palliat Care. 2006;23(3):229–35.
353. Cherny N, Ripamonti C, Pereira J, Davis C, Fallon M, McQuay H, et al. Strategies to manage the adverse effects of oral morphine: an evidence-based report. J Clin Oncol. 2001;19(9):2542–54.
354. Razvi Y, Chan S, McFarlane T, McKenzie E, Zaki P, DeAngelis C, et al. ASCO, NCCN, MASCC/ESMO: a comparison of antiemetic guidelines for the treatment of chemotherapy-induced nausea and vomiting in adult patients. Support Care Cancer. 2019;27(1):87–95.
355. Grunberg SM, Osoba D, Hesketh PJ, Gralla RJ, Borjeson S, Rapoport BL, et al. Evaluation of new antiemetic agents and definition of antineoplastic agent emetogenicity--an update. Support Care Cancer. 2005;13(2):80–4.
356. Jordan K, Chan A, Gralla RJ, Jahn F, Rapoport B, Warr D, et al. 2016 updated MASCC/ESMO consensus recommendations: emetic risk classification and evaluation of the emetogenicity of antineoplastic agents. Support Care Cancer. 2017;25(1):271–5.
357. Grunberg SM, Deuson RR, Mavros P, Geling O, Hansen M, Cruciani G, et al. Incidence of chemotherapy-induced nausea and emesis after modern antiemetics. Cancer. 2004;100(10):2261–8.
358. Aapro M, Zhang L, Yennu S, LeBlanc TW, Schwartzberg L. Preventing chemotherapy-induced nausea and vomiting with netupitant/palonosetron, the first fixed combination antiemetic: current and future perspective. Future Oncol. 2019;15(10):1067–84.
359. Navari RM, Qin R, Ruddy KJ, Liu H, Powell SF, Bajaj M, et al. Olanzapine for the prevention of chemotherapy-induced nausea and vomiting. N Engl J Med. 2016;375(2):134–42.
360. Berger MJ, Ettinger DS, Aston J, Barbour S, Bergsbaken J, Bierman PJ, et al. NCCN guidelines insights: antiemesis, Version 2.2017. J Natl Compr Cancer Netw. 2017;15(7):883–93.
361. Hesketh PJ, Kris MG, Basch E, Bohlke K, Barbour SY, Clark-Snow RA, et al. Antiemetics: ASCO guideline update. J Clin Oncol. 2020;38:JCO2001296.
362. Herrstedt J, Roila F, Warr D, Celio L, Navari RM, Hesketh PJ, et al. 2016 updated MASCC/ESMO consensus recommendations: prevention of nausea and vomiting following high emetic risk chemotherapy. Support Care Cancer. 2017;25(1):277–88.
363. Einhorn LH, Rapoport B, Navari RM, Herrstedt J, Brames MJ. 2016 updated MASCC/ESMO consensus recommendations: prevention of nausea and vomiting following multiple-day chemotherapy, high-dose chemotherapy, and breakthrough nausea and vomiting. Support Care Cancer. 2017;25(1):303–8.
364. Hardy J, Skerman H, Glare P, Philip J, Hudson P, Mitchell G, et al. A randomized open-label study of guideline-driven antiemetic therapy versus single agent antiemetic therapy in patients with advanced cancer and nausea not related to anticancer treatment. BMC Cancer. 2018;18(1):510.
365. Davis MP, Hallerberg G. Palliative medicine study group of the multinational association of supportive care in c. a systematic review of the treatment of nausea and/or vomiting in cancer unrelated to chemotherapy or radiation. J Pain Symptom Manag. 2010;39(4):756–67.
366. Navari RM, Pywell CM, Le-Rademacher JG, White P, Dodge AB, Albany C, et al. Olanzapine for the treatment of advanced cancer-related chronic nausea and/or vomiting: a randomized pilot trial. JAMA Oncol. 2020;6(6):895–9.
367. Davis MP. Cannabinoids for symptom management and cancer therapy: the evidence. J Natl Compr Cancer Netw. 2016;14(7):915–22.
368. Winston AW, Rinehart RS, Riley GP, Vacchiano CA, Pellegrini JE. Comparison of inhaled isopropyl alcohol and intravenous ondansetron for treatment of postoperative nausea. AANA J. 2003;71(2):127–32.
369. Verma DK, Bansal S, Sharma P, Sundararaman P. Control of postoperative nausea and vomiting in oral and maxillofacial surgery patients with isopropyl alcohol: a prospective randomized clinical trial. J Maxillofac Oral Surg. 2018;17(4):576–81.
370. Teran L, Hawkins JK. The effectiveness of inhalation isopropyl alcohol vs. granisetron for the prevention of postoperative nausea and vomiting. AANA J. 2007;75(6):417–22.

371. Schwartz A. Comparison of inhalation of isopropyl alcohol vs promethazine in the treatment of postoperative nausea and vomiting (PONV) in patients identified as high risk for developing PONV. AANA J. 2009;77(6):417–8. author reply 8
372. Radford KD, Fuller TN, Bushey B, Daniel C, Pellegrini JE. Prophylactic isopropyl alcohol inhalation and intravenous ondansetron versus ondansetron alone in the prevention of postoperative nausea and vomiting in high-risk patients. AANA J. 2011;79(4 Suppl):S69–74.
373. Pellegrini J, DeLoge J, Bennett J, Kelly J. Comparison of inhalation of isopropyl alcohol vs promethazine in the treatment of postoperative nausea and vomiting (PONV) in patients identified as at high risk for developing PONV. AANA J. 2009;77(4):293–9.
374. Beadle KL, Helbling AR, Love SL, April MD, Hunter CJ. Isopropyl alcohol nasal inhalation for nausea in the emergency department: a randomized controlled trial. Ann Emerg Med. 2016;68(1):1–9 e1.
375. Dupuis LL, Roscoe JA, Olver I, Aapro M, Molassiotis A. 2016 updated MASCC/ESMO consensus recommendations: anticipatory nausea and vomiting in children and adults receiving chemotherapy. Support Care Cancer. 2017;25(1):317–21.
376. Zeltzer LK, Dolgin MJ, LeBaron S, LeBaron C. A randomized, controlled study of behavioral intervention for chemotherapy distress in children with cancer. Pediatrics. 1991;88(1):34–42.
377. Varejao CDS, Santo F. Laser acupuncture for relieving nausea and vomiting in pediatric patients undergoing chemotherapy: a single-blind randomized clinical trial. J Pediatr Oncol Nurs. 2019;36(1):44–54.

# 15 Rehabilitation Medicine

Jack B. Fu, George J. Francis, Shinichiro Morishita, and Julie K. Silver

## Introduction

The field of cancer rehabilitation is relatively new having its roots tracing back to the late 1960s and early 1970s [1]. Interest in cancer rehabilitation has grown tremendously in the past 10 years, propelled by the tremendous growth in survivors, the resulting increase in oncology-related functional impairments, and their impact on quality of life in survivorship [2]. Cancer survivors can suffer from a variety of impairments related to cancer and its treatment that rehabilitation can address, including cancer-related fatigue, chemotherapy-induced peripheral neuropathy, lymphedema, shoulder dysfunction, and muscle imbalances. More recently, the concept of exercise as cancer medicine (e.g., prehabilitation and exercise in advanced recovery) and its potential impact on survival has propelled a new and exciting era to the field.

The field of rehabilitation focuses on improving patient function and consists of multiple disciplines including physical therapists, occupational therapists, speech language pathologists, recreational therapists, music therapists, neuropsychologists, social workers, case managers, and physical medicine and rehabilitation (PMR) physician specialists (also known as physiatrists). There are numerous other clinicians that may be involved as well. Physical therapy typically focuses on increasing endurance, strength, and mobility. Occupational therapy focuses on improving activities of daily living (ADLs) such as bathing and dressing, instrumental ADLs (IADLs) such as performing chores and work or community activities, recommending adaptive equipment for home or work including durable medical equipment and wheelchairs. Speech language pathologists work on improving swallowing (e.g., dysphagia after head and neck cancer treatment), verbal communication (including dysarthria and aphasia), and cognition. Recreational therapists seek to find feasible hobbies and activities based on patient function that provide joy and meaning. Neuropsychologists provide cognitive testing that can be useful for therapists and physicians to determine the ability to return to certain basic ADLs and higher-level activities such as returning to work. In particular, cancer physiatrists contribute to rehabilitation by prescribing therapies and functional testing, performing electrodiagnostic testing, overseeing patient management on inpatient rehabilitation, assisting with return to work and disability, prescribing medications to reduce patient symptoms, and performing injections and other procedures to reduce pain and improve function [3, 4].

In 1980, Dr. J. Herbert Dietz, a physiatrist and surgeon at Memorial Sloan Kettering Cancer Center, published an influential review article on cancer rehabilitation. Dietz described four stages of cancer rehabilitation which continue to describe cancer rehabilitation interventions (Table 15.1). The stages include preventative, restorative, supportive, and palliative cancer rehabilitation. Palliative cancer rehabilitation was initially defined by Dietz as "rehabilitation efforts to increase functional independence and emotional support to reduce discomfort of patients with advanced disease where relentless disease progression and death can be expected" [5]. In practice, palliative cancer rehabilitation focuses on efficiently improving patient function, but also informed by expected prognosis and survival time. In 2017, Cheville et al.

J. B. Fu (✉)
Department of Palliative, Rehabilitation and Integrative Medicine, University of Texas MD Anderson Cancer Center, Houston, TX, USA
e-mail: jfu@mdanderson.org

G. J. Francis
Department of Clinical Neurosciences, Cumming School of Medicine, University of Calgary, Calgary, AB, Canada
e-mail: george.francis@ahs.ca

S. Morishita
Department of Physical Therapy, School of Health Sciences, Fukushima Medical University, Fukushima, Japan
e-mail: morishit@fmu.ac.jp

J. K. Silver
Department of Physical Medicine and Rehabilitation, Harvard Medical School, Massachusetts General Hospital, Boston, MA, USA
e-mail: julie_Silver@hms.harvard.edu


C. K. Ullrich, E. J. Roeland (eds.), *Palliative Care in Hematologic Malignancies and Serious Blood Disorders*, https://doi.org/10.1007/978-3-031-38058-7_15

**Table 15.1** Dietz's cancer rehabilitation stages [5]

| Stage | Definition | Example |
|---|---|---|
| Preventative | Rehabilitation and education prior to a significant cancer intervention (e.g., surgery, hematopoietic stem cell transplant, CAR-T treatment) to minimize the expected effects of the treatment and mitigate functional deterioration. | Prehabilitation before Whipple procedure or allogeneic stem cell transplant. Education regarding neurogenic bowel/bladder prior to sacrectomy. Shoulder range of motion prior to mastectomy or radiation. |
| Restorative | Rehabilitation after an intervention with expectation of no evidence of disease or ongoing | Inpatient neurorehabilitation after craniotomy and neurosurgical resection of a grade I meningioma with low risk of recurrence Rehabilitation may be focused on recovering strength, balance, and mild cognitive deficits. |
| Supportive | Rehabilitation during ongoing cancer treatment with expectation of continued cancer presence or progression. | Outpatient rehabilitation efforts in a patient with glioblastoma multiforme who completed chemoradiation, then experienced radiation necrosis, tumor recurrence, and then transitioned to bevacizumab. This patient is expected to have permanent and likely progressive neurologic deficits. |
| Palliative | End of life. Emphasis can be on family training and getting the patient home | No additional cancer treatments are being offered by the oncology team in a patient who has suffered a recent functional decline. |

*CAR-T* chimeric antigen receptor thymocyte

defined palliative cancer rehabilitation as "function-directed care delivered in partnership with other disciplines and aligned with the values of patients who have serious and often incurable illness in contexts marked by intense and dynamic symptoms, psychological stress, and medical morbidity, to realize potentially time-limited goals" [6].

## Challenges to Rehabilitating Hematologic Malignancy Patients

The significant co-morbidities associated with advanced cancers can make palliative rehabilitation challenging. Multiple studies have demonstrated that cancer patients, and in particular hematologic malignancy patients, are at significantly increased risk of experiencing medical complications hindering rehabilitation efforts. Infections have repeatedly been found to be the most common reason for transfer off of acute inpatient rehabilitation units to the acute care service, with other reasons including progression of disease requiring further chemotherapy, profound fatigue, or respiratory decompensation [7–12].

Pancytopenia is a common finding in cancer rehabilitation patients due to the cancer itself, chronic disease, chemotherapy/radiation-related marrow suppression, or during the engraftment period after hematopoietic cell transplantation. A number of pancytopenia exercise precautionary guidelines have been proposed over time [13]. Unfortunately, the research in this area has been sparse. MD Anderson Cancer Center therapy guidelines used for pancytopenia are described in Table 15.2.

Leukopenia/neutropenia may increase the risk of patient infections. Neutropenic precautions may be utilized to minimize the risk of potentially catastrophic infection in these severely immunosuppressed patients. Anemia is also a concern due to the risk of syncope, pre-syncope, and increased cardiac burden. Hemoglobin should be checked frequently in patients with myelosuppression so appropriate physical activity adjustments and transfusions can be provided. Additionally, thrombocytopenia can be worrisome due to the

**Table 15.2** MD Anderson cancer center institutional exercise precautions for cancer-related pancytopenia [14]

| Precaution | Definition | MD Anderson precautions |
|---|---|---|
| Neutropenia | Absolute neutrophil count <500/μL | 1. Therapist wears mask/ gloves in room<br>2. Patient wears mask/ gloves outside of room<br>3. Clean equipment<br>4. Avoid group therapy or close proximity to other patients |
| Anemia | Hemoglobin <13.5 grams/100 mL in males<br>Hemoglobin <12.0 grams/100 mL in females | 1. Hemoglobin <8, transfuse<br>2. Hemoglobin <7, no therapy<br>3. Therapy can be considered if blood transfusion running |
| Thrombocytopenia | Platelet count <150,000/μL | 1. 20,000/μL—No additional restrictions<br>2. 10,000-20,000/μL—No resistive exercise. If a high fall risk, avoid standing/ambulating.<br>3. 5000–10,000/μL—No resistive exercises and minimal activity (limit the exercises to in bed or chair)<br>4. < 5000/μL—Discuss with medical team or consider deferring treatment |

*μL* microliter, *mL* milliliter

potential risk of exercise associated bleeding such as intramuscular hematomas, intracranial hemorrhages, and trauma/fall-related bleeding. A recently published study demonstrated a low risk of physical activity-related bleeding complications in profoundly thrombocytopenic acute inpatient rehabilitation patients using the MD Anderson institutional guidelines [15].

Inpatient rehabilitation can be delivered in a number of settings including the acute care oncology service, an acute inpatient rehabilitation facility (IRF), skilled nursing facility (SNF), and long-term acute care facility (LTAC). These inpatient cancer rehabilitation settings are defined by differing levels of rehabilitation, medical stability, ability to participate in rehabilitation treatment, and intensity of medical/nursing care. Acute inpatient rehabilitation, frequently called an IRF, is the most intensive rehabilitation setting with 3 h Monday through Friday including a combination of physical therapy, occupational therapy, and/or speech language pathology. In order to qualify, patients must be able to medically and physically tolerate all 3 h of daily therapy. They also require a medical doctor or advanced practice practitioner to evaluate the patient at least five times a week. However, in many cancer acute inpatient units, patients are seen seven times a week due in part to concern of their medical complexity. Subacute inpatient rehabilitation is a term used to describe SNFs and LTACs. The biggest difference between LTAC and SNF is the medical/nursing component. LTAC patients typically receive daily physician visits and more intensive nursing care for issues including prolonged mechanical ventilation, wound care, intravenous antibiotics, dialysis, or total parental nutrition. Therapy is usually 1-h per day (but can be up to 3-h per day in some facilities). Lastly, physicians or advanced practice providers evaluate SNF patients one to two times per week with 24-h nursing care. Therapies are usually 1–2-h per day. The presence or absence of IRFs and SNFs in various geographic regions may result in rehabilitation being delivered in acute care hospitals or LTACs until these units or centers are established.

Studies on the return to primary acute care of some acute inpatient rehabilitation cancer populations have shown increased medical complications compared to non-cancer patients [7, 8]. In a study of acute inpatient rehabilitation hematopoietic stem cell transplant patients, 41% of patients transferred back to the primary acute care service due to medical complications. Of those, 38% died in the hospital after subsequent transfer [12]. Data show a return to the primary acute care service rate of 26–37% in other hematologic malignancy populations [9–11].

Given the medical complexity of oncology patients, clinicians manage the risks of complications creatively during inpatient rehabilitation. One solution is having an internist or the oncology team continue to follow the patient while on inpatient rehabilitation. This arrangement, however, may not be possible due to distance from the acute care hospital, physician hospital privileges, or time constraints [11]. Another potential model is to provide increased and more intensive physiatrist-supervised rehabilitation on the inpatient acute care service. The Mayo Clinic uses this type of model for decades, and more recently, the University of Michigan utilizes this model [16, 17].

In the United States (US), cancer rehabilitation can be administered at home (e.g., via in person home health therapy visits or virtually with telemedicine), at an outpatient ambulatory therapy facility or in some cases, inpatient hospice. In the US, the maximum frequency covered by most insurance payers is three times per week for each discipline. Total covered outpatient therapy visits per year may also have a cap by the insurer. For home health therapy, patients must be considered "home bound" and thus unable to receive therapy at an outpatient facility due to medical or transportation reasons. Telemedicine is becoming an increasingly available option and patients may have virtual visits with a variety of clinicians including physicians, rehabilitation therapists, and mental health clinicians. Of course, virtual visits have limitations, but a recent study demonstrated feasibility specifically for rehabilitation interventions in oncology patients and in the COVID era are increasingly utilized [18].

## Palliative Care and Cancer Rehabilitation: Treating a Common Patient Population

The two disciplines of rehabilitation and palliative care share many commonalities. Both specialties utilize multidisciplinary teams and both are predominantly focused on improving quality of life rather than prolonging survival [19]. A rehabilitation team can include a combination of team members as previously mentioned, including physiatry, physical therapy, occupational therapy, speech language pathology, neuropsychology, social work, and case management.

In the US, physiatrists are one of several physician specialties that are able to pursue palliative care fellowships and seek board certification in palliative care. Due to the interplay of cancer-related symptoms and function, many cancer physiatrists have pursued this dual board certification.

Cancer rehabilitation and palliative care frequently see the same patients with advanced cancer suffering from considerable symptom burden. Reduced physical function often triggers a rehabilitation consultation. Oftentimes, the patients' functional decline is due to cancer-related symptoms in patients with advanced cancer such as cancer-related fatigue, cancer pain, or failure to thrive secondary to nausea, anorexia, and cachexia. Several models of collaboration between rehabilitation and palliative care have been proposed [6, 19–21]. At MD Anderson Cancer Center, palliative care and physiatry are two sections within the same department and share the same outpatient clinic space. Cross consultation between the two specialties is common. Examples of physiatry involvement in palliative care patients include assessing the appropriateness of inpatient or outpatient rehabilitation for patients receiving palliative care, strategies for energy conservation including caregiver training and appropriate equipment, and interventional pain management.

Cancer rehabilitation utilization is common in patients with advanced cancer. During inpatient acute care admissions, rehabilitation is frequently consulted to prepare a patient for potential hospital discharge. If a patient is unable to be safely discharged home due to functional/safety concerns, transfer to post-acute inpatient rehabilitation facilities (e.g., acute inpatient rehabilitation, SNF, or LTAC) may be needed. Early involvement of palliative care has demonstrated improved quality of life and coping for patients and caregivers leading to goal aligned care and healthcare cost reductions [22].

Another frequent situation found in patients with advanced cancer is the need to improve physical performance status in order to qualify for additional cancer treatment. Oncologists may require patients to be mobile with specific functional abilities (e.g., a minimum Eastern Cooperative Oncology Group [23] or Karnofsky Performance Score [24]) and ask patients to pause cancer treatments with the goal of building enough strength to enroll in experimental protocols or for an additional cycle of chemotherapy. The potential that ineffective rehabilitation could perhaps lead to a patient not receiving life-prolonging treatment can be stressful for patients and the rehabilitation team [25]. Similarly, clinicians advocate for cancer rehabilitation involvement earlier in the oncology trajectory [19, 26].

Exercise is safe in patients with advanced cancer and improves quality of life and function (though caution is always warranted and clinical judgment is important). Benefits in physical outcome measures such as the 6-min walk test as a result of aerobic exercise are used in patients with metastatic cancer patients [27]. Besides improving functional status, multiple randomized control trials demonstrate physical activity and exercise decrease cancer-related symptoms in patients with early and advanced stage cancer. Exercise interventions improve quality of life, cancer-related fatigue, insomnia, and dyspnea in patients with advanced cancer. Physical activity may help minimize the need for medications and their associated side effects [28]. In summary, exercise may be a useful tool for any oncology clinician treating cancer-related symptoms.

Many clinicians utilize the American College of Sports Medicine Exercise Guidelines for Cancer Survivors clinicians to advise patients on exercise participation most recently updated in 2019. The new guidelines emphasize targeted exercise prescriptions but also proposed at least 30-min of moderate-intensity exercise three times per week and resistance exercise two to three times per week for 30 min per session (targeting large muscle groups in 2–3 sets) [29]. Physiatry can help in determining the ability of palliative care patients to participate in an exercise program, utilizing exercise prescriptions taking into account the time, dose, and appropriate facilitative equipment such as stationary ergometers and walking programs.

The goal of the cancer physiatrist is to maximize function. Cancer-related symptoms can impact functions, such as excessive fatigue, nausea, vomiting, and cachexia. Cancer symptoms can also affect rehabilitation participation which is an important issue for physiatrists. To receive acute inpatient rehabilitation, patients must be able to participate in 3-h of therapy daily. In order to achieve these goals, many cancer physiatrists are experienced in treating cancer-related symptoms. Two studies on the acute inpatient rehabilitation unit at MD Anderson have demonstrated significant improvements in Edmonton Symptom and Assessment Scores (ESAS) from admission to discharge [30, 31]. The effects of increased physical activity and resolution of acute medical conditions are likely contributors to this symptomatic improvement; however, physiatrist interventions such as medication or injections likely also contributed.

Pain management is a prominent subspecialty within physiatry. The use of systemic analgesic medications and the use of injections are common within physiatry residency training programs. Therefore, most physiatrists are comfortable managing pain in cancer patients including both nociceptive and neuropathic pain. The physiatrist's knowledge of neurologic and musculoskeletal anatomy and related ailments are useful for treating non-cancer-related pain. For example, the use of focal injections to alleviate non-cancer-related pain could potentially reduce the need for opioids with their associated side effects [3, 4]. Additionally, the ability to utilize both neuromuscular knowledge and electrodiagnostic testing to identify comorbid sources of pain (e.g., compressive neuropathy, plexopathy, radiculopathy, chemotherapy-induced peripheral neuropathy) help to diagnose and further treat previously unidentified sources of pain [32].

The rehabilitation goals of a patient at the end of life are quite different from an individual with a long-life expectancy. Important and meaningful future events such as the wedding of a child, graduation of a relative, or upcoming family reunion should be considered. Near the end of life, time becomes an important and limited resource for the patient and thus becomes an important consideration for rehabilitation interventions. If a patient has a few weeks to live, spending 2 weeks on acute inpatient rehabilitation may be a poor use of that time if getting home is not a realistic goal. The quickest, yet safest way, to get patients home should be taken into consideration. This may require caregiver training to give the extra help needed or extra equipment (e.g., Hoyer Lift) to manage patients at home. For example, for most patients with newly diagnosed paraplegia multiple tasks must be performed, including performing transfers, bowel program, bladder intermittent catheterizations, and wheelchair mobility independently. However, in someone with advanced cancer with new spinal cord compression-related paraplegia, many of these goals may need to be done at home by caregivers or home care, or through outpatient services. While the outpatient/home setting is typically not the optimal setting to address these goals, it may be necessary to get the patient closer to family, friends, and the important people in their lives.

Yet, accurately predicting survival time is incredibly challenging for physicians. Studies demonstrate the objective predictors (e.g., the palliative prognostic score [PAP]) significantly more accurate than subjective physician prediction [33–35]. In a study of 2700 patients with metastatic brain lesions, 45% of estimations were inaccurate by 6 or more months, including 18% off by 12 months or more [36]. Prognostic inaccuracy makes discussions regarding the appropriate choice for rehabilitation in the palliative setting quite difficult at times, given the unpredictable nature of some patients' tumors and rate of disease progression. Clearly discussing the goals of rehabilitation interventions openly with patients and their caregivers is recommended in the setting of advanced cancer and potentially limited prognosis. Hopefully, a balance between spending time at home and the beneficial effects of rehabilitation can be achieved including reduced caregiver burden and increased patient independence.

Psychologically, palliative care patients may want to focus on maintaining function and maximum independence while still orienting to their disease and prognosis [37]. Physical function and the ability to perform ADLs have been found to be one of the greatest unmet needs for patients with terminal cancer [38, 39]. Worsening dependency can be a distressing concern at the end of life [40–42]. Studies have shown that patients receiving palliative care felt less abandonment, anxiety, and loss of control through participation in rehabilitation programs [43]. In a study of Japanese inpatient hospice rehabilitation, patients made demonstrable functional gains (mean Barthel Mobility Index [44] increased from 12.4 to 19.9). In addition, patients and their caregivers reported increased satisfaction with their care when rehabilitation was incorporated into their inpatient hospice care. This study demonstrated that 46/355 hospice inpatients were able to discharge to home hospice from inpatient hospice because of their functional improvement. In that study, 68% of families participated in the patients' rehabilitation [45]. In another randomized control trial of hospice patients receiving daily multidisciplinary rehabilitation, those that received rehabilitation had fewer unmet needs at the end of life and utilized fewer resources than the usual care control group [46].

Low rate of referral to cancer rehabilitation has been a chronic issue for the subspecialty. Movsas et al. demonstrated that 87% of an oncology inpatient cohort had motor/functional needs, however, only 18% received a physiatry consult [47]. Cheville et al. found 92% of patients with metastatic breast cancer in the outpatient setting had at least one physical impairment (with a total of 530 impairments identified); yet, only 30% received rehabilitation treatment [48]. Additionally, while patients with cancer experience benefits from rehabilitation, cancer patients themselves are often unaware of the potential benefits of rehabilitation. In a study of patients with late-stage cancer, only 31.8% expressed interest in rehabilitation services [49].

While rehabilitation efforts in palliative care patients may lead to functional improvements and patients and caregivers describe its integration as useful, quality studies specifically focused on the palliative oncology population are lacking. One noted that obstacle may include physician attitudes regarding palliative rehabilitation interventions particularly among oncologists. In a comparative survey of medical oncologists and physiatrists, only 8% of medical oncologists compared to 35% of physiatrists would recommend inpatient rehabilitation to patients with advanced cancer [50]. In a study of palliative care physicians, many reported concerns that rehabilitation would provide false hope and that palliative care services often lack the ability to provide high-quality rehabilitation [51, 52].

## Advancing Cancer Rehabilitation

While both cancer rehabilitation and palliative care have historically experienced low rates of referral and under-recognition by referring oncologists, over the past decade, palliative care has made great strides toward becoming an integrated component of the oncology standard of care compared to rehabilitation. Palliative care's journey has been proposed as a model for cancer rehabilitation's advancement [53].

One of the glaring deficiencies for cancer rehabilitation is the amount of quality research; in particular in the areas of survival and cost effectiveness. Physiatry is a relatively small field, and admittedly the research output (while increasing) has been inadequate [54]. Physical activity and exercise likely have a role in improving cancer survival and outcomes through programs like prehabilitation. While improvements in function and quality of life may not resonate with some referring clinicians, the life-prolonging impact of physical activity likely will. Furthermore, cost effectiveness of integration of cancer rehabilitation needs to be better demonstrated. Can cancer rehabilitation interventions such as injectable procedures result in cost savings due to reduced need for opioids and related side effects resulting in reduced admissions and treatments? Can intensive inpatient cancer rehabilitation interventions reduce 30-day hospital readmissions due to improved patient physical resilience and other outcomes such as reduced falls? We require more randomized controlled trials published in high impact oncology journals [53].

The need (while not always recognized) for cancer rehabilitation is tremendous, but the number of cancer rehabilitation clinicians with experience or qualified to treat oncology patients is inadequate, and cancer rehabilitation experience is lacking in medical training. In physiatry, for example, cancer rehabilitation exposure during physiatry residency is highly variable and the Accreditation Council for Graduate Medical Education residency guidelines for physiatry mention the word "oncologic" only once in a paragraph with miscellaneous medical conditions [53, 55]. Other areas of noted action including shaping public opinion regarding cancer rehabilitation, influencing public policy, and increased integration into clinical practice guidelines.

## Conclusion

Cancer rehabilitation and palliative care can be complementary services in the treatment of patients with advanced cancer. Rehabilitation interventions are generally safe in this population and can improve cancer-related symptoms, function, and quality of life, while potentially reducing hospital admissions, length of inpatient stays, and medical complications. A number of opportunities exist in the growth of cancer rehabilitation including referrer knowledge/attitudes, patient awareness of cancer rehabilitation benefits, and inadequate high-quality research.

## References


1. Kevorkian CG. The history of cancer rehabilitation. In: Stubblefield MD, editor. Cancer rehabilitation principles and practice. 2nd ed. New York: Demos Medical; 2019. p. 4–5.
2. Cancer Facts & Figures 2017. American Cancer Society. https://www.cancer.org/research/cancer-facts-statistics/all-cancer-facts-figures/cancer-facts-figures-2017.html Accessed 31 May 2020.
3. Fu JB, Dhah SS, Bruera E. Corticosteroid injections for knee pain at the end of life. J Palliat Med. 2015;18(7):570–1.
4. Fu J, Ngo A, Shin K, Bruera E. Botulinum toxin injection and phenol nerve block for reduction of end-of-life pain. J Palliat Med. 2013;16(12):1637–40.
5. Dietz JH. Adaptive rehabilitation of the cancer patient. Curr Probl Cancer. 1980;5(5):1–56.
6. Cheville AL, Morrow M, Smith SR, Basford JR. Integrating function-directed treatments into palliative care. PM R. 2017;9(9S2):S335–46.
7. Alam E, Wilson RD, Vargo MM. Inpatient cancer rehabilitation: a retrospective comparison of transfer back to acute care between patients with neoplasm and other rehabilitation patients. Arch Phys Med Rehabil. 2008;89(7):1284–9.
8. Guo Y, Persyn L, Palmer JL, Bruera E. Incidence of and risk factors for transferring cancer patients from rehabilitation to acute care units. Am J Phys Med Rehabil. 2008;87(8):647–53.
9. Fu JB, Lee J, Shin BC, Silver JK, Smith DW, Shah JJ, Bruera E. Return to the primary acute care service among patients with multiple myeloma on an acute inpatient rehabilitation unit. PM R. 2017;9(6):571–8.
10. Fu JB, Lee J, Smith DW, Shin K, Guo Y, Bruera E. Frequency and reasons for return to the primary acute care service among patients with lymphoma undergoing inpatient rehabilitation. PM R. 2014;6(7):629–34.
11. Fu JB, Lee J, Smith DW, Bruera E. Frequency and reasons for return to acute care in patients with leukemia undergoing inpatient rehabilitation: a preliminary report. Am J Phys Med Rehabil. 2013;92(3):215–22.
12. Fu JB, Lee J, Smith DW, Guo Y, Bruera E. Return to primary service among bone marrow transplant rehabilitation inpatients: an index for predicting outcomes. Arch Phys Med Rehabil. 2013;94(2):356–61.
13. Maltser S, Cristian A, Silver JK, Morris GS, Stout NL. A focused review of safety considerations in cancer rehabilitation. PM R. 2017;9(9S2):S415–28.
14. Morishita S, Nakano J, Fu JB, Tsuji T. Physical exercise is safe and feasible in thrombocytopenic patients with hematologic malignancies: a narrative review. Hematology. 2020;25:95–100.
15. Fu JB, Tennison JM, Rutzen-Lopez IM, Silver JK, Morishita S, Dibaj SS. Bruera E bleeding frequency and characteristics among hematologic malignancy inpatient rehabilitation patients with severe thrombocytopenia. Support Care Cancer. 2018;26(9):3135–41.
16. Sabers SR, Kokal JE, Girardi JC, Philpott CL, Basford JR, Therneau TM, Schmidt KD, Gamble GL. Evaluation of consultation-based rehabilitation for hospitalized cancer patients with functional impairment. Mayo Clin Proc. 1999;74(9):855–61.
17. Ragnarsson KT, Thomas DC. The cancer rehabilitation and adaptation team. In: Kufe DW, Pollock RE, Weichselbaum RR, et al., editors. Holland-Frei cancer medicine. 6th ed. Hamilton (ON): BC Decker; 2003; http://www.ncbi.nlm.nih.gov/books/NBK13112/.
18. Myers JS, Cook-Wiens G, Baynes R, Jo MY, Bailey C, Krigel S, Klemp J, Asher A. Emerging from the Haze: a multi-center, controlled pilot study of a multi-dimensional, psycho-education-based cognitive rehabilitation intervention for breast cancer survivors delivered with telehealth conferencing. Arch Phys Med Rehabil. 2020;101(6):948–59. https://doi.org/10.1016/j.apmr.2020.01.021.
19. Silver JK, Raj VS, Fu JB, Wisotzky EM, Smith SR, Kirch RA. Cancer rehabilitation and palliative care: critical components in the delivery of high-quality oncology services. Support Care Cancer. 2015;23(12):3633–43.
20. Barawid E, Covarrubias N, Tribuzio B, Liao S. The benefits of rehabilitation for palliative care patients. Am J Hosp Palliat Care. 2015;32(1):34–43.
21. Hopkins KF, Tookman AJ. Rehabilitation and specialist palliative care. Int J Palliat Nurs. 2000;6(3):123–30.
22. Ferrell B, Temel J, Temin S, Alesi E, Balboni T, Basch E, Firn J, Paice J, Peppercorn J, Phillips T, Stovall E, Zimmermann C, Smith T. Integration of palliative care into standard oncology care: American Society of Clinical Oncology clinical practice guideline update. J Clin Oncol. 2017;35:96–110.
23. Oken M, Creech R, Tormey D, et al. Toxicity and response criteria of the eastern cooperative oncology group. Am J Clin Oncol. 1982;5:649–55.

24. Karnofsky D, Burchenal J. The clinical evaluation of chemotherapeutic agents in cancer. In: MacLeod C, editor. Evaluation of chemotherapeutic agents. New York, NY: Columbia University Press; 1949. p. 191–205.
25. Temel JS, Greer JA, Muzikansky A, Gallagher ER, Admane S, Jackson VA, Dahlin CM, Blinderman CD, Jacobsen J, Pirl WF, Billings JA, Lynch TJ. Early palliative care for patients with metastatic non-small-cell lung cancer. N Engl J Med. 2010;363(8):733–42.
26. Veloso AG, Sperling C, Holm LV, Nicolaisen A, Rottmann N, Thayssen S, Christensen RD, Lehmann Knudsen J, Hansen DG. Unmet needs in cancer rehabilitation during the early cancer trajectory--a nationwide patient survey. Acta Oncol. 2013;52(2):372–81.
27. Nadler MB, Desnoyers A, Langelier DM, Amir E. The effect of exercise on quality of life, fatigue, physical function, and safety in advanced solid tumor cancers: a meta-analysis of randomized control trials. J Pain Symptom Manag. 2019;58(5):899–908.e7.
28. Chen YJ, Li XX, Ma HK, Zhang X, Wang BW, Guo TT, Xiao Y, Bing ZT, Ge L, Yang KH, Han XM. Exercise training for improving patient-reported outcomes in patients with advanced-stage cancer: a systematic review and meta-analysis. J Pain Symptom Manag. 2020;59(3):734–749.e10.
29. Campbell KL, Winters-Stone KM, Wiskemann J, May AM, Schwartz AL, Courneya KS, Zucker DS, Matthews CE, Ligibel JA, Gerber LH, Morris GS, Patel AV, Hue TF, Perna FM, Schmitz KH. Exercise guidelines for cancer survivors: consensus statement from international multidisciplinary roundtable. Med Sci Sports Exerc. 2019;51(11):2375–90.
30. Fu JB, Lee J, Tran KB, Siangco CM, Ng AH, Smith DW, Bruera E. Symptom burden and functional gains in a cancer rehabilitation unit. Int J Ther Rehabil. 2015;22(11):517–23.
31. Guo Y, Young BL, Hainley S, Palmer JL, Bruera E. Evaluation and pharmacologic management of symptoms in cancer patients undergoing acute rehabilitation in a comprehensive cancer center. Arch Phys Med Rehabil. 2007;88(7):891–5.
32. Baima JA, Silver JK, Most M. Neuromuscular dysfunction in the cancer patient: evaluation and treatment. Muscle Nerve. 2018;58(3):335–43.
33. Hui D, Ross J, Park M, Dev R, Vidal M, Liu D, Paiva CE, Bruera E. Predicting survival in patients with advanced cancer in the last weeks of life: how accurate are prognostic models compared to clinicians' estimates? Palliat Med. 2020;34(1):126–33.
34. Hui D, Park M, Liu D, Paiva CE, Suh SY, Morita T, Bruera E. Clinician prediction of survival versus the palliative prognostic score: which approach is more accurate? Eur J Cancer. 2016;64:89–95.
35. Alsirafy SA, Zaki O, Sakr AY, Farag DE, El-Sherief WA, Mohammed AA. The use of the Chuang's prognostic scale to predict the survival of metastatic colorectal cancer patients receiving palliative systemic anticancer therapy. Indian. J Palliat Care. 2016;22(3):312–6.
36. Venur VA, Ahluwalia MS. Prognostic scores for brain metastasis patients: use in clinical practice and trial design. Chin Clin Oncol. 2015;4(2):18.
37. Coyle N. The hard work of living in the face of death. J Pain Symptom Manag. 2006;32:266–74.
38. Morasso G, Capelli M, Viterbori P, Di Leo S, Alberisio A, Costantini M, Fiore M, Saccani D, Zeitler G, Verzolatto N, Tirelli W, Lazzari L, Partinico M, Borzoni G, Savian C, Obertino E, Zotti P, Ivaldi GP, Henriquet F. Psychological and symptom distress in terminal cancer patients with met and unmet needs. J Pain Symptom Manag. 1999;17(6):402–9.
39. Houts PS, Yasko JM, Harvey HA, Kahn SB, Hartz AJ, Hermann JF, et al. Unmet needs of persons with cancer in Pennsylvania during the period of terminal care. Cancer. 1988;62:627–34.
40. Rahman H. Journey of providing care in hospice: perspectives of occupational therapists. Qual Health Res. 2000;10:806–18.
41. Chochinov HM, Kristjanson LJ, Hack TF, Hassard T, McClement S, Harlos M. Burden to others and the terminally ill. J Pain Symptom Manag. 2007;34:463–71.
42. McPherson CJ, Wilson KG, Murray MA. Feeling like a burden to others: a systematic review focusing on the end of life. Palliat Med. 2007;21:115–28.
43. Belchamber CA, Gousy MH. Rehabilitative care in a specialist palliative day care center: a study of patients' perspectives. Int J Ther Rehabil. 2004;1:425–34.
44. Mahoney FI, Barthel D. Functional evaluation: the Barthel index. Md State Med J. 1965;14:56–61.
45. Yoshioka H. Rehabilitation for the terminal cancer patient. Am J Phys Med Rehabil. 1994;73:199–206.
46. Jones L, Fitzgerald G, Leurent B, Round J, Eades J, Davis S, Gishen F, Holman A, Hopkins K, Tookman A. Rehabilitation in advanced, progressive, recurrent cancer: a randomized controlled trial. J Pain Symptom Manag. 2013;46(3):315–325.e3.
47. Movsas SB, Chang VT, Tunkel RS, Shah VV, Ryan LS, Millis SR. Rehabilitation needs of an inpatient medical oncology unit. Arch Phys Med Rehabil. 2003;84(11):1642–6.
48. Cheville AL, Troxel AB, Basford JR, Kornblith AB. Prevalence and treatment patterns of physical impairments in patients with metastatic breast cancer. J Clin Oncol. 2008;26(16):2621–9.
49. Cheville AL, Rhudy L, Basford JR, Griffin JM, Flores AM. How receptive are patients with late stage cancer to rehabilitation services and what are the sources of their resistance? Arch Phys Med Rehabil. 2017;98(2):203–10.
50. Spill GR, Hlubocky FJ, Daugherty CK. Oncologists' and physiatrists' attitudes regarding rehabilitation for patients with advanced cancer. PM R. 2012;4(2):96–108.
51. Runacres F, Gregory H, Ugalde A. Restorative care for palliative patients: a retrospective clinical audit of outcomes for patients admitted to an inpatient palliative care unit. BMJ Support Palliat Care. 2016;6(1):97–100.
52. Smith SR, Zheng JY. The intersection of oncology prognosis and cancer rehabilitation. Curr Phys Med Rehabil Rep. 2017;5(1):46–54.
53. Lyons KD, Padgett LS, Marshall TF, Greer JA, Silver JK, Raj VS, Zucker DS, Fu JB, Pergolotti M, Sleight AG, Alfano CM. Follow the trail: using insights from the growth of palliative care to propose a roadmap for cancer rehabilitation. CA Cancer J Clin. 2019;69(2):113–26.
54. Stout NL, Alfano CM, Belter CW, Nitkin R, Cernich A, Lohmann Siegel K, Chan L. A bibliometric analysis of the landscape of cancer rehabilitation research (1992-2016). J Natl Cancer Inst. 2018;110(8):815–24.
55. Raj VS, Balouch J, Norton JH. Cancer rehabilitation education during physical medicine and rehabilitation residency: preliminary data regarding the quality and quantity of experiences. Am J Phys Med Rehabil. 2014;93(5):445–52.

# 16 Psychosocial Considerations and Assessment of Patients with Hematological Malignancies and Serious Blood Disorders

Kristin Drouin, Nicholas Purol, Sarah J. Tarquini, Darcy E. Burgers, and Kristen Uhl

## Introduction

It has long been held that all persons are intrinsically tied to a network of family, society, culture, and community [1]. No person exists in a vacuum. It is incumbent on clinicians to remember that a patient is a person first and not merely an accumulation of diagnoses to be treated. A person's unique identity directly relates to how that individual navigates and copes with a challenging, life-altering diagnosis and impacts the development, delineation, and evolution of their goals throughout the illness.

One classic paradigm that illuminates this person-in-environment perspective is Maslow's hierarchy of needs [2]. While debated, edited, summarized, and modified throughout the years, this model provides a context in which persons must navigate certain needs in a prioritized fashion: physiological/concrete needs, safety needs, sense of belonging, self-actualization needs, and transcendental needs (Fig. 16.1). Serious illness disrupts nearly all aspects of this conceptual framework of basic human need. Any number of psychosocial needs or factors can relate to the treatment and support of patients, caregivers, and families facing a hematologic malignancy or serious blood disorder. A comprehensive plan of care that addresses these needs, and how they are shaped by serious illness, is an essential component of healing a person, rather than merely treating a patient with a disease. The psychosocial assessment is the cornerstone of understanding the full breadth of a person's needs.

Moreover, the assessment serves the multimodal role of building rapport between patient and provider, identifying both strengths and potential indicators for recurring challenges, and pointing to interventional strategies.

This chapter provides an overview of the goals and practicalities of such an assessment, including when it is done and whom should be present; key areas for assessment and empirical tools that can be utilized throughout the assessment process, and how psychosocial assessment informs the use of specific interventions or therapeutic modalities to improve patient and family function. Knowledge of the psychosocial assessment as a whole will help all clinicians, regardless of their role in the patient's care, to understand better the unique needs of patients and families throughout the continuum of care.

K. Drouin (✉)
Grief and Trauma Psychotherapist, The Wendt Center for Loss and Healing, Washington, DC, USA
e-mail: kdrouin@wendtcenter.org

N. Purol
Department of Psychosocial Oncology and Palliative Care, Boston Children's Hospital and Dana-Farber Cancer Institute, Boston, MA, USA
e-mail: Nicholas_purol@dfci.harvard.edu

S. J. Tarquini · K. Uhl
Department of Psychosocial Oncology and Palliative Care, Dana-Farber Cancer Institute, Boston, MA, USA
e-mail: sarah_tarquini@dfci.harvard.edu; Kristen_Uhl@dfci.harvard.edu

D. E. Burgers
Division of Pediatric Psychosocial Oncology, Department of Psychosocial Oncology and Palliative Care, Dana-Farber Cancer Institute, Boston, MA, USA


C. K. Ullrich, E. J. Roeland (eds.), *Palliative Care in Hematologic Malignancies and Serious Blood Disorders*,
https://doi.org/10.1007/978-3-031-38058-7_16

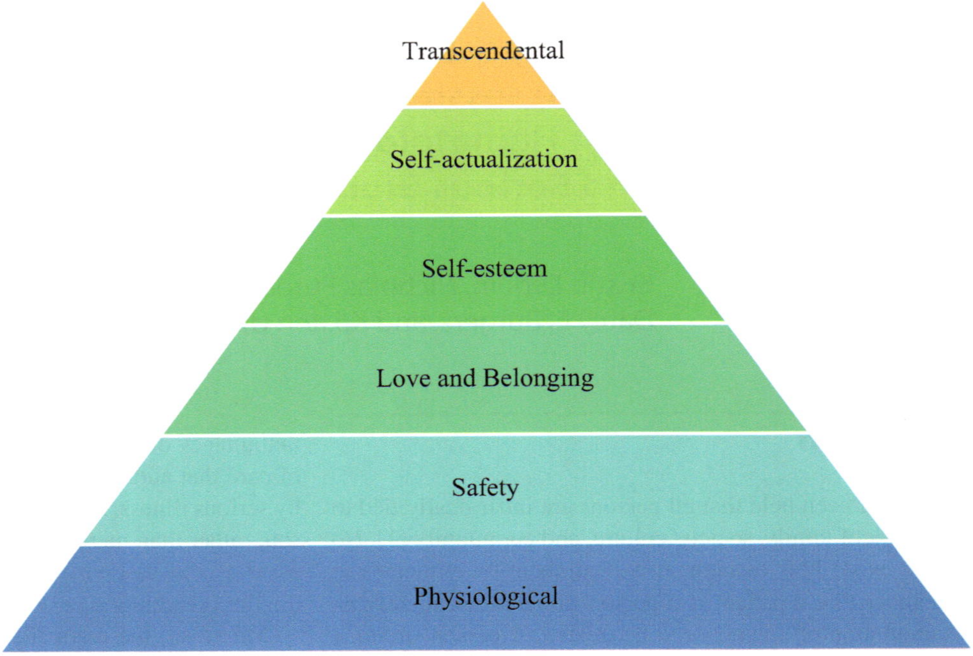


**Fig. 16.1** Adapted and expanded Maslow's hierarchy of needs [2]. (Adapted from Maslow, A. H. (1970b). *Religions, values, and peak experiences*. New York: Penguin. (Original work published 1966))

## Approaching Assessment: Setting the Stage

### Timing

While medical teams should consider the inclusion of a psychosocial clinician in diagnostic conversations to offer support, a full psychosocial assessment may wait until after the diagnosis and treatment options have been shared and, at least to some extent, processed by the patient and family. The postponement of assessment until after such a meeting can increase the likelihood of patient and caregiver engagement, while also offering the clinician opportunity to assess how patients and families are interpreting and acting upon the diagnostic and treatment information that was received. Timing of assessment should be reevaluated, however, in cases of prolonged diagnostic uncertainty, as patients and families can benefit from psychosocial support throughout such a tenuous period. Regardless of the initial timing, psychosocial assessments are best considered to be ongoing processes that change in correlation with the continued evolution of patient and family needs.

### Integration of Palliative Care

Given the intensity, duration, and prognostic uncertainty associated with hematologic conditions, early integration of palliative care is recommended and is appropriate at any stage of care. The involvement of palliative care specialists representing multiple disciplines maximizes support available to patients, their caregivers, family members, and primary oncology team members, critical care colleagues, and clinicians on other consulting services. Early integration of palliative care allows for ongoing assessment of patient and family values and treatment goals, which are particularly dynamic in the context of disease progression and/or increasing prognostic uncertainty. In such circumstances, patients and families benefit from creating a safe and empathic environment to explore decision-making processes that consider the prioritization of comfort, pain control, and symptom management. As sub-specialty palliative care teams function both alongside and separate from primary teams, they are well-situated to provide this support while engaging around the delineation and actualization of evolving goals of care as a patient's condition changes.

### Primary and Consultative Psychosocial Collaboration

For the purposes of this chapter, *primary* psychosocial clinician refers to the oncology or transplant social worker, psychologist, therapist, etc. who is likely first known to patients and their families as a key part of upfront treatment. Many hospitals and clinics additionally have sub-specialty palliative care social workers who work primarily as part of an interdisciplinary palliative care consultation team. In many settings these clinicians may be one and the same, as primary and palliative care psychosocial clinicians share many overlapping skillsets. However, there are some unique differences in training and approach that highlight the benefit of involvement and collaboration between primary and palliative care psychosocial clinicians when available.

For instance, primary psychosocial clinicians often are the first point of contact and support for patients and families, allowing for the development of a unique, longitudinal, and deep relationship. The primary psychosocial clinician may focus on assessment, development of rapport, creation of conceptual framework, and provision of direct support and interventions geared toward the complex coping and concrete needs of patients throughout treatment.

Palliative care psychosocial clinicians often meet patients and families further along in the disease trajectory as part of a palliative care consultation. The palliative care psychosocial clinician seeks to focus on the delineation of patient and family goals around the specific point of care at which they are introduced, explore patient and family understandings of prognosis, and work with existing psychosocial clinician(s) to enact and enhance quality of life and meaning-making resources within the lens and long-term conceptual framework of grief and bereavement.

The division of primary and consultative roles can be complex, nuanced and affected by availability of institutional resources, often necessitating a case-by-case delineation of psychosocial roles. Coordination of ongoing assessments, frequent communication, and shared understanding of said delineation can minimize confusion for patients, caregivers, and medical teams and eliminate duplicative interventions, allowing for the delivery of a deeper, more comprehensive level of psychosocial care.

## Stakeholders

Who is present for an initial psychosocial assessment may vary depending on the age, developmental capacity, and function of the patient, the availability of the primary caregiver, and the psychosocial clinician's practice. If conducted as part of a palliative care consultation, a physician and/or nurse practitioner may also be present as psychosocial information is gathered. Often, psychosocial clinicians—be they a member of the palliative care team or a psychosocial clinician embedded within the primary medical team—will meet with the patient and/or family again to follow up on aspects of the assessment that were not discussed during the first encounter with the broader respective teams; indeed, that initial meeting may be the setting in which diagnosis is shared, which is an inherently challenging time to ask the patient and/or caregivers to reflect on anything outside of the immediate, distressing news they have just received.

The number of stakeholders present should be determined within the context of confidentiality and the patient's right to privacy. Psychosocial clinicians can play a key role in ensuring that only the minimum relevant information needed for medical treatment or safety purposes is shared with the broader team. Creating a safer, smaller space within which to discuss topics that are not "need-to-know" for the broader team allows for development of rapport, trust, and a stronger therapeutic relationship.

The psychosocial assessment itself can also indicate areas where referral to or involvement of additional psychosocial clinicians may be beneficial. For instance, the distress of a pediatric patient in learning their diagnosis or the coping of pediatric siblings throughout the treatment process may be mitigated by the involvement of a Certified Child Life Specialist (CCLS), whose training in child development, procedural support, and medical play/psychoeducation could allow for more specialized intervention. Similarly, expression of significant spiritual distress in an initial psychosocial assessment could warrant the involvement of a chaplain or pastoral care provider, many of whom have received training in theology, faith traditions, and the interplay of grief, loss, and crises of faith within the context of life-threatening or chronic illness.

All psychosocial providers involved in a patient's case bear responsibility for updating their psychosocial colleagues about the level and role of their involvement. A primary psychosocial "point person"—perhaps the clinician who is most frequently in contact with the patient and/or caregivers—can alert other members of the care team when additional psychosocial disciplines are consulted and ensure that the entirety of the psychosocial care team is aware of major developments in treatment or changes in level of support that may be deemed necessary through the ongoing assessment process. Consistent, clear communication between all psychosocial clinicians involved in the care ensures that members of the care team continue to complement each other's work and adapt in concert to meet patient and family needs, which are often as organic and dynamic as the disease itself.

## Strengths-Based Approach

Regardless of specific psychosocial assessment paradigms and content, the focus of such assessments, particularly with patients facing serious illness, must always strive to incorporate the strengths and protective factors of patients, their families, and their caregivers. "Strengths-based" assessments and interventions have long been part of social work theory and literature and remain central to the holistic support of patients and families regardless of setting [3]. Such approaches seek to find a balance between acknowledging the complex and often devastating realities of serious illness, suffering, and grief with the competencies, resources, adaptive coping, empowerment, and resiliency that patients bring to their understanding and navigation of illness (Fig. 16.2).

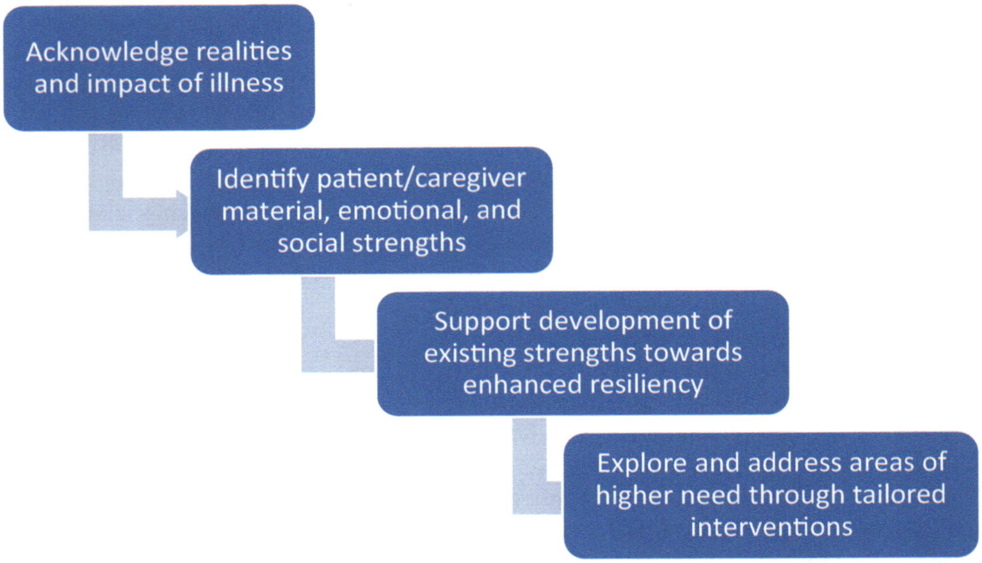


**Fig. 16.2** Strengths-based framework

Knowing and framing the material, emotional, systematic, familial, self-narrative, and spiritual strengths of patients provides a framework for addressing future areas of need and tailoring specific interventions. Only by gathering an inventory of strengths can the medical team best support patients through illness and treatment course, while also reinforcing the therapeutic relationship so crucial to the long-term health and well-being of patients and their caregivers.

## Key Areas of Assessment

A quality psychosocial assessment includes demographic information, internal and external resources, coping styles, relationships, and spirituality, with the ultimate goal of understanding and supporting patient and family adaptation to serious illness [4]. In pediatric populations, assessment of resources, family support, history of stressors, family functioning, and family structure is of heightened importance given the interdependent nature of children and their caregivers [5]. Gathering details of the physical/socioeconomic resources, emotional/behavioral health histories, social support networks, socially and individually-prescribed identities, and spiritual or value-oriented contexts of patients, all within a strengths-based framework, are essential total-person treatment and care.

### Concrete/Material Resources

The diagnosis of a serious hematologic condition affects and alters families' material needs, which, in turn, can have far-reaching impact on their illness experiences and treatment outcomes. For example, patients with lower socioeconomic status are associated with higher rates of morbidity for cancer-related disorders such as multiple myeloma, even after controlling for other demographics and treatment [6]. Additionally, several studies highlight the direct financial cost of patients and families facing hematologic conditions, as well as the associated and simultaneous loss of income [7, 8]. For example, individuals pursuing therapies not covered by insurance, such as some cellular therapies, may bear significant out-of-pocket costs.

Additional factors may further complicate the patient and family's financial stability. For example, an adult patient may be the primary or sole source of income for the family. The patient's healthy partner may, by necessity, transition from caring full-time for their children to entering the commercial workforce; the cost of out-of-home childcare can be significant and even prohibitive for families. Individuals pursuing hematopoietic cell therapy (HCT), cellular or experimental therapies, or treatments requiring rare expertise also incur travel or relocation expenses. Patients and families may also encounter new expenses associated with the acquisition of in-home nursing and supportive care, particularly as an increasing number of oral agents allow for in-home treatment. Table 16.1 highlights some of the resources available to patients and families to navigate some of these changes and challenges (Table 16.1).

Access to financial means, secure and safe housing, reliable transportation, adequate nutrition, and medical care have an inherent impact on patient and caregiving functioning, coping, adherence to treatment, and treatment outcomes. It is therefore essential that these areas be explored as part of a comprehensive psychosocial assessment. Knowledge of patients and their families' socioeconomic resources allows

**Table 16.1** HCT financial and educational resources for patients, families, and caregivers. (Adapted from *Leukemia and Lymphoma Society*: https://www.lls.org/support/other-helpful-organizations/financial-resources/blood-and-marrow-transplantation-finances)

| Organization | Website | Target population |
|---|---|---|
| Be the Match | https://bethematch.org | Patients, caregivers, and families before, during, and after a blood or marrow transplant (BMT); healthcare professionals; researchers |
| BMT InfoNet | https://www.bmtinfonet.org/ | Bone marrow transplant patients, survivors and their caregivers in the U.S. |
| Children's Leukemia Research Association (CLRA) | https://www.childrensleukemia.org/ | Children and adults with leukemia in the U.S.; healthcare professionals and researchers |
| Childrens Organ Transplant Association (COTA) | https://cota.org | Patients 21 and under who require a life-saving organ, bone marrow, cord blood or stem cell transplant *(United States)* |
| Cord Blood Registry | https://cordblood.com/ | Patients, families, caregivers |
| Family Reach | https://familyreach.org/ | Patients with cancer and their families *(United States including Puerto Rico and U.S. territories)* |
| HelpHOPELive | https://helphopelive.org/ | Patients in need of financial help for a stem cell transplant |
| Icla da Silva Foundation | https://icla.org | Those in need of a stem cell transplant or anyone looking to be a bone marrow donor |
| Live Like Bella Childhood Cancer Foundation | https://livelikebella.org/ | Families whose child is under the age of 21 and diagnosed with a pediatric cancer before age 18 |
| National Foundation for Transplants (NFT) | https://transplants.org/ | Patients needing tissue, bone marrow or other transplants, and their loved ones *(United States)* |
| The Andrew McDonough B+ Foundation | https://bepositive.org | Families of children with cancer *(United States)* |
| The Bone Marrow and Cancer Foundation | https://bonemarrow.org | Transplant patients and families; caregivers, survivors *(United States)* |

for the anticipatory identification of potential areas of need. It helps set the stage for the holistic assessment and care of patients within their larger family and social systems.

## Behavioral Health/Safety

Comprehensive psychosocial assessments must also account for mental and behavioral health history and supports. While patients with advanced cancer face psychiatric conditions at nearly the same prevalence as the general population, they are less likely to receive emotional and behavioral health interventions—or even assessment—by their care team [9]. At the same time, untreated psychiatric conditions can negatively impact treatments and lengthen hospital stays during interventions such as HCT [10].

This evidence underscores the importance of identifying existing behavioral health concerns and histories. This background will enable clinicians to better support individuals during their adjustment to serious or advanced illness. For example, having identified a patient with a previous history of a substance use disorder, providers could work with the patient to develop a safety plan around pain management while also connecting the patient and/or caregiver with appropriate supports within the health system and the community.

Indeed, early identification and anticipation of mental or behavioral health challenges a patient may encounter throughout their medical treatment can minimize the cumulative medical trauma a patient might experience as part of their diagnostic or treatment course. In the particularly vulnerable patient population of pediatrics, clinical trials have highlighted the benefit of tailored interventions in lowering posttraumatic stress symptoms in children and their caregivers [11, 12].

Ultimately, an early, comprehensive psychosocial assessment holds the key to enhancing patient resiliency and outcomes, as clinicians can implement supports and interventions near the beginning of the disease trajectory, which can mitigate complications that might arise down the road.

## Caregivers and Family Systems

In the setting of serious illness, patient well-being is often closely correlated to their caregiver's well-being (s) [14]. Therefore, understanding and supporting the individual's needs while providing informal care and formal support must also be prioritized.

Understanding this key component of the patient's illness experience may begin by engaging the patient around their understanding of their direct and indirect caregivers, their family, and their social networks, as well as their assessment of whom within these networks provides the most support—or adds another layer of complexity to their caregiver constellation. Assessment may then include direct or indirect evaluation of caregivers' functional coping and behavioral health needs. The knowledge that specific treatment courses may lend themselves to increased caregiver challenges can aid in this investigation. For instance, in caregivers of HCT recipients, negative financial impact, increased social isolation, and higher rates of depression were all common [13]. Awareness of these commonalities and desire to understand the caregiver's unique needs and challenges may lead to a more thorough assessment.

Like many assessment domains, caregiver and familial coping and needs have a symbiotic relationship with the needs and coping of the patients themselves. Wadhwa et al. found that the symptom management, coping, and quality of life (QOL) of patients facing advanced cancer were strongly associated with caregivers' QOL and mental health [14]. Similar data derived from pediatric patients with oncological/hematological disease and their parents/caregivers indicate a correlation between pain experienced by the patient and emotional distress of and perceived burden on caregivers [15]. The association of the patient and caregiver/family experience speaks to the importance of developing an understanding—and ongoing, interconnected assessment—of the patient and caregiver's social systems.

Inclusion of the caregiver(s) and family system(s) within initial and ongoing psychosocial assessments offers an opportunity, particularly in the setting of poor prognosis, to indirectly explore areas of higher need or potential risk factors that could affect anticipatory grief and bereavement. Obtaining this initial understanding, and revising as needed across the treatment trajectory, can enable more immediate implementation of bereavement interventions should the patient's death occur suddenly.

It is perhaps doubly important to include a caregiver, sibling, or family member in ongoing psychosocial assessment if they are the patient's stem cell donor. Research indicates that, similar to stem cell recipients, donors can experience a range of emotions throughout the donation and transplant process. Special consideration should be taken of donors who are minors (e.g., pediatric sibling donors), who may report that they do not feel they have a choice in donating due to expectations within the family system [16]. So, too, should specific attention be paid to donor coping and support in the setting of failed engraftment or post-transplant relapse, as donors may endorse failings of guilt or blame, which can be particularly acute if the patient does not survive [17].

## Identity

Equally important and intimately tied to the systems in which people live are the identities that they inherit and develop. Age, gender, race, ethnicity, and sexual orientation both outwardly and inwardly affect how the individual navigates the healthcare system. Racial minorities, for instance, must often contend with the well-documented historical and contemporary realities of disparities in access to and outcomes from cancer-directed and symptom management therapies and interventions [18–20]. Such demographically informed identities impact everything from trust in and expectation of members of the medical community personal to lived experience throughout treatment, and even how a healthcare system interacts with an individual or family.

Beyond demographic attributes are those more nebulous roles with which patients identify. Mother, father, child, "provider," "nurturer," "peacemaker," "warrior": these subjective roles may be as developed and as central to an individual as their race or age. Introduction of serious illness, complex treatment, and increasingly present reminders of one's own mortality may directly challenge such self-images or ascribed roles, and may further complicate the integration of various—sometimes competing—identities in a patient's life.

Exploring patients' and caregivers' demographic and subjective identities within the context of a psychosocial assessment may offer insight into deeply held values, the dissection of which could illuminate the patient's perception of QOL, what makes life meaningful, and how these views are shaped by their priorities and decisions. Whether grappling with a new diagnosis, complex symptoms, prolonged or challenging treatment, anticipatory grief, or impact on family and friends, a person's identity and the struggle to maintain or redefine that identity remains an integral part of psychosocial assessment and care. Developing a deeper appreciation for how patients define themselves allows for the anticipation of potential barriers to care and provides potential opportunities for maximization and support of the things that matter most to them.

## Spirituality and Meaning-Making

Though a patient may not subscribe to a particular faith or religious doctrine, a serious illness often represents a significant threat to a patient's understanding of the universe and their place within it. Incorporating spirituality and meaning-making into the psychosocial assessment provides space for the patient to begin to navigate and integrate their prior conceptions of faith and spirituality with the medical reality in which they unexpectedly find themselves. Indeed, the search for meaning within the patient population of individuals with serious hematologic conditions is known to be an important component of adaptive coping [21]. Even pediatric patients have demonstrated a desire to search for understanding and meaning in ways that correspond to their socioemotional development, particularly when they are facing advanced cancer or otherwise life-limiting illness [22, 23].

Endeavoring to understand these elements of a patient's experience builds rapport with them and offers insight into and context to better understand how they incorporate meaning-making into their daily lives. Exploring and knowing the patient's spiritual and/or religious scaffolding—and the existential questions that may emerge from such exploration—can also indicate to primary psychosocial providers when referral to a chaplain or pastoral care provider would be helpful.

Delving into spirituality, faith, and meaning-making with the patient's primary caregiver(s) or family system can provide a pathway to promote support, resiliency, and healing during bereavement. Consideration of the post-mortem meaning a caregiver or loved one ascribes to the patient's illness experience—and their own experience in it—provides an avenue through which to define the patient's legacy. This experience, in turn, can be an important component of adjusting to a world in which the deceased no longer physically exists [24].

## Assessment Models and Tools

Information obtained in a comprehensive assessment can be synthesized by applying psychosocial models designed to inform the level of intervention needed to best support a patient and family. Similarly, standardized screening and assessment tools can provide a structured way to translate information into intervention or indicate the need for reassessment.

### Pediatric Population

Drawing from Bronfenbrenner's work [1], a social-ecological framework is central to understanding and assessing psychosocial risk and resilience in a pediatric population [25, 26]. Social ecology places the child at the core of surrounding concentric circles representing the many microsystems (e.g., family, medical condition, social network, school, culture, religion) that, in turn, interact with one another to impact the child's well-being [25, 26]. For a child with serious illness, the surrounding concentric circles offer a visual representation of the factors that impact that child's ability to adapt and cope with illness and treatment [27]. In conjunction with conversation with the patient and family, the social-ecological framework can help identify potential targets for psychosocial intervention.

Kazak's Pediatric Psychosocial Preventative Health Model (PPPHM) draws from a public health framework to identify three distinct levels of psychosocial risk, and corresponding psychosocial interventions, for pediatric patients and their families [5, 26]. Within the pyramid-like structure of the PPPHM, most children and families fall at the base or Universal Level. This tier indicates that the family's experience of temporary distress in the context of the child's illness is mitigated by minimal risk factors, adequate resources, and skills enabling them to adapt to their current situation. Because of this, psychosocial interventions beyond basic, preventative support are likely unnecessary at the Universal Level [25].

Families with some identified risk factors and/or moderate resource needs who would benefit from targeted psychosocial intervention present in the middle—or Targeted Level—of the PPPHM. Families occupy the pyramid's apex (Clinical Level) when there are preexisting psychological morbidities or chronic, complex psychosocial issues that will likely require immediate and intensive psychosocial support.

Both the social-ecological framework and the PPPHM incorporate the myriad contexts and systems that interact within a child's world. As mentioned at the beginning of the chapter, assessment of these domains is necessary to adequately understand the patient and family's current psychosocial functioning, as well as the potential risk and protective factors that may impact the patient and family's functioning over time.

In addition to these frameworks, pediatric-specific screening measures have been developed to capture a snapshot of patient and family psychosocial functioning at a single moment in time. Kazak's Psychosocial Assessment Tool (PAT) draws from the PPPHM and serves as a brief caregiver screening tool to identify a family's risk stratification on the PPPHM pyramid [26, 28]. Additional screening tools, such as the PROMIS assessments, can be administered directly to pediatric patients as well as their caregivers to measure parent and child-reported medical symptoms, functioning, behavior, and emotions [29]. The Distress Thermometer [30, 31] is also a brief screening tool used to capture a one-item rating of distress.

Assessment of a patient and family's psychosocial functioning can be used to guide potential interventions through a combination of screening tools and clinical assessment.

### Adult Population

Psychosocial assessment and care models in the adult patient population may follow a tiered approach similar to Kazak's PPPHM. Watson, Dunn, and Holland [32] proposed altering an earlier model created by Great Britain's National Institute of Health and Clinical Excellence [33] to include four tiers in which escalation of psychosocial needs increases with each level. Level 1 indicates the need for a general level of support provided by all staff. Level 4 reflects the need for psychosocial clinicians trained to support individuals with moderate to severe behavioral and mental health challenges [32, 33].

A later version of the model [34] uses the pyramid to illustrate a five-tiered approach that specifies which psychosocial clinicians may be most beneficial at each tier. At the base of this stepped psychosocial care model lies "minimal to mild distress," for which the authors recommend a "universal care" approach to psychosocial need, with any member of the healthcare team providing "brief emotional support" and community resources. Subsequent tiers include suggestions of "supportive care" from peers, social workers, and other psychosocial clinicians for mild to moderate distress; "extended care," incorporating counseling and time-limited therapy from a psychologist or social worker for moderate distress, and "specialist care," with targeted/focused therapy from a psychologist or psychiatrist to address moderate to severe distress. As in Kazak's model, the apex of the pyramid signifies the level of greatest distress or need for intervention; at this pinnacle of severe distress, the authors suggest an "acute care" approach with intensive, comprehensive therapeutic intervention from a psychiatrist or team of mental health providers.

As in the pediatric patient population, myriad evidence-based screening tools have been developed to inform assessment and guide interventions. Often, it is the use of such a screening tool, administered with regularity across the illness trajectory, that indicates a need for more in-depth and comprehensive reassessment. The National Comprehensive Cancer Network's (NCCN) Distress Thermometer, for example, incorporates a checklist of symptoms, psychosocial stressors, relationship issues, emotional problems, and spiritual concerns to determine the level of patient distress and need for further assessment and intervention. NCCN recommends that the Distress Thermometer be administered at every healthcare visit and at intervals when increased distress may be expected (i.e., change in the treatment plan related to disease progression) [35]. Because of the standardization of questions on the tool, any member of the patient's team—including nurses or medical assistants—could administer it, though the analysis of results and subsequent formulation of interventions should be completed by the psychosocial clinician.

The interconnectedness of patient and caregiver well-being underscored earlier in this chapter highlights the necessity of ongoing screening of caregiver coping. Several tools exist for this purpose, including the Perceived Support Measure [36]—which assesses tangible, emotional and informational support, satisfaction with support, and negative social interaction—and the Cultural Justification for Caregiving Scale [37], which asks caregivers to assess their own reasons for and expectations in providing care. Table 16.2 provides an overview of these and other screening tools that may help initial and ongoing psychosocial assessment of adult patients and caregivers (Table 16.2).

**Table 16.2** Selection of validated instruments to incorporate into assessment

| Assessment Tool | Areas of assessment | Domains |
|---|---|---|
| Sickness Impact Profile (SIP) [38] | Physical and psychosocial functioning | Sleep and rest, eating, work, home management, recreation and pastimes, ambulation, mobility, body care and movement, social interaction, alertness behavior, emotional behavior, communication |
| Nottingham Health Profile (NHP) [39] | Physical and psychosocial functioning | Physical mobility, social isolation, emotional reactions, pain, sleep, energy |
| EQ-5D [40] | Physical and psychosocial functioning | Mobility, self-care, usual activities, pain/discomfort, anxiety/depression |
| QLQ-C30 [41] | Functioning, symptoms, global health, QOL | Functionality (physical, role, cognitive, emotional, and social); symptoms (fatigue, pain, nausea, and vomiting) |
| Hospital Anxiety and Depression Scale (HADS) [42] | Psychosocial Well-being | Anhedonia, energy, psychiatric coping |
| Mental Adjustment to Cancer (MAC) [43] | Psychosocial functioning and coping post-diagnosis | "Fighting spirit," "helpless/hopeless," "anxious preoccupation," "fatalism," "avoidance" |
| Experiences in Close Relationships Scale (ECR-M16) [44] | Psychosocial functioning and attachment style | Self-esteem, social support, depressive symptoms |
| FICA Spirituality Assessment [45] | Psychosocial functioning and spiritual well-being | Faith and belief, importance of spirituality, religious or spiritual community, assessment |

**Table 16.2** (continued)

| Assessment Tool | Areas of assessment | Domains |
|---|---|---|
| *Caregiver/family* | | |
| Caregiver Reaction Scale [46] | Caregiver psychosocial well-being and functioning of a family system | Role captivity, overload, relational deprivation, competence, personal gain, family beliefs and conflict, job conflicts, financial disruption |
| Picot Caregiver Rewards Scale [47] | Caregiver psychosocial well-being | Caregiver demands, coping, burden, and depression |
| Perceived Support Scale [36] | Caregiver psychosocial functioning and coping | Tangible, emotional, and informational support, satisfaction with support, negative social interaction |
| Cultural Justification for Caregiving Scale [37] | Caregiver well-being and functioning of a family system | Reasons and expectations for providing care |
| Parenting Stress Index (pediatric patient population) [48] | Caregiver well-being and functioning of a family system | Child characteristics, parent characteristics, situational stressors |
| Impact on Family Scale (pediatric patient population) [49] | The functioning of a family system | Financial impact, familial-social impact, personal strain, mastery |

## Translating Assessment to Intervention

Psychosocial assessment may identify psychosocial domains warranting further intervention, including areas pertaining to caregiver and patient functioning in a medical setting. As seen in Table 16.3, numerous empirically-supported interventions exist to address common psychosocial needs present for patients and their families (Table 16.3).

Patients with serious hematological malignancies may face unique challenges necessitating specific types of intervention. For instance, prolonged hospitalizations, such as those experienced by patients undergoing HCT, can generate increased concrete, financial, and socioemotional need due to distance traveled to the transplant center. On the converse, however, the cause of such challenges can create new opportunities as well, as the longer hospitalization may lend itself to more frequent therapeutic check-ins and interventions. To address social isolation, psychosocial clinicians can think creatively about incorporating peer-based support, utilizing institutional resources or community-based organizations such as Leukemia and Lymphoma Society and Imerman Angels to link patients and caregivers with other patients or caregivers who can relate in a manner beyond the scope and role of the psychosocial clinician.

Regardless of each patient and/or families' circumstances, social workers, psychologists, psychiatrists, spiritual care providers, child life specialists, and other psychosocial clinicians are vital to the multidisciplinary management of patients and their caregivers' emotional and behavioral functioning in the inpatient and outpatient medical settings.

**Table 16.3** Empirically supported psychosocial interventions for chronic illness

| Domain | Intervention target(s) | Psychosocial intervention |
|---|---|---|
| *Pediatric* | | |
| Child physical functioning [50, 51] | Pain<br>Nausea<br>Sleep | Cognitive behavioral therapy (CBT)<br>Hypnosis<br>Behavioral interventions |
| Child behavioral functioning [52] | Treatment adherence | Behavior management<br>Combined behavior Management/psychoeducation |
| Child emotional functioning [53, 54] | Psychological adjustment<br>Anxiety/depression<br>Procedural distress | Cognitive behavioral therapy (CBT)<br>Mindfulness-based interventions |
| *Adult* | | |
| Adult physical functioning [55, 56] | Pain<br>Nausea<br>Sleep | Cognitive behavioral therapy-insomnia (CBTi)<br>Hypnosis |
| Adult behavioral functioning [57] | Treatment adherence | Motivational interviewing (MI)<br>Psychoeducation |
| Adult emotional functioning [58] | Psychological adjustment<br>Anxiety/depression | Cognitive behavioral therapy (CBT)<br>Acceptance and commitment therapy (ACT)<br>Mindfulness-based cancer recovery (MBCR) |
| *Caregiver* | | |
| Parent/pediatric caregiver functioning [59] | Emotional distress<br>Maladaptive parenting behaviors | Cognitive behavioral therapy (CBT)<br>Problem-solving therapy |
| Adult caregiver functioning [60, 61] | Burnout<br>Emotional distress | Cognitive behavioral therapy (CBT)<br>Dialectical behavior therapy (DBT) |

## Assessment and the Patient–Provider–Primary Caregiver Relationship

As has been outlined, learning about a patient's history, values, strengths, vulnerabilities, and individual experiences is essential to understanding how diagnosis and associated treatment impact the patient's functioning and overall well-being. The comprehensive assessment also helps guide the medical team in their support of the patient, caregiver(s), and other key stakeholders in the patient's family or support system. Through communication grounded in clinical expertise, compassion, and attention to the longitudinal nature of the illness experience, the relationships between the patient, caregiver, and medical provider can be leveraged in such a way as to enhance the well-being of all three.

### Communication

Effective communication skills are essential for all clinicians, their caregivers, and their family members. These skills are contribute to overall satisfaction with medical care, increase adherence to medical regimens, and foster an open environment for complex decision-making processes [62, 63]. Clinicians can utilize this skillset by sharing their medical knowledge and expertise while also actively listening, acknowledging emotions, and responding with empathy as often as possible. To maintain a patient and family-focused perspective throughout the working relationship, clinicians should incorporate their understanding of patient goals and values into each clinical interaction, effectively creating a connection characterized by honest, respectful, and non-judgmental communication.

The SPIKES model [64] is an approach that enables clinicians to build and maintain such a relationship. The model's steps include **s**etting up the conversation, assessing patient **p**erceptions, obtaining the patient's **i**nvitation to enter into the conversation, sharing **k**nowledge and information with the patient, naming their **e**motions, and offering a **s**ummary of the conversation and **s**trategy for next steps (Table 16.4).

An important component of this model - one that encourages patient autonomy and control of communication in an otherwise uncontrollable situation—is seeking a patient's permission to share specific information. Clinicians can offer options for patients about what information they want to hear ("Would it be helpful for me to share more about what to expect during the procedure, or would you like to wait until your next visit?") and, as in the case of adolescent patients and parents/caregivers, whom they want to hear the information ("Would you like me to share this with all of you together, or would you prefer to speak one-on-one first?"). These types of questions implicitly communicate that a

**Table 16.4** The SPIKES model for Sharing Bad News. (Adapted from Baile et al. [64])

| | Description | Example question(s) to ask |
|---|---|---|
| Set up | Ensure a private setting is available and prepared for such a conversation, with adequate seating for all participants and supportive materials within reach (e.g., boxes of tissues) | "Who do you want present for this conversation?" *Invite family, primary caregiver(s) and other social support, as specified by patient.* |
| Perception of patient | Begin by establishing patient (and family/caregiver) understanding of illness and purpose of this meeting by asking open-ended questions | "What do you understand about your illness?" "What have the doctors been telling you?" "What is your understanding of why we're meeting today?" |
| Invitation to share information | Elicit patient/family preferences for and limitations on receiving difficult information. Obtain their permission to proceed with the conversation | "How would you like to have difficult information communicated to you?" "Are you someone who prefers to have all the details, or would you rather know the big picture?" "Would it be alright for me to share with you the results of your test now?" |
| Knowledge | Provide challenging information, in keeping with communication preferences ascertained as above. Check for understanding | "I know this is a lot of information to digest right now. What questions do you have?" |
| Exploration of emotions | Name the emotions you are observing and empathize | "I can only begin to imagine how you are feeling" "Tell me what is going through your mind right now" |
| Strategy and summary | Summarize main points. Make a plan for next steps, including future decision points and additional support services available | "We are waiting on the results of these next tests. Would it be helpful to meet again?" "You've mentioned how important your faith is to you. In light of our conversation today, would it be helpful to meet with one of our spiritual care providers?" |

patient's preference matters and explicitly acknowledge a patient's emotions. This approach offers the clinician a space to normalize and validate the emotional experience, which is key in establishing and maintaining the relational bond between the patient and clinician.

## Longitudinal Care

The establishment and maintenance of a positive working relationship with patient and caregiver is a proactive strategy that can enhance well-being by promoting trust and confidence in the medical team. Continuity clinicians can build this trust by demonstrating their understanding of the patient as both an individual and an integrated part of their family and social systems. Familiarity with the patient's narrative and needs before diagnosis and throughout the illness trajectory enables clinicians to navigate complicated conversations and complex emotional responses more deftly. Knowledge of patient preferences and values can help clinicians approach interactions in such a way as to minimize anxiety and distress.

## End-of-Life Care

When a patient's condition continues to progress through therapy and cure is unlikely, despite the best efforts of caregivers and care teams, patients and their caregivers must begin to more actively balance goals and burdens of disease-directed interventions with hopes, values, and psychosocial considerations beyond their illness. Knowledge of a patient's larger psychosocial context assists primary and palliative care teams alike in navigating shifting priorities for patients and their families and making goals-based recommendations accordingly. What hopes or worries arise with the knowledge that death may be relatively certain? Is the ability to engage with family members or participate in certain activities as important to a patient as the possibility of life prolongation? Does the patient have a preference around the location or circumstances of their final days? In what ways would the patient's death affect their family system (emotionally, economically, spiritually)? What goals would a patient have if they knew that time was short?

The answers to these questions, among many others, may be gleaned from prior knowledge of patients and their psychosocial realities gleaned through existing relationships. This further demonstrates how the process of psychosocial assessment extends well beyond initial diagnosis and continues to unfold and shape interventions and recommendations through end-of-life and even bereavement care of families and caregivers. Ultimately, as goals of care shift away from curative treatment toward maximizing QOL and/or minimizing pain and suffering, primary psychosocial clinicians and palliative care teams work collaboratively to incorporate relevant psychosocial, practical, and value-oriented information to provide essential emotional, psychological, and logistical support to patients and family members.

## Bereavement

This support also extends beyond the death of a patient. Everything from care received in the EOL period to economic factors may influence the long-term bereavement outcomes of families [65, 66]. Evidence suggests that connection with health care teams following a death is strongly desired and beneficial to families and needs to be considered as part of the care that teams provide [67]. Ongoing assessment of families undergoing treatment for hematological conditions and HCT provides foundational knowledge of strengths, challenges, and areas of need that can be instrumental in identifying and providing optimal bereavement support. For psychosocial and palliative care clinicians, the early establishment of rapport with families and caregivers creates a more natural pathway through which to provide support and resources in the acute bereavement period. The continuation of support beyond a patient's death is the true embodiment of family-centered care.

## Summary

Far beyond diagnosing and treating their serious hematologic and oncologic conditions, patients exist as complex beings, deeply tied to their social relationships, personal identities, and material resources or needs. The psychosocial circumstances of patients, their dynamics with the people and the world, and their sense of self and values inform their understanding of a serious medical condition and affect their decision-making, coping, and utilization of various supports. Therefore, medical, psychosocial, and palliative care clinicians must work together through effective communication and thoughtful, collaborative engagement to support a patient's physical, material, emotional, social, and spiritual needs. Regardless of the course of an illness, it behooves the entire healthcare team to develop an appreciation of their patients as people outside of a diagnosis to best align with their priorities, make goal-concordant recommendations, and identify when specialized supportive psychosocial care may be necessary. Only through this intentional, strengths-based, iterative psychosocial assessment of patients, their caregivers, and their families can truly holistic care of the total person be accomplished.

## References


1. Bronfenbrenner U. The ecology of human development. Cambridge, MA: Harvard University Press; 1979.
2. Maslow AH. Religions, values, and peak experiences. New York: Penguin; 1970. (Original work published 1966)
3. Saleebey D. The strengths perspective in social work practice: extensions and cautions. Soc Work. 1996;41(3):296–305.
4. Nicholas DR, Veach TA. The psychosocial assessment of the adult cancer patient. Prof Psychol Res Pract. 2000;31(2):206–15.
5. Kazak AE, Brier M, Alderfer MA, Reilly A, Parker SF, Rogerwick S, Ditaranto S, Barakat LP. Screening for psychosocial risk in pediatric cancer. Pediatr Blood Cancer. 2012;59(5):822–7. https://doi.org/10.1002/pbc.24166.
6. Fiala MA, Finney JD, Liu J, Stockerl-Goldstein KE, Tomasson MH, Vij R, Wildes TM. Socioeconomic status is independently associated with overall survival in patients with multiple myeloma. Leuk Lymphoma. 2015;56(9):2643–9.
7. Liou SY, Stephens JM, Carpiuc KT, Feng W, Botteman MF, Hay JW. Economic burden of haematological adverse effects in cancer patients: a systematic review. Clin Drug Investig. 2007;27:381–96.
8. Stump TK, Eghan N, Egleston BL, Hamilton O, Pirollo M, Sanford Schwartz J. Cost concerns of patients with cancer. J Oncol Pract. 2013;9:251–7.
9. Kadan-Lottick NS, Vanderwerker LC, Block SD, Zhang B, Prigerson HG. Psychiatric disorders and mental health service use in patients with advanced cancer: a report from the coping with cancer study. Cancer. 2005;104(12):2872–81.
10. Prieto JM, Blanch J, Atala J, Carreras E, Rovira M, Cirera E, Gasto C. Psychiatric morbidity and impact on hospital length of stay among hematologic cancer patients receiving stem-cell transplantation. J Clin Oncol. 2002;20(7):1907–17.
11. Kazak AE, Alderfer MA, Streisand R, Simms S, Rourke MT, Barakat LP, Gallagher P, Cnaan A. Treatment of posttraumatic stress symptoms in adolescent survivors of childhood cancer and their families: a randomized clinical trial. J Fam Psychol. 2004;18(3):493–504.
12. Stuber ML, Shemesh E. Post-traumatic stress response to life-threatening illnesses in children and their parents. Child Adolesc Psychiatr Clin N Am. 2006;15:597–609.
13. Applebaum A, Bevans M, Son T, Evans K, Hernandez M, Giralt S, DuHamel K. A scoping review of caregiver burden during allogeneic HSCT: lessons learned and future directions. Bone Marrow Transplant. 2016;51:1416–22.
14. Wadhwa D, Burman D, Swami N, Rodin G, Lo C, Zimmermann C. Quality of life and mental health in caregivers of outpatients with advanced cancer. Psycho-Oncology. 2013;22(2):403–10.
15. Edmond SN, Graves PE, Whiting SE, Karlson CW. Emotional distress and burden among caregivers of children with oncological/hematological disorders. Fam Syst Health. 2016;34(2):166–171.s.
16. MacLeod KD, Whitsett SF, Mash EJ, Pelletier W. Pediatric sibling donors of successful and unsuccessful hematopoietic stem cell transplants (HSCT): a qualitative study of their psychosocial experience. J Pediatr Psychol. 2003;28(4):223–30. https://doi.org/10.1093/jpepsy/jsg010.
17. Wanner M, Bochert S, Schreyer IM, et al. Losing the genetic twin: donor grief after unsuccessful unrelated stem cell transplantation. BMC Health Serv Res. 2009;9:2. https://doi.org/10.1186/1472-6963-9-2.
18. Kahn JM, Keegan TH, Tao L, Abrahão R, Bleyer A, Viny AD. Racial disparities in the survival of American children, adolescents, and young adults with acute lymphoblastic leukemia, acute myelogenous leukemia, and Hodgkin lymphoma. Cancer. 2016;122(17):2723–30.
19. Ward E, Jemal A, Cokkinides V, Singh GK, Cardinez C, Ghafoor A, Thun M. Cancer disparities by race/ethnicity and socioeconomic status. CA Cancer J Clin. 2004;54(2):78–93.
20. Kirtane K, Lee SJ. Racial and ethnic disparities in hematologic malignancies. Blood. 2017;130(15):1699–705.
21. Adelstein KE, Anderson JG, Taylor AG. Importance of meaning-making for patients undergoing hematopoietic stem cell transplantation. Oncol Nurs Forum. 2014;41(2):E172–84.

22. Bluebond-Langner M. The private worlds of dying children. Princeton, NJ: Princeton University Press; 1978.
23. Heilferty C. Spiritual development and the dying child: the pediatric nurse practitioner's role. J Pediatr Health Care. 2004;18(6):271–5.
24. Worden JW. Grief counseling and grief therapy: a handbook for the mental health practitioner. 4th ed. New York: Springer Publishing Company; 2008.
25. Kazak AE. Pediatric psychosocial preventative health model (PPPHM): research, practice, and collaboration in pediatric family systems medicine. Fam Syst Health. 2006;24(4):381–95.
26. Kazak AE, Didonato S, Schneider SJ, Pai ALH. Assessing family psychosocial risks in pediatric cancer. In: Abrams AN, Muriel AC, Wiener L, editors. Pediatric psychosocial oncology: textbook for multidisciplinary care. Cham: Springer; 2016. p. 51–65.
27. Burgers DE, Tarquini SJ, Kazak AE, Muriel AC. Screening and assessment in pediatric psycho-oncology. In: Breitbart MD, Butow PN, Jacobsen PB, Lam W, Lazenby M, Loscalzo MJ, editors. Psycho-oncology. 4th ed. Oxford; forthcoming.
28. Kazak AE, Hwang WT, Chen FF, et al. Screening for family psychosocial risk in pediatric cancer: validation of the psychosocial assessment tool (PAT) version 3. J Pediatr Psychol. 2018;43(7):737–48. https://doi.org/10.1093/jpepsy/jsy012.
29. Hinds P, et al. PROMIS pediatric measures in pediatric oncology: valid and clinically feasible indicators of patient-reported outcomes. Pediatr Blood Cancer. 2013;60(3):402–8. https://doi.org/10.1002/pbc.24233.
30. Patel SK, Mullins W, Turk A, Dekel N, Kinjo C, Sato JK. Distress screening, rater agreement, and services in pediatric oncology. Psycho-Oncology. 2011;20(12):1324–33.
31. Wiener L, Battles H, Zadeh S, Widemann BC, Pao M. Validity, specificity, feasibility and acceptability of a brief pediatric distress thermometer in outpatient clinics. Psycho-Oncology. 2017;26(4):461–8.
32. Watson M, Dunn J, Holland JC. Review of the history and development in the field of psychosocial oncology. Int Rev Psychiatry. 2014;26(1):128–35.
33. NICE. Guidance on cancer services improving supportive and palliative care for adults with cancer. London: National Institute of Health and Clinical Excellence; 2004.
34. Hutchison SD, Steginga SK, Dunn J. The tiered model of psychosocial intervention in cancer: a community-based approach. Psychooncology. 2005;15:541–6.
35. National Comprehensive Cancer Center. (2020). Distress during cancer care [brochure]. https://www.nccn.org/patients/guidelines/content/PDF/distress-patient.pdf.
36. Krause N, Borawski-Clark E. Social class differences in social support among older adults. The Gerontologist. 1995;35:498–508.
37. Dilworth-Anderson P, Brummett BH, Goodwin P, Williams SW, Williams RB, Siegler IC. Effect of race on cultural justifications for caregiving. J Geronol Series B. 2005;60(5):257–62.
38. Beckham JC, Burker EJ, Feldman ME, Costakis MJ. Self-efficacy and adjustment in cancer patients: a preliminary report. Behav Med. 1997;23(3):138–42.
39. Hunt SM, McEwen J, McKenna SP. J R Coll Gen Pract. 1985;35(273):185–8.
40. Vrettos I, Konstantinos K, Kontodimopoulos N, Pappa E, Georgiadou E, Haritos D, Papadopoulos A, Niakas D. Comparing health-related quality of life of cancer patients under chemotherapy and of their caregivers. Sci World J. 2012;2012:135283. https://doi.org/10.1100/2012/135283.
41. Aaronson NK, Ahmedzai S, Bergman B, Bullinger M, Cull A, Duez NJ, Filiberti A, Flechtner H, Fleishman SB, de Haes JCJM, Kaasa S, Klee M, Osoba D, Razavi D, Rofe PB, Schraub S, Sneeuw K, Sullivan M, Takeda E. The European Organization for Research and Treatment of cancer QLQ-C30: a quality-of-life instrument for use in international clinical trials in oncology. J Natl Cancer Inst. 1993;85(5):365–76.
42. Carroll BT, Kathol RG, Noyes R, Wald TG, Clamon GH. Screening for depression and anxiety in cancer patients using the hospital anxiety and depression scale. Gen Hosp Psychiatry. 1993;15(2):69–74.
43. Watson M, Greer S, Young J, Inayat Q, Burgess C, Robertson B. Development of a questionnaire measure of adjustment to cancer: the MAC scale. Psychol Med. 1988;18:203–9.
44. Lo C, Walsh A, Mikulincer M, Gagliese L, Zimmermann C, Rodin G. Measuring attachment security in patients with advanced cancer: psychometric properties of a modified and brief experiences in close relationships scale. Psycho-Oncology. 2008;18:490–9.
45. Puchalski C, Romer AL. Taking a spiritual history allows clinicians to understand patients more fully. J Palliat Med. 2000;3(1):129–37.
46. Pearlin LI, Mullan JT, Semple SJ, Skaff MM. Caregiving and the stress process: an overview of concepts and their measures. The Gerontologist. 1990;30:583–94.
47. Picot SJF, Youngblut J, Zeller R. Development and testing of a measure of perceived caregiver rewards in adults. J Nurs Meas. 1997;5(1):33–52.
48. Abidin RR. Parenting stress index. 4th ed. Lutz, FL: PAR; 2012.
49. Stein REK, Riessman CK. The development of the impact on family scale: preliminary findings. Med Care. 1980;18:465–72.
50. Meltzer LJ, Mindell JA. Systematic review and meta-analysis of behavioral interventions for pediatric insomnia. J Pediatr Psychol. 2014;39(8):932–48.
51. Uman LS, Chambers CT, McGrath PJ, Kisely S. A systematic review of randomized controlled trials examining psychological interventions for needle-related procedural pain and distress in children and adolescents: an abbreviated Cochrane review. J Pediatr Psychol. 2008;33(8):842–54.
52. Dean AJ, Walters J, Hall A. A systematic review of interventions to enhance medication adherence in children and adolescents with chronic illness. Arch Dis Child. 2010;95(9):717–23.
53. Bennett S, Shafran R, Coughtrey A, Walker S, Heyman I. Psychological interventions for mental health disorders in children with chronic physical illness: a systematic review. Arch Dis Child. 2015;100(4):308–16.
54. Ahola Kohut S, Stinson J, Davies-Chalmers C, Ruskin D, van Wyk M. Mindfulness-based interventions in clinical samples of adolescents with chronic illness: a systematic review. J Altern Complement Med. 2017;23(8):581–9.
55. Zhou ES, Suh S, Youn S, Chung S. Adapting cognitive-behavior therapy for insomnia in cancer patients. Sleep Med Res. 2017;8(2):51–61.
56. Richardson J, Smith JE, McCall G, Richardson A, Pilkington K, Kirsch I. Hypnosis for nausea and vomiting in cancer chemotherapy: a systematic review of the research evidence. Eur J Cancer Care. 2006;16:402–12.
57. Spencer JC, Wheeler SB. A systematic review of motivational interviewing interventions in cancer patients and survivors. Patient Educ Couns. 2016;99(7):1099–105.
58. Carlson L, Speca M, Segal Z. Mindfulness-based cancer recovery: a step-by-step MBSR approach to help you cope with treatment and reclaim your life. Oakland, CA: New Harbinger Publications; 2011.
59. Law E, Fisher E, Eccleston C, Palermo TM. Psychological interventions for parents of children and adolescents with chronic illness. Cochrane Database Syst Rev. 2019;3:1–171.
60. Toledo T, Akinyemi E. Caregiver burnout: application of dialectical behavior therapy. Am J Geriatr Psychiatry. 2017;25(3):88–9.
61. Secinti E, Tometich DB, Johns SA, Mosher CE. The relationship between acceptance of cancer and distress: a meta-analytic review. Clin Psychol Rev. 2019;71:27–38.
62. Meyer EC, Sellers DE, Browning DM, McGuffie K, Solomon MZ, Truog RD. Difficult conversations: improving communication

skills and relational abilities in health care. Pediatr Crit Care Med. 2009;10(3):352–9.
63. Spinetta JJ, Masera G, Eden T, Oppenheim D, Martins AG, van Dongen-Melman J, Weyl M. Refusal, non-compliance, and abandonment of treatment in children and adolescents with cancer. A report of the SIOP working committee on psychosocial issues in pediatric oncology. Med Pediatr Oncol. 2002;38(2):114–7.
64. Baile WF, Buckman R, Lenzi R, Glober G, Beale EA, Kudelka AP. SPIKES-A six-step protocol for delivering bad news: application to the patient with cancer. Oncologist. 2000;5(4):302–11.
65. Kim Y, Carver CS, Spiegel D, Mitchell HR, Cannady RS. Role of family caregivers' self-perceived preparedness for the death of the cancer patient in long-term adjustment to bereavement. Psycho-Oncology. 2017;26(4):484–92.
66. McCarthy MC, Clarke NE, Ting CL, Conroy R, Anderson VA, Heath JA. Prevalence and predictors of parental grief and depression after the death of a child from cancer. J Palliat Med. 2010;13(11):1321–6.
67. Lichtenthal WG, Sweeney CR, Roberts KE, Corner GW, Donovan LA, Prigerson HG, Wiener L. Bereavement follow-up after the death of a child as a standard of care in pediatric oncology. Pediatr Blood Cancer. 2015;62(S5):S834–69.

# Multicultural and Spiritual Considerations

# 17

Allison Kestenbaum, Portia Howard, and Yuko Abbott

## Introduction

Hematologic malignancies and blood disorders impact physical, emotional, and spiritual well-being in various ways [1]. While these illnesses impact individual patients differently, the interdisciplinary guidance and focus of palliative care can help clinicians identify, address, and refer appropriately to address spiritual and multicultural considerations. This chapter highlights how cultural and spiritual beliefs and practices may serve as a source of comfort and resources that can improve well-being [2].

## Overlap of Multicultural and Spiritual Care

A holistic approach to clinical care includes patients' multicultural and spiritual needs and resources for reducing suffering. This approach aligns with palliative care's focus on quality of life by reducing the emotional, mental, physical, social, and spiritual distress of individuals with serious illnesses and their family members [3].

Culturally competent clinical care begins with a heightened awareness of one's own multicultural and spiritual framework and how it intersects with the patient. Multicultural care is a person-centered approach that invites a clinician to see the patient as they see themselves and allows that to inform their medical decision-making for their disease process. This approach also supports positive coping while facing a new diagnosis or prognosis [4]. Does the patient see *themselves* as old or young, male, female or non-binary, a part of an ethnic group, or a part of a religious or spiritual community? If so, what importance does the aforementioned have on providing competent person-centered care? For instance, a patient identifies as a young, non-gender binary, European-American who is non-religious yet spiritual. The patient would like to appoint *their* partner as their medical decision-maker in a suburban Christian hospital despite the patient's family's disapproval. Or another instance: a patient identifies as a middle-aged, Arabic male who is Muslim and is greeted by a female clinician that extends her hand, and the patient draws back as per his custom to not touch a person of the opposite sex. The patient's anxiety is heightened because his multicultural identity is not understood or honored, and he requests to be transferred to another facility. The two examples highlight that a heightened awareness of a patient's multicultural identity is normative in providing culturally competent care.

Regarding religious/spiritual identity, 27% of Americans no longer ascribe to a religious preference but to a spiritual preference; therefore, defining the difference is important [5]. Religion is a specific set of organized beliefs and practices, usually shared by a community or group. Spirituality is more of an individual practice and has to do with having a sense of peace and purpose, among many aspects [5]. One prevalent model in healthcare is to recognize spirituality as being divided into seven pathways that can bring dignity and meaning-making as a person suffers: Connect to the soul, the deeper self; connect through the body; connect to another person; connect to a community and make a contribution to that community; connect to earth/nature; connect through art/music; connect to God or a Higher Power [6] (Table 17.1).

The overlap of multicultural and spiritual care has vital implications regarding understanding a person as they receive a new diagnosis or functional decline. With the

A. Kestenbaum (✉)
Spiritual Care Services/Howell Palliative Care, UC San Diego Health, La Jolla, CA, USA
e-mail: akestenbaum@health.ucsd.edu

P. Howard
Volunteer and Spiritual Care Services, University of California, San Diego Health, San Diego, CA, USA
e-mail: pohoward@health.ucsd.edu

Y. Abbott
Moores Cancer Center Radiation Oncology, UC San Diego Health, La Jolla, CA, USA
e-mail: yabbott@health.ucsd.edu


C. K. Ullrich, E. J. Roeland (eds.), *Palliative Care in Hematologic Malignancies and Serious Blood Disorders*,
https://doi.org/10.1007/978-3-031-38058-7_17

**Table 17.1** Spirituality pathways [6]

| 7 Pathways of spirituality | Examples |
|---|---|
| Connect to the soul, the deeper self | Meditation, prayer |
| Connect through the body | Exercise, massage, human contact |
| Connect to another person | Fully known and fully loved by at least one individual |
| Connect to a community and make a contribution to that community | Fully known and fully loved by a group of people |
| Connect to earth/nature | Pets, natural landscapes |
| Connect through art/music | Deciphering what fosters positive coping |
| Connect to God or a higher power | Optional yet individual meaning-making approach |

person-centered framework in mind, the healthcare team needs to integrate the patient's deepest need as they suffer and process that they are a person that happens to have cancer and/or another hematological disease. Clinicians should consider which of the following represents their deepest needs: medical, existential, spiritual, emotional, or cultural practice and if their needs can be met through spirituality. Another important consideration is the impact of medical or psychosocial treatment on the patient and family's quality of life. Clinicians can elevate their cultural sensitivity by establishing a therapeutic alliance with the patient, family, and the interdisciplinary team and considering how the patient's deepest needs can be met. When treatment itself is no longer beneficial to the patient, how can the interdisciplinary team maintain a therapeutic alliance? All of these considerations are accessible to all interdisciplinary team members and are emphasized in palliative care. They will inform the plan of care regarding goals of care, advance care planning, meaning-making, and make appropriate referrals to members of the interdisciplinary team, such as the social worker and the spiritual care clinicians/chaplains.

## Interdisciplinary Integrated Palliative Care for Hematologic Malignancies and Serious Blood Disorders

Coordination of healthcare is critical to achieve and deliver optimal outcomes for patients with complex healthcare needs. While a patient is at the center of any healthcare provision, it is important to remember that everyone involved in patient care impacts and plays a critical role in the outcome. The term "interdisciplinary" will be used in this chapter to reflect the patient-focused, coordinated care provided by professionals from various disciplines to achieve an optimal outcome—in this case, specifically related to attending to spiritual and cultural aspects of care [7].

This chapter's authorship is purposeful because it reflects both a social worker and chaplain's availability in assessing and addressing spiritual and cultural needs in people living with serious blood disorders. Patients' psychosocial needs are best met by an interdisciplinary care team, such as a fully staffed palliative care consultation or embedded team [8]. Social workers and chaplains have distinct yet overlapping roles, and thus, close communication and consultation can positively impact patient care [9]. Both roles assess and address cultural and spiritual concerns. The chaplain is the expert in addressing spiritual distress once it is diagnosed [10, 11]. For social workers, an initial assessment is a start of a relationship with patients and their families, guiding them to navigate changing and emerging *bio-psycho-social-spiritual* issues as they begin the continuum of care. For example, certified oncology social workers are expected to possess such skills because any conversations and interactions with patients and their loved ones could lead to a more in-depth and personal conversation about their cultural and spiritual beliefs as they face life with cancer [12] (Fig. 17.1).

The reality is that most care teams for hematologic malignancies and blood disorders do not have the benefit of a spiritual counselor or professional chaplain dedicated to the team. Rather, spiritual care may fall to the social worker on the front line caring for patients. Amid their screening and assessments, the social worker also identifies religious/spiritual and cultural needs and resources [13]. This social worker may be part of the specialty/primary team or palliative care team consulted to assist with symptoms, quality of life, and whole-person care. Social workers advocate for the involvement of a professional chaplain at the institution, and if one is not available, may collaborate with community clergy.

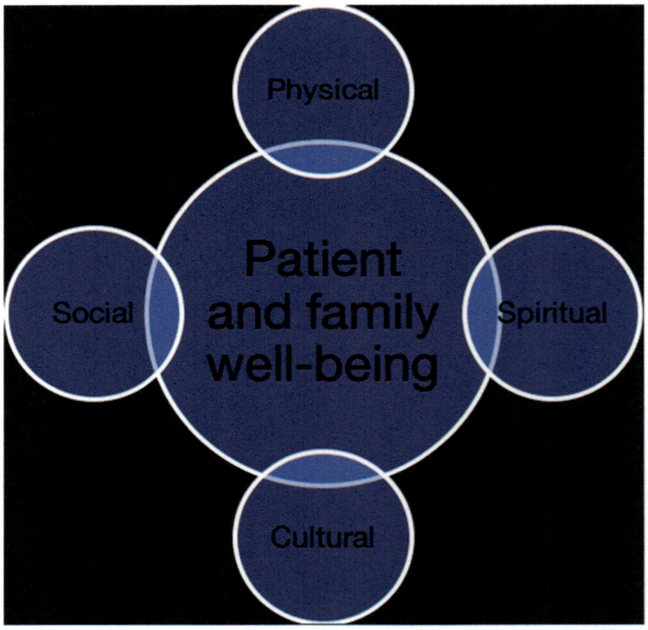


**Fig. 17.1** Palliative care

Short of a best-case scenario where both a chaplain and social worker with palliative care training are available to assist patients with serious blood illnesses, collaborations with psychosocial staff available to the care team are crucial to whole-person care [14].

## Spiritual and Cultural Screening and Assessment

Several guidelines for blood cancer and other hematological illnesses emphasize the importance of screening patients for distress and psychosocial needs as a critical first step to providing high-quality care [15]. Distress is defined as an uncomfortable feeling that can influence a patient's thoughts and actions [16]. Early detection and treatment of such distress are important in overall care. Accrediting and regulating bodies' practice guidelines and accreditation requirements include a psychosocial distress screening program as an indicator of quality care. Oncology program standards and practice guidelines, such as The Joint Commission, National Comprehensive Cancer Network (NCCN), The Quality Oncology Practice Initiative (QOPI), and Commission on Cancer (CoC), have been updated to include screening for psychosocial distress. Distress screening and assessment identify the presence of physical, psychological, social, spiritual, and financial support needs and identify the appropriate referrals as needed. Nursing and Social Work professionals are often on the front line to routinely screen, assess, address, and/or refer patients with/without a screening tool. A short screening tool is often used and preferred to lengthier questionnaires to avoid negative impact on clinic operations. For example, NCCN Distress Thermometer is commonly used as a part of the check-in process at pivotal oncology visits. It is a one-page screening tool with a visual graphic of a thermometer to indicate distress level 1–10. The tool also contains a problem list which includes physical, practical, family, emotional, and spiritual/religious concerns. NCCN has made it accessible by not requiring permission for using the tool with patients. Some adaptation is also permitted.

A formal or informal distress screening of patients is just the first step in assessing patients' coping, needs, and understanding of illness and treatment throughout the care continuum. Clinicians must also recognize and assess the influence of various dimensions of a patient, especially cultural and spiritual. It is important to consider how blood disorder diagnosis and treatment impact a patient as a whole person and her/his family, which belongs to a larger society and a system. The lens through which one views the world is based on her/his experiences and perspectives, which are learned and shaped by multiple factors such as socioeconomic status, educational and professional background, ethnic and racial background, religious and spiritual orientation, and family and community traditions and practices. Clinicians must remain humble enough to pause and ask patients/families for information, clarification, and/or confirmation of how they understand their diagnoses and what it might mean for them. According to the 2017 US Census, 40% of Americans identify as racial or ethnic minorities in the United States [17]. Each interaction with patients can potentially be an intercultural interaction leading to unintentional misunderstanding, false assumptions, and prejudgment of healthcare decisions. Understanding how the history, culture, and tradition impacts a patient is helpful, but even more important is a healthcare professional's ability to listen and learn from a patient in a respectful and nonjudgmental way while being aware of one's own biases [18].

The interdisciplinary practice of palliative care and the standards of practice for social work and spiritual care further addresses the importance of screening and assessing patients and their support system to develop an evidence-informed care plan [12]. Furthermore, identifying a patient's priorities and goals is a foundation of care planning. Assessment is an ongoing process and an opportunity to revisit previously identified concerns and goals and to respond to changing and emerging concerns and needs of patients and families. Bio-psycho-social-spiritual assessment (Fig. 17.2) is a model often used in patient assessment by spiritual caregivers, social workers, and other mental health clinicians in healthcare settings to understand how these dimensions of a patient's life contribute to the patient's current functioning.

Spiritual and religious resources and concerns are a subset of cultural needs [19]. Often conducted by a social worker or a spiritual caregiver or any interdisciplinary team member, bio-psycho-social-spiritual screening is used to assess needs, resources, and goals, including spiritual issues [20, 21]. "Spiritual" is a subjective concept and can be based on personal interpretation and understanding of the patient and the family. However, a consensus definition of spirituality in palliative care is "Spirituality is the aspect of humanity that refers to the way individuals seek and express meaning and purpose and the way they experience their connectedness to the moment, to self, to others, to nature, and to the significant or sacred" [22]. An initial goal of spiritual screening is to understand how a patient sees and values her/his religious/spiritual life and preferences for clinicians to respond to spiritual distress and suffering. Spiritual assessment involves a chaplain assessing a patient's sense of self, meaning, purpose, and significant relationships. It also involves considering what her/his value base is and religious life and to what extent these play a role in healthcare decisions [20, 23].

Spirituality can be a valuable source of coping, strength, hope, and peace, as well as a means through which patients articulate or demonstrate distress, suffering, and negative coping [23, 24]. At baseline, clinicians' role in the spiritual-

**Fig. 17.2** Bio-psycho-social-spiritual assessment model

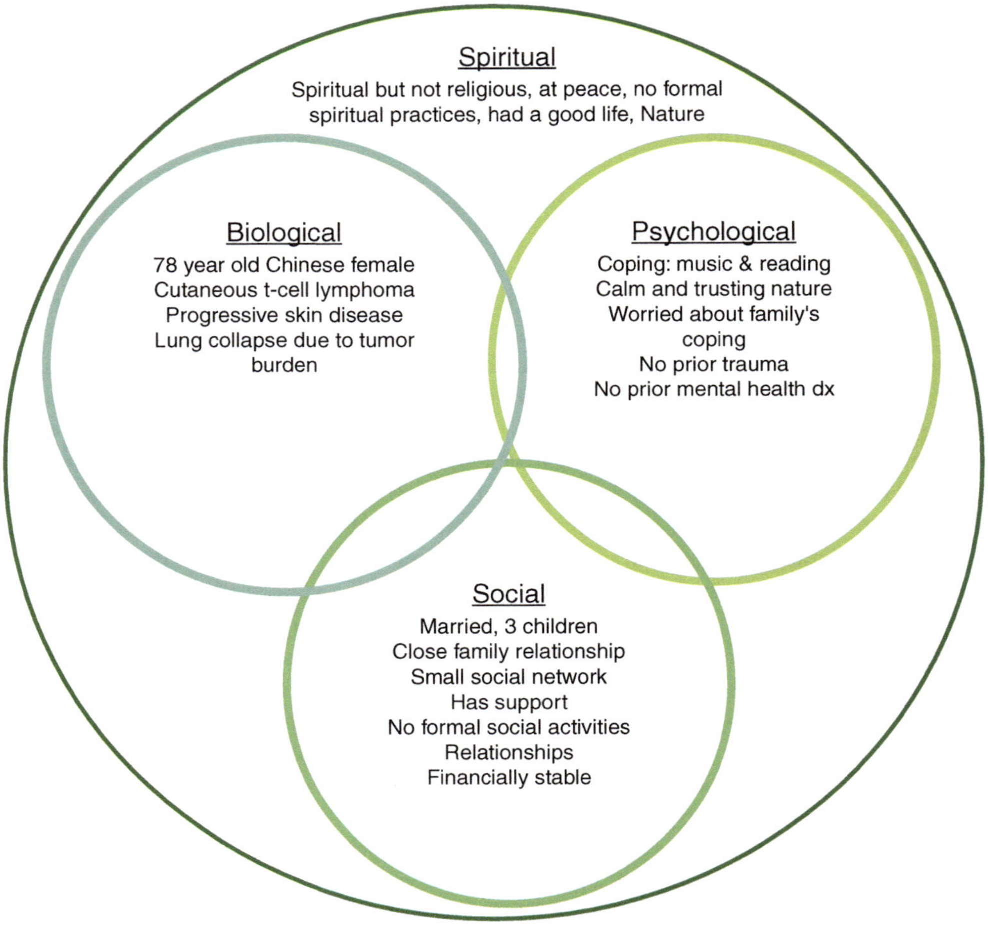


ity of patients is to simply be open-minded, respectful, and to encourage a patient's desire to access spiritual support and resources. Early identification of faith, spiritual and religious beliefs, strengths, and values by clinicians often promotes open and ongoing conversations through all phases of blood cancer/disorders and treatment [25]. Clinicians can refer to healthcare chaplains for further consultation and to conduct a more in-depth spiritual assessment and intervention plan [26]. Collaboration with community clergy may also be hugely beneficial to the patient in finding alignment between their treatment goals, values, and overall beliefs. In some cases, non-chaplain clinicians asking about a patient's spirituality and what it means can be a bit like learning to ask a question in a language in which you are not fluent—you may not be able to fully understand the answer you receive or know how to respond effectively, so it is recommended that you have a plan for follow-up on spiritual needs [27].

Ideally, screening a patient by any clinician should include spiritual and religious dimensions because it could help or hinder a patient's coping with a new diagnosis of a hematologic disorder or living with a chronic illness. In patients with blood cancer, spiritual and religious foundations help find meaning, solace, and prayer to comfort and promote healthy coping with challenges [28]. Patients may feel conflicted as if their illness is a test of faith. They may feel guilty or even blame themselves due to not living a life consistent with faith. It is important to understand how spirituality functions in the patient's life, from their perspective, and to avoid making assumptions. Meaning-making occurs when patients are engaging in reflection and internal dialogue to accept the reality of being diagnosed. Meaning-making and finding purpose is an important process. It helps them understand being diagnosed in a way that makes sense to them, based on how they have lived their lives thus far, put it in a context they understand, and see connections to their faith and values [29]. For a patient who feels that the diagnosis puts their identity and legacy into question, meaning-making may be a fraught and painful process that can benefit from empathy on the part of all caregivers and the skillful guidance of a psychosocial-spiritual professional.

Culture also influences how patients view diagnosis as a health problem and how symptoms are experienced and expressed. Healthcare decisions are influenced by culture and how medical information is received and understood. Clinicians face different ways of navigating and managing patients' and families' care from non-native US patients [30]. A family spokesperson and a decision-maker might not always be a patient. An expression of their emotional distress might be very dramatic or stoic. It is also common to observe varying degrees of acculturation and assimilation into US culture within a family system. These differences are based on the years spent in the US, generational differences, and other demographic factors such as level of education, socioeconomic status, and employment status in the United States [18]. At times, there is a clash of culture and beliefs within a family system, complicating a patient's care. A family spokesperson of the younger generation might simply say, "She is from the old generation," referring to how a patient might perceive her cancer or how a decision is being made based on cultural beliefs.

Clinicians must recognize and acknowledge diversity as well as respect patients' and families' cultural preferences and practices when providing care. Culturally sensitive interventions could be as simple as encouraging patients to discuss and integrate spiritual, religious, cultural, and health practices into their care plan [18].

## Impact of Underlying Emotional/Spiritual Suffering on Care

An initial screening may point to physical or emotional distress. While some patients are truly experiencing physical pain, discomfort, and emotional struggle due to their diagnosis, it might be just the tip of a larger iceberg. Patients with hematologic disorders bring their whole selves, including all of their past and current issues as well as their hopes and fears for the future. These could manifest in unexpected ways during treatment. However, any biopsychosocial spiritual dimension of a patient could act as a resource or barrier to care, and therefore it must be understood and addressed [31]. Intractable pain, missed appointments, or avoidance could be due to past traumatic and violent experiences with physical exams. These memories trigger overwhelming feelings of sadness and remind them of loved ones who died from the same illness. Some are scared that they would cease to exist after physical death—being forgotten, to darkness and nothingness after life. Only further conversation and a willingness to explore with patients, with respect and a nonjudgmental approach, can reveal the true underlying causes of distress impacting a patient's ability to participate in care. Whether these are real or imagined, clinicians must address the patient's reality.

## Spiritual Care in Palliative Care

All palliative care, whether or not it is for hematological disorders, includes spiritual care. Palliative and spiritual care have always been congruent because of the shared emphasis on whole-patient care (i.e., the goal of supporting patients' and their loved ones' spiritual, psychosocial, physical, and existential needs). Therefore, the importance of the inclusion of spiritual care in all palliative care is implicit for hematological disorders. Yet, palliative care itself and overcoming the myths surrounding it have grown exponentially in the last 10 years in clinicians' awareness and understanding. The existence of this volume demonstrates the ever-present need to describe the healing potential of palliative care integrated into hematology [32, 33]. Similarly, professional spiritual care provided by adequately educated, clinically trained, and credentialed chaplains or spiritual counselors is becoming more prominent in healthcare [5]. This awareness is still growing, and it is important to highlight what spiritual care in palliative care for this population does and can entail.

The fourth edition of the National Consensus Project of Clinical Practice Guidelines for Palliative Care represents the multi-professional and discipline perspectives criteria for palliative care. It explicitly recognizes the spiritual, religious, and existential along with cultural aspects of care (i.e., Domains 5 and 6). The guidelines designate that professionally trained chaplains are the specialists in addressing this domain, particularly with regard to conducting a spiritual assessment, as discussed above. Cultural aspects overlap with religious/spiritual needs and are often key to understanding patients' and families' values and beliefs. Awareness of these aspects may also help clinicians acknowledge and address their own biases about cultural aspects such as race, ethnicity, gender, immigration, refugee status, religion, and spirituality.

Although spiritual needs are universal and important to consider in all health crises and chronic illnesses, there are several special considerations for patients with hematologic malignancies and serious blood disorders. Being attentive to these may help clinicians be more attuned to symptoms of spiritual distress that may be masked by behaviors that are often attributed to a patient's challenge, non-compliance, anger, etc. [34–37]. Specifically in addressing the spiritual needs of blood cancer patients, one thing to consider is the staggering expanse of information there is to learn about their disease. Mystery and uncertainty are spiritual considerations at their very core [38, 39]. Patients seek to make meaning, which facilitates their understanding of the diagnosis, how it might impact them and what it might mean for them and their family in the future. Meaning-making could also help to cultivate a sense of hope and purpose. Being diagnosed and living with an illness can be a traumatic experience for which no one is fully prepared.

Blood cancers pose particular challenges to meaning because comprehending a solid tumor or cancer in a more "concrete" part of their body provides a target and clearer goals. There is a lot to learn about blood cancers, including the array and complexity of short-term and long-term treatment [35]. There is a vast network of support programs and communities. Patients may initially and periodically feel overwhelmed and, as a result, isolated, which is itself a spiritual concern. If spiritual and emotional concerns are identified and addressed proactively through interdisciplinary palliative care intervention, patients may benefit from an overall improvement in well-being. One example is that patients may experience post-traumatic growth, which is defined as one's subjective perception of positive changes in the aftermath of dealing with a critical life event such as cancer [40]. A stronger sense of meaning may also relate to lower levels of anxiety and depression, a higher level of satisfaction with life, and better health-related functioning [41]. Cancer patients who have had post-traumatic growth have enhanced appreciation in life, open to possibilities, reevaluation of priorities and goals in life, a sense of personal strength, closeness with loved ones, and positive changes in spiritual beliefs. This growth is particularly significant in patients with blood cancers because lengthy remissions are possible, and seeking emotional and spiritual well-being wherein one is not overwhelmed by the trauma of treatment and fear of remission is key to good quality of life [42]. One way to address this challenge is that palliative care-informed social workers and chaplains can engage patients in a meaningful conversation about their hopes and fears based on uncertainty about the illness.

Many patients receiving palliative care for blood cancers, particularly long-term, may be receiving proactive pain management and may have fears about addiction. The reverse of that scenario are patients whose pain is undertreated because clinicians fear the patient will abuse, misuse, or chemically cope with pain medication [43]. Addressing and preventing addiction through a bio-psycho-social-spiritual approach, with interdisciplinary clinicians regularly discussing and advising on the patient's case where these concerns are present, removes the stigma. It cultivates trust in the relationship while improving outcomes for the patient and decreasing frustration for clinicians. Culture also plays a role in treating pain. Due to unconscious bias, it has been shown that patients from some cultural backgrounds are less likely to receive pain medication [44]. Another scenario is for non-native or non-English speakers to find themselves in misunderstandings about symptom management with caregivers, thereby leading to isolation and a sense of powerlessness and hopelessness. Appropriate use of professional medical interpreters is imperitive.

Sensitivity to spiritual and multicultural considerations is essential with blood disorders that have a genetic component and disproportionately impact patients from particular cultural, ethnic, and religious backgrounds. Patients may logically understand a disease process has nothing to do with them personally. However, feeling that one is part of a disproportionately impacted group can raise several spiritual issues. Some patients may experience their sense of self-worth negatively impacted, resulting in a tendency not to prioritize their well-being and become isolated [20, 24, 45]. For others, the situation's unfairness may spark sadness and grief that is masked as anger and result in challenges and brokenness in interpersonal relationships. Culture can influence how grief is expressed. Patients experience numerous losses due to hematologic malignancies and disorders, even if death is not imminent. Historic health disparities further exacerbate this experience. Even clinicians who are educated about this dynamic may feel helpless or untrained about responding and propagating a sense of spiritual and moral injury within themselves. The intentional psychosocial and spiritual aspects of palliative care can help patients and caregivers substantially address these concerns.

Palliative care's proactive and skilled approach to exploring and regularly revisiting patients' goals of care and beliefs about what constitutes sufficient quality of life is an important way to mitigate suffering related to chronic conditions and/or targeted treatment. There is also abundant wisdom offered by faith, spiritual and cultural traditions about suffering. Resilience and dignity are enhanced for patients when these are actively allowed into the care plan for patients. The experience of living either with chronic pain (e.g., patient with sick-cell anemia) or living through the acute agony accompanying hematopoietic cell transplantation (HCT) or other treatment (e.g., radiation or chemotherapy) raises enormous existential concerns about survival and quality of life. Although the metaphor of "fighting" a disease at all costs to stay alive is present in popular medical discourse about hematologic illness, posing the question to a patient about their wishes may alleviate distress. For instance, discussing an elderly patient's wishes who is internally and secretly weighing the costs and benefits of pursuing aggressive treatment for a blood cancer may relieve existential distress.

## Case Studies

These case studies provide examples of how palliative care's involvement and leadership address the intersection of cultural and spiritual considerations. These scenarios demonstrate situations related to hematological disorders and malignancy care.

### Case #1 Culture and Decision-Making

A 78-year-old Chinese female with Cutaneous T-cell Lymphoma was referred to social work for assistance with communication about goals of care. Her lymphoma has progressed through treatment, and now she is experiencing respiratory failure due to the tumor burden in her right lung. The oncology social worker completed an assessment using the bio-psycho-social-spiritual model. She is psychologically fairly stable and seems to have effective coping skills. Her temperament is calm and trusting, and she has no prior history of trauma or mental health issues. She has strong family ties and support. Her husband and three adult children are very much involved in her care and are concerned for her well-being. Although she has not been engaging in social activities outside of her home for several weeks, she seems to be very content with her current social engagement level. Spiritual screening found that she is very spiritual but not religious. She gets in touch with her spirituality through nature and music, which brings her calm and inner peace. She feels she has had a good life, is at peace, and accepts that the end of her life is approaching simply as a part of a life cycle. Despite her progressively worsening disease, she seems to be accepting failing health and appears peaceful. However, she is worried about her husband's endurance being with her at the bedside daily and her adult children putting their lives on hold for so long for her. The oncological social worker observes that psychological and social well-being appear to be possible for her because of her strong spiritual foundation, despite worsening biological health.

Despite the patient's acceptance of death and dying, her husband and adult children could not initially agree to transition her to comfort care after she could no longer make her own decisions. The adult children have a high education level in the United States and understand the patient is gravely ill. The family and patient met with outpatient oncological palliative care on one occasion, thanks to a referral from their oncologist, and were educated about what it means to receive comfort care. Yet, the husband is committed to doing everything possible for his wife instead of "giving up on her." He expresses his sense of responsibility and duty to care for her and make sure she receives what she needs to get better. Her adult children were able to gently facilitate a conversation with the oncologist and palliative care clinicians to help the husband understand that there is no treatment available to treat her cancer. Once the discussion shifted and reframed her needs related to quality of life, the husband was able to see his role and duty to make sure she was getting what she needed to be comfortable.

In this case example, it appeared that the patient did not explicitly discuss her wishes with her family in advance nor had advance directives. This situation is typical in Asian families in which a decision tends to be made by the family, not by an individual patient. She probably did not see the need [13]. However, this resulted in disagreement about her care among family members. It would be understandable for clinicians to look to her husband to make healthcare decisions as next of kin and as her surrogate decision-maker. However, culturally speaking, it was a family decision.

Fulfilling duty and avoiding the larger community's disapproval (for giving up on her) often drive medical decision-making among Chinese families. This example shows how families with various acculturation and assimilation levels created different decisions for the patient and resulted in, at least temporarily, tension within the family. By understanding the family's sense of duty, the oncologist and palliative care team could reframe providing comfort care as they fulfilled their duty to her. Biopsychosocial spiritual assessment identified the conflict in a complex situation and how to bridge the gap to move toward a shared goal (Fig. 17.2).

A conversation in a family meeting also proved to be a valuable tool, as cultural, religious, and spiritual issues enriched and complicated the family's decision-making. The role of clinicians is to help families understand and embrace the concept that medical conditions change and new issues could emerge. Therefore, it is healthy for hope and wishes for a patient to change accordingly. This model is true not just at the end of life but with any new diagnosis regardless of expected mortality or morbidity rates. This type of conversation can begin to cultivate psychological flexibility and resilience. The interdisciplinary palliative care approach engaged in supportive counseling to facilitate the ability to hold two seemingly conflicting views simultaneously—wanting to deny but accepting the diagnosis. This concept is similar to "hope for the best while preparing for the worst."

### Case #2 Cultural and Spiritual Distress and Collaboration with the Care Team

A 28-year-old Christian, African-American woman was born with sickle-cell anemia and subsequently has spent her life facing repeat hospitalizations. The patient's intersectionality and identity are key in this case study as it helps identify areas of distress that clinicians can integrate into healthcare delivery. The patient became extremely medically literate about her symptoms and pain management to feel more empowered about her physical distress. Emotional and spiritual distress arose as she struggled with how to communicate with clinicians who appeared not to have the capacity to provide empathetic clinical care, or in other words, a culturally competent bedside manner. The patient remained acutely aware of interpersonal dynamics between her and the clinicians, and since she was a child, she has actively prayed for wisdom and well-being for them.

In speaking with a palliative-care-trained chaplain, the patient admitted she suspected that an "us vs. them" approach was attributed to emotional distress regarding how she was engaging with the clinicians. This approach was increasing her suffering because she saw "entitled men" telling her what her plan of care should be, i.e., pain and symptom management in a vacuum from the whole picture of who she is. Anger and becoming verbally combative rather than positive, therapeutic coping from her sources of strength resulted in a clinician terminating her hospitalization and discharging her during a sickle cell pain crisis. This example raised several questions. How can a clinician lean in and fully see a patient while also not experiencing maltreatment from a patient? What was this patient's most profound need? The patient desired to be fully seen and fully heard, and without that, the clinical plan of care is not achievable. Conversely, what therapeutic alliance is possible in an acute care setting? What were the clinicians' needs?

Interdisciplinary palliative support expressed in part through the chaplain's role allowed for a unique aspect of the coordination of care to be realized. A significant role of the chaplain is to help the patient process this blood disorder and to encourage reliance on spiritual coping. A nurse, in this case, invited a chaplain to the bedside with the clinical team. The chaplain's engagement fostered the support in actively listening to the patient, creating a therapeutic reliance, and supporting the return of the patient's pain to baseline levels.

Pain is inevitable as a sickle cell patient, but the chaplain helped the patient consider how she can rely on her Christian faith to address pain. The patient owned that she was more spiritual than religious. Rituals such as having essential oils concentrated in her diffuser were hospital approved, and it helped her manage her grief and anger, which was, in turn, helpful to the clinical team. When the patient met the palliative care team that recognized her distress at every level, she remarked: "I thank God there is a team that takes care of me beyond my medical care. They communicate with the hospitalists and empower me to feel that I have the tools to empower myself not to be solely dependent on other people or medical interventions."

As clinicians, it is crucial to identify when we are augmenting physical suffering or providing healing in nonphysical means. This case raises questions about how clinicians can transform their approach to an angry patient amid a sickle-cell pain crisis and invite the patient to build rapport with the clinical team members. As soon as the patient got in touch with her vulnerability and fear, she could extend trust to those assuaging her suffering through IV/PCA pain management. The patient feared that since her pain is not always visibly shown in vital signs or other metrics, she would be dismissed as "pain medication-seeking" and having a psychiatric decline from the care team's perspective. The patient's deepest need, as articulated by her, is as follows: "If the doctor could just sit down with me, it would lower my anxiety. I just want to be treated like a human being." Both the chaplain and social worker were equipped to take the initiative to reframe with the patient and the clinicians to foster dignity and guidance to all involved.

**Case #3 Engaging with Spiritual Struggle**

A religiously observant Jewish man in his 70s immigrated to the United States from Iran in the 1970s. He has a history of myeloma dating back 3 years. He initially complained of chronic fatigue and pain, which ultimately was diagnosed, along with compression fractures and lesions in his spine, consistent with his illness. Likely, his illnesses dated back further, but because of the stigma of cancer diagnosis in his cultural background, the patient was reluctant to seek medical attention at the onset of his symptoms. He initially kept his symptoms hidden from his family and friends.

He ultimately underwent an HCT 2 years ago and has received oncological care at a cancer center throughout. During his diagnosis and HCT hospitalization, the patient was referred to outpatient palliative care for assistance with symptom management, goals of care, and emotional/spiritual support. The primary reasons for referral to palliative care were pain and anxiety expressed through frequent and lengthy online communications with his primary care and oncologist through the online patient communication portal. Throughout his illness, the patient has received outpatient palliative care through which his pain has been well managed, and his cultural and spiritual-cultural beliefs have been assessed on an ongoing basis. For example, his wife's buy-in and presence through treatment and remission have been key to the patient remaining open and honest about his symptoms and concerns. He developed a positive rapport with a chaplain during BMT and has been forthcoming about his theological hopes and questions. As he has felt more bolstered and encouraged by remission, he has also been more willing to share information about his illness with his rabbi and faith community, again breaking the stigma and cultivating support.

During HCT, the patient's anxiety and mental health were being addressed by a psychologist specializing in patients with cancer, collaborating with his primary and palliative care clinicians. The patient expressed several aspects of spiritual need and cultural beliefs to the palliative team and chaplain. The patient was initially private about his concerns, but when he and his wife allowed the chaplain to visit when the patient was experiencing the most challenging HCT symptoms in the hospital, he opened up about his faith and spiritual distress. "I have always felt my life is in God's gracious hands, and I count my blessings. But I don't know if I can make it through this treatment. I have been good to my family and worked hard—where is God now, and how could my gracious God watch me suffer like this?" The spiritual care intervention was to develop trust with the patient, who could express his lament, history of faith, and current struggle given the extent of his suffering. The chaplain allowed him to express all this without being shut down or reassured. Rather, he was validated and reminded of his spiritual distress's universality given his situation and that he is not alone in asking such questions. In expressing this fully without shame, the patient ultimately found his spiritual healing during treatment. About a third of the way through his hospitalization, he told the chaplain, "I've been having dreams. My parents are coming to me, and they are telling me I'm not alone, that they are bringing God to me. These dreams mean everything to me—my father was very religious, and he died when I was ten. Somehow he is back with me now." Within his culture, the presence and support of family to alleviate cancer's stigma is the key to healing. Given the opportunity to articulate his spiritual needs and wisdom, the patient could derive and create this support for himself.

After 2 years of remission, the patient remains on a waitlist and eligible for various trials expected to have slots opening within the coming 6 months. However, due to the patient's increasing frailty and limited remission period, the oncologist has indicated to the patient that she does not recommend a second BMT. Anticipated remission time benefit does not outweigh the risk of treatment. Circumstances are different for the patient this time as he faces likely progression and decreasing treatment options. Thanks to the collaboration between his oncologist and his interdisciplinary palliative care nurse practitioner, social worker, chaplain, and psychologist, he expressed confidence that his most distressing symptoms—pain, anxiety, spiritual and social isolation, are being addressed. He can now express sadness about his increased frailty and limited treatment options and genuine gratitude for the quality of time that he has had with his family.

## Conclusion

Addressing religious/spiritual and cultural issues competently helps to avoid further suffering for patients, families, and medical clinicians. Doing so can promote positive coping, well-being, and post-traumatic growth. Integrating an interdisciplinary and whole-person focus with palliative care in the care of patients with blood cancers and hematologic disorders decreases suffering.

## References


1. Lesko LM, Holland JC. Psychological issues in patients with hematological malignancies. Recent Results Cancer Res. 1988;108:243–70.
2. Astrow AB, Kwok G, Sharma RK, Fromer N, Sulmasy DP. Spiritual needs and perception of quality of care and satisfaction with care in hematology/medical oncology patients: a multicultural assessment. J Pain Symptom Manag. 2018;55(1):56–64 e1.
3. Cain CL, Surbone A, Elk R, Kagawa-Singer M. Culture and palliative care: preferences, communication, meaning, and mutual decision making. J Pain Symptom Manag. 2018;55(5):1408–19.
4. Givler A, Maani-Fogelman PA. The importance of cultural competence in pain and palliative care. 2020.
5. A Joint Publication of ACPE A, CASC, NACC, NAJC. The Impact of Professional Spiritual Care. 2019.
6. O'Hanlon B, Bertolino B. The Therapist's notebook on positive psychology. New York, NY: Routledge; 2012.
7. Delgado-Guay MO. Spirituality and religiosity in supportive and palliative care. Curr Opin Support Palliat Care. 2014;8(3):308–13.
8. Crawford GB, Price SD. Team working: palliative care as a model of interdisciplinary practice. Med J Aust. 2003;179(S6):S32–4.
9. Harr C, Openshaw L, Moore B. Interdisciplinary relationships between chaplains and social workers in health care settings. J Health Care Chaplain. 2009;16(1–2):13–23. https://doi.org/10.1080/08854720903451048.
10. Handzo G, Koenig HG. Spiritual care: whose job is it anyway? South Med J. 2004;97(12):1242–4.
11. Fitchett G, Hisey Pierson AL, Hoffmeyer C, Labuschagne D, Lee A, Levine S, et al. Development of the PC-7, a quantifiable assessment of spiritual concerns of patients receiving palliative care near the end of life. J Palliat Med. 2020;23(2):248–53.
12. Workers NAoS. Standards for social work practice in health care settings 2016. https://www.socialworkers.org/practice/standards/index.asp.
13. Hughes, Brian & Wintz, Sue & Carbonell, Ellen & Hall, Eric & Hodge, David R. & Mulvaney, Elizabeth & Nelson-Becker, Holly & Shim, Soo & Sormanti, Mary & Stepney, Lois. Spiritual care and social work: integration into practice. Health care chaplaincy network. 2018.
14. Wolcott DL. The role of psychosocial supportive services in palliative care: a conversation with Deane L. Wolcott, MD. In: Cavallo J, editor. The ASCO Post; 2014.
15. Adler N, Page A. Cancer care for the whole patient. Washington, D.C.: National Academies Press; 2008.
16. Managing Stress and Distress. Nccn.org. 2020 [cited 14 May 2020]. https://www.nccn.org/patients/resources/life_with_cancer/distress.aspx.
17. Governing.com. State population by race, ethnicity data. 2020. https://www.governing.com/gov-data/census/state-minority-population-data-estimates.html. Accessed 7 Feb 2020.
18. Colón Y. Ethnic diversity and cultural competency in cancer care. Oncol Issues. 2007;22(5):28–31.
19. Shields M, Joseph D. Spiritual care in the ICU. In: Rocker G, Puntillo KA, Azoulay E, Nelson JE, editors. End of life care in the ICU: from advanced disease to bereavement. New York: Oxford University Press; 2010. p. 140–9.
20. Shields M, Kestenbaum A, Dunn LB. Spiritual AIM and the work of the chaplain: a model for assessing spiritual needs and outcomes in relationship. Palliat Support Care. 2015;13(1):75–89.
21. Fitchett G, Risk JL. Screening for spiritual struggle. J Pastoral Care Counsel. 2009;63(1-2):4-1-12:1.
22. Puchalski C, Ferrell B, Virani R, Otis-Green S, Baird P, Bull J, et al. Improving the quality of spiritual care as a dimension of palliative care: the report of the consensus conference. J Palliat Med. 2009;12(10):885–904.
23. Puchalski CM. The role of spirituality in health care. Proc (Baylor Univ Med Cent). 2001;14(4):352–7.
24. Kestenbaum A, Shields M, James J, Hocker W, Morgan S, Karve S, et al. What impact do chaplains have? A pilot study of spiritual AIM for advanced cancer patients in outpatient palliative care. J Pain Symptom Manag. 2017;54:707.
25. Clark E, Lauria M, Stearns N. Social work in oncology. Chicago: American Cancer Society; 2012.
26. Jankowski KR, Handzo GF, Flannelly KJ. Testing the efficacy of chaplaincy care. J Health Care Chaplain. 2011;17(3–4):100–25.
27. Ernecoff NC, Curlin FA, Buddadhumaruk P, White DB. Health care Professionals' responses to religious or spiritual statements by sur-

rogate decision makers during goals-of-care discussions. JAMA Intern Med. 2015;175(10):1662–9.
28. Farsi Z. The meaning of disease and spiritual responses to stressors in adults with acute leukemia undergoing hematopoietic stem cell transplantation. J Nurs Res. 2015;23(4):290–7.
29. Park CL. Meaning making and psychological adjustment following cancer: the mediating roles of growth, life meaning, and restored just-world beliefs. J Consult Clin Psychol. 2008;76:863–75.
30. Taira DA. Improving the health and health care of non-English-speaking patients. J Gen Intern Med. 1999;5:322–3.
31. Novy DM, Aigner CJ. The biopsychosocial model in cancer pain. Curr Opin Support Palliat Care. 2014;8(2):117–23.
32. Odejide OO, Uno H, Murillo A, Tulsky JA, Abel GA. Goals of care discussions for patients with blood cancers: association of person, place, and time with end-of-life care utilization. Cancer. 2020;126(3):515–22.
33. Wilkie DJ, Johnson B, Mack AK, Labotka R, Molokie RE. Sickle cell disease: an opportunity for palliative care across the life span. Nurs Clin North Am. 2010;45(3):375–97.
34. Bergman EJ, Diamond NJ. Sickle cell disease and the "difficult patient" conundrum. Am J Bioeth. 2013;13(4):3–10.
35. Kretchy I, Owusu-Daaku F, Danquah S. Spiritual and religious beliefs: do they matter in the medication adherence behaviour of hypertensive patients? BioPsychoSoc Med. 2013;7(1):15.
36. Abbas SQ, Dein S. The difficulties assessing spiritual distress in palliative care patients: a qualitative study. Ment Health Relig Cult. 2011;14(4):341–52.
37. Bhatnagar S, Gielen J, Satija A, Singh SP, Noble S, Chaturvedi SK. Signs of spiritual distress and its implications for practice in Indian palliative care. Indian J Palliat Care. 2017;23(3):306–11.
38. Hatamipour K, Rassouli M, Yaghmaie F, Zendedel K, Majd HA. Spiritual needs of cancer patients: a qualitative study. Indian J Palliat Care. 2015;21(1):61–7.
39. Puchalski CM. Making health care whole: integrating spirituality into patient care. West Conshohocken, PA: Templeton Press; 2010.
40. Loeffler S, Poehlmann K, Hornemann B. Finding meaning in suffering?-meaning making and psychological adjustment over the course of a breast cancer disease. Eur J Cancer Care. 2018;27(3):e12841.
41. Tedeschi R, Calhoun L. Posttraumatic growth: conceptual foundations and empirical evidence. Psychol Inq. 2004;15(1):1–18.
42. Simard S, Thewes B, Humphris G, Dixon M, Hayden C, Mireskandari S, et al. Fear of cancer recurrence in adult cancer survivors: a systematic review of quantitative studies. J Cancer Surviv. 2013;7(3):300–22.
43. Mundt-Leach R. End of life and palliative care of patients with drug and alcohol addiction. Ment Health Pract. 2016;20:17–21.
44. Mossey JM. Defining racial and ethnic disparities in pain management. Clin Orthop Relat Res. 2011;469(7):1859–70.
45. Leite MA, Nogueira DA, Terra FS. Evaluation of self-esteem in cancer patients undergoing chemotherapy treatment. Rev Lat Am Enfermagem. 2015;23(6):1082–9.

# Ethical Considerations in Palliative Care

# 18

Jonathan M. Marron and Melissa K. Uveges

## Introduction

The National Cancer Institute defines palliative care as "an approach to care that addresses the person as a whole, not just their disease" [1]. Palliative care aims to treat, or preferably, to prevent, the symptoms and side effects of disease and its treatment, including the physical, psychosocial, and other considerations related to these. The American Society of Clinical Oncology supports early integration of palliative care into the care of all patients with advanced cancers [2], and the American Society of Hematology has affirmed the palliative care guidelines developed by the National Consensus Project for Quality Palliative Care [3]. In the pages that follow, we will describe the ethical considerations in palliative care. Ethics and palliative care certainly are closely related, and many hospitals have combined ethics/palliative care services. Similarly, numerous individuals practice simultaneously as palliative care providers and ethicists for their institutions. There are, however, unique ethical features of palliative practice that warrant particular focus. In the following section, we describe several common methods of ethical analysis, particularly as it relates to palliative care. In the remainder of this chapter, we will provide an overview of some of the unique ethical considerations in palliative care for individuals with hematologic malignancies and serious blood disorders, including ethical issues surrounding uncertainty, the ethics of healthcare decision-making and symptom management, special considerations regarding withholding/withdrawing (the latter term often referenced as "discontinuing" so as to not convey that a treatment is being taken away from a patient) treatments, and ethical issues related to medical aid in dying. We also briefly explore unique ethical considerations with vulnerable populations and in palliative care research. Throughout, we include brief cases with important but challenging questions to ground the concepts introduced in this chapter. Many of these questions do not have simple answers and/or the answers vary according to case-specific circumstances, but pondering these questions will assist readers in understanding clinical applications of these complex ethical considerations.

## Ethical Analysis

Within the field of ethics, many different ethical theories or frameworks have been developed for identifying and analyzing situations where clinical ethics issues arise, or where ethical principles might come into conflict. One of the most well-known ethical frameworks is that of principlism, which looks to fundamental principles to examine ethical questions [4]. The goals from the standpoint of principlism include maximizing patient benefits (beneficence), minimizing harms (non-maleficence), respecting an individual's right to make decisions about their care (autonomy), and ensuring equal treatment for all (justice). These goals overlap considerably with the goals of palliative care, given palliative care goals focus on optimally balancing the risks and benefits of interventions, supporting patient/surrogate decision-making, and focusing on both quantity and quality of life. However, ethics encourages us to ask challenging, pointed questions about how we come to healthcare decisions, who should make these decisions, and how to manage disagreements when they arise. Principlism, as a framework, offers some guidance in terms of how to resolve conflicts that may arise among these four principles, but leaves a considerable amount of discretion to the person deliberating about the dilemma as to how to judge which moral action ought to be prioritized [4].

J. M. Marron (✉)
Department of Pediatric Oncology, Dana-Farber Cancer Institute and the Harvard Medical School Center for Bioethics, Boston, MA, USA
e-mail: Jonathan_Marron@dfci.harvard.edu

M. K. Uveges
Boston College Connell School of Nursing, Chestnut Hill, MA, USA
e-mail: uveges@bc.edu


C. K. Ullrich, E. J. Roeland (eds.), *Palliative Care in Hematologic Malignancies and Serious Blood Disorders*,
https://doi.org/10.1007/978-3-031-38058-7_18

Other ethical theories/frameworks besides principlism have developed over time. In addition to ethical theories/frameworks, which serve as a scaffolding for how to approach an ethical question, several ethical modes of analysis have been developed. Ethical modes of analysis offer practical tools for helping the clinician to analyze ethically complex cases. A non-exhaustive list of a few well-known ethical theories/frameworks and ethical modes of analysis are included in Table 18.1.

**Table 18.1** Example ethical theories/frameworks and modes of ethical analysis

| Select ethical theories and frameworks | |
|---|---|
| Theory or framework | Defining features |
| Principlism [4] | The use of fundamental *prima facie* principles (which may ultimately come into conflict) to address ethical issues/conflicts. |
| Casuistry [5] | A moral approach that draws on outcomes of previous cases for comparison and analogy to reach moral conclusions in new cases. |
| Virtue ethics [4, 6] | An ethical approach that emphasizes positive character traits and virtues (i.e., compassion, respect, trustworthiness), which promote caring and caregiving. This approach offers clinicians an aspirational, enduring basis for their actions. |
| Narrative ethics [7, 8] | An ethical approach focused on personal identity, meaning, and moral decision-making achieved through eliciting and understanding unfolding stories. |
| Feminist ethics [9] | In healthcare, this approach aims to uncover assumptions about power in relationships and situations. Originally focused on the experience of women, acknowledging their history of oppression and domination, it has expanded to encompass concerns associated with race, class, disability, and sexual orientation. |
| **Select ethical modes of analysis** | |
| Mode of analysis | Description |
| Four Box Method [10] | A case-based approach to decision-making, whereby analysis involves consideration of the patient's medical indications, personal preferences, quality of life, and contextual features, which might distinguish the case from other similar cases. |
| CASES [11] | An approach designed for ethics consultants who respond to active clinical cases involving ethical components or dilemmas. Analysis involves clarifying the case consultation request, assembling relevant information, synthesizing information, explaining the synthesis, and supporting the consultation process |
| Rest Framework [12] | A moral action approach that focuses on the interaction of affective and cognitive processes. Moral decision-making in a specific case can be approached by considering how one interprets a situation, how one determines the morally ideal course of action, how one decides what to do, and how one perseveres to implement this action. |

## Ethics and Uncertainty

A fundamental challenge in healthcare is that of the uncertainty of patient outcomes—rarely do we know with certainty what will happen and when [13, 14]. This is particularly relevant in palliative care, given the great prognostic uncertainty that exists for many conditions. It is impossible to tell, for example, whether a child newly diagnosed with sickle cell disease will eventually demonstrate mild or severe disease-related sequelae. Similarly, a patient with advanced leukemia may have only days left to live or may survive for many months. This uncertainty has important implications for advance care planning and discussions of goals of care, both of which are discussed in greater detail elsewhere in this text.

Importantly, informed decision-making about advanced illness requires accurate—or at least the best available—information about that illness. While complete and comprehensive disclosure to patients/surrogates was not always standard, today this is the standard of care with very few exceptions [4, 15]. Only following comprehensive disclosure of clinical factors including, but not limited to, diagnosis and prognosis can a patient/surrogate begin to make informed decisions about their care. Clinicians sometimes express concern that prognostic disclosure may have unintended consequences, such as diminishing hope, harming the clinician–patient relationship, or adding unnecessary stress or anxiety [16, 17]. Research in this area, however, demonstrates that communication about prognosis may actually support hope, trust, and peace of mind, and strengthen the clinician–patient relationship in both pediatric and adult settings [18–20]. It is unclear how best to ensure prognostic awareness (particularly in the face of significant uncertainty [21]), but various strategies have been developed to assist clinicians in leading conversations about prognosis and support informed decision-making [2, 22–25].

Recent and forthcoming advances in technology make prognostication only more complex. For example, immunotherapies, targeted agents, and other promising novel therapeutics provide a new source of hope for many patients, but they simultaneously add further layers of prognostic uncertainty [26, 27]. The wide breadth of possible outcomes—from non-responder to "exceptional responder"—makes clear and comprehensive communication about the entire range of possibilities of utmost importance. (See Box 18.1) Improved supportive therapies, including new antimicrobials, extracorporeal membrane oxygenation (ECMO), and advances such as next-generation sequencing provide similar challenges in providing precise and reliable prognostic information. It is likely that future innovations in gene therapy, proteomics, and other advances will improve the quality and length of life for some, but not all, patients with hematologic malignancies and blood disorders. Advances such as these will only make communication about prognosis, including fundamental discussions about underlying uncertainty, more important.

**Box 18.1: Mr. A**
Mr. A is a 45-year-old man who has been diagnosed with acute myeloid leukemia with very poor prognosis. His clinician tells him about various treatment options, including an early-phase clinical trial of a targeted agent. The clinician explains that it appears that some individuals have extraordinary responses to this investigational agent, but many do not respond at all.

1. What questions should Mr. A ask about this drug?
2. What standards are there about informed consent in this setting?

## Ethical Considerations in Healthcare Decision-Making

### Identifying the Appropriate Decision-Maker

At the core of the intersection of ethics and palliative care is the question of who has the authority to make healthcare decisions on behalf of a patient. In the modern era of healthcare, there is general consensus that any person of sound mind has the right to self-determination (i.e., to make autonomous decisions about their healthcare) [4]. However, this becomes more complicated when considering patients unable to make choices for themselves and in the setting of disagreements about healthcare decisions.

In order to support those capable of making their own decisions and protect individuals incapable of doing so, it is imperative to identify whether a patient is legally and ethically (the law and ethics here are inextricably intertwined) able to make their own healthcare decisions. Described in greater detail in Chaps. 9 and 10, and elsewhere in this text, the ability of an individual to make decisions about their healthcare is typically described as decisional capacity or competence. While some distinguish between these, due to inconsistencies in these distinctions in the legal and medical literature, we will here use these terms interchangeably but refer primarily to capacity in this discussion. For a patient to have decisional capacity, they must be able to demonstrate a) an understanding of the information communicated to them about their condition and care option(s); b) appreciation of the potential consequences of their situation and possible care option(s); c) the ability to weigh the risks/benefits of treatment and come to a decision that is consistent with their stated values/preferences; and d) communicate their chosen care option [28]. Importantly, decisional capacity is specific to the healthcare decision under consideration. Most commonly, clinicians assess a patient's capacity based on a "sliding scale approach"—the greater the complexity/risk of the decision, the greater degree of capacity that is required [28, 29]. Various assessment instruments are available for assistance in capacity assessment, and frameworks are available to guide clinicians in identifying those at elevated risk of having diminished capacity and performing and acting upon a capacity assessment [30].

In some circumstances, a patient is deemed not to have capacity to make a particular decision about their care. This could be related to age (minors by definition in most cases do not have legal capacity [31]), due to their primary disease (e.g., a patient with a large CNS bleed that affects their mental status), comorbidities (e.g., an elderly patient with lymphoma and age-related cognitive decline), treatment-related sequelae (e.g., a patient with decreased mental status due to severe cytokine release syndrome after CAR T-cell therapy for leukemia), or other causes. In such cases, it is necessary to identify who should make decisions on behalf of the patient.

How to identify a patient's surrogate is beyond the scope of this review, but for minors (those under age 18 in most jurisdictions in the United States) the designated surrogate is most commonly the pediatric patient's parent/guardian [31]. For adults, legal statutes regarding surrogacy vary by jurisdiction [32], including how to prioritize possible decision-makers in absence of an advance directive. The surrogate should not make the healthcare decision they would want for themselves or the one that they would prefer the patient make. Rather, in most cases, they are tasked with making decisions according to a "substituted judgment" standard, meaning they are to support the healthcare decision(s) best aligned with the previously stated values and preferences of the patient [33].

### Navigating Decisional Conflict

Occasionally, stakeholders disagree about the best approach to healthcare decisions; such disagreements can be stressful and ethically complex. Ideally, such disagreements can be addressed via a process of engagement, communication, and negotiation, whenever time, clinical, and psychosocial considerations allow for this. It is generally preferable to work toward consensus among stakeholders—or at least a plan that is deemed acceptable, if not ideal, to all involved—rather than proceeding despite significant objections of one stakeholder or another. In nearly all cases of decisional conflict, an important first step is to engage in a process of shared decision-making, whereby the patient/surrogate's goals, values, and preferences are explored, with the clinician(s) describing the available therapeutic options in order to maximally support informed decision-making [34].

One common conflict is between a patient (or their surrogate) and the clinical team. As described above, patients have the authority to accept or decline medical interventions, even one that is life-saving and/or life-prolonging, assuming that they have decisional capacity and are fully informed; this same authority is ascribed to duly appointed surrogates [4]. Care should be taken, however, to ensure that such declinations of interventions are well-informed. Another situation that can create conflict is when patients/surrogates request an intervention that is not recommended by the clinical team. Clinicians may choose to support such a request after consideration of the risks, benefits, and alternatives. That is not to say, however, that clinicians have an obligation to provide any therapy requested. Clinicians are not obligated, for example, to provide interventions that would be clinically ineffective [35]. Though the term has largely fallen out of favor, conflicts about potentially "futile" interventions are one such type of disagreement [36]. (Box 18.2) We will discuss this particular type of disagreement further below.

**Box 18.2: Ms. B**

Ms. B has relapsed lymphoma and was recently diagnosed with a pulmonary embolism. Her clinical team recommends a course of anticoagulation, which she declines, stating that this is a sign that this is "her time." Her clinicians are quite distressed.

1. Does Ms. B have the authority to decline this potentially life-saving intervention?
2. How can the clinicians determine if Ms. B has the capacity to make this decision?

Conflicts also can arise between the patient and their surrogate. How to navigate this type of conflict depends, in part, on whether the patient has capacity. If the patient lacks capacity, their surrogate has legal authority to make healthcare decisions on their behalf; however, lack of capacity does not mean that an individual should not have a voice in their healthcare decisions, despite not having legal decisional authority. Rather, incapacitated patients should be involved in their healthcare decision-making to the greatest extent possible. In pediatrics, for example, minors are encouraged to be integrated into decisions about their care [31]. The perspectives and preferences of adults lacking capacity should be integrated into decisions in a similar fashion whenever possible. Conflicts between patients without capacity and their surrogates may best be approached with discussions among stakeholders. It is important to confirm that, as described above, the surrogate is supporting the plan they believe the patient themselves would support, if they had capacity. A full discussion of the challenges presented when an incapacitated patient expresses different preferences than they did before they became incapacitated is beyond the scope of this chapter, but such situations are particularly challenging (Box 18.3) [37]. Consultation with ethics and/or legal experts is recommended in such cases.

**Box 18.3: Mr. C**

Mr. C is an 85-year-old man who has advanced dementia but is quite happy and has an excellent quality of life. He had previously stated that he never wanted to "be put on machines." He develops sepsis and now requires intubation and ventilatory support.

1. Should Mr. C's prior wishes still apply in this current state, even though Mr. C's clinical status (and preferences) is quite different than that imagined when he previously expressed his wishes?
2. Who should make this decision, since Mr. C cannot?

Conflicts between family members of a patient sometimes can arise regarding treatment decisions on behalf of their incapacitated loved one. Though the individual designated as the patient's healthcare proxy or authorized decision-maker based on legal statute [32] has the legal authority to ultimately make decisions in this case, an important and worthwhile step is to facilitate thoughtful discussion among all involved stakeholders to assist in solving these disagreements. Support from psychosocial clinicians and/or those with expertise in communication and/or conflict resolution may also be beneficial.

A final noteworthy type of decisional conflict involves patient or family requests for treatments thought by the healthcare team to be potentially inappropriate. Such conflicts are of particular importance in those with chronic and/or life-limiting disease. In the past, such interventions were often referred to as "futile," but this term is now thought by many to be ill-defined and subjective [36]. Recent work has suggested describing these as "potentially inappropriate" or "likely non-beneficial," rather than futile (reserving "futile" only for those interventions whose goals would be physiologically impossible to achieve) [38, 39], but such changes may be more semantic than consequential. Disagreements about potentially inappropriate therapies remain very controversial, but most agree upon the importance of a procedural approach to intractable conflicts [36, 38]. Commonly, disagreements about potentially inappropriate (or even potentially "futile") interventions will revolve around a patient's resuscitation status and whether a do-not-attempt-resuscitation (DNAR) order should be placed in the patient's chart over their objections (Box 18.4). Some have argued that "unilateral" DNAR orders, those instituted over the objections of the patient/surrogate, are rarely—if ever—appropriate in pediatric [40] and adult [41] settings, but practices vary widely [42]. In the setting of conflict about the appropriateness of intensive care, cardiopulmonary resuscitation, and/or other requested interventions, it is always important to refer to institutional ethics policies and local law. Institutional ethics services may also help negotiate resolutions when such conflicts arise.

**Box 18.4: Mrs. D**

Mrs. D is a 44-year-old woman with sickle cell disease who has had a severe stroke and is in the intensive care unit. The clinical team believes that, if her heart were to stop, performing cardiopulmonary resuscitation would not be in her best interest. They encourage Mrs. D's husband (her healthcare proxy) to sign a DNAR order, but he states that he wants them to continue to "do everything" to support her.

1. Does Mrs. D's husband have the authority to decline the DNAR order in this scenario?
2. How should the clinical team proceed?

## Ethical Considerations in Symptom Management

### Disagreements about Symptom Management

In general, disagreements about symptom management are navigated similarly to those about other treatments and aspects of care. Patients, caregivers, and members of the healthcare team may occasionally disagree about such considerations as goals of care, the perception of benefit of parts of the care plan, and the use of specific medications/treatments for pain and other symptoms. Anecdotally, most disagreements can be solved with the tincture of time and further communication, but these scenarios can be very difficult, and time is often in short supply. Assistance from those with expertise in communication and/or conflict resolution may prove beneficial, and legal and/or ethics teams may be of assistance for particularly intractable conflicts. One particularly controversial area is that of the use of morphine and similar analgesics in light of the opioid epidemic (Box 18.5). If a patient with capacity declines/refuses treatment with opioids, such a declination by should be respected in the same fashion as declinations/refusals of other potential treatments, as described above, and healthcare teams should examine, via shared decision-making, why the patient prefers not to receive opioid treatment. If patients have capacity and are fully informed, they have the legal and ethical right to decline opioid treatment, just as they do any medical intervention. There is less clarity, however, regarding refusal of pain medications by surrogates on behalf of incapacitated adults [43] and children [44]. In the setting of disagreement, ethics and/or legal consultation may be beneficial.

**Box 18.5: Mr. E**

Mr. E is a 29-year-old man with sickle cell disease who comes to the emergency department with a severe pain crisis. Among other interventions, the clinicians recommend a dose of morphine, but he declines this, concerned about its potentially addictive properties.

1. Can Mr. E decline this recommended treatment?
2. Would this situation be different if Mr. E were refusing the morphine on behalf of his child?

### Palliative Sedation

Palliative sedation, described more fully in Chap. 24, is one particularly noteworthy aspect of symptom management with ethical relevance. Used somewhat infrequently, palliative sedation is considered only when symptoms cannot be adequately controlled despite maximal supportive therapies. Its intent is to alleviate the symptoms of the dying patient, understanding that doing so may unintentionally hasten their death [45]. The doctrine of double effect (DDE), generally first attributed to Thomas Aquinas, a Catholic priest in the Middle Ages, provides justification for palliative sedation in children and adults [46, 47]. According to the DDE, an intervention such as palliative sedation is considered ethically permissible if it meets each of four conditions (see Table 18.2).

Importantly, palliative sedation has legal backing in addition to the aforementioned ethical support. In 1997, the US Supreme Court invoked the DDE in stating that it is legal to provide medication to alleviate suffering to a dying patient "even to the point of causing unconsciousness and hastening death" [48]. Of note, hastened death is not a certain outcome of palliative sedation. In fact, at least some patients receiving

**Table 18.2** The doctrine of double effect and its application to palliative sedation

| Requisite element of the doctrine of double effect | Application to palliative sedation |
|---|---|
| The act is morally good (or at very least morally neutral). | In palliative sedation, the act is administration of a sedating medication such as a benzodiazepine, which is a morally neutral act. |
| The clinician intends for the "good" effect of the intervention but does not intend for the possible "bad" effect (though the latter may be foreseen). | In palliative sedation, the good (intended) effect is relief of the patient's pain/suffering. The bad (unintended) effect is the potential hastening of death. |
| The bad effect cannot be the means for achievement of the good effect. | Pain/symptom relief in palliative sedation cannot be because of death but rather due to the primary or off-target action of the medication provided. |
| The benefit of the good effect must outweigh the harms of the bad effect. | It is generally agreed that the relief of intractable pain/suffering outweighs the possibility of hastened death, but this condition is subjective and occasionally a point of contention when considering palliative sedation. |

palliative sedation have been reported to have similar or even greater survival than those not receiving palliative sedation [49]. Therefore, though the DDE highlights the *possibility* of hastened death when utilizing palliative sedation, this outcome is not always seen in clinical practice.

## Ethical Considerations Regarding Withholding and Withdrawing/Discontinuing Treatment

Among the most ethically complex decisions in palliative care are those related to withholding and withdrawing (or discontinuing) treatment. Notably, in palliative care, when a previously initiated treatment or intervention is stopped, this is typically referred to as "discontinuing," while in clinical ethics this is often called "withdrawing." Here, we will use the former term, but it is worthwhile to be aware of both terms in this setting. Importantly, as described elsewhere in this text, *care* is never withheld. Rather, decisions are made on occasion to withhold or discontinue certain aspects of treatment, such as mechanical ventilation, dialysis, antimicrobial therapy, or transfusions. No matter what individual therapies are withheld or discontinued, *the same is never said for care itself* [50].

In the United States, well-known court cases surrounding Karen Ann Quinlan (1976) and Nancy Cruzan (1990) established that individuals (or their surrogates) have the right to refuse therapy, even that which might be life-prolonging [51, 52]. In parallel, the Patient Self-Determination Act of 1990 and similar laws codify this right, requiring healthcare organizations to provide written information to all patients about advance directives and their right to accept or refuse life-sustaining therapies [53]. Advance directives, discussed more comprehensively in Chap. 10, have great legal and ethical importance. They (and their application by surrogates) certainly have limitations, including that patient preferences are inconsistent over time [54] and surrogates frequently inaccurately predict patients' end-of-life preferences, but they simultaneously help to support provision of desired interventions and avoidance of those not desired [55].

Physician orders for life-sustaining treatment (often referred to by the acronym POLST, these sometimes go by other names including MOLST, MOST, etc.) supplement advance directives by summarizing the patient's end-of-life preferences. Ultimately entered into a standardized form, POLST orders start with a conversation between the patient/surrogate and their clinician to identify end-of-life treatment preferences [56, 57]. Whereas do-not-attempt-resuscitation (DNAR) orders only address whether the patient wishes to receive cardiopulmonary resuscitation, POLST orders address a wide variety of potential interventions and whether the patient/surrogate wishes for these to be initiated or withheld. Most states now have POLST programs, but it is advisable to be familiar with standards in your local jurisdiction, given POLST's legal standing [57].

Many have argued that there is no ethically significant difference between withholding (i.e., not starting) and withdrawing (i.e., discontinuing) a given treatment [4, 58, 59]. They posit that small, arbitrary differences could lead to one patient having a treatment initiated and another not. Both, as described above, should have the opportunity to decline unwanted treatment, so it should not matter whether the treatment has already been initiated (and thus would be withdrawn/discontinued) or not (and thus would be withheld). Many clinicians, however, report discontinuing therapies to be both more psychologically difficult and more ethically fraught than not initiating it at all [60, 61]. A comprehensive review of these issues is beyond the scope of this chapter, but it is important to recognize that patients and clinicians may feel differently about this distinction, so it is a point that warrants thoughtful discussion. It is also important to be aware that some religious denominations recognize a distinction between withholding and withdrawing/discontinuing, while others do not [4, 61].

One particularly ethically complex category of treatment refusals is that of nutrition and hydration. There is consensus that competent individuals may decline "extraordinary" measures (e.g., mechanical ventilation, dialysis, etc.) [62], but some express hesitancy about the ethical acceptability of withholding more "ordinary" measures like medically administered (parenteral or via NG/G-tube) nutrition and hydration.[1] Notably, however, there is consensus among most professional healthcare organizations that it is ethically permissible to withhold or discontinue medically-administered nutrition and hydration at the request of adult patients or their surrogates [35, 62, 64, 65] and under certain circumstances, from children [66] at the end of life (Box 18.6). Voluntarily stopping eating and drinking (VSED)—when a competent patient intentionally stops taking food and liquid by mouth as a way to hasten their death—is a rare but ethically distinct form of withholding nutrition/hydration [67]. Notably, VSED is considered both ethically and legally distinct from Medical Aid in Dying (MAiD), as VSED involves refusal of an intervention, while MAiD involves active request for a lethal medication [67].

**Box 18.6: Ms. F**

Ms. F is a 76-year-old woman with relapsed aplastic anemia despite several prior lines of therapy and allogeneic transplantation. She is not imminently dying but has no curative treatment options. She receives tube feedings through a gastrostomy tube and wishes to discontinue these in order to hasten her death. Her clinicians are unsure of the legality of this request.

1. Is it legally and ethically acceptable for the clinicians to discontinue Ms. F's feedings?
2. If they are unsure, how should the clinicians determine if they can fulfill this request?

## Ethical Issues Related to Medical Aid in Dying (MAiD)

One debate about palliative care is whether it is always sufficient in addressing an individual's pain and suffering. Those who argue that palliative care can fall short of these aims may support the option of medical aid in dying (MAiD), also termed physician aid in dying, physician-assisted suicide, patient-administered hastened death, and death with dignity. Here, for simplicity, we will use the term MAiD [68, 69]. MAiD is a controversial topic, both where it is legal and where it is not. Those who support MAiD argue that an individual's autonomous right to govern healthcare decisions, informed by personal beliefs, values, and choices, ought to extend to requests for MAiD [68]. Proponents argue that MAiD can alleviate unbearable pain and suffering and support the terminally ill patient's wish to control the details of their death, without unnecessarily burdening family [70]. Some opponents of MAiD state that MAiD destroys an individual's autonomy by eradicating the possibility of future autonomous acts, and it is thus impermissible [71, 72]. Similarly, another opposition to MAiD is that MAiD violates the sanctity of human life [73]. Others argue that legalization of MAiD may precipitate a slippery slope, leading to the allowance of voluntary euthanasia [68, 69, 72]. Still other opponents are concerned that legalizing MAiD may lead to inequitable care, with vulnerable or marginalized patients disproportionately opting for MAiD; however, the data do not currently support this concern [74].

Another ethical concern held by some regarding MAiD is that it conflicts with professional core values [75, 76]. For example, the American Nurses Association and American Medical Association both recently revised their policies on aid in dying. Both policies denounce the participation of clinicians in MAiD [77, 78], but notably, at the time of this work's writing, the AMA Code of Medical Ethics includes two different statements, one expressing the opinion of those who oppose physician-assisted suicide, and another the position of those physicians who may support it [79]. In recent years, several state and national medical organizations have shifted to a neutral position on MAiD, including the American Academy of Hospice and Palliative Medicine [80].

In the United States, at the time of this chapter's writing, 7 states and Washington, D.C. have statutes allowing MAiD, and it is allowable following court decisions in Montana and California [81]. But even states where MAiD is legal, it is often not accessible, raising questions about justice. For example, in 2019, a Colorado physician was fired from a faith-based hospital for planning to help a terminally ill patient end his life at home. The hospital stated that the physician was fired because she encouraged an act that she knew was "morally unacceptable to her employer." [82] MAiD may also be inaccessible in states where it is legal due to voluntary refusal of providers to participate and high costs of the medications used, which may not be covered by insurance [83].

## Ethical Considerations with Special Populations

Individuals with chronic and/or critical illnesses are vulnerable in their own right, but certain situations may compound a patient's vulnerability. In this section, we discuss unique ethical considerations for certain populations that may require access to palliative care. This is not intended to be a comprehensive discussion of all categories of vulnerable

[1]The phrasing "ordinary" versus "extraordinary" is important here, as this distinction has been made in Catholic teachings, which do not obligate "extraordinary means of preserving life" (see reference 63: Ball H. The right to die: a reference handbook. Santa Barbara, California: ABC-CLIO; 2017) and was cited in the official ruling in the case of Karen Ann Quinlan (see reference 51: In Re Quinlan, 355 A.2d 647 (1976)).

patients but rather to introduce this important but challenging topic as it relates to ethics and palliative care.

## Individuals with Physical/Intellectual Disabilities

Persons with disabilities represent one such vulnerable population in palliative care. In the United States, one in four adults has some type of disability; 14% of the US population is impacted by a physical disability and 10% is impacted by a cognitive disability [84]. Persons with disabilities experience, on average, 4 to 13 secondary conditions per year, some of which are life threatening [85]. Those with intellectual disabilities have twice the number of health issues as the general population and many have fragile health and palliative care needs from birth onward [86]. At the same time, they may not recognize changes indicating ill health; communication challenges can further complicate symptom recognition for individuals with intellectual disabilities [87]. As a result of these and other barriers, those with disabilities often experience delays in accessing timely and appropriate palliative care [88], compounded only further by the fact that clinicians caring for persons with intellectual disabilities may lack knowledge or confidence in providing care to this population. A recent study reported that 82% of U.S. physicians surveyed perceived that people with disabilities have worse quality of life than those without disabilities [89], though prior work has shown that external observers—including clinicians—often perceive the quality of life of those with disabilities as lower than do those with disabilities themselves [90]. Together, these observations raise important questions about the provision of equitable and patient-centered care for this population. Clinicians may benefit from education about how implicit and/or explicit biases can influence their views of people with disabilities. Clinicians should also be familiar with the use of supplementary communication formats such as signs, symbols, or pictorial tools to capture the input of persons with physical and/or intellectual disabilities and sensory impairments, who have self-reported good quality of life [89, 91]. Overall, it is crucial to work collaboratively with experts to ensure that clinicians can meet the care needs of individuals with disabilities in the palliative setting [87, 88].

## Patients with Mental Illness

For individuals with mental illness, particularly severe mental illness, under-detection and under-treatment of somatic disease and late access to palliative care are common [92]. This is thought to stem from a tendency for individuals with severe mental illness to have a small social network and symptoms that impair communication, leading to underreporting of somatic symptoms and delayed access to healthcare. Further, organizational factors unfortunately often create barriers to timely palliative care interventions. For example, in many areas, palliative care expertise around somatic issues for those with mental illness is lacking, and there often is a stark separation between inpatient mental healthcare and general medicine settings, with poor collaboration between clinicians [92]. Additionally, because mental healthcare is not necessarily the purview of one discipline, it can be difficult to determine who is responsible for tending to these needs of patients [93]. Facilitating access to palliative care in this vulnerable population is an important ethical (justice) issue, which may require further advocacy work by various clinicians. Given that patients with mental illness (particularly severe mental illness) may not have full decisional capacity, special consideration regarding their healthcare decision-making is warranted, as described earlier in this chapter.

## Incapacitated, Unrepresented Patients

Particular ethical considerations are relevant for "unbefriended" or unrepresented individuals—those who lack capacity to provide informed consent for a specified medical treatment, lack a healthcare surrogate or other representative, and have no advance directive offering guidance on decision-making, particularly in the palliative care setting [94–96]. Many unrepresented patients have a history of psychiatric illness, substance abuse, trauma, and/or homelessness [97]. Moreover, unrepresented older adults often have dementia or other cognitive impairments, along with multiple chronic diseases, and they frequently reside in nursing homes [95, 98]. Given the vulnerability of unrepresented patients to overtreatment, undertreatment, or treatment inconsistent with their values, they are owed a special duty of care and procedural fairness in seeking out care options [94–96, 98]. The American Geriatrics Society recommends that clinicians work as a team and use a systematic process to synthesize all available evidence when determining unrepresented individuals' healthcare treatment plan [94, 96].

## Children

Child mortality continues to decline, reflecting, in part, the ability of advanced technology to prolong the lives of children with complex and/or chronic conditions [99, 100]. With this prolongation of life comes the increasing need for palliative care in the pediatric setting. As mentioned above, parents are most often the appropriate decision-making surrogate for their children [31]. Closely aligned with this reality is the centrality of family-centered care in pediatric palliative care. Family-centered care, described more fully in Chaps. 19 and 20, revolves around the idea that the family is the primary source of strength, support, information, and perspective in clinical decision-making for a child [100]. However, there may be times when parents and clinicians do not align in their approach to palliative care for a child, as discussed earlier in the section on decisional conflict. In some such cases, questions arise regarding whether the parent is appropriately looking out for the child's interests versus their own [31].

For example, pediatric palliative care interventions sometimes involve the consideration of the child's welfare in light of parent's religious values, which may inform the type of intervention the parent is willing to accept [101]. Courts generally become involved when parents decline recommended life-saving treatments for their child, such as when a parent of the Jehovah's Witness faith declines a life-saving blood transfusion for their child [101, 102]. In *Prince v. Massachusetts*, the US Supreme Court ruled that parental authority is not absolute and can be restricted in certain circumstances [103]. In 1952, transfusion of a Witness's child was further clarified through *Morrison v. State*, which ruled that if parental religious beliefs put a child's life in danger, the state could intervene to protect the child [104, 105]. However, the practice of overriding parental preference to transfuse children is not universal or without controversy [106]. Overriding the parent's preference to decline transfusion should be done in a way that seeks to preserve the clinician–parent relationship, understanding that for Witnesses, blood transfusions have not only personal spiritual ramifications but can result in dissociation and shunning by others in the Witness community [106].

Another point of possible contention between parents and clinicians occurs at/near the end of a child's life. One particularly challenging situation involves the use of cardiopulmonary resuscitation (CPR) on a child with a terminal illness and no known curative options (Box 18.7) [40]. Some institutions have developed "unilateral DNAR" policies that allow for clinicians to place a DNAR order in cases where they deem cardiopulmonary resuscitation to not be an appropriate intervention. While some view these policies as appropriate under the condition that providers deem resuscitation to not be in the child's best interests, others argue that such a policy should only be utilized in situations where the parent clearly has malicious intent or performing CPR is an obvious violation of the child's well-being [40].

**Box 18.7: Gail**

Gail is a 7-year-old girl with multiply-relapsed leukemia without any further curative options available. She is receiving palliative care, and her clinicians recommend placement of a DNAR order, in case her heart were to stop. Gail's parents state that they would like Gail to receive CPR in such a situation and decline the DNAR order.

1. Do Gail's parents have the authority to decline the DNAR order in this scenario?
2. How should the clinical team proceed?

## Pregnant Women

One rare but important population to consider in palliative care is that of pregnant women who are dying. Pregnant women, like other patients at the end of life, may have an advance directive or an identified surrogate decision-maker; however, in many jurisdictions of the United States, the condition of pregnancy can invalidate a person's wishes or efforts by surrogates to honor such wishes, citing an interest in protecting rights of the fetus when these conflict with those of the mother [107]. Therefore, clinicians of dying pregnant patients may face challenging dilemmas about how to handle their care. For instance, clinicians might be forced to choose between following the legal restrictions on a state advance directive form and fulfilling their ethical duties to uphold patient preferences [107]. Becoming familiar with any restrictions to honoring advance directives for pregnant women in one's jurisdiction and identifying potential contingencies in advance care planning can help optimally care for this vulnerable population. This is only more important—and more challenging—following recent legal rulings regarding access to abortion, though a full discussion of these complex issues is beyond the scope of this chapter.

## Prisoners

Increasingly, prisoners are being recognized as a vulnerable population. Worldwide, the number of incarcerated individuals with multiple, complex health conditions is growing, with the United States having the largest prison population [108]. Prisoners face a number of factors that can negatively impact health, including a decreased level of activity, substandard hygiene, suboptimal nutrition, exposure to stress, social isolation, and violence [109]. Additionally, prisoners face negative perceptions or attitudes toward them by the public. Due to these factors, prisoners are at high risk of accelerated aging, and prisoner mortality rates are at an all-time high, with prisoners frequently dying in community hospitals after receiving poor palliative care prior to death [110]. With these shortcomings in mind, it is particularly important to involve family in inmate healthcare decisions whenever possible, in order to optimally provide care that promotes of quality of life and relief of suffering for this vulnerable group [108, 109].

## Moral Distress and Conscience-Based Objections in Palliative Care

Professionals who provide palliative care to patients and their families may encounter cases where internal/external conflicts cause them moral distress. Moral distress is a term originally coined in the 1980s and describes the negative feelings that arise when an individual decides on an action they feel to be morally correct in a given situation, but is prevented from taking that action [111]. Although moral distress was originally attributed to external (or institutional) constraints, it is now understood to involve either external or internal (personal) constraints [112]. Persistent and/or recurrent experiences of moral distress can be associated with loss of moral identity and other adverse responses [112]. Common sources of moral distress include witnessing harm (pain and suffering) to patients, inadequate staffing, and institutional or wider policy constraints [113]. Moral distress is more common in certain settings, including settings where prolonged treatment or EOL decisions occur [112].

A number of strategies for addressing or minimizing moral distress have been proposed. These include: interdisciplinary dialogue that involves naming moral distress, establishing professional support networks that allow professionals to voice moral distress, focusing on institutional changes that contribute to moral distress, educational activities targeted toward the impact of or ways to address moral distress, and preventive approaches, such as regular involvement of ethics committees or consultation services on units where moral distress is prevalent [112, 114]. Personal approaches involving promotion of individual physical and mental health have also been suggested and are consistent with professional codes of ethics [35, 115].

While moral distress is a feeling of constraint or the inability to act appropriately, which arises when generally and professionally recognized ethical norms are violated, another type of response, termed conscience-based objections (or conscientious objection), involves the refusal to perform or participate in an activity associated with an individual's professional role because doing so would violate their personal moral conscience [113, 116]. Although clinicians may object to providing treatment on many bases, refusal is only termed conscience-based if the reason for refusal is grounded in one's moral conscience. Conscience-based objections can derive from religious or secular principles, beliefs, or convictions [113]. Provision of palliative sedation and organ donation after cardiac or brain death are two examples of activities/procedures in palliative care that might elicit conscientious objection for some palliative care clinicians [113]. Importantly, however, conscientious objection only applies to an activity (e.g., performing palliative sedation), not to an individual or group of individuals (e.g., of a given background) [116]. Although state and federal laws have long-established "conscience clauses" protecting the professional's right to decline to provide a particular service, these conscience clauses have sometimes been called an over-protected right because equal attention to ensuring patient access to care has not been undertaken [117].

## Ethical Considerations in Palliative Care Research

Many common ethical considerations in palliative care research are quite similar to those in other types of clinical research, including such issues as informed consent, therapeutic misconception, and protection of vulnerable human subjects [118–122]. As discussed elsewhere in this chapter and throughout this text, high-quality communication is of utmost importance in making the decision to participate in palliative care research. The patient or their surrogate should be fully informed about the risks and benefits of the research, and it should be made clear how/whether the research interventions (if applicable) are different from standard clinical care [118]. Those performing research in palliative care should be familiar with the requirements for determining whether a clinical research study is ethical. Ethically sound research must have social or scientific value as well as scientific validity, utilize fair subject selection, have a favorable risk-benefit ratio, undergo independent review, provide informed consent to potential subjects, and ensure respect for all potential and enrolled subjects [121].

## References

1. National Cancer Institute. Palliative care in cancer. Last updated 20 Oct 2017. Last viewed 07 Jul 2020. https://www.cancer.gov/about-cancer/advanced-cancer/care-choices/palliative-care-fact-sheet.

2. Ferrell BR, Temel JS, Temin S, Alesi ER, Balboni TA, Basch EM, et al. Integration of palliative care into standard oncology care: American Society of Clinical Oncology clinical practice guideline update. J Clin Oncol. 2017;35(1):96–112.
3. National Coalition for Hospice and Palliative Care. Clinical practice guidelines for quality palliative care. 4th ed. Richmond, VA: National Coalition for Hospice and Palliative Care; 2018.
4. Beauchamp TL, Childress JF. Principles of biomedical ethics. 6th ed. New York: Oxford University Press; 2009.
5. Jonsen AR, Toulmin S. The abuse of casuistry: a history of moral reasoning. Berkeley: University of California Press; 1988.
6. Donovan GK, Pellegrino ED. Virtues and goals in pediatrics. In: Miller G, editor. Pediatric bioethics. London, England: Cambridge University Press; 2009.
7. Charon R, Montello M. Stories matter : the role of narrative in medical ethics. New York: Routledge; 2002.
8. Montello M. Narrative ethics. Hast Cent Rep. 2014;44(1 Suppl):S2–6.
9. Jaggar AM. Feminist ethics. In: The Blackwell guide to ethical theory; 2013. p. 433–60.
10. Jonsen AR, Siegler M, Winslade WJ. Clinical ethics: a practical approach to ethical decisions in clinical medicine. Eighth edition. ed. New York: McGraw-Hill Education; 2015.
11. National Center for ethics in health care. Ethics consultation: responding to ethics questions in health care. Last viewed 26 Jun 2020. https://www.ethics.va.gov/ECprimer.pdf.
12. Grace PJ. Nursing ethics and professional responsibility in advanced practice. Third edition. ed. Burlington, Massachusetts: Jones & Bartlett Learning; 2018.
13. O'Brien JM Jr, Aberegg SK, Ali NA, Diette GB, Lemeshow S. Results from the national sepsis practice survey: predictions about mortality and morbidity and recommendations for limitation of care orders. Crit Care. 2009;13(3):R96.
14. Curtis JR, Park DR, Krone MR, Pearlman RA. Use of the medical futility rationale in do-not-attempt-resuscitation orders. JAMA. 1995;273(2):124–8.
15. Novack DH, Plumer R, Smith RL, Ochitill H, Morrow GR, Bennett JM. Changes in physicians' attitudes toward telling the cancer patient. JAMA. 1979;241(9):897–900.
16. The AM, Hak T, Koëter G, van der Wal G. Collusion in doctor-patient communication about imminent death: an ethnographic study. West J Med. 2001;174(4):247–53.
17. Lamont EB, Christakis NA. Prognostic disclosure to patients with cancer near the end of life. Ann Intern Med. 2001;134(12):1096–105.
18. Enzinger AC, Zhang B, Schrag D, Prigerson HG. Outcomes of prognostic disclosure: associations with prognostic understanding, distress, and relationship with physician among patients with advanced cancer. J Clin Oncol. 2015;33(32):3809–16.
19. Marron JM, Cronin AM, Kang TI, Mack JW. Intended and unintended consequences: ethics, communication, and prognostic disclosure in pediatric oncology. Cancer. 2018;124(6):1232–41.
20. Chhabra KR, Pollak KI, Lee SJ, Back AL, Goldman RE, Tulsky JA. Physician communication styles in initial consultations for hematological cancer. Patient Educ Couns. 2013;93(3):573–8.
21. Smith AK, White DB, Arnold RM. Uncertainty — The other side of prognosis. N Engl J Med. 2013;368(26):2448–50.
22. Baile WF, Buckman R, Lenzi R, Glober G, Beale EA, Kudelka AP. SPIKES-A six-step protocol for delivering bad news: application to the patient with cancer. Oncologist. 2000;5(4):302–11.
23. Kissane DW, Bultz BD, Butow PN, Noble S, Wilkinson S. Oxford textbook of communication in oncology and palliative care. Oxford University Press; 2017.
24. LeBlanc TW, Marron JM, Ganai S, McGinnis MM, Spence RA, Tenner L, et al. Prognostication and communication in oncology. J Oncol Pract. 2019;15(4):208–15.
25. Jackson VA, Jacobsen J, Greer JA, Pirl WF, Temel JS, Back AL. The cultivation of prognostic awareness through the provision of early palliative care in the ambulatory setting: a communication guide. J Palliat Med. 2013;16(8):894–900.
26. Temel JS, Shaw AT, Greer JA. Challenge of prognostic uncertainty in the modern era of cancer therapeutics. J Clin Oncol. 2016;34(30):3605–8.
27. LeBlanc TW, Temel JS, Helft PR. "How much time do I have?": communicating prognosis in the era of exceptional responders. Am Soc Clin Oncol Educ Book. 2018;38:787–94.
28. Appelbaum PS. Clinical practice. Assessment of patients' competence to consent to treatment. N Engl J Med. 2007;357(18):1834–40.
29. Drane JF. Competency to give an informed consent. A model for making clinical assessments. JAMA. 1984;252(7):925–7.
30. Marron JM, Kyi K, Appelbaum PS, Magnuson A. Medical decision-making in oncology for patients lacking capacity. Am Soc Clin Oncol Educ Book. 2020;40:e186–e96.
31. Katz AL, Webb SA, Committee on Bioethics. Informed consent in decision-making in pediatric practice. Pediatrics. 2016;138(2):e20161485.
32. DeMartino ES, Dudzinski DM, Doyle CK, Sperry BP, Gregory SE, Siegler M, et al. Who decides when a patient Can't? Statutes on alternate decision makers. N Engl J Med. 2017;376(15):1478–82.
33. Buchanan AE, Brock DW. Deciding for others: the ethics of surrogate decision making. Cambridge England; New York: Cambridge University Press; 1989.
34. Elwyn G, Frosch D, Thomson R, Joseph-Williams N, Lloyd A, Kinnersley P, et al. Shared decision making: a model for clinical practice. J Gen Intern Med. 2012;27(10):1361–7.
35. American Medical Association. Council on ethical and judicial affairs. Code of medical ethics of the American Medical Association. Chicago: American Medical Association; 2017.
36. Burns JP, Truog RD. Futility: a concept in evolution. Chest. 2007;132(6):1987–93.
37. Nuffield Council on Bioethics. Dementia: ethical issues 2009. Published 01 Oct 2009. Last viewed 07 Jul 2020. https://www.nuffieldbioethics.org/publications/dementia.
38. Bosslet GT, Pope TM, Rubenfeld GD, Lo B, Truog RD, Rushton CH, et al. An official ATS/AACN/ACCP/ESICM/SCCM policy statement: responding to requests for potentially inappropriate treatments in intensive care units. Am J Respir Crit Care Med. 2015;191(11):1318–30.
39. Kon AA, Shepard EK, Sederstrom NO, Swoboda SM, Marshall MF, Birriel B, et al. Defining futile and potentially inappropriate interventions: a policy statement from the Society of Critical Care Medicine ethics Committee. Crit Care Med. 2016;44(9):1769–74.
40. Marron JM, Jones E, Wolfe J. Is there ever a role for the unilateral do not attempt resuscitation order in pediatric care? J Pain Symptom Manag. 2018;55(1):164–71.
41. Biegler P. Should patient consent be required to write a do not resuscitate order? J Med Ethics. 2003;29(6):359–63.
42. Courtwright AM, Brackett S, Cadge W, Krakauer EL, Robinson EM. Experience with a hospital policy on not offering cardiopulmonary resuscitation when believed more harmful than beneficial. J Crit Care. 2015;30(1):173–7.
43. Blinderman CD. Do surrogates have a right to refuse pain medications for incompetent patients? J Pain Symptom Manag. 2012;43(2):299–305.
44. Moreno-Galvan A, Marron JM, Marsiglio AM. How should we approach parental refusals of opioids on behalf of children in the perioperative setting? A practical approach based on ethical theory. Paediatr Anaesth. 2020;30:852.
45. Olsen ML, Swetz KM, Mueller PS. Ethical decision making with end-of-life care: palliative sedation and withholding

or withdrawing life-sustaining treatments. Mayo Clin Proc. 2010;85(10):949–54.
46. Quill TE, Dresser R, Brock DW. The rule of double effect—a critique of its role in end-of-life decision making. N Engl J Med. 1997;337(24):1768–71.
47. McIntyre A. Doctrine of double effect. In: Zalta EN, ed. The Stanford encyclopedia of philosophy. Last updated 24 Dec 2018. Last viewed 07 Jul 2020. https://plato.stanford.edu/entries/double-effect/.
48. Vacco v. Quill. United States Supreme Court; 1997.
49. Mercadante S, Porzio G, Valle A, Fusco F, Aielli F, Costanzo V. Palliative sedation in patients with advanced cancer followed at home: a systematic review. J Pain Symptom Manag. 2011;41(4):754–60.
50. Fine RL. Language matters: "sometimes we withdraw treatment but we never withdraw care". J Palliat Med. 2007;10(6):1239–40.
51. In Re Quinlan, 355 A.2d 647, 1976.
52. Cruzan v Director, Missouri Department of Health, 497 US, 110 S. Ct, 2841,1990.
53. Omnibus Budget Reconciliation Act of 1990, 1991.
54. Fried TR, O'Leary J, Van Ness P, Fraenkel L. Inconsistency over time in the preferences of older persons with advanced illness for life-sustaining treatment. J Am Geriatr Soc. 2007;55(7):1007–14.
55. Patrick DL, Pearlman RA, Starks HE, Cain KC, Cole WG, Uhlmann RF. Validation of preferences for life-sustaining treatment: implications for advance care planning. Ann Intern Med. 1997;127(7):509–17.
56. Meier DE, Beresford L. POLST offers next stage in honoring patient preferences. J Palliat Med. 2009;12(4):291–5.
57. National POLST. POLST. National POLST Paradigm. Last updated 2020. Last viewed 07 Jul 2020. https://polst.org/.
58. Brock DW. Death and dying. In: Veatch R, editor. Medical ethics. 2nd ed. Sudbury, MA: Jones and Bartlett Publishers; 1997.
59. Wilkinson D, Butcherine E, Savulescu J. Withdrawal aversion and the equivalence test. Am J Bioeth. 2019;19(3):21–8.
60. Chung GS, Yoon JD, Rasinski KA, Curlin FA. US Physicians' opinions about distinctions between withdrawing and withholding life-sustaining treatment. J Relig Health. 2016;55(5):1596–606.
61. Sulmasy DP, Sugarman J. Are withholding and withdrawing therapy always morally equivalent? J Med Ethics. 1994;20(4):218–22.
62. President's Commission for the Study of ethical problems in medicine and biomedical and behavioral research. Deciding to forego life-sustaining treatment: a report on the ethical, medical, and legal issues in treatment decisions. Washington, DC: US Government Printing Office; 1983.
63. Ball H. The right to die: a reference handbook. Santa Barbara, California: ABC-CLIO, LLC; 2017.
64. American Academy of hospice and palliative medicine. Statement on artificial nutrition and hydration near the end of life. Last updated 13 Sep 2013. Last viewed 07 Jul 2020. http://aahpm.org/positions/anh.
65. ANA Center for Ethics and Human Rights. position statement: nutrition and hydration at the end of life silver springs, MD. Last updated 2017. Last viewed 07 Jul 2020. https://www.nursingworld.org/~4af0ed/globalassets/docs/ana/ethics/ps_nutrition-and-hydration-at-the-end-of-life_2017june7.pdf.
66. Diekema DS, Botkin JR. Forgoing medically provided nutrition and hydration in children. Pediatrics. 2009;124(2):813.
67. Rubin EB, Bernat JL. Voluntarily stopping eating and drinking. In: Quill TE, Miller FT, editors. Palliative care and ethics. New York, NY: Oxford University Press; 2014.
68. Dugdale LS, Lerner BH, Callahan D. Pros and cons of physician aid in dying. Yale J Biol Med. 2019;92(4):747–50.
69. O'Rourke MA, O'Rourke MC, Hudson MF. Reasons to reject physician assisted suicide/physician aid in dying. J Oncol Pract. 2017;13(10):683–6.
70. Dees M, Vernooij-Dassen M, Dekkers W, van Weel C. Unbearable suffering of patients with a request for euthanasia or physician-assisted suicide: an integrative review. Psychooncology. 2010;19(4):339–52.
71. Sjostrand M, Helgesson G, Eriksson S, Juth N. Autonomy-based arguments against physician-assisted suicide and euthanasia: a critique. Med Health Care Philos. 2013;16(2):225–30.
72. Materstvedt LJ. Palliative care on the 'slippery slope' towards euthanasia? Palliat Med. 2003;17(5):387–92.
73. Death with Dignity. Religion and Spirituality. 2020. https://www.deathwithdignity.org/learn/religion-spirituality/.
74. Gopal AA. Physician-assisted suicide: considering the evidence, existential distress, and an emerging role for psychiatry. J Am Acad Psychiatry Law. 2015;43(2):183–90.
75. Olsen DP, Chan R, Lehto R. Ethical nursing care when the terminally ill patient seeks death. Am J Nurs. 2017;117(7):50–5.
76. Sulmasy DP, Finlay I, Fitzgerald F, Foley K, Payne R, Siegler M. Physician-assisted suicide: why neutrality by organized medicine is neither neutral nor appropriate. J Gen Intern Med. 2018;33(8):1394–9.
77. ANA Center for Ethics and Human Rights. ANA position statement: The Nurse's role when a patient requests medical aid in dying. Online J Issues Nurs. 2019;24(3)
78. Frieden J. Physician-assisted suicide once again divides AMA members: MedPage today. Last updated 11 Jun 2019. 2020. https://www.medpagetoday.com/meetingcoverage/ama/80384.
79. American Medical Association. Physician-assisted suicide. Last updated 14 Nov 2016. Last viewed 26 Jun 2020. https://www.ama-assn.org/delivering-care/ethics/physician-assisted-suicide.
80. Position statement on physician-assisted death. J Pain Palliat Care Pharmacother. 2007;21(4):55–7.
81. CNN Editorial research. Physician-assisted suicide fast facts: CNN. Last updated 11 Jun 2020. Last viewed 07 Jul 2020. https://www.cnn.com/2014/11/26/us/physician-assisted-suicide-fast-facts/index.html.
82. Law T. Colorado doctor fired after suing to provide patient with aid-in-dying medication: time. Last updated 03 Sep 2019. Last viewed 26 Jun 2020. https://time.com/5666225/colorado-doctor-fired-after-suing-to-provide-patient-with-aid-in-dying-medication/.
83. Aleccia J. Terminally ill, he wanted aid-in-dying. His Catholic hospital said no. Kaiser Health News. Last updated 29 Jan 2020. Last viewed 26 Jun 2020. https://khn.org/news/when-aid-in-dying-is-legal-but-the-medicine-is-out-of-reach/.
84. National Center on Birth Defects and Developmental Disabilities. Disability impacts all of us. Centers for Disease Control and Prevention. Last updated 09 Sep 2019. Last viewed 26 Jun 2020. https://www.cdc.gov/ncbddd/disabilityandhealth/infographic-disability-impacts-all.html.
85. Mitchell SE, Weigel GM, Stewart SK, Mako M, Loughnane JF. Experiences and perspectives on advance care planning among individuals living with serious physical disabilities. J Palliat Med. 2017;20(2):127–33.
86. Voss H, Vogel A, Wagemans AMA, Francke AL, Metsemakers JFM, Courtens AM, et al. Advance care planning in palliative care for people with intellectual disabilities: a systematic review. J Pain Symptom Manag. 2017;54(6):938–60 e1.
87. Read S. Palliative care for people with intellectual disabilities: pitfalls and potential. Palliat Med. 2013;27(1):3–4.
88. Dunkley S, Sales R. The challenges of providing palliative care for people with intellectual disabilities: a literature review. Int J Palliat Nurs. 2014;20(6):279–84.

89. Iezzoni LI, Rao SR, Ressalam J, Bolcic-Jankovic D, Agaronnik ND, Donelan K, et al. Physicians' perceptions of people with disability and their health care. Health Aff (Millwood). 2021;40(2):297–306.
90. Albrecht GL, Devlieger PJ. The disability paradox: high quality of life against all odds. Soc Sci Med. 1999;48(8):977–88.
91. Smith AK, Ritchie CS, Wallhagen ML. Hearing loss in hospice and palliative care: a National Survey of providers. J Pain Symptom Manag. 2016;52(2):254–8.
92. den Boer K, de Veer AJE, Schoonmade LJ, Verhaegh KJ, van Meijel B, Francke AL. A systematic review of palliative care tools and interventions for people with severe mental illness. BMC Psychiatry. 2019;19(1):106.
93. Kozlov E, Niknejad B, Reid MC. Palliative care gaps in providing psychological treatment: a review of the current state of research in multidisciplinary palliative care. Am J Hosp Palliat Care. 2018;35(3):505–10.
94. Farrell TW, Widera E, Rosenberg L, Rubin CD, Naik AD, Braun U, et al. AGS position statement: making medical treatment decisions for Unbefriended older adults. J Am Geriatr Soc. 2017;65(1):14–5.
95. Effiong A, Harman S. Patients who lack capacity and lack surrogates: can they enroll in hospice? J Pain Symptom Manag. 2014;48(4):745–50 e1.
96. Pope TM, Bennett J, Carson SS, Cederquist L, Cohen AB, DeMartino ES, et al. Making medical treatment decisions for unrepresented patients in the ICU. An official American Thoracic Society/American Geriatrics Society policy statement. Am J Respir Crit Care Med. 2020;201(10):1182–92.
97. Connor DM, Elkin GD, Lee K, Thompson V, Whelan H. The Unbefriended patient: an exercise in ethical clinical reasoning. J Gen Intern Med. 2016;31(1):128–32.
98. Chamberlain S, Baik S, Estabrooks C. Going it alone: a scoping review of Unbefriended older adults. Can J Aging. 2018;37(1):1–11.
99. American Academy of Pediatrics. Committee on bioethics and Committee on hospital care. Palliative care for children. Pediatrics. 2000;106(2 Pt 1):351–7.
100. Hellsten MB, Berg S. Symptom management in paediatric palliative care. In: Ferrell BR, Coyle N, Paice J, editors. Oxford textbook of palliative nursing. 3rd ed. Oxford: Oxford University Press; 2010.
101. Paul SR. Child welfare vs. parental religious views. AAP News. 2011;32(5):20.
102. Religious Objections to Medical Care. Pediatrics. 1997;99(2):279.
103. Prince v. Massachusetts, 321 US 158, 1944.
104. Woolley S. Children of Jehovah's witnesses and adolescent Jehovah's witnesses: what are their rights? Arch Dis Child. 2005;90(7):715–9.
105. Morrison v. State, 252 S.W.2d 97. Kansas City Court of Appeals, Missouri, 1952.
106. Ukachi N, Morrison W, Vanhorn S, Sundaram R, Lantos JD. A young adult Jehovah's witness with severe anemia. Pediatrics. 2013;132(3):547–51.
107. Lyerly AD. Statutory restrictions on advance care planning and pregnancy. JAMA. 2019;321(16):1574–5.
108. Turner M. Editorial. Palliat Med. 2018;32(1):4–5.
109. Pazart L, Godard-Marceau A, Chassagne A, Vivot-Pugin A, Cretin E, Amzallag E, et al. Prevalence and characteristics of prisoners requiring end-of-life care: a prospective national survey. Palliat Med. 2018;32(1):6–16.
110. Rothman A, McConville S, Hsia R, Metzger L, Ahalt C, Williams BA. Differences between incarcerated and non-incarcerated patients who die in community hospitals highlight the need for palliative care services for seriously ill prisoners in correctional facilities and in community hospitals: a cross-sectional study. Palliat Med. 2018;32(1):17–22.
111. Jameton A. Nursing practice : the ethical issues. Englewood Cliffs, N.J: Prentice-Hall; 1984.
112. Epstein EG, Hamric AB. Moral distress, moral residue, and the crescendo effect. J Clin Ethics. 2009;20(4):330–42.
113. Wicclair MR. Conscientious objection in health care: an ethical analysis. Cambridge: Cambridge University Press; 2011.
114. Rushton CH, Caldwell M, Kurtz M. CE: moral distress: a catalyst in building moral resilience. Am J Nurs. 2016;116(7):40–9.
115. American Nurses Association. Code of ethics for nurses with interpretive statements. 2nd ed. Silver Spring, MD: American Nurses Association; 2015.
116. Sulmasy DP. Conscience, tolerance, and pluralism in health care. Theor Med Bioeth. 2019;40(6):507–21.
117. Giubilini A. Conscientious objection in healthcare: neither a negative nor a positive right. J Clin Ethics. 2020;31(2):146–53.
118. Emanuel EJ. The Oxford textbook of clinical research ethics. Oxford; New York: Oxford University Press; 2008.
119. Henderson GE, Churchill LR, Davis AM, Easter MM, Grady C, Joffe S, et al. Clinical trials and medical care: defining the therapeutic misconception. PLoS Med. 2007;4(11):e324.
120. Williams MA, Haywood C Jr. Critical care research on patients with advance directives or do-not-resuscitate status: ethical challenges for clinician-investigators. Crit Care Med. 2003;31(3 Suppl):S167–71.
121. Emanuel EJ, Wendler D, Grady C. What makes clinical research ethical? JAMA. 2000;283(20):2701–11.
122. Casarett DJ, Knebel A, Helmers K. Ethical challenges of palliative care research. J Pain Symptom Manag. 2003;25(4):S3–5.

# 19 Advancing the Field through Research

Oreofe O. Odejide

## Introduction

Although the World Health Organization recognized palliative care as a distinct specialty in 1990, little palliative care research focused on patients with hematologic malignancies, much less serious blood disorders, until recently. In randomized controlled trials of integrated palliative and oncologic care published prior to 2016, only ten patients with hematologic malignancies were included out of well over a thousand enrollees [1–4]. Moreover, early retrospective analyses demonstrated a clinical gap in palliative care for this population with low rates of subspecialty palliative care involvement and a high likelihood of experiencing intensive healthcare utilization close to death (e.g., chemotherapy in the last 2 weeks of life, intensive care unit admission in the last month of life, and hospital death) [5, 6]. Accordingly, in their 2012 publication, Epstein and colleagues called for effective collaboration between palliative care and hematologic oncology [7].

There has been a steady growth of palliative care research in hematologic oncology in the past decade. By sheer numbers, the number of original research publications focused on this population increased from only about one in 2010 to more than ten new publications in the year 2019. This progress has likely been galvanized by collaborations between investigators clinically trained in hematologic oncology and those trained in palliative medicine. Collaboration has bolstered critical knowledge transfer between both specialties. Palliative care specialists have a greater understanding of the unique challenges of caring for patients with blood cancers; hematologic oncologists also have a greater awareness, understanding, and acceptance of palliative care. This transfer is illustrated by educational and research sessions on palliative care now being featured at national hematology conferences that gather thousands of hematologic oncologists from all over the world.

O. O. Odejide (✉)
Department of Medical Oncology, Harvard Medical School, Dana-Farber Cancer Institute, Boston, MA, USA
e-mail: Oreofe_Odejide@dfci.harvard.edu

On the other hand, palliative care research focusing on patients with serious blood disorders that are not malignant (e.g., sickle cell disease) is very sparse. A recent retrospective cohort study of patients with sickle cell disease demonstrated high intensity of healthcare utilization near the end of life, highlighting the need for palliative care integration and additional palliative care research for this population [8].

This chapter will discuss the evolution of palliative care research for individuals with blood cancers and highlight research methods that investigators have applied in this field. We will also review major research themes that have emerged over the past decade. Finally, we will highlight future research directions to promote continued advancement in the field and further close the gap between hematology/oncology and optimal palliative care.

## Evolution of Palliative Care Research in Hematologic Oncology

As palliative care research in hematologic oncology has grown, the types of research questions being studied have also evolved. Investigators have gradually transitioned from asking "what" (i.e., what is the state of palliative care in hematologic oncology?) to "why" (i.e., why are there barriers to palliative care?) to "how" (i.e., how do we optimize palliative care for patients with hematologic malignancies?). Along with this transition, study methods being employed by investigators are also growing in sophistication. Early studies in this field were largely qualitative or single-institution based; however, in the last 3–4 years, investigators are engaging in more multicenter and national studies. In addition, the first randomized controlled trial of palliative care in this population was published in 2016. This section will discuss some of the study designs employed to advance knowledge in this field, including retrospective cohort studies, qualitative and mixed-methods studies, survey studies, and randomized controlled trials (Table 19.1).



C. K. Ullrich, E. J. Roeland (eds.), *Palliative Care in Hematologic Malignancies and Serious Blood Disorders*,
https://doi.org/10.1007/978-3-031-38058-7_19

**Table 19.1** Palliative care research study designs that have been used in hematologic oncology

| Study type | Applications | Benefits | Challenges |
|---|---|---|---|
| Retrospective cohort studies | • Characterize rates and predictors of palliative care use<br>• Characterize association of palliative care with quality of end-of-life care<br>• Characterize rates and predictors of hospice use<br>• Characterize intensity of healthcare utilization near the end-of-life care<br>• Characterize rates and predictors of documented goals of care discussions | • Granular data can be abstracted from electronic medical records<br>• Large claims-based datasets (e.g., SEER-Medicare) consist of large, nationally representative datasets, boosting generalizability<br>• Large claims-based datasets enable robust multivariable analyses | • Inability to capture patient preferences<br>• Variables limited to those already collected in dataset<br>• Causality cannot be determined from analyses |
| Qualitative and mixed methods studies | • Characterize hematologic oncologists' perspectives regarding palliative care, end-of-life care, and hospice care<br>• Characterize perspectives of patients with blood cancers regarding quality of life<br>• Characterize perspectives of patients with blood cancers regarding hospice care | • Generates comprehensive data<br>• Ideal for building initial evidence base to guide additional research in areas with absence of empiric data | • Time-intensive<br>• Recruiting seriously ill patients with high symptom burden and multiple clinic appointments may be difficult |
| Survey studies | • Characterize perspectives and practices of hematologic oncologists related to palliative care<br>• Characterize perspectives and practices of hematologic oncologists related to hospice care<br>• Characterize perspectives of hematologic oncologists regarding end-of-life care | • Postal or electronic survey distribution allows a large target population to be reached<br>• Generalizability is high if survey samples widely | • Based on self-report, which may not always be congruent with true practice<br>• Susceptible to social desirability bias<br>• Physician surveys more likely to have lower response rates than other populations |
| Randomized controlled trials | • Test impact of integrated palliative care on quality of life for patients undergoing hematopoietic stem cell transplant<br>• Test impact of integrated palliative care on quality of life for patients with acute myeloid leukemia | • Use of randomization removes biases that may be introduced by investigators in selecting participants for intervention versus control arm<br>• Allows causality to be established regarding effect of palliative care | • Recruitment and retention can be difficult<br>• Typically resource intensive |

## Retrospective Cohort Studies

Retrospective cohort studies have been widely used to characterize the state of palliative care for patients with hematologic malignancies [6, 9–22]. Retrospective cohort studies have been instrumental in quantifying rates of palliative care engagement, hospice use, and intensity of end-of-life care. Early retrospective studies often relied on data from single institutions. For example, Hui and colleagues' large single-center retrospective study provided important and detailed data demonstrating low rates of subspecialty palliative care consultation for individuals with blood cancer as well as high intensity of care near the end of life [6, 19]. Moreover, this study and others have the strength of including a comparator arm and provided crucial data suggesting associations between palliative care and EOL outcomes [6, 22]; however, prospective randomized controlled trials are still needed to demonstrate causality. Although single-center studies have the benefit of providing granular data abstracted from electronic medical records, they suffer from limited generalizability. Reassuringly, the findings from Hui and colleagues have been replicated in several other retrospective cohort studies [9, 15, 20].

Over the past 4 years, retrospective studies in this field have evolved from analyzing single-institution data to secondary analyses of large claims-based datasets such as the Surveillance Epidemiology and End-Results (SEER)-Medicare dataset [12, 13, 16–18]. This evolution presents multiple benefits. First, such analyses often consist of large, nationally representative cohorts, which boost results' generalizability. Second, the large cohort sizes available in these datasets provide the ability to study diagnostic groups separately (e.g., lymphoma, leukemia, myelodysplastic syndromes, myeloma) as opposed to combining these heterogeneous diseases as one single analytic category. Third, the large sample sizes provide the opportunity to build robust multivariable models to characterize patient- or disease-related characteristics that influence hospice use or end-of-life care. For example, the use of large datasets led to the evidence that transfusion-dependence is a significant predictor of hospice use among blood cancer patients [12, 16]. Finally, secondary analysis of large longitudinal datasets enables close examination of trends in palliative care over time [13, 16, 18].

Despite the strengths of using these large datasets, it is essential to note that claims data are proxies of care and are not perfect representations of the actual quality of care. The lack of granular data (e.g., communication patterns) and the inability to understand clinician or patient preferences are also important limitations. In addition, the typical anchoring of palliative care retrospective cohort studies—whether single-center or claims-based—on the time of death inherently assumes that clinicians providing care are aware that their patients are *dying*. This anchoring is problematic as *prospectively* identifying death can be challenging, and some patients may have died unexpectedly in the context of curative-intent treatment. Investigators have attempted to address this limitation by including only patients with poor prognosis such as relapsed/refractory disease or by excluding patients who died within a few months after diagnosis from such analyses.

## Qualitative and Mixed-Methods Studies

Qualitative and mixed-methods studies have been vital in building a rich evidence base regarding perspectives and attitudes that influence palliative care for this population [23–28]. Early studies using these designs focused on characterizing the perspectives and attitudes of hematologic oncologists [23, 24]. Investigators have employed various modes of data collection, including focus groups and in-depth interviews. These studies have resulted in a detailed understanding of clinician-related barriers to primary palliative care, subspecialty palliative care, and end-of-life care. Also, they uncovered misperceptions that hematologic oncologists harbor regarding palliative care and their concerns regarding hospice. In the past year, investigators have begun to expand qualitative work to directly engage patients with blood cancers and their caregivers [25, 26]. This progression is beginning to provide vital data about how patients perceive palliative care, hospice services, and what matters to them as they conceptualize quality of life in the context of serious illness.

Qualitative and mixed-methods studies have the strength of providing rich, comprehensive data. Moreover, in the stark absence of empiric data, which was the case for many palliative care topics in hematologic oncology just a few years ago, these studies are ideal for building an initial evidence base before transitioning to quantitative studies. Investigators who want to embark on these studies must note that they are typically very time-intensive, especially concerning data collection and analysis. Besides, it may be challenging to recruit blood cancer patients who are sick and have multiple medical appointments to participate in interviews or focus groups. For example, in a focus group study of blood cancer patients with an estimated life expectancy of 6 months or less, most patients who initially agreed to participate but subsequently declined did so because they were too sick [25]. Strategies such as flexible modes of data collection (phone versus in-person interviews) or scheduling in-person interviews to coincide with the day of in-person clinic appointments to minimize travel time burden may help address recruitment challenges.

## Survey Studies

Survey studies have been integral in understanding hematologic oncologists' perspectives and practices concerning palliative care and end-of-life care [29–35]. Indeed, the empiric evidence regarding hematologic oncologists' practices regarding goals of care discussions and hospice referrals as well as their perception of palliative care, hospice care, and end-of-life quality measures has been largely garnered from surveys. Researchers conducting surveys of hematologic oncologists have either sampled from single institutions or national professional organizations (e.g., the American Society of Hematology and the American Society for Transplantation and Cellular Therapy). Surveys have broad generalizability to the extent that different participant characteristics are represented in the sample.

Understanding the challenges of surveys is important to conduct or interpret such studies successfully. First, surveys are based on self-report and self-reported practices may not necessarily align with actual practices. Second, social desirability bias—a situation where participants choose a response because they think it is the more socially acceptable response—may lead to respondents overestimating their engagement rates in practices such as goals of care discussions. Another challenge is the ability to obtain high response rates, particularly with physician-targeted surveys. Indeed, response rates for physician surveys are estimated to be about 14% lower than non-physicians [36]. Strategies that may boost response rates for national physician surveys include creating brief surveys, adding incentives with survey administration (rather than sending incentives only after survey completion), sending paper surveys (rather than web or emails), and physician-to-physician follow-up telephone calls [36].

### Randomized Controlled Trials

Although randomized controlled trials provide the highest level of evidence, this study design for palliative care research has been sparse in hematologic oncology. The only published randomized controlled trial focusing solely on this population tested the effect of integrated palliative care versus usual care in a cohort of 160 patients who were hospitalized for autologous or allogeneic hematopoietic stem cell transplant (HCT) [37, 38]. The study established that integrated palliative care has significant and clinically meaningful benefits on quality of life and mood for this patient population. More randomized controlled trials are needed to further develop the evidence base for palliative care for hematologic malignancies. Yet, challenges associated with these studies must be carefully considered to design rigorous and feasible studies. For example, recruitment and retention of study participants can be particularly difficult for palliative care trials. This challenge can be secondary to clinicians or caregivers being concerned that research is burdensome or upsetting, thus discouraging patients' enrollment (i.e., gatekeeping). Early engagement of stakeholders (e.g., hematologic oncologists, hematology nurses) to obtain buy-in is critical to successful recruitment [39]. It is also important to avoid overly restrictive eligibility criteria, as this can hamper recruitment and limit the generalizability of study findings.

## Palliative Care Research Themes in Hematologic Oncology

Four major themes have emerged from palliative care research in the past decade: 1) Palliative care needs of patients with hematologic malignancies, 2) Palliative care for patients with hematologic malignancies, 3) Barriers to optimal palliative care, and 4) Models of palliative care for patients with hematologic malignancies. Each of these themes is discussed in detail below.

### Theme 1: Palliative Care Needs of Patients with Hematologic Malignancies

Patients with blood cancers experience substantial physical and psychological symptom burden throughout their disease trajectory, negatively affecting their overall quality of life [40–44]. Physical symptoms include but are not limited to fatigue, dyspnea, drowsiness, difficulty sleeping, delirium, lack of appetite, anorexia, and pain. Multiple studies suggest that fatigue or tiredness is the most prevalent physical symptom for blood cancer patients [40–42]. For example, in a single-institution study, 69% of 180 patients with blood cancer at various stages of illness (diagnosis, treatment, remission, relapse) reported fatigue [40]. In addition, 51% of individuals with blood cancers in a multicenter study reported clinically significant tiredness [41]. Severity of fatigue also escalates as patients draw closer to death [42].

Individuals with blood cancers also experience extensive psychological burden. More than 75% have psychological symptoms such as feeling nervous, irritable, sad, or worried [40]. Such psychological morbidity often worsens in the context of treatment. For example, in a longitudinal study of 90 patients with hematologic malignancies hospitalized for HCT, the percentage who met diagnostic criteria for major depression or other depressive syndrome increased by more than fourfold from baseline (8%) to the eighth-day post-transplant (37%) [43]. Additionally, HCT recipients experienced a steep decline in their quality of life along with a concurrent reduction in their caregivers' quality of life [43]. Unfortunately, psychological symptoms and decline in quality of life during the acute transplant hospitalization have long-lasting effects as affected patients are significantly more likely to be still suffering from depression and post-traumatic stress disorder at 6 months after their transplant [45].

Although the extensive symptom burden of patients with blood cancers is largely comparable to those with solid malignancies, some data suggest that patients with blood cancer have higher prevalence and severity of fatigue, delirium, and drowsiness [10, 41, 44]. In a multicenter study of 1235 patients with cancer, those with hematologic malignancies had higher rates of clinically significant tiredness (51% vs. 42%; $p = 0.03$) than did those with solid tumors, and in multivariable models had significantly higher odds of drowsiness. It is hypothesized that higher disease and treatment-related anemia rates for patients with blood cancers may contribute to increased fatigue and drowsiness. In addition, hospice enrollees with blood cancers have significantly worse functional status at the time of enrollment compared to those with other cancers [10]. Deconditioning is a known risk factor for fatigue [46]. In sum, individuals with blood cancers suffer from a broad and severe range of symptoms, emphasizing the critical need to optimize palliative care throughout their illness trajectory.

## Theme 2: Palliative Care for Patients with Hematologic Malignancies

Although patients with hematologic malignancies have substantial palliative care needs, several studies have demonstrated low palliative care and hospice use rates for this population [6, 9–12, 16, 17, 19, 47]. Rates of palliative care consultation for those who die of hematologic malignancies range from 16% to 33% [6, 9, 19]. Compounding the problem of low rates of palliative care consultation is the fact that even when consultation is sought, this typically occurs late, with the median time from consultation to death ranging from only 7 days to 12 days [6, 9]. Such low and late levels of palliative care engagement limit the ability of patients to experience associated benefits of improved quality of life, mood, and opportunities to prepare appropriately for EOL that are more likely with earlier palliative care [2, 3].

The pattern of low and late engagement with subspecialty palliative care is also mirrored in hospice use. Single-center and large claims-based studies have repeatedly shown that patients with hematologic malignancies have the lowest rates of hospice use in oncology [5, 9, 17, 47]. In a retrospective cohort study of 209 patients who died of hematologic malignancies, only 25% enrolled in hospice [47]. Moreover, a substantial proportion of enrollees do so in the last 3 days of life, thus precluding meaningfully benefit from hospice care [5, 10, 11]. For example, in a large study of 64,264 patients with a primary diagnosis of cancer who enrolled in 12 US-based hospices, patients with hematologic malignancies had 52% higher odds of enrolling in hospice in the last 3 days of life compared to solid malignancies [11]. Although recent studies suggest a rising trend in hospice use for blood cancer patients [12, 13, 16–18], there has been a concurrent and significant rise in rates of late enrollment [13, 16, 17].

In contrast to low palliative and hospice care rates for individuals with hematologic malignancies, intensive healthcare utilization near the end of life is high. Compared to patients with solid malignancies, blood cancer patients are more likely to receive chemotherapy in the last 2 weeks of life, be admitted to the intensive care unit in the last month of life, and die in hospitals [5, 6]. In a cohort of 816 cancer decedents, the proportion of patients with hematologic malignancies admitted to the ICU in the last month of life (39% vs. 8%, $p < 0.001$) or who had a hospital death (47% vs. 16%, $p < 0.001$) exceeded twice the proportion for those with solid malignancies [6]. Additionally, a large population-based study of older adults who died of acute myeloid leukemia showed significantly rising trends in chemotherapy use and ICU admission close to death between 1999 and 2012 [13]. Such intense healthcare utilization is often considered to reflect suboptimal end-of-life care. Research demonstrating the underuse of palliative and hospice care alongside high intensive healthcare utilization rates laid important groundwork for the subsequent investigation to identify and overcome barriers to palliative care for blood cancer patients.

## Theme 3: Barriers to Optimal Palliative Care

As data emerged regarding the extensive palliative care needs for patients with hematologic malignancies alongside low palliative and hospice care rates, the imperative to identify barriers to optimal palliative care became clear. Multiple studies suggest that barriers to palliative care are multifactorial and span the entire palliative care spectrum from early palliative care to hospice and end-of-life care. These barriers can be divided into four broad categories: 1) Disease-based, 2) Patient-based, 3) Clinician-based, and 4) System-based (Table 19.2).

### Disease-Based Barriers

The hematologic malignancies are a heterogeneous group of diseases with distinct features that contribute to low palliative care and hospice engagement rates. One unique feature of hematologic malignancies is a heightened level of prognostic uncertainty compared to solid malignancies. Unlike most solid malignancies where stage IV disease is synonymous with incurability, many hematologic malignancies (e.g., aggressive lymphomas) are potentially curable even at advanced stages. More so, patients with relapsed/refractory diseases may still have the potential of cure with HCT or

**Table 19.2** Barriers to optimal palliative care for patients with hematologic malignancies

| |
|---|
| Disease factors |
| • *High prognostic uncertainty* |
| • *Unpredictable disease course* |
| • *Cytopenias with the need for transfusion support* |
| Patient factors |
| • *Prognostic misunderstanding* |
| • *Misperceptions about palliative care* |
| • *Perspective that hospice is inadequate for patients' needs* |
| Clinician factors |
| • *Misperceptions about palliative care* |
| • *Untimely goals of care discussions* |
| • *Perspective that hospice is inadequate for patients' needs* |
| System factors |
| • *Lack of universal standardized primary palliative care training* |
| • *Specialty palliative care workforce not enough to meet demand* |
| • *Limited transfusion access in hospices* |

other novel therapies such as chimeric antigen receptor T-cell therapy [48, 49]. On the other hand, hematologic malignancies such as follicular lymphoma or myeloma, which are incurable at diagnosis, can respond to multiple lines of treatment, and patients may experience prolonged remissions measured in several years. In the context of such high levels of prognostic uncertainty, sole dependence on prognosis-based triggers to determine specialty palliative care timing often results in delayed or no referrals. Indeed, in a qualitative study of 20 palliative care specialists in the UK, participants felt that the most significant barrier to palliative care was the unpredictable prognoses associated with hematologic malignancies [28]. High levels of prognostic uncertainty also contribute to late hospice referrals and transition to end-of-life care, as over 50% of hematologic oncologists consider this a barrier to high-quality end-of-life care [23, 30].

The often-rapid trajectory of death associated with hematologic malignancies, especially for aggressive diseases (e.g., acute leukemia, aggressive lymphoma), also contributes to the underuse of palliative care for this population [23, 27, 28]. In focus groups with hematologic oncologists, many reported that the paradigm of sometimes being able to predict death months ahead for some solid malignancies seldom works for several blood cancers. Participants recounted instances of patients with acute leukemia previously thought to be cured having recurrence with rapid decline and death within few days to weeks [23]. This rapid decline near death limits the time available for transition to hospice care and may contribute to low rates of timely hospice use.

The high prevalence of low blood counts among blood cancer patients and the need for transfusion support is another important disease-based barrier for timely hospice use. Patients with hematologic malignancies often suffer from dyspnea, fatigue, and bleeding because of disease- and treatment-related anemia and thrombocytopenia. Although red blood cell and platelet transfusions may help to palliate these symptoms, many patients are not able to access these services in hospice, thus leading to never enrolling or only doing so late [12, 16, 18].

## Patient-Based Barriers

Patient-based determinants of optimal palliative care include expectations regarding prognosis and perceptions about specialty palliative care and hospice. Individuals with hematologic malignancies often have an overly optimistic view of their prognosis. In a study of older adults with acute myeloid leukemia, 90% reported that they were "somewhat" or "very likely" to be cured of their disease, whereas only 31% of their hematologic oncologists concurred with this chance of cure [50]. High rates of prognostic discordance between patients and hematologic oncologists have also been identified as a problem among other types of hematologic malignancies [51, 52]. Misperceptions about prognosis likely influence choices that patients make about palliative and end-of-life care and may contribute to lower rates of palliative care involvement and higher rates of intense healthcare utilization near death.

Although there is a paucity of studies directly assessing blood cancer patients regarding palliative care, survey studies of hematologic oncologists suggest that some patients may harbor misconceptions about hospice [34, 35]. For example, almost two-third of respondents in a survey of HCT physicians reported that they felt that their patients would think that nothing more could be done for their disease if palliative care referral were suggested. In addition, 82% of transplant physicians reported that blood cancer patients feel scared when they hear the term "palliative care." [35] These findings suggest that palliative care may be conflated with end-of-life care, resulting in a reluctance to utilize palliative care services.

Dying at home with hospice care has generally been viewed as a good death; however, recent data suggest that over one-quarter of patients with hematologic malignancies may prefer a hospital death [53]. Patients with hematologic malignancies, especially those with acute leukemia, receive a large proportion of their treatment in hospital settings and develop strong relationships with their hematology team while receiving round-the-clock support. This comfort with hospital-based care coupled with perceptions that hospice care may not provide the level of care needed likely contributes to low hospice use rates. In a focus group with bereaved caregivers of patients who died of hematologic malignancies, many viewed a hospital death as appropriate and acceptable because of expert nursing care, symptom relief, and the sense of being safe and secure in a familiar environment with people they knew and trusted [26].

## Clinician-Based Barriers

As hematologic oncologists typically initiate palliative care referrals, their perspectives regarding palliative care are central to whether patients with blood cancers receive optimal palliative care. Both qualitative and survey-based studies have demonstrated substantial misperceptions about palliative care among hematologic oncologists [24, 32, 34, 35]. In a multicenter mixed-methods study, most hematologic oncologists viewed ongoing cancer-directed therapy as a contraindication to palliative care involvement. Moreover, they were more likely to view palliative care as synonymous with end-of-life care as compared to solid tumor specialists (61% vs. 16%, $p < 0.001$) [24]. These findings have been confirmed in surveys of hematologic specialists and transplant clinicians, where over 50% consider the term "palliative care" to be synonymous with "hospice and end-of-life care." [34, 35] Equating palliative care with end-of-life care substantially reduces hematologic oncologists' propensity to refer patients to specialty palliative care in a timely fashion.

Hematologic oncologists' concerns and discomfort with having goals-of-care discussion also significantly influences care for blood cancer patients. The most commonly reported clinician-based barrier to such discussions in a hematologic oncologist survey was concern about taking away hope (71.3%) [30]. Hematologic oncologists are also significantly more likely to feel a sense of failure when their patients' disease progresses and are less comfortable discussing death and dying than solid tumor specialists [32]. These concerns about taking away patients' hope, sense of failure, and discomfort deter hematologic specialists from engaging in timely goals of care discussions. Indeed, over half of hematologic oncologists report that conversations about goals of care typically occur "too late." [29]

Clinician perspectives about the adequacy of hospice services influence their propensity to recommend or refer patients to hospice. In a focus group of 20 hematologic oncologists, most participants acknowledged the importance of hospice; however, many felt that the prevalent hospice model, wherein transfusions are often unavailable, was not sufficient to meet the needs of patients with blood cancer [23]. Similar findings emerged from a survey of 349 hematologic oncologists. Although over 90% agreed or strongly agreed that hospice care was helpful for their patients, 46% felt that home hospice was inadequate for their patients' needs [31]. These concerns about the relevance of hospice care for this patient population's needs likely contribute to hematologic specialists either avoiding hospice discussions or waiting until death is imminent before initiating such discussions [15, 29].

### System-Based Barriers

There are important system-based barriers that influence primary palliative care provision by hematologic oncologists, specialty palliative care, and hospice use. Lack of universal and standardized training in palliative care competencies is problematic. Less than half of hematologic oncology trainees report having ever completed a palliative care rotation, and only about one-quarter report feeling adequately trained to make timely hospice care referrals or conduct family meetings [54, 55]. The majority of hematologic oncologists also report that they learned how to provide end-of-life care through trial and error in clinical practice [23], and only 19–30% report any formal rotation on a palliative care service [23, 35]. Moreover, over 50% of hematologic oncologists report that "not knowing the right thing to say" is a barrier to goals-of-care discussions [30]. Limited training and skills in primary palliative care diminish the likelihood of providing high-quality primary palliative care and reduce the likelihood of referral to specialty palliative care [33, 35].

Although there has been a growth in specialty palliative care programs in the past decade, a significant number of hospitals still do not have any palliative care service. In a recent survey of US hospitals, almost one-third of hospitals with more than 50 beds did not have any palliative care service [56]. This shortage limits access to specialty palliative care for many patients with blood cancers. This barrier is especially compounded for blood cancer patients treated in rural or community settings, where the penetration of specialty palliative care services is less robust.

A significant system-based barrier to hospice use that has been the subject of recent studies is limited access to blood transfusions in hospice settings [12, 13, 16, 18, 31]. Although transfusions can palliate dyspnea, fatigue, and bleeding, most hospices do not provide this service due to reimbursement constraints. This barrier affects hospice use and length of stay. In a large SEER-Medicare study of older adults who died of myelodysplastic syndromes, transfusion-dependent patients were significantly less likely to enroll in hospice [12]. Another study of leukemia decedents demonstrated that transfusion-dependent patients had significantly shorter hospice stays with a median of 6 vs. 11 days for those not transfusion-dependent [16]. Moreover, among leukemia decedents who disenroll from hospice, the majority (62%) do so specifically to receive transfusions [13]. These studies combined suggest that transfusion access impacts the entire hospice trajectory from enrollment, length of stay, to disenrollment.

## Theme 4: Models of Palliative Care for Patients with Hematologic Malignancies

Despite multiple challenges to palliative care for patients with blood cancer, data show that optimizing palliative care for this population is feasible and has substantial benefits [37, 38, 57–61]. Published data include two main specialty palliative care models (consultative versus integrated) in multiple settings (inpatient versus outpatient). In an outpatient pre-transplant palliative care consultation study for patients scheduled to undergo allogeneic HCT, 69% of patients who were approached enrolled in the study and 82% of participants reported that they were very comfortable with early palliative care [57]. Another analysis of a consultative inpatient palliative care model in an HCT unit instituted as a quality improvement project resulted in a substantial increase in hospice referral rates from a 5% pre-implementation baseline to 41% during the program. These studies illustrate the feasibility and benefits of consultative models of palliative care.

Integrating palliative care with hematologic care is also a successful model. For example, an outpatient palliative care clinic for patients with multiple myeloma jointly established by palliative care and hematology departments at a comprehensive cancer center was associated with a significant decrease in pain, and significant improvement in overall physical and emotional burden among patients was seen in the integrated system [59]. Of note, the palliative care clinic was physically embedded within the hematology outpatient clinic, thus promoting a seamless integration model. The integrated palliative care model was also proven to be efficacious in a randomized controlled trial of patients undergoing HCT [37]. Study participants were randomized to receive inpatient integrated palliative care (twice-weekly visits) or standard transplant care. Intervention patients experienced significant improvements in quality of life, symptom burden, and emotional symptoms 2 weeks after transplant compared to patients receiving usual transplant care [37]. Although the intervention was limited to the acute transplant hospitalization, patients had sustained improvement in depression and posttraumatic symptoms at 6-month follow-up compared to the standard care arm [38]. These findings emphasize that integrated palliative care benefits for individuals with blood cancer are clinically meaningful and long-lasting.

## Future Directions

Although there has been substantial advancement in palliative care research for patients with hematologic malignancies, there is still ample room for growth. Most palliative care evidence based on hematologic oncology has entailed describing the unmet palliative care needs and barriers to optimal care for this population. To move the field to the next phase, there is a critical need for well-designed intervention studies to optimize palliative care. We especially need intervention studies that focus on the entire spectrum of palliative care from primary palliative care to hospice care (Fig. 19.1).

Primary palliative care interventions to improve prognostic and goals of care discussions by hematologic oncologists are needed. Existing data shows that hematologic oncologists' rates of timely goals-of-care discussions are low and often occur late, with a median of only 15 days between the first documented discussion and death [15]. At the same time, hematologic oncologists' involvement in the first goals-of-care discussion (as opposed to other clinicians) is significantly associated with higher rates of timely hospice use and low rates of intensive cancer-directed care near death for blood cancer patients [15]. This highlights the need for goals of care interventions that specifically engage *hematologic oncologists*. Inclusion of hematologic oncologists in early phases of intervention development and inclusion of strategies to effectively handle heightened prognostic uncertainty will be important considerations for such interventions.

Rigorously designed randomized controlled trials to test various specialty palliative care models are vital to advance the field. The only published randomized controlled trial of specialty palliative care in this field included patients undergoing autologous or allogeneic HCT. To build on this, we need studies of palliative care that engage patients with hematologic malignancies at other points in their disease trajectory aside from transplantation. The ideal time to integrate specialty palliative care interventions may vary by disease. Integrating specialty palliative care at diagnosis may be most beneficial for diseases with high symptom burden and mortality like acute myeloid leukemia. On the other hand, this strategy is not likely to be ideal for indolent diseases like follicular lymphoma, where patients have low symptom burden and mortality and may not need cancer-directed treatment for years. For such indolent diseases, testing a specialty palliative care intervention in a high-risk population (e.g., early disease progression, refractory disease) may be more appropriate. In addition, research testing different modes of palliative care delivery (e.g., telehealth delivery) to broaden access to palliative care and to alleviate transportation burden is another critical area of inquiry. Finally, identifying triggers for specialty palliative care integration (that are not solely prognosis-based) is vital for intervention studies,

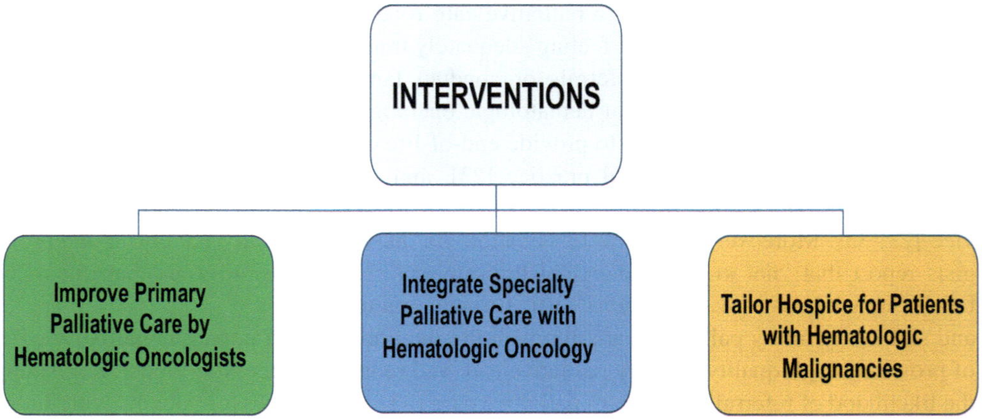


**Fig. 19.1** Focus areas for future intervention research to advance palliative care for hematologic malignancies

given the degree of heterogeneity and prognostic uncertainty in hematologic oncology.

Another critical aspect of advancing palliative care in hematologic oncology is testing interventions to improve hospice use. Although effective primary and specialty palliative care interventions are likely to enhance the use of hospice use for patients with blood cancers, they do not address the barrier of lack of transfusion access in many hospice settings. Therefore, we need intervention studies that will actively engage hospice organizations and payers to test hospice delivery models and innovative payment models that enable access to palliative transfusions in hospice.

Palliative care research in hematologic oncology has burgeoned in the past 10 years; yet, there is strong potential for even more growth in this new decade. Multiple randomized controlled trials to test various specialty palliative care integration models are recruiting participants in the US and Europe (NCT03743480, NCT03800095, NCT03641378). Leaders of large hematology associations highlight the need for optimal palliative care research and research engagement toward this end [35, 51, 57]. As research advances, we hope to see the "promise of collaboration between palliative care and hematologic oncology" [7] fully realized.DisclosuresNo relevant financial conflicts of interest.

## References


1. Zimmermann C, Swami N, Krzyzanowska M, et al. Early palliative care for patients with advanced cancer: a cluster-randomised controlled trial. Lancet. 2014;383:1721–30.
2. Temel JS, Greer JA, Muzikansky A, et al. Early palliative care for patients with metastatic non-small-cell lung cancer. N Engl J Med. 2010;363:733–42.
3. Bakitas M, Lyons KD, Hegel MT, et al. Effects of a palliative care intervention on clinical outcomes in patients with advanced cancer: the project ENABLE II randomized controlled trial. JAMA. 2009;302:741–9.
4. Bakitas MA, Tosteson TD, Li Z, et al. Early versus delayed initiation of concurrent palliative oncology care: patient outcomes in the ENABLE III randomized controlled trial. J Clin Oncol. 2015;33:1438–45.
5. Earle CC, Landrum MB, Souza JM, Neville BA, Weeks JC, Ayanian JZ. Aggressiveness of cancer care near the end of life: is it a quality-of-care issue? J Clin Oncol. 2008;26:3860–6.
6. Hui D, Didwaniya N, Vidal M, et al. Quality of end-of-life care in patients with hematologic malignancies: a retrospective cohort study. Cancer. 2014;120:1572–8.
7. Epstein AS, Goldberg GR, Meier DE. Palliative care and hematologic oncology: the promise of collaboration. Blood Rev. 2012;26:233–9.
8. Johnston EE, Adesina OO, Alvarez E, et al. Acute care utilization at end of life in sickle cell disease: highlighting the need for a palliative approach. J Palliat Med. 2020;23:24–32.
9. El-Jawahri AR, Abel GA, Steensma DP, et al. Health care utilization and end-of-life care for older patients with acute myeloid leukemia. Cancer. 2015;121:2840–8.
10. LeBlanc TW, Abernethy AP, Casarett DJ. What is different about patients with hematologic malignancies? A retrospective cohort study of cancer patients referred to a hospice research network. J Pain Symptom Manag. 2015;49:505–12.
11. O'Connor NR, Hu R, Harris PS, Ache K, Casarett DJ. Hospice admissions for cancer in the final days of life: independent predictors and implications for quality measures. J Clin Oncol. 2014;32:3184–9.
12. Fletcher SA, Cronin AM, Zeidan AM, et al. Intensity of end-of-life care for patients with myelodysplastic syndromes: findings from a large national database. Cancer. 2016;122:1209–15.
13. Wang R, Zeidan AM, Halene S, et al. Health care use by older adults with acute myeloid leukemia at the end of life. J Clin Oncol. 2017;35:3417–24.
14. Wang WS, Ma JD, Nelson SH, et al. Transfusion practices at end of life for hematopoietic stem cell transplant patients. Support Care Cancer. 2018;26:1927–31.
15. Odejide OO, Uno H, Murillo A, Tulsky JA, Abel GA. Goals of care discussions for patients with blood cancers: association of person, place, and time with end-of-life care utilization. Cancer. 2020;126:515–22.
16. LeBlanc TW, Egan PC, Olszewski AJ. Transfusion dependence, use of hospice services, and quality of end-of-life care in leukemia. Blood. 2018;132:717–26.
17. Odejide OO, Cronin AM, Earle CC, LaCasce AS. Abel GA, vol. 108. Hospice Use Among Patients With Lymphoma: Impact of Disease Aggressiveness and Curability. J Natl Cancer Inst; 2016. p. 108.
18. Odejide OO, Li L, Cronin AM, et al. Meaningful changes in end-of-life care among patients with myeloma. Haematologica. 2018;103:1380–9.
19. Hui D, Kim SH, Kwon JH, et al. Access to palliative care among patients treated at a comprehensive cancer center. Oncologist. 2012;17:1574–80.
20. Beaussant Y, Daguindau E, Chauchet A, et al. Hospital end-of-life care in haematological malignancies. BMJ Support Palliat Care. 2018;8:314–24.
21. Johnston EE, Alvarez E, Saynina O, Sanders L, Bhatia S, Chamberlain LJ. Disparities in the intensity of end-of-life Care for Children with Cancer. Pediatrics. 2017;140(4):e20170671.
22. Ullrich CK, Lehmann L, London WB, et al. End-of-life care patterns associated with pediatric palliative care among children who underwent hematopoietic stem cell transplant. Biol Blood Marrow Transplant. 2016;22:1049–55.
23. Odejide OO, Salas Coronado DY, Watts CD, Wright AA, Abel GA. End-of-life care for blood cancers: a series of focus groups with hematologic oncologists. J Oncol Pract. 2014;10:e396–403.
24. LeBlanc TW, O'Donnell JD, Crowley-Matoka M, et al. Perceptions of palliative care among hematologic malignancy specialists: a mixed-methods study. J Oncol Pract. 2015;11:e230–8.
25. Henckel C, Revette A, Huntington SF, Tulsky JA, Abel GA, Odejide OO. Perspectives regarding hospice services and transfusion access: focus groups with blood cancer patients and bereaved caregivers. J Pain Symptom Manag. 2020;59:1195.
26. McCaughan D, Roman E, Smith AG, et al. Perspectives of bereaved relatives of patients with haematological malignancies concerning preferred place of care and death: a qualitative study. Palliat Med. 2019;33:518–30.
27. McCaughan D, Roman E, Smith AG, et al. Determinants of hospital death in haematological cancers: findings from a qualitative study. BMJ Support Palliat Care. 2018;8:78–86.
28. McCaughan D, Roman E, Smith AG, et al. Palliative care specialists' perceptions concerning referral of haematology patients to their services: findings from a qualitative study. BMC Palliat Care. 2018;17:33.
29. Odejide OO, Cronin AM, Condron N, Earle CC, Wolfe J, Abel GA. Timeliness of end-of-life discussions for blood cancers: a

National Survey of hematologic oncologists. JAMA Intern Med. 2016;176:263–5.
30. Odejide OO, Cronin AM, Condron NB, et al. Barriers to quality end-of-life Care for Patients with Blood Cancers. J Clin Oncol. 2016;34:3126–32.
31. Odejide OO, Cronin AM, Earle CC, Tulsky JA, Abel GA. Why are patients with blood cancers more likely to die without hospice? Cancer. 2017;123:3377–84.
32. Hui D, Bansal S, Park M, et al. Differences in attitudes and beliefs toward end-of-life care between hematologic and solid tumor oncology specialists. Ann Oncol. 2015;26:1440–6.
33. Hui D, Cerana MA, Park M, Hess K, Bruera E. Impact of Oncologists' attitudes toward end-of-life care on patients' access to palliative care. Oncologist. 2016;21:1149–55.
34. Hui D, Park M, Liu D, Reddy A, Dalal S, Bruera E. Attitudes and beliefs toward supportive and palliative care referral among hematologic and solid tumor oncology specialists. Oncologist. 2015;20:1326–32.
35. El-Jawahri A, LeBlanc TW, Burns LJ, et al. What do transplant physicians think about palliative care? A national survey study. Cancer. 2018;124:4556–66.
36. Martins Y, Lederman RI, Lowenstein CL, et al. Increasing response rates from physicians in oncology research: a structured literature review and data from a recent physician survey. Br J Cancer. 2012;106:1021–6.
37. El-Jawahri A, LeBlanc T, VanDusen H, et al. Effect of inpatient palliative care on quality of life 2 Weeks after hematopoietic stem cell transplantation: a randomized clinical trial. JAMA. 2016;316:2094–103.
38. El-Jawahri A, Traeger L, Greer JA, et al. Effect of inpatient palliative care during hematopoietic stem-cell transplant on psychological distress 6 months after transplant: results of a randomized clinical trial. J Clin Oncol. 2017;35:3714–21.
39. LeBlanc TW, Lodato JE, Currow DC, Abernethy AP. Overcoming recruitment challenges in palliative care clinical trials. J Oncol Pract. 2013;9:277–82.
40. Manitta V, Zordan R, Cole-Sinclair M, Nandurkar H, Philip J. The symptom burden of patients with hematological malignancy: a cross-sectional observational study. J Pain Symptom Manag. 2011;42:432–42.
41. Hochman MJ, Yu Y, Wolf SP, Samsa GP, Kamal AH, LeBlanc TW. Comparing the palliative care needs of patients with hematologic and solid malignancies. J Pain Symptom Manag. 2018;55:82–88.e81.
42. LeBlanc TW, Smith JM, Currow DC. Symptom burden of haematological malignancies as death approaches in a community palliative care service: a retrospective cohort study of a consecutive case series. Lancet Haematol. 2015;2:e334–8.
43. El-Jawahri AR, Traeger LN, Kuzmuk K, et al. Quality of life and mood of patients and family caregivers during hospitalization for hematopoietic stem cell transplantation. Cancer. 2015;121:951–9.
44. Fadul NA, El Osta B, Dalal S, Poulter VA, Bruera E. Comparison of symptom burden among patients referred to palliative care with hematologic malignancies versus those with solid tumors. J Palliat Med. 2008;11:422–7.
45. El-Jawahri AR, Vandusen HB, Traeger LN, et al. Quality of life and mood predict posttraumatic stress disorder after hematopoietic stem cell transplantation. Cancer. 2016;122:806–12.
46. Dirou S, Chambellan A, Chevallier P, et al. Deconditioning, fatigue and impaired quality of life in long-term survivors after allogeneic hematopoietic stem cell transplantation. Bone Marrow Transplant. 2018;53:281–90.
47. Sexauer A, Cheng MJ, Knight L, Riley AW, King L, Smith TJ. Patterns of hospice use in patients dying from hematologic malignancies. J Palliat Med. 2014;17:195–9.
48. Philip T, Guglielmi C, Hagenbeek A, et al. Autologous bone marrow transplantation as compared with salvage chemotherapy in relapses of chemotherapy-sensitive non-Hodgkin's lymphoma. N Engl J Med. 1995;333:1540–5.
49. Neelapu SS, Locke FL, Bartlett NL, et al. Axicabtagene Ciloleucel CAR T-cell therapy in refractory large B-cell lymphoma. N Engl J Med. 2017;377:2531–44.
50. El-Jawahri A, Nelson-Lowe M, VanDusen H, et al. Patient-clinician discordance in perceptions of treatment risks and benefits in older patients with acute myeloid leukemia. Oncologist. 2019;24:247–54.
51. Loh KP, Xu H, Back A, et al. Patient-hematologist discordance in perceived chance of cure in hematologic malignancies: a multicenter study. Cancer. 2020;126:1306–14.
52. El-Jawahri A, Traeger L, Kuzmuk K, et al. Prognostic understanding, quality of life and mood in patients undergoing hematopoietic stem cell transplantation. Bone Marrow Transplant. 2015;50:1119–24.
53. Howell DA, Wang HI, Roman E, et al. Preferred and actual place of death in haematological malignancy. BMJ Support Palliat Care. 2017;7:150–7.
54. Buss MK, Lessen DS, Sullivan AM, Von Roenn J, Arnold RM, Block SD. Hematology/oncology fellows' training in palliative care: results of a national survey. Cancer. 2011;117:4304–11.
55. Thomas RA, Curley B, Wen S, Zhang J, Abraham J, Moss AH. Palliative care training during fellowship: a National Survey of U.S. hematology and oncology fellows. J Palliat Med. 2015;18:747–51.
56. Dumanovsky T, Augustin R, Rogers M, Lettang K, Meier DE, Morrison RS. The growth of palliative Care in U.S. hospitals: a status report. J Palliat Med. 2016;19:8–15.
57. Loggers ET, LeBlanc TW, El-Jawahri A, et al. Pretransplantation supportive and palliative care consultation for high-risk hematopoietic cell transplantation patients. Biol Blood Marrow Transplant. 2016;22:1299–305.
58. Selvaggi KJ, Vick JB, Jessell SA, Lister J, Abrahm JL, Bernacki R. Bridging the gap: a palliative care consultation service in a hematological malignancy-bone marrow transplant unit. J Community Support Oncol. 2014;12:50–5.
59. Porta-Sales J, Guerrero-Torrelles M, Moreno-Alonso D, et al. Is early palliative care feasible in patients with multiple myeloma? J Pain Symptom Manag. 2017;54:692–700.
60. Roeland E, Mitchell W, Elia G, et al. Symptom control in stem cell transplantation: a multidisciplinary palliative care team approach. Part 1: physical symptoms. J Support Oncol. 2010;8:100–16.
61. Roeland E, Mitchell W, Elia G, et al. Symptom control in stem cell transplantation: a multidisciplinary palliative care team approach. Part 2: psychosocial concerns. J Support Oncol. 2010;8:179–83.

# Part IV

# The Intersection of Palliative Care and Hematologic Malignancies and Serious Blood Disorders: Special Populations

# Palliative Care for Special Populations: Pediatrics

# 20

Danielle Faye Jonas, Angela Steineck, Joshua A. Johnson, Mallory Fossa, Julienne Brackett, Erica Carmen Kaye, and Deena R. Levine

The field of pediatrics encompasses care provided from the time of birth through early adulthood across a diverse spectrum of pathophysiology. The provision of palliative care within pediatrics requires fluidity, creativity, and flexibility to optimize care for patients representing a vast range of ages, developmental abilities, and disease processes. Individuals with comorbidities diagnosed during childhood, particularly those with developmental delays, often continue to receive care at pediatric centers into early adulthood [1]. Due to the prognostic uncertainty intrinsic to many serious pediatric illnesses, pediatric patients frequently are followed by specialized palliative care teams over extended periods, thus setting pediatric palliative care apart from palliative care in the adult world [1].

Within pediatrics, hematologic malignancies comprise more than a third of cancer diagnoses, and many of these patients experience critical illness requiring intensive interventions and support [2, 3]. For adolescent and young adult (AYA) patients, the underlying biology of hematologic malignancies often relates more closely to neoplasms diagnosed in young children than older adults; accordingly, young adults are often referred to pediatric centers for evaluation and treatment. Young adults with relapsed hematologic malignancies also often continue to receive care at the pediatric center where they initially were treated, rather than transferring care to an adult center, particularly in the context of an anticipated poor prognosis when care continuity becomes paramount.

Pediatric blood and cancer programs also provide care to large numbers of patients with benign hematologic disorders. Severe and life-threatening benign hematologic disorders that manifest during childhood typically require close chronic disease management, including Sickle Cell Disease, Thalassemia, Bone Marrow Failure Syndromes, Hemophilia, and other bleeding and clotting disorders. Although categorized as "benign," these diseases and their respective therapies can yield significant morbidity and mortality. As such, palliative care and other supportive services are integral to providing optimal, holistic patient- and family-centered care. More specifically, in an illness like Sickle Cell Disease where symptom severity often waxes and wanes, palliative care services may be useful episodically. Diagnoses with progressive or relapsing trajectories, such as Hemophilia or Bone Marrow Failure disorders, respectively, often require escalation of treatment intensity and carry greater prognostic uncertainty, necessitating closer palliative care involvement. Given the unpredictable nature of many severe benign hematologic disorders, early integration of palliative care should be considered to provide an additional layer of support to patients and families across a stressful and uncertain illness arc [4].

D. F. Jonas (✉)
Silver School of Social Work, New York University, New York, NY, USA
e-mail: DFJ215@NYU.EDU

A. Steineck
Department of Pediatrics, Seattle Children's Hospital, Seattle, WA, USA
e-mail: angela.steineck@seattlechildrens.org

J. A. Johnson
Department of Spiritual Care, Carondelet St. Joseph's Hospital, Tucson, AZ, USA

M. Fossa
Department of Pain and Palliative Medicine, Connecticut Children's Medical Center, Hartford, CT, USA
e-mail: MFOSSA@CONNECTICUTCHILDRENS.ORG

J. Brackett
Department of Pediatrics, Section of Hematology-Oncology, Baylor College of Medicine, Texas Children's Cancer Center, Houston, TX, USA
e-mail: jxbracke@texaschildrens.org

E. C. Kaye
Hospice and Palliative Medicine Fellowship Program, Department of Oncology, St. Jude Children's Research Hospital, Memphis, TN, USA
e-mail: erica.kaye@stjude.org

D. R. Levine
Department of Oncology, Division of Quality of Life and Palliative Care, St. Jude Children's Research Hospital, Memphis, TN, USA
e-mail: Deena.Levine@stjude.org


C. K. Ullrich, E. J. Roeland (eds.), *Palliative Care in Hematologic Malignancies and Serious Blood Disorders*,
https://doi.org/10.1007/978-3-031-38058-7_20

Integration of palliative care into the management of children with hematologic malignancies and serious blood disorders requires an interdisciplinary approach as standard practice [5, 6]. Optimizing the wellbeing of children with malignant and serious non-malignant hematologic diagnoses encompasses many facets of care, including the assessment and management of pain and other symptoms, psychological distress, caregiver and sibling distress, sociocultural and financial concerns, and spiritual suffering. Altogether, the primary objective of pediatric palliative care integration is to provide holistic support and reduce suffering [7]. Collaborative efforts from interdisciplinary clinicians are essential to meet the unique physical, psychosocial, and spiritual needs of each patient and family [5]. Important stakeholders include, but are not limited to: the primary medical team, specialized pediatric palliative care clinicians, psychosocial support services (e.g., psychology, social work, chaplaincy), and allied health professionals (e.g., physical and occupational therapists, child-life therapists, art and music therapists, pain specialists) [8, 9].

At the intersection of pediatric palliative care and blood disorders, the ideal timing for integrating specialty palliative care remains a moving target [10, 11]. Certain hematologic malignancies and severe benign blood disorders may carry a "good" prognosis, contributing to primary clinicians' reluctance to involve palliative care clinicians. Prognostication is increasingly challenging in the developing era of immunotherapy, molecularly targeted therapies, and gene therapy [12]. However, a compelling case can be made for early integration of pediatric palliative care into pediatric cancer care in the setting of prognostic uncertainty and high burden of illness to assist patients and families with stressful and complicated decision-making [13]. Certain transition points also represent natural opportunities for introducing a specialized palliative care team, including evidence of relapsed or refractory disease [11, 14].

Perhaps most unique to the intersection of palliative care and serious blood disorders in the field of pediatrics is the focus on the care triad encompassing patient-parent-clinician. Family-centered care is defined as the engagement of the patient and family as collaborative partners of the care team, respecting their strengths and cultural values in medical decision-making [15, 16]. Striving for family-centered care is considered essential to the practice of pediatric medicine and palliative care [6, 16, 17]. Balancing patient and caregiver input in decision-making relies on assessing developmental status, patient–family relationships, sociocultural factors, and therapeutic alliance with the clinician. Palliative care involvement can help empower AYA patients to find their voice or may enable them to defer information receipt and decision-making to parental caregivers based on their individualistic and cultural preferences [18, 19]. Palliative care clinicians can assist primary teams with exploring the communication and decision support preferences of a given patient and family [20].

## Models of Palliative Care Integration

Palliative care integration for pediatric patients with serious illness should begin early in the course of therapy whenever possible. Elements of primary palliative care can be delivered by the primary treating clinician, incorporating comprehensive symptom assessment and management, open communication, and goal-directed care to optimize quality of life. Secondary subspecialty palliative care services also can benefit many patients and families, especially those with complex or refractory symptoms, psychosocial complexity, and/or high-risk disease. Although pediatric hematology-oncology clinicians often worry about introducing palliative care services, patients and families express receptivity to the integration of palliative care as early as the time of diagnosis [21]. Models of palliative care integration include consults at the primary team's discretion, triggered consults, and universal palliative care consultation. Within the latter models exist subsets of integration that include a tiered approach to service delivery to maximize resources and deliver optimal individualized care [22].

Figure 20.1 illustrates multiple described palliative care integration models specific to pediatric hematopoietic cell transplant (HCT) [22]. Many pediatric patients with hematologic malignancies and serious blood disorders may consider or undergo HCT and/or cellular therapies, and the proposed models of palliative care integration can be highly beneficial for this population. Extrapolating these models to other care settings for pediatric patients with a serious illness can be successfully implemented by tailoring timepoints, triggers, and interventions to each clinic and patient population's unique needs [23].

Multidisciplinary collaboration is key to providing comprehensive care for pediatric patients, including members of the primary team, palliative care team, child life, social work, spiritual care, and others [24] (Fig. 20.2). It is imperative for care collaboration to span across multiple settings to maintain continuity across outpatient clinics, inpatient settings, and the home environment [24]. Home hospice programs can provide essential services to pediatric patients in the community while patients receive concurrent disease-directed

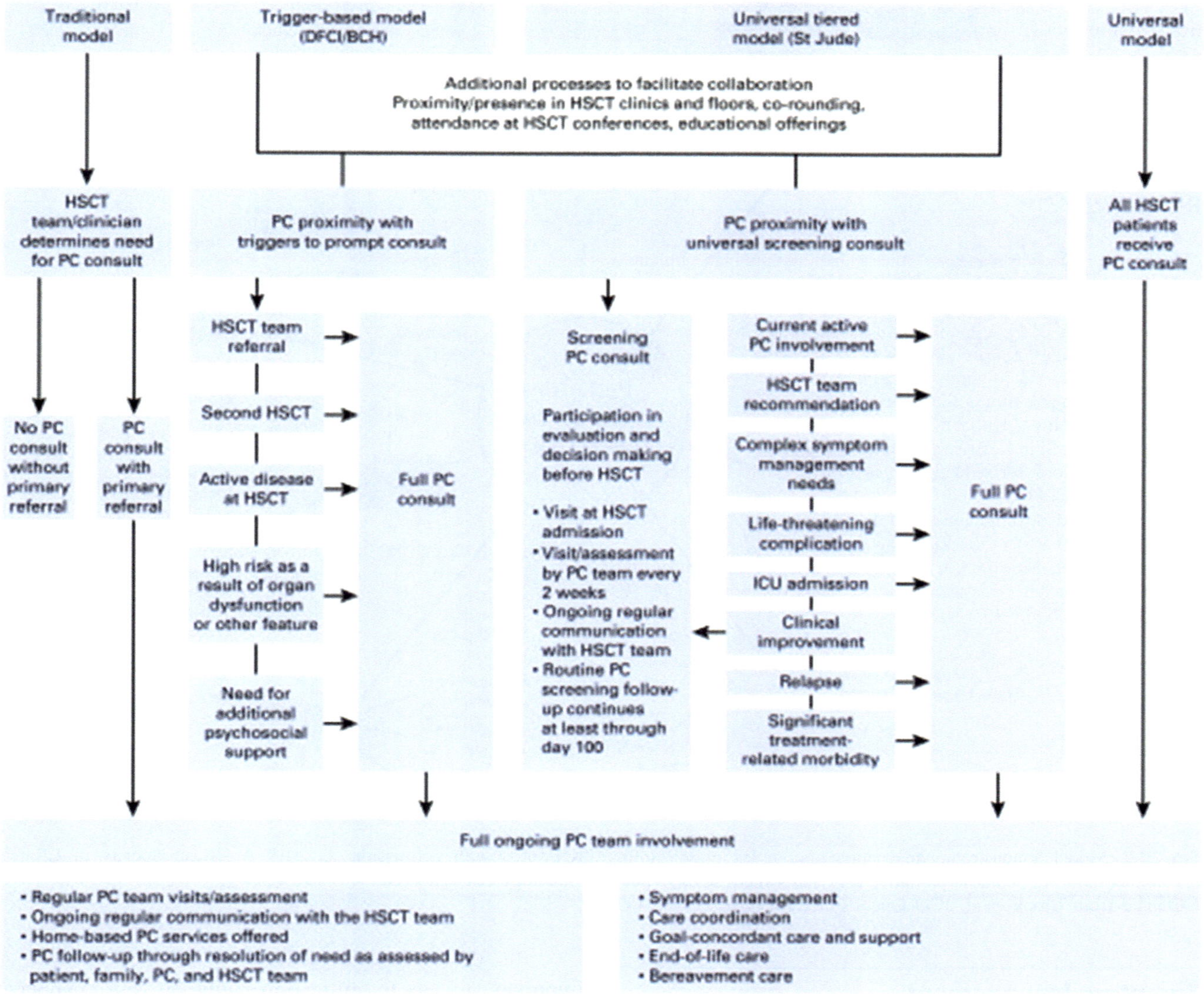


**Fig. 20.1** Models of palliative care integration in pediatric HCT with application to patients with hematologic malignancies and serious blood disorders [22]. (Adapted from Levine D et al. J Oncol Pract 13 (9), 2017:569–577. Reprinted with permission. ©2017 American Society of Clinical Oncology. All rights reserved)

therapy [25]. Barriers to optimal care delivery may include confusion around roles and responsibilities in the context of multi-team collaboration. Interdisciplinary team meetings can help this respect, including as many representative clinicians as possible to promote clear communication, designate roles, and delineate tasks. Within the pediatric hematology and oncology population, a common barrier to care delivery in the home setting is the availability of and access to blood product transfusions. Creative care coordination in conjunction with the concurrent care provision for pediatric patients can maximize home-based resource utilization and support while enabling access to supplemental services as well.

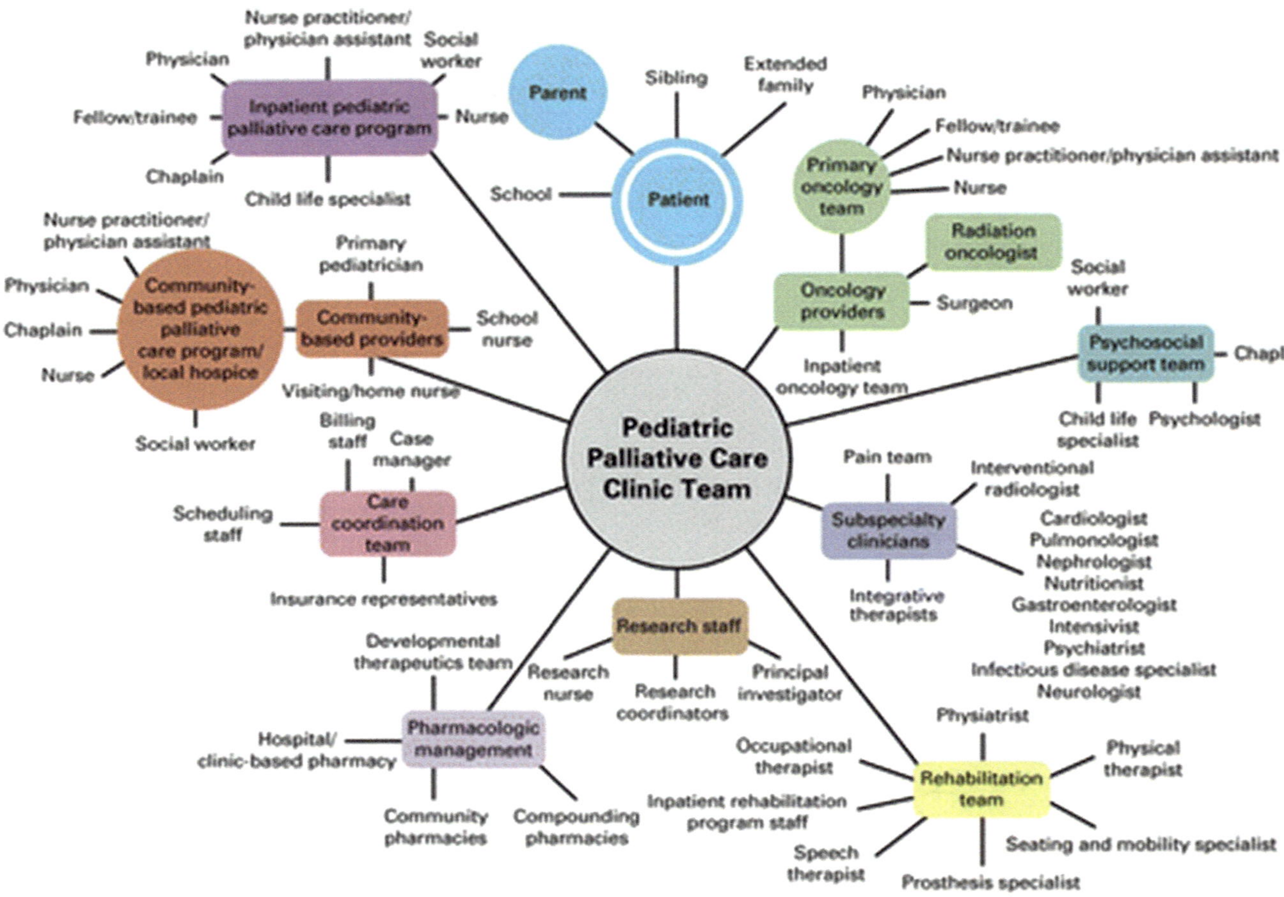


**Fig. 20.2** Model demonstrating an example of complex interdisciplinary collaboration in pediatric palliative care across care settings [24]. (Adapted from Brock et al. JCO Oncol Pract 15(9), 2019:476–487. Reprinted with permission. )

## Symptom Management

Pediatric patients with hematologic malignancies and other serious blood disorders may experience a significant symptom burden across their illness trajectory. Unfortunately, despite their high risk for suffering, this population is not regularly referred to specialized palliative care services early in the illness course [26, 27]. Even in the context of a high symptom burden at the end of life, pediatric hematologic malignancy patients do not consistently receive referrals to hospice or receive comfort-focused care [26, 28–31]. Symptom management in this patient population is critical; however, a greater symptom burden in children is associated with increased suffering and poorer quality of life (QOL) [32, 33]. Moreover, parents who perceive greater suffering in their child at the end of life suffer from increased anxiety and decreased QOL themselves, further emphasizing the need for optimizing symptom management [34–37]. Early integration of specialized palliative care services offers an important strategy for mitigating symptoms as a component of comprehensive family-centered care in pediatric hematology-oncology [5].

Common symptoms experienced by children with serious blood disorders are similar to those seen in adults, including pain, dyspnea, nausea, vomiting, abdominal discomfort, diarrhea, constipation, pruritis, fatigue, mental status changes, anxiety, and depression, among others [21, 38, 39]. However, in caring for pediatric patients, developmental considerations are essential to the practice of symptom assessment and management. Specifically, one's ability to express the presence and/or severity of symptoms relies on developmental stage and cognitive abilities [40]. For children unable or unwilling to describe symptoms, physiologic and behavioral signs of discomfort (e.g., tachycardia, hypertension, tachypnea, grimacing, crying, restlessness) are vital for guiding symptom management [9]. Additionally, parental caregivers are experts in their child's symptom experience, and healthcare professionals should value and prioritize caregiver insights and concerns when developing a symptom management strategy [6, 9]. In synergy with honoring parental reports, patient-reported symptom experiences should be elevated as much as possible to the extent that it is developmentally possible. Patient-reported outcome tools should be integrated into routine clinical care to aid in the guidance of symptom management for children, adolescents, and young adults with malignant and non-malignant hematologic diagnoses [12, 41–47].

Additional developmental considerations must be considered for the successful management of pediatric symptoms, including mechanisms and modalities of treatment delivery. Younger children often are unable to take pills by mouth; in these cases, creative and flexible approaches are needed, along with an interdisciplinary plan that emphasizes child life and psychology services to assist with behavioral interventions [9]. When pills are not possible, certain medications may be crushed or available in suspension; notably, this may exclude extended-release preparations, and collaboration with local compounding pharmacies may be necessary. Weight-based dosing is standard in pediatrics, and close partnerships with pediatric pharmacist experts are recommended to consider age-specific variation in drug metabolism, which may be compounded by disease-related hepatic or renal dysfunction in the setting of chemotherapy or diseases with a high likelihood of organ dysfunction such as Sickle Cell Disease [48].

For pediatric patients who suffer from disease relapse or progression, access to palliative care services and resources in the community can be helpful. Existing legislation, including the Patient Protection and Affordable Care Act (ACA), enable children enrolled on Medicaid or the Children's Health Insurance Program (CHIP) to receive disease-directed therapies and hospice services concurrently [6, 49]. The Concurrent Care Provision of the ACA allows pediatric patients (up to age 21 years) to receive disease-directed chemotherapy and radiation, as well as blood product transfusions while receiving palliative care and hospice resources and services simultaneously. Specific available resources vary by state; generally, concurrent care services are more widely available for pediatric patients than adults [50]. While the Concurrent Care Provision does expand access to hospices for some children, some challenges remain. For example, it is limited to children enrolled on Medicaid or CHIP. In addition, some hospice agencies may not accept pediatric patients and others may lack pediatric-specific expertise, highlighting the value of partnerships between hospice agencies and primary pediatric hematology-oncology and specialized palliative care clinician [51].

Availability of and access to hospice and concurrent care services for children and young adults varies considerably depending on location, coverage, age, and diagnosis. For example, one study found that older children who resided near a pediatric hospice and had a serious health condition with multiple comorbidities were more likely to access hospice services [52]. Further, it is estimated that only about 10 percent of children with serious/life-limiting illnesses are enrolled in hospice care nationally [53]. Clinicians should be mindful when considering access to and the quality of hospice and concurrent care services in their areas before discussing care plans with families instead of offering scenarios that are not logistically feasible.

For pediatric patients with hematologic malignancies at the end of life, the use of blood products for the management of anemia-associated fatigue or thrombocytopenia-associated bleeding may be considered when benefits are felt to outweigh risks. Families can be made aware of the availability of radiation and chemotherapy for the primary purpose of pain or symptom control in the setting of progressive disease, while also benefiting from hospice services. Families may also benefit from the knowledge that participation in early phase clinical trials may remain a possibility while their child is enrolled in hospice services, if that is most consistent with their goals of care. However, careful discussion regarding goals of care is recommended in these instances to avoid receipt of interventions that may be detrimental to QOL without realistic hope for therapeutic benefit [54].

## Communication

Open communication is critical to the care of pediatric patients and their families. A therapeutic relationship built upon mutual respect begins with clear and accurate information sharing. Open-ended questions help clinicians explore goals, preferences, beliefs, and values with pediatric patients and caregivers. In a developmentally appropriate way, addressing pediatric patients directly can help build therapeutic partnerships and foster trust. Clinicians can support families by responding to emotional cues, normalizing concerns, and providing reassurance in clinical communication. Maintaining open lines of communication and reassessing preferences and levels of understanding at regular intervals is essential, as pediatric patient and parent informational needs, goals, and values often evolve. Figure 20.3 describes communication and decision-making in pediatric oncology across a potential disease trajectory.

For pediatric patients with hematologic malignancies and serious blood disorders, straightforward and compassionate communication is a fundamental pillar of care. In the context of both hematologic malignancies and serious blood disorders, the therapeutic path often begins with cure-oriented and/or disease-directed therapy; however, as the illness progresses, goals may evolve, and high-quality communication is essential to help patients and families navigate newly stressful and difficult terrain. The therapeutic options for both pediatric hematologic malignancy and benign hematol-

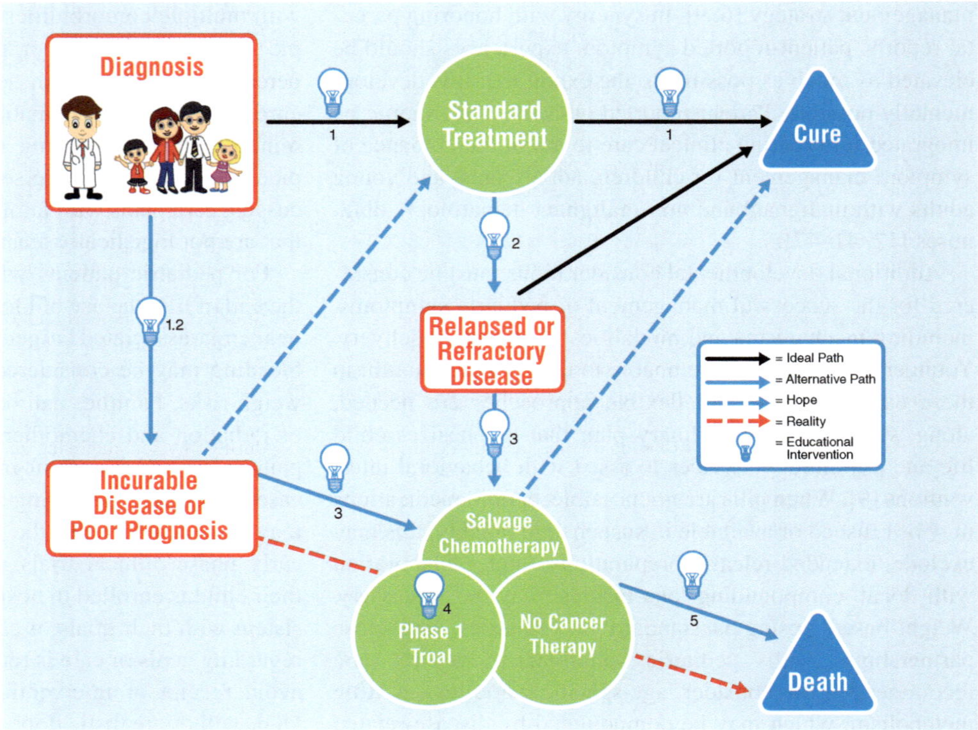


**Fig. 20.3** Communication model as an example of strategies to enhance patient and family understanding for informed decision-making across the disease trajectory [55]. (Adapted from Baker J et al. Practical communication guidance to improve phase I informed consent conversations and decision-making in pediatric oncology. Cancer 121(14), 2015)

ogy patient populations may also include HCT, cellular therapy, and investigational agents at multiple phases of research, either as standard or experimental therapies. At each stage of treatment, critical opportunities exist for clinicians to provide clear information, education, recommendations, and support to pediatric patients and their caregivers [55].

Exploring each patient's and family's definition of QOL and their sources of support can allow a clinician to tailor holistic care to the patient and family unit. Understanding the parents' conception of a "good parent" can also provide valuable insights into the factors that drive their goals, priorities, and actions [56]. "What if" conversations can be a valuable tool for advance care planning and can aid in goal-directed decision-making [57].

Goal-directed communication and decision-making are predicated upon a shared understanding of the pediatric patient and family's operational and therapeutic priorities. In a goal of cure, patients and parents may be willing to accept a higher degree of risk of therapy and symptom burden in the hope of disease eradication. Children with cancer and their families have been found to prioritize QOL while simultaneously pursuing cure-directed therapy [21]. Patients and families, in fact, often maintain overlapping goals, and high-quality communication can help normalize awareness that they need not be mutually exclusive [58]. In the setting of a goal of prolonging life, therapy is aimed at disease stabilization, and good communication centers on weighing the risks and benefits of balancing quality versus quantity of life. When patients and families transition to a goal of comfort, communication emphasizes the value of symptom palliation instead of disease control, focusing on improving QOL through every means possible.

Hope serves as a common thread across communication around evolving goals for patients and families. Hopes vary widely for individual patients and family units, and pediatric patients and parents often hold multiple hopes simultaneously [59]. Preserving and nurturing hope is a valuable, normative coping mechanism for patients and families facing the stressor of serious illness, and clinicians should explore and support their patient's and family's unique hopes while encouraging realistic goal-directed decision-making [60]. Open lines of communication around providing clear prognostic and therapeutic information create the requisite infrastructure for exploring hopes and goals [61]. Because hopes often evolve in parallel with an advancing illness trajectory, clinicians should gently readdress patient and family hopes, fears, and specific goals when new information or transitions arise and throughout the disease trajectory to ensure the maximal provision of support to patients and families [62].

## Decision-Making

Medical decision-making within pediatric and AYA patient populations often presents a unique set of challenges. Legal implications are important to consider, as patients under 18 years of age are minors under parents or guardians' legal jurisdiction. However, given that the child or adolescent is directly affected by the illness and treatment, the transmission of age-appropriate, honest information and acquisition of consent are essential to the ethical provision of high-quality care [63]. When working with the pediatric population, clinicians should not assume to know patient preferences; particularly when caring for AYA patients, clinicians should always ask how much and what types of information patients wish to receive regarding medical updates, prognosis, and decision-making. Querying preferences helps to engender trust and therapeutic alliance with the medical team and provides a sense of control and personhood for the AYA patient [64].

Decisional involvement for AYA patients spans the spectrum from passive or disengaged to highly active, autonomous, and engaged. Offering patients the ability to choose when and how much they wish to participate in medical decision-making can promote respect and trust within the therapeutic alliance. Clinicians should offer AYA patients options (e.g., "Would you like to hear information alone?", "Do you want your parents to be present when we talk about the next steps?", or "Would you rather for your parents to hear all the information, and they can share it with you when you feel ready?").

Once a preference is established, clinicians are encouraged to probe more deeply to gain insights into how and why certain decisions are reached. For example, is the AYA patient perceived by the family as the "ultimate" decision-maker, or does a shared decision-making model exist within the family unit? Preferences should also be revisited periodically, as patients' wishes and needs often evolve across the illness course.

Importantly, pediatric patients with hematologic malignancies or serious blood disorders often have long-standing relationships with their care clinician, and this partnership is essential to nurture [65]. A critical strategy for building trust towards shared decision-making entails consistent provision of honest, transparent information about prognosis, treatment options, risks and benefits, and alternatives, with intentional space created to allow patients the opportunity to weigh options and share their opinions and wishes through the lens of their personal values and lived experiences [19]. Clear and consistent documentation of and advocacy for stated preferences can foster improved understanding, communication, and shared decision-making between patients, families, and clinicians [65].

In the context of end-of-life planning for pediatric patients, tools such as My Wishes, Voicing My Choices, and 5Wishes may help clinicians and families to navigate difficult conversations [66]. When properly documented, the 5Wishes tool is a legal document for patients over 18 years of age [66]. Each state has different tools and policies regarding the completion of other decision-making guides, including advance directives. It is important to be aware of the laws and regulations specific to one's region.

## Prognostic Uncertainty: Treatment Options for Relapsed or Refractory Hematologic Malignancies

The prognosis for pediatric hematologic malignancies has improved over the past few decades, particularly for acute lymphoblastic leukemia (ALL), the most common pediatric hematologic malignancy [2, 67, 68]. However, relapsed and refractory disease remains challenging, both in terms of treatment and prognostication [68]. A variety of therapeutic regimens with differing success rates and the potential for HCT or immunotherapy enable patients and families to continue the pursuit of cure-directed therapy in the face of advancing disease. Even when the chance of cure is small in hematologic malignancies, treatment for relapsed or refractory disease is often provided with curative intent until options are exhausted. In the setting of prognostic uncertainty, patients may pursue multiple sequential attempts at achieving disease remission with a focus on getting to curative intent-therapy and less emphasis on QOL. These patterns and goals of treatment may contribute to delayed referral for subspecialty palliative care, compared to other pediatric malignancies [27, 69].

In the last decade, the advent of chimeric antigen receptor (CAR) T-cell therapy and other immunotherapies has further compounded prognostic uncertainty for patients with relapsed or refractory hematologic malignancies [12, 68]. These therapies use the patient's own immune system to specifically target cancer cells, often yielding fewer traditional toxicities than conventional chemotherapy. CAR T-cell therapy, in particular, has revolutionized therapy for patients with relapsed or refractory leukemia, offering a curative potential to some who would have previously been incurable [68] [70, 71]. Ongoing research suggests the efficacy of this therapy; however, not all patients are eligible for CAR-T cell therapy and these novel therapies are not successful for all patients [67, 72, 73].

Novel therapies, including CAR-T cell therapy and other experimental agents, often are available at a limited number of institutions, requiring patients and families to be willing and able to travel to access these interventions. When patients travel to seek experimental therapy, family members may be separated geographically at a critical time in the child's disease course, leaving patients and families particularly vulnerable and needing psychosocial support. Additionally, patients and families must adapt to new medical teams, and communication becomes particularly critical to aid in continuity of care and support for the family. Palliative care teams are both referring and treating centers that can help support patients and families as they transition through different treatment phases [12].

Although traditional toxicities occur less commonly with CAR T-cell therapies than with traditional chemotherapy or HCT, immunomodulatory therapies may still yield severe toxicities that can be more unpredictable in occurrence and severity. The risk factors that predispose certain patients to complications, such as neurotoxicity or severe inflammatory response, remain unknown. Anticipatory guidance around these potential toxicities is essential to preparing families for all possible outcomes.

Compounding the prognostic uncertainty inherent to CAR-T cell therapy, patients who experience a relapse following CAR T-cell administration may be given the option to use previously collected cells to make new CAR T-cell products or use the remaining manufactured CAR-T cells for another infusion. These options provide patients and families with ongoing hope for a cure, which historically had not been available [68]. In this case, clinicians less familiar with the curative potential of immunotherapy may not understand that prognosis could remain optimistic, leading to conflicts in treatment recommendations between clinicians and confusion for families. Additionally, because CAR T-cell therapy is a relatively new practice, the data on which to base prognostication is limited, further complicating prognostication efforts.

In the setting of prognostic uncertainty and differing views about what is reasonable between services such as oncology, HCT, and critical care clinicians [74], the involvement of a palliative care team can be beneficial in helping patients and families to discuss "what if" situations and ensuring clear and transparent dialogue between care teams and with the patient and family [14].

When curative therapies such as HCT or CAR T-cell therapy are an option, opportunities to explore phase I studies might offer some benefit in terms of disease stabilization or symptom control. Phase I trials can offer benefits with respect to disease stabilization or symptom control; however, the primary goal of a phase I trial is to study drug toxicities and determine the maximum tolerated dose of a novel agent. Although some phase I studies have demonstrated disease-related efficacy and life-prolongation, this is uncommon [75]. In the era of more targeted therapies and immunotherapy, certain phase I trials in hematologic malignancies have shown higher response rates than previously seen, contributing to difficulties with accurate prognostication. Informed consent documents for phase I studies specify the trial's goals; however, providing detailed information during consent discussions occurs at the primary oncology team's discretion, who may not be directly involved in the phase I studies. Even after participating in informed consent, families may overestimate a phase I trial's potential efficacy or underestimate the risks involved in participation [76]. As with CAR-T cell therapy and HCT, phase I studies are limited to specialized referral centers, so families must decide if traveling to other sites aligns with their goals of care, particularly if therapy necessitates separation from family, loss of support system and peers, or excessive financial burdens. For patients and families exploring these experimental options, a palliative care team's involvement can assist with determining goals of care, understanding treatment options, managing symptoms, and reframing hopes along an advancing illness course [77].

In advancing illness, patients and parents may develop different perspectives related to goals of care and therapy options. For minor patients (aged 17 years or younger), unique challenges arise when opinions and goals differ from their parents. Even when patients are legally minors, assent for therapy remains essential, and collaborative involvement of medical and psychosocial teams is paramount. Maturity level, development, and prior experiences may affect patients' views on therapy and their understanding of the consequences of their decisions. Patients may formulate a narrative about their condition, which may or may not be accurate, and exploring patient and parent perceptions is critical to provide goal-concordant care [78]. Research suggests that parents who discuss prognosis with their child rarely regret this decision, while parents who withhold information about impending death more often regret their decision [79]. Palliative care teams can support parents in navigating how and when to discuss prognosis and treatment options with their children and make decisions about future courses of action [20].

## Psychosocial Care for Children

A family-centered model of care approach improves care for pediatric patients and families, and psychosocial clinicians are integral to achieving this care model. A trained psychosocial clinician should conduct a full psychosocial assessment for each child and family. Depending on the patient's age, developmental level, personality, needs, and family patterns, an individualized approach for psychosocial care can be developed and implemented [80]. Table 20.1 describes developmentally appropriate communication strategies for children according to age/developmental stage. In creating an individualized plan, each patient's developmental needs should be considered, in conjunction with parental preferences for how information is shared with their child, to optimize communication and decision-making. Given that psychosocial clinicians often treat patients across extended periods, clinicians should consider reevaluating psychosocial care plans and communication needs serially as development and processing needs evolve.

Psychosocial clinicians contribute directly to the pediatric patient's management plan by integrating developmental level assessments with recommendations for communicating effectively with a patient, given their individual needs and comprehension potential [81]. In particular, developmental considerations should be factored into symptom management care plans. For example, assessment of an acute vaso-occlusive pain episode in a patient with Sickle Cell Disease will be different for a 3-year-old versus a 15-year-old; when toddlers lack the requisite language and communication skills to articulate their physical experience and needs, psychosocial clinicians can help provide strategies and tools to assist young patients with articulating their needs.

Another aspect of psychosocial care specific to pediatrics involves how and when to include patients and/or siblings in discussions about diagnosis, treatment options, legacy building, and prognosis. Prognostic uncertainty and prolonged illness trajectories within this population require nuanced communication and inclusion of the entire family unit, to the extent desired by the child and family members. Psychosocial clinicians can assist with assessing patient and/or sibling needs to ensure that each child receives the necessary psychological and social supports [82]. Just as pediatric patients should be included in discussions around illness progression, siblings also should be invited to join conversations and/or granted opportunities to process and receive support from psychosocial clinicians [81]. Additionally, psychosocial clinicians may assist by engaging various community-based supportive systems such as school, religious communities, and other community-family partnerships to bolster supportive measures available to children and families.

Psychosocial clinicians also play a critical role in supporting parents and other caregivers across a pediatric patient's illness course. Clinicians should assess how, where, and when parents prefer to receive information about their child's care. In synergy with considering parents' educational, social, financial, and cultural needs concerning medical decision-making, clinicians should reflect on caregivers' abilities to be present, both physically and emotionally. Psychosocial staff should be readily available to answer questions and support parents and families in processing challenging information and decisions [81]. Additionally, parents of children with serious and prolonged illness benefit from preserving their parental relationship and role [81]. Particularly at the end of life, psychosocial clinicians can help caregivers assume parental tasks and responsibilities as a proactive strategy for bonding with their children and creating memories and legacy building during a challenging time.

Transitions between pediatric and adult care practices can also be quite challenging for young adults with serious illnesses and their families. Psychosocial clinicians within palliative care teams are well-positioned to play an important role in easing this process when possible [83]. Interdisciplinary clinicians are encouraged to familiarize themselves with the transition processes unique to their respective institutions and begin communication about the process early and often, allowing for ample time and space to navigate complex systems and optimize care along the way [83].

Lastly, when a child is seriously ill or approaching the end of life, the illness experience can induce rippling effects across an entire community [84]. Children and families are often a part of a layered community consisting of extended family members, friends, neighbors, religious community members, school systems, athletic/activity communities, and various others. As part of their psychosocial assessment, clinicians should be mindful of the sources of support available to the patient and family, as well as the various members of the community who may benefit from additional resources to optimize coping. For example, a child's peers and teachers may be deeply influenced by the patient's illness and may benefit from resources to discuss the child's illness and death. Furthermore, extended family members may be deeply impacted by the loss, yet they often do not receive access to bereavement resources nor age-appropriate psycho-educational tools. Pediatric clinicians should be mindful of the larger community within which a child lives and dies and work to educate families about resources available locally.

## Social Disparities

When caring for children with serious illness, clinicians should consider how social disparities impact holistic care provision [85]. The impact of race and ethnicity on the medical care of children with cancer remains understudied, with conflicting findings regarding the ways that race/ethnicity affect advance care planning, interventions, access to palliative care and hospice services, and end-of-life care [26, 86–88]. Disparities related to socioeconomic status also raise concerns in the management of children with hematologic malignancies and serious blood disorders [89].

Additionally, access to pediatric palliative care services may be influenced further by social components such as cultural values, religious or spiritual beliefs, environment, and past familial experiences [90]. Recognition of the individual patient's and family's total identity is central to providing high-quality health care [85]. Clinicians should be aware of how power imbalances and cultural differences may impact shared decision-making and affect trust between clinicians, patients, and caregivers. Increasing evidence demonstrates that patients and families who identify with a racial or ethnic minority group may experience mistrust of medical clinicians rooted in past personal or historical experiences with the medical system, and clinicians must meet these families with humility, respect, patience, and compassion [91].

Within the philosophy of cultural humility exists a clinical approach encouraging clinicians to embrace a framework guided by genuine curiosity and openness to learn about how an individual family's unique background, culture, religious beliefs, and lived experiences intersect with their clinical questions, values, and needs [92]. Cultural humility invites clinicians to be kind, curious, thoughtful listeners in lieu of making assumptions based on stereotypes, implicit biases, or past personal or professional experiences [92]. Approaching clinical care with a cultural humility framework can assist clinicians in bridging care gaps associated with social disparities in medicine and can improve trust, build a therapeutic alliance, and overall enhance patient and family experiences [93].

## Nursing Considerations

In partnership with other interdisciplinary team members, nurses play a vital role in providing holistic care to pediatric patients. During a child's critical illness, bedside nurses often serve as a sounding board for parents and offer ongoing opportunities to explore thoughts and feelings following difficult conversations and/or decision-making with medical clinicians [94]. Within the care team, nurses have a unique position to assess and clarify how family members interpret and process information shared by the larger medical team [95]. Recognizing that nurses and clinicians may have their own worries for the patient is important in navigating their role in these often difficult conversations [96].

Nursing care for children with hematologic malignancies or serious blood disorders necessitates comprehension of and comfort with the concept of "total pain" management. Nurses comprise the first line in holistic pain assessment and intervention to promote comfort for patients and support for families. In this capacity, nurses must understand how "total pain" represents a combination of physical, psychological, emotional, social, and spiritual sources of discomfort or distress. For example, a nurse who cares for a child with relapsed leukemia may need to manage manifestations of bony pain through the administration of different medications targeting nociceptive and neuropathic pain; at the same time, the nurse is well-positioned to ascertain whether additional factors may be contributing to or exacerbating the child's pain: yearning for a sibling who is unable to visit, existential questioning of faith-based support systems, anxiety around the loss of peer interactions or school involvement, depression over the loss of self-identity or autonomy, guilt at leaving behind grieving parents. The nurse plays an important role in acknowledging and addressing "total pain" to prevent inappropriate and incomplete pain management that exclusively focuses on pharmacotherapeutic regimens [97].

Pediatric nurses also have an opportunity to empower patients and families to nourish the pediatric patient [98]. In many cultures, food and meals have a social connection with "caring" and share meaning and symbolism with select traditions and rituals. Medical teams may introduce conversations around withholding or withdrawing artificial nutrition in the setting of approaching the end of life; often, nurses play an important role in partnering with families to help navigate how this will look for each patient and their family. Nurses may offer valuable insights to help families understand the evolution of appetite and nutritional needs at the end of life and suggest or redirect families towards alternative caregiving and legacy-building activities [99].

Nurses are particularly critical in managing children with hematologic malignancies at the end of life when real-time symptom management and support at the bedside becomes paramount to facilitating a good death. Specifically, controlling bleeding becomes an increasing concern for children with hematologic malignancies as death approaches [100]. Nursing interventions may help reduce stress and mitigate the shock from visible bleeding at the end of life, including intentional and strategic placement of dark towels or sheets to decrease the trauma from visualizing acute blood loss. Administration of stool softeners and a consistent bowel regimen may mitigate constipation and decrease rectal bleeding risk. For hospitalized patients, infusions of platelets may help to decrease bleeding events [95]. Importantly, patients who wish to remain at home may still receive blood products in the clinic. Nursing can help coordinate these interventions in collaboration with home care or hospice agencies [101].

Ultimately, nursing remains integral to the care of children with hematologic malignancies and serious blood disorders across illness course and particularly at the end of life. Often, nurses are uniquely positioned to partner with both the patient/family and the medical teams to bridge communication and create space for further processing. Nurses also offer invaluable support through their frequent presence at the bedside, allowing for managing total pain and other considerations as the disease progresses.

## Spiritual Care

The word spirituality is derived from the Latin root *spirare*, to breathe. Spirituality encompasses the human drive to explore, question, and find meaning in one's relationship with self, loved ones, community, nature, and existential forces larger than our comprehension [102, 103]. Organized religion comprises rituals, traditions, and community to demonstrate faith and codify spirituality [104]. Patients with serious illness and their families may find their religious/spiritual beliefs challenged in the face of stressful medical circumstances. Individuals often process and interpret the illness experience through the lens of personal religious/spiritual beliefs [105], and unmet religious/spiritual needs may adversely impact mental health and lead to existential distress [106, 107]. When religious/spiritual needs are acknowledged and affirmed, religious/spiritual practices can benefit seriously ill children and their families, through enhancing connections with support networks, improving one's sense of self-efficacy, bolstering resilience, and even mitigating symptoms [108, 109].

Spiritual care clinicians are trained to assess the religious/spiritual strengths and needs of patients and families to provide a foundation upon which to maximize the use of spirituality as a source of resilience [105]. Children have unique spiritual needs, and spirituality in the pediatric context tends to be experiential and immediate [106]. Typically, the most effective spiritual care for infants and toddlers is an effective support for their caregivers. High-quality support of parental religious/spiritual needs likely indirectly benefits children of all ages. Spiritual care of preschoolers may cater to their fascination with and immersion in a story; for school-aged children, it may involve engaging with the relationship of logic to the imagination; for adolescents, it often centers on identity and self-efficacy.

Chaplains provide in-depth spiritual assessments and insight into how a patient-family's spiritual resources and needs interface with their other healthcare needs. They may assist families in adapting religious practices within the healthcare environment, which is particularly important in the context of lengthy and/or repeated hospitalizations associated with pediatric hematologic malignancies and serious blood disorders. Given the complexities of care coordination across multiple teams, a stable and trusting relationship with a chaplain can promote continued and effective therapeutic communication between patients/families and medical clinicians. Chaplains may help healthcare professionals better consider and interpret how individual religious/spiritual beliefs may influence decision-making, allowing further opportunities to deepen the integration of family values into care [103]. Chaplains also play a valuable role in educating and empowering community clergy to care for families before, during, and after a child's death. From diagnosis through bereavement support, spiritual conversations offer a vital avenue for patients and families to seek meaning, experience comfort, and find hope across the illness journey.

## End-of-Life Considerations

As illness advances and therapeutic options transition from cure-oriented to comfort-oriented, patients and families often benefit from conversations with clinicians about their goals and preferences for location of care as the end-of-life approaches. Patients with hematologic malignancies often receive therapy with curative intent until late in the disease-trajectory, which may contribute to a greater likelihood of dying in the hospital than patients with other malignancies. Death is also more likely to occur in the intensive care unit for these patients although the involvement of a palliative care team may decrease the odds of dying in the intensive care unit compared to patients without palliative care consultation [3, 31, 110] Unfortunately, patients with hematologic malignancies often experience high levels of treatment intensity with significant symptom burden, further increasing the need for palliative care involvement as the end-of-life approaches.

For patients with relapsed or refractory hematologic malignancies, the desire for ongoing transfusion support may limit the feasibility of going home or palliation with or without hospice. Home transfusions are not possible in most cases, requiring patients to travel to a healthcare facility to receive blood products in the hopes of providing symptomatic relief for anemia-related fatigue, dyspnea, headaches, and prevention of bleeding. Fortunately, ongoing transfusion support, chemotherapy, or radiation does not need to delay or preclude hospice referral for patients with hematologic malignancies. Under the auspices of Concurrent Care legislation, pediatric patients are eligible to receive insurance coverage for disease-directed therapy and transfusion support in conjunction with hospice services [49].

Because patients with pediatric hematologic malignancies typically require therapy over an extended period with prolonged hospitalizations due to severe neutropenia and risk of infection or treatment complication, families commonly develop strong attachments to their child's medical team and to nursing and ancillary staff. These relationships may provide comfort to families and may influence the decision for hospitalization at the end of life. Visitor inpatient restrictions, however, may limit the ability of a family to receive the full extent of their extended family and community support in the hospital setting. In pediatrics, the preferred location of death may also be influenced by the intensity of supportive care needs or concern for the impact on siblings or other family members in the home.

Anticipatory guidance and support from the primary oncology team, palliative care team, and hospice team are critical as the end-of-life approaches, whether at home or inpatient. Discussion of signs and symptoms signifying the dying process can help families understand what is occurring and how the child's needs are changing (e.g., diminishing appetite or the hazards of continuing fluids/transfusions). An interdisciplinary team also can support family members as they cope with a child's impending death. Social workers, chaplains, psychologists, child life specialists, and music therapists play a significant role in supporting the family as they navigate anticipatory grief and create memories as the end-of-life approaches [111, 112].

## Bereavement

Parental loss of a child is one of the most challenging events that a person can experience during their lifetime [84]. Family members and loved ones continue to require specialized support, and palliative care clinicians are trained to provide grief and bereavement care for this population [113, 114]. Additionally, the loss of a sibling during childhood can have life-long impacts on development, emotional regulation, and maturity and identity [84]. Psychological, physical, and spiritual factors should be considered when evaluating the bereavement needs of a family network following a child's death [84]. For the families of children with hematologic malignancies and serious blood disorders, the bereavement process also may be complicated by the impact of prolonged illness trajectories, complex decision-making, and intensive involvement of long-term relationships with healthcare clinicians [35, 115].

After the death of a child, parental grief is intense, penetrating every facet of a family's life, and can result in a prolonged bereavement process [114]. Parents may experience various psychological and physical symptoms, including but not limited to anxiety, depression, social isolation, or changes in appetite or sleep [114]. Bereaved parents often report experiences of guilt, shame, self-blame, and regret following their child's death [84]. Additionally, parents may report feeling abandoned by their child's medical team as a factor contributing to feelings of social isolation [116]. This experience further highlights the importance of bereavement follow-up care.

To provide optimal bereavement support to parents following a child's death, pediatric clinicians should be familiar with basic supportive interventions. Such interventions may include sending a bereavement card with a personal message inscribed or making a bereavement phone call during the days or weeks following the child's death. Clinicians should be aware of local services and referrals as well as basic safety protocols when making contact with bereaved family members who are at higher risk for severe grief responses. Mental health clinicians and chaplains can serve as additional sources of support and education during the grieving process [9]. Interdisciplinary clinicians may find it helpful to make joint bereavement calls to families, especially in the setting of newer clinicians learning this process. Additionally, depending on comfort, availability, clinical relationship, and organizational policies, clinicians may also consider attending patient funerals when invited by parents. Given that this population's care often involves long-term, intense relationships with patients and families, clinicians should be particularly mindful about boundary setting and awareness of their personal grief reactions. At the same time, some evidence suggests that bereaved families experience an additional loss of the clinical team after their child's death, thus highlighting the importance of bereavement follow-up from these valued team members [117].

When providing bereavement support in pediatrics, it is also crucial to consider the bereavement needs of siblings and other grieving children [114]. The loss of a sibling during childhood can have life-long impacts on development, emotional regulation, maturity, and identity [84]. Specifically, siblings of pediatric patients often experience significant long-term impacts such as separation from parents and sibling for prolonged periods, instability in housing location or caregivers, and reliance upon other adults in their lives for support [84]. Pediatric clinicians are trained to consider and care for the needs of children, including emotional processing, developmental conceptualization, and behavioral response patterns [84].

Interventions for supporting bereaved children may include collaboration with schools, consideration of social media usage, engaging peer support networks, and formal referrals to resources such as support groups, bereavement camps, and counseling services [84]. Bibliotherapy, or the use of books in a therapeutic manner, can also benefit and support children's grief processing [118]. Storytelling can promote healing, foster connection, and affect behavior, helping children feel less isolated in their intense feelings of grief [118]. When it makes sense to do so, some children benefit from the opportunity to see and interact with their sibling, even if they are very ill. Child life specialists and other psychosocial clinicians are well-positioned to support healthy siblings as they interact with and create memories of those precious moments [119, 120].

## Self-Care in Pediatric Palliative Care

Clinicians who care for children with hematologic malignancies and serious blood disorders often develop long-term relationships with patients and families. These experiences, while deeply meaningful, can also yield stress and sadness. Burnout and compassion fatigue are well-established collateral damage for healthcare professionals who care for children with life-limiting illnesses [121]. When providing pediatric palliative care, the practice of intentional self-care is essential to sustaining career longevity and satisfaction. Self-awareness and self-compassion are key pillars for maintaining wellbeing in the field, in synergy with a team culture that models and promotes practices that optimize clinician mental health [121].

For busy clinicians, practicing self-care can feel overwhelming and impractical. One pragmatic and facile place to start is by creating space for self-awareness. Self-awareness can be defined as one's subjective perception of and reaction to one's surrounding environment and lived experiences. Optimization of self-awareness can be fostered through regular opportunities for reflection and group discussion. Clinicians in leadership positions can promote self-awareness by creating a culture of transparency around emotional responses to challenging clinical experiences. Greater self-awareness has been shown to lead to greater job satisfaction, enhanced self-care, and compassion satisfaction allowing for improved patient care and satisfaction [121].

Self-compassion is another critical component to optimizing self-care and minimizing burnout. Self-compassion involves the idea of turning compassion that one readily gifts to others inward, offering the same kindness and grace to oneself [122]. Practicing self-compassion can involve positive self-talk, forgiveness, grace, and regular reminders about the aspects of patient care within one's control versus those out of one's individual control. An example of this may include permitting oneself to acknowledge that an aggressive disease cannot be cured, despite best efforts. Allowing oneself the permission to grieve is also an essential aspect of self-compassion, whether the death of a specific patient or the cumulative impact of micro-losses, personal loss, or changes within the medical team. When caring for children with hematologic malignancies or serious blood disorders across many months or years, clinicians often develop deeply meaningful relationships with patients and families. It is important to recognize that more complicated grief and bereavement reactions may arise for clinicians who become intimately connected to a child and family across time. Interdisciplinary teams can help remind individuals to practice self-compassion, holding one another accountable by debriefing difficult conversations or experiences in real-time and following stressful situations.

Much like the care of patients with life-limiting illnesses, self-care for clinicians should be considered through a whole-person lens, including physical, emotional/psychological, spiritual/existential, social, and environmental perspectives. For example, clinicians should be mindful of how events in one's personal life may impact their experiences at work and visa-versa. Generally speaking, self-awareness and self-compassion practices can take time to develop and hone and may evolve over time depending on the individual and team needs. However, concrete initial actions can be incorporated into daily life, such as physical exercise, mindfulness/meditation practices, reflective writing/journaling, meaningful connection with loved ones, and time in nature.

## Conclusion

Pediatric and AYA patients with hematologic malignancies and serious blood disorders benefit from the early integration of palliative care. Comprehensive care for this patient population encompasses individualized communication, symptom management, goal-directed care, and interdisciplinary support throughout the trajectory, taking into account the physiological, developmental, psychosocial, and familial dynamic. Pediatric palliative care services extend across care settings, in partnership with primary medical teams, to deliver holistic support to pediatric patients and their families throughout the course of illness.

## References


1. Feudtner C, Kang TI, Hexem KR, et al. Pediatric palliative care patients: a prospective multicenter cohort study. Pediatrics. 2011;127(6):1094–101. https://doi.org/10.1542/peds.2010-3225.
2. Howlader NNA, Krapcho M, Miller D, Brest A, Yu M, Ruhl J, Tatalovich Z, Mariotto A, Lewis DR, Chen HS, Feuer EJ, Cronin KA. SEER Cancer Statistics Review, 1975–2017. National Cancer Institute; 2019; https://seer.cancer.gov/csr/1975_2017.
3. Snaman JM, Kaye EC, Lu JJ, Sykes A, Baker JN. Palliative care involvement is associated with less intensive end-of-life Care in Adolescent and Young Adult Oncology Patients. J Palliat Med. 2017;20(5):509–16. https://doi.org/10.1089/jpm.2016.0451.
4. Benjamin L. Pain Management in Sickle Cell Disease: palliative care begins at birth? Hematology. 2008;2008(1):466–74. https://doi.org/10.1182/asheducation-2008.1.466.
5. Weaver MS, Heinze KE, Kelly KP, et al. Palliative care as a standard of Care in Pediatric Oncology. Pediatr Blood Cancer. 2015;62(S5):S829–33. https://doi.org/10.1002/pbc.25695.
6. American Academy of Pediatrics. Section on hospice and palliative medicine and committee on hospital care. Pediatric palliative care and hospice care commitments, guidelines, and recommendations. Pediatrics. 2013;132(5):966–72. https://doi.org/10.1542/peds.2013-2731.
7. Ananth P, Ma C, Al-Sayegh H, et al. Provider perspectives on use of medical marijuana in children with cancer. Pediatrics. 2018;141(1):e20170559. https://doi.org/10.1542/peds.2017-0559.
8. Anderson C, Lund JL, Weaver MA, Wood WA, Olshan AF, Nichols HB. Noncancer mortality among adolescents and young adults with cancer. Cancer. 2019;125(12):2107–14. https://doi.org/10.1002/cncr.32063.
9. Jordan M, Keefer PM, Lee Y-LA, et al. Top ten tips palliative care clinicians should know about caring for children. J Palliat Med. 2018;21(12):1783–9. https://doi.org/10.1089/jpm.2018.0482.
10. Weaver MS, Rosenberg AR, Tager J, Wichman CS, Wiener L. A summary of pediatric palliative care team structure and services as reported by centers caring for children with cancer. J Palliat Med. 2018;21(4):452–62. https://doi.org/10.1089/jpm.2017.0405.
11. Thienprayoon R, LeBlanc T. Early integration of palliative care into the care of patients with cancer. Hematology. 2015;2015(1):479–83. https://doi.org/10.1182/asheducation-2015.1.479.
12. Steineck A, Wiener L, Mack JW, Shah NN, Summers C, Rosenberg AR. Psychosocial care for children receiving chimeric antigen receptor (CAR) T-cell therapy. Pediatr Blood Cancer. 2020;67(5):e28249. https://doi.org/10.1002/pbc.28249.
13. Kaye EC, Friebert S, Baker JN. Early integration of palliative Care for Children with high-risk cancer and their families. Pediatr Blood Cancer. 2016;63(4):593–7. https://doi.org/10.1002/pbc.25848.
14. Humphrey L, Kang TI. Palliative care in pediatric patients with hematologic malignancies. Hematology. 2015;2015(1):490–5. https://doi.org/10.1182/asheducation-2015.1.490.

15. Committee on Hospital Care. American Academy of Pediatrics. Family-centered care and the pediatrician's role. Pediatrics. 2003;112(3 Pt 1):691–7.
16. Committee on hospital care and institute for patient- and family-centered care. Patient- and family-centered care and the pediatrician's role. Pediatrics. 2012;129(2):394–404. https://doi.org/10.1542/peds.2011-3084.
17. Brousseau DC, Hoffmann RG, Nattinger AB, Flores G, Zhang Y, Gorelick M. Quality of primary care and subsequent pediatric emergency department utilization. Pediatrics. 2007;119(6):1131–8. https://doi.org/10.1542/peds.2006-3518.
18. Mack JW, Wolfe J, Cook EF, Grier HE, Cleary PD, Weeks JC. Parents' roles in decision making for children with cancer in the first year of cancer treatment. J Clin Oncol Off J Am Soc Clin Oncol. 2011;29(15):2085–90. https://doi.org/10.1200/JCO.2010.32.0507.
19. Mack JW, Fasciano KM, Block SD. Adolescent and Young adult cancer patients' experiences with treatment decision-making. Pediatrics. 2019;143(5):e20182800. https://doi.org/10.1542/peds.2018-2800.
20. Mack JW, Feudtner C, Hinds PS. Communication and decision support for children with advanced cancer and their families. Am Soc Clin Oncol Educ Book. 2012:637–43. https://doi.org/10.14694/EdBook_AM.2012.32.164.
21. Levine DR, Mandrell BN, Sykes A, et al. Patients' and parents' needs, attitudes, and perceptions about early palliative care integration in pediatric oncology. JAMA Oncol. 2017;3(9):1214–20. https://doi.org/10.1001/jamaoncol.2017.0368.
22. Levine DR, Baker JN, Wolfe J, Lehmann LE, Ullrich C. Strange bedfellows no more: how integrated stem-cell transplantation and palliative care programs can together improve end-of-life care. J Oncol Pract. 2017;13(9):569–77. https://doi.org/10.1200/JOP.2017.021451.
23. Moynihan KM, Snaman JM, Kaye EC, et al. Integration of pediatric palliative care into cardiac intensive care: a champion-based model. Pediatrics. 2019;144(2):e20190160. https://doi.org/10.1542/peds.2019-0160.
24. Brock KE, Snaman JM, Kaye EC, et al. Models of pediatric palliative oncology outpatient care—benefits, challenges, and opportunities. J Oncol Pract. 2019;15(9):476–87. https://doi.org/10.1200/JOP.19.00100.
25. Keim-Malpass J, Hart T, Miller J. Coverage of palliative and hospice care for pediatric patients with a life-limiting illness: a policy brief. J Pediatr Health Care. 2013;27(6):511–6. https://doi.org/10.1016/j.pedhc.2013.07.011.
26. Brock KE, Steineck A, Twist CJ. Trends in end-of-life Care in Pediatric Hematology, oncology, and stem cell transplant patients. Pediatr Blood Cancer. 2016;63(3):516–22. https://doi.org/10.1002/pbc.25822.
27. Kaye EC, Jerkins J, Gushue CA, et al. Predictors of late palliative care referral in children with cancer. J Pain Symptom Manag. 2018;55(6):1550–6. https://doi.org/10.1016/j.jpainsymman.2018.01.021.
28. Pritchard M, Burghen E, Srivastava DK, et al. Cancer-related symptoms most concerning to parents during the last week and last day of their child's life. Pediatrics. 2008;121(5):e1301–9. https://doi.org/10.1542/peds.2007-2681.
29. Kassam A, Sutradhar R, Widger K, et al. Predictors of and trends in high-intensity end-of-life care among children with cancer: a population-based study using health services data. J Clin Oncol Off J Am Soc Clin Oncol. 2017;35(2):236–42. https://doi.org/10.1200/JCO.2016.68.8283.
30. Snaman JM, Talleur AC, Lu J, et al. Treatment intensity and symptom burden in hospitalized adolescent and young adult hematopoietic cell transplant recipients at the end of life. Bone Marrow Transplant. 2018;53(1):84–90. https://doi.org/10.1038/bmt.2017.187.
31. Kaye EC, DeMarsh S, Gushue CA, et al. Predictors of location of death for children with cancer enrolled on a palliative care service. Oncologist. 2018;23(12):1525–32. https://doi.org/10.1634/theoncologist.2017-0650.
32. Wolfe J, Orellana L, Ullrich C, et al. Symptoms and distress in children with advanced cancer: prospective patient-reported outcomes from the PediQUEST study. J Clin Oncol. 2015;33(17):1928–35. https://doi.org/10.1200/JCO.2014.59.1222.
33. Rosenberg AR, Orellana L, Ullrich C, et al. Quality of life in children with advanced cancer: a report from the PediQUEST study. J Pain Symptom Manag. 2016;52(2):243–53. https://doi.org/10.1016/j.jpainsymman.2016.04.002.
34. Rosenberg AR, Baker KS, Syrjala K, Wolfe J. Systematic review of psychosocial morbidities among bereaved parents of children with cancer. Pediatr Blood Cancer. 2012;58(4):503–12. https://doi.org/10.1002/pbc.23386.
35. McCarthy MC, Clarke NE, Ting CL, Conroy R, Anderson VA, Heath JA. Prevalence and predictors of parental grief and depression after the death of a child from cancer. J Palliat Med. 2010;13(11):1321–6. https://doi.org/10.1089/jpm.2010.0037.
36. Dussel V, Joffe SJ, Hilden JM, Watterson-Schaeffer J, Weeks JC, Wolfe J. Considerations about hastening death among parents of children who die of cancer. Arch Pediatr Adolesc Med. 2010;164(3):231–7. https://doi.org/10.1001/archpediatrics.2009.295.
37. van der Geest IMM, Darlington A-SE, Streng IC, Michiels EMC, Pieters R, van den Heuvel-Eibrink MM. Parents' experiences of pediatric palliative care and the impact on long-term parental grief. J Pain Symptom Manag. 2014;47(6):1043–53. https://doi.org/10.1016/j.jpainsymman.2013.07.007.
38. Wolfe J, Grier HE, Klar N, et al. Symptoms and suffering at the end of life in children with cancer. N Engl J Med. 2000;342(5):326–33. https://doi.org/10.1056/NEJM200002033420506.
39. Wolfe J, Hammel JF, Edwards KE, et al. Easing of suffering in children with cancer at the end of life: is care changing? J Clin Oncol Off J Am Soc Clin Oncol. 2008;26(10):1717–23. https://doi.org/10.1200/JCO.2007.14.0277.
40. Bevans KB, Riley AW, Moon J, Forrest CB. Conceptual and methodological advances in child-reported outcomes measurement. Expert Rev Pharmacoecon Outcomes Res. 2010;10(4):385–96. https://doi.org/10.1586/erp.10.52.
41. Wolfe J, Orellana L, Cook EF, et al. Improving the care of children with advanced cancer by using an electronic patient-reported feedback intervention: results from the PediQUEST randomized controlled trial. J Clin Oncol Off J Am Soc Clin Oncol. 2014;32(11):1119–26. https://doi.org/10.1200/JCO.2013.51.5981.
42. Dussel V, Orellana L, Soto N, et al. Feasibility of conducting a palliative care randomized controlled trial in children with advanced cancer: assessment of the PediQUEST study. J Pain Symptom Manag. 2015;49(6):1059–69. https://doi.org/10.1016/j.jpainsymman.2014.12.010.
43. Chakraborty R, Sidana S, Shah GL, Scordo M, Hamilton BK, Majhail NS. Patient-reported outcomes with chimeric antigen receptor T cell therapy: challenges and opportunities. Biol Blood Marrow Transplant. 2019;25(5):e155–62. https://doi.org/10.1016/j.bbmt.2018.11.025.
44. Efficace F, Gaidano G, Lo-Coco F. Patient-reported outcomes in hematology: is it time to focus more on them in clinical trials and hematology practice? Blood. 2017;130(7):859–66. https://doi.org/10.1182/blood-2017-03-737403.
45. Recht M, Konkle BA, Jackson S, Neufeld EJ, Rockwood K, Pipe S. Recognizing the need for personalization of haemophilia

patient-reported outcomes in the prophylaxis era. Haemophilia. 2016;22(6):825–32. https://doi.org/10.1111/hae.13066.
46. Knisely MR, Pugh N, Kroner B, et al. Patient-reported outcomes in sickle cell disease and association with clinical and psychosocial factors: report from the sickle cell disease implementation consortium. Am J Hematol. 2020;95(9):1066–74. https://doi.org/10.1002/ajh.25880.
47. Brock KE, Wolfe J, Ullrich C. From the Child's word to clinical intervention: novel, new, and innovative approaches to symptoms in pediatric palliative care. Children. 2018;5(4):45. https://doi.org/10.3390/children5040045.
48. Horst J, Frei-Jones M, Deych E, Shannon W, Kharasch ED. Pharmacokinetics and analgesic effects of methadone in children and adults with sickle cell disease. Pediatr Blood Cancer. 2016;63(12):2123–30. https://doi.org/10.1002/pbc.26207.
49. Strokoff SL, Grossman EG. Compilation of Patient Protection and Affordable Care Act: As Amended Through November 1, 2010 Including Patient Protection and Affordable Care Act Health-Related Portions of the Health Care and Education Reconciliation Act of 2010, vol. 2010; 2010. p. 974.
50. Zebrack BJ, Stuber ML, Meeske KA, et al. Perceived positive impact of cancer among long-term survivors of childhood cancer: a report from the childhood cancer survivor study. Psychooncology. 2012;21(6):630–9. https://doi.org/10.1002/pon.1959.
51. Lindley LC, Mark BA, Daniel Lee S-Y, Domino M, Song M-K, Jacobson VJ. Factors associated with the provision of hospice care for children. J Pain Symptom Manag. 2013;45(4):701–11. https://doi.org/10.1016/j.jpainsymman.2012.03.010.
52. Lindley LC, Shaw S-L. Who are the children using hospice care? J Spec Pediatr Nurs JSPN. 2014;19(4):308–15. https://doi.org/10.1111/jspn.12085.
53. Lindley LC, Lyon ME. A profile of children with complex chronic conditions at end of life among Medicaid beneficiaries: implications for health care reform. J Palliat Med. 2013;16(11):1388–93. https://doi.org/10.1089/jpm.2013.0099.
54. Kang TI, Hexem K, Localio R, Aplenc R, Feudtner C. The use of palliative chemotherapy in pediatric oncology patients: a national survey of pediatric oncologists. Pediatr Blood Cancer. 2013;60(1):88–94. https://doi.org/10.1002/pbc.24329.
55. Johnson L-M, Leek AC, Drotar D, et al. Practical communication guidance to improve phase I informed consent conversations and decision-making in pediatric oncology. Cancer. 2015;121(14):2439–48. https://doi.org/10.1002/cncr.29354.
56. Feudtner C, Walter JK, Faerber JA, et al. Good-parent beliefs of parents of seriously ill children. JAMA Pediatr. 2015;169(1):39–47. https://doi.org/10.1001/jamapediatrics.2014.2341.
57. Snaman J, Feraco A, Wolfe J, Baker J. "What if?": addressing uncertainty with families. Pediatr Blood Cancer. 2019;66:66. https://doi.org/10.1002/pbc.27699.
58. Wolfe J, Klar N, Grier HE, et al. Understanding of prognosis among parents of children who died of cancer: impact on treatment goals and integration of palliative care. JAMA. 2000;284(19):2469. https://doi.org/10.1001/jama.284.19.2469.
59. Feudtner C. The breadth of hopes. N Engl J Med. 2009;361(24):2306–7. https://doi.org/10.1056/NEJMp0906516.
60. Folkman S. Stress, coping, and hope. Psychooncology. 2010;19(9):901–8. https://doi.org/10.1002/pon.1836.
61. Mack JW, Wolfe J, Cook EF, Grier HE, Cleary PD, Weeks JC. Hope and prognostic disclosure. J Clin Oncol Off J Am Soc Clin Oncol. 2007;25(35):5636–42. https://doi.org/10.1200/JCO.2007.12.6110.
62. Granek L, Barrera M, Shaheed J, et al. Trajectory of parental hope when a child has difficult-to-treat cancer: a prospective qualitative study. Psychooncology. 2013;22(11):2436–44. https://doi.org/10.1002/pon.3305.
63. Levetown M, Academy A, of Pediatrics Committee on Bioethics. Communicating with children and families: from everyday interactions to skill in conveying distressing information. Pediatrics. 2008;121(5):e1441–60. https://doi.org/10.1542/peds.2008-0565.
64. Wiener L, Zadeh S, Battles H, et al. Allowing adolescents and young adults to plan their end-of-life care. Pediatrics. 2012;130(5):897–905. https://doi.org/10.1542/peds.2012-0663.
65. Weaver MS, Baker JN, Gattuso JS, Gibson DV, Sykes AD, Hinds PS. Adolescents' preferences for treatment decisional involvement during their cancer. Cancer. 2015;121(24):4416–24. https://doi.org/10.1002/cncr.29663.
66. Five Wishes. Pediatrics, adolescents & young adults. https://fivewishes.org/five-wishes/individuals-families/individuals-and-families/children-and-adolescents. Accessed 17 Nov 2020.
67. Hunger SP, Lu X, Devidas M, et al. Improved survival for children and adolescents with acute lymphoblastic leukemia between 1990 and 2005: a report from the children's oncology group. J Clin Oncol Off J Am Soc Clin Oncol. 2012;30(14):1663–9. https://doi.org/10.1200/JCO.2011.37.8018.
68. Hunger SP, Raetz EA. How I treat relapsed acute lymphoblastic leukemia in the pediatric population. Blood. 2020;136(16):1803–12. https://doi.org/10.1182/blood.2019004043.
69. Manitta V, Zordan R, Cole-Sinclair M, Nandurkar H, Philip J. The symptom burden of patients with hematological malignancy: a cross-sectional observational study. J Pain Symptom Manag. 2011;42(3):432–42. https://doi.org/10.1016/j.jpainsymman.2010.12.008.
70. Grupp SA, Kalos M, Barrett D, et al. Chimeric antigen receptor-modified T cells for acute lymphoid leukemia. N Engl J Med. 2013;368(16):1509–18. https://doi.org/10.1056/NEJMoa1215134.
71. Grady D. In Girl's Last Hope, Altered immune cells beat leukemia (2012). The New York Times. https://wwwnytimescom/2012/12/10/health/a-breakthrough-against-leukemia-using-altered-t-cellshtml. Published 09 Dec 2012. Accessed 17 Nov 2020.
72. Maude SL, Frey N, Shaw PA, et al. Chimeric antigen receptor T cells for sustained remissions in leukemia. N Engl J Med. 2014;371(16):1507–17. https://doi.org/10.1056/NEJMoa1407222.
73. Whittington MD, McQueen RB, Ollendorf DA, et al. Long-term survival and value of chimeric antigen receptor T-cell therapy for pediatric patients with relapsed or refractory leukemia. JAMA Pediatr. 2018;172(12):1161–8. https://doi.org/10.1001/jamapediatrics.2018.2530.
74. Odeniyi F, Nathanson PG, Schall TE, Walter JK. Communication challenges of oncologists and intensivists caring for pediatric oncology patients: a qualitative study. J Pain Symptom Manag. 2017;54(6):909–15. https://doi.org/10.1016/j.jpainsymman.2017.06.013.
75. Kim A, Fox E, Warren K, et al. Characteristics and outcome of pediatric patients enrolled in phase I oncology trials. Oncologist. 2008;13(6):679–89. https://doi.org/10.1634/theoncologist.2008-0046.
76. Cousino MK, Zyzanski SJ, Yamokoski AD, et al. Communicating and understanding the purpose of pediatric phase I cancer trials. J Clin Oncol. 2012;30(35):4367–72. https://doi.org/10.1200/JCO.2012.42.3004.
77. Cuviello A, Boss R, Shah N, Battles H, Beri A, Wiener L. Utilization of palliative care consultations in pediatric oncology phase I clinical trials. Pediatr Blood Cancer. 2019;66(8):e27771. https://doi.org/10.1002/pbc.27771.
78. The private worlds of dying children. 1980. https://press.princeton.edu/books/paperback/9780691028200/the-private-worlds-of-dying-children. Accessed 18 Nov 2020.

79. Kreicbergs U, Valdimarsdóttir U, Onelöv E, Henter J-I, Steineck G. Talking about death with children who have severe malignant disease. N Engl J Med. 2004;351(12):1175–86. https://doi.org/10.1056/NEJMoa040366.
80. Jankovic M, Spinetta J, Riva L, Conter V, Masera C. Telling young children with leukemia their diagnosis: the flower garden as analogy. Pediatr Hematol Oncol. 1994;11(1):75–81.
81. McSherry M, Kehoe K, Carroll JM, Kang TI, Rourke MT. Psychosocial and spiritual needs of children living with a life-limiting illness. Pediatr Clin N Am. 2007;54(5):609–29; ix–x. https://doi.org/10.1016/j.pcl.2007.08.002.
82. Jones B, Currin-Mcculloch J, Pelletier W, Sardi-Brown V, Brown P, Wiener L. Psychosocial standards of care for children with cancer and their families: a national survey of pediatric oncology social workers. Soc Work Health Care. 2018;57(4):221–49. https://doi.org/10.1080/00981389.2018.1441212.
83. Ajayi TA, Edmonds KP. Palliative care answers the challenges of transitioning serious illness of childhood to adult medicine. J Palliat Med. 2014;17(4):469–71. https://doi.org/10.1089/jpm.2013.0263.
84. Jonas D, Scanlon C, Rusch R, Ito J, Joselow M. Bereavement after a Child's death. Child Adolesc Psychiatr Clin N Am. 2018;27(4):579–90. https://doi.org/10.1016/j.chc.2018.05.010.
85. Wiener L, McConnell DG, Latella L, Ludi E. Cultural and religious considerations in pediatric palliative care. Palliat Support Care. 2013;11(1):47–67. https://doi.org/10.1017/S1478951511001027.
86. Kaye EC, Gushue CA, DeMarsh S, et al. Impact of race and ethnicity on end-of-life experiences for children with cancer. Am J Hosp Palliat Care. 2019;36(9):767–74. https://doi.org/10.1177/1049909119836939.
87. Thienprayoon R, Lee SC, Leonard D, Winick N. Racial and ethnic differences in hospice enrollment among children with cancer. Pediatr Blood Cancer. 2013;60(10):1662–6. https://doi.org/10.1002/pbc.24590.
88. Ilowite MF, Cronin AM, Kang TI, Mack JW. Disparities in prognosis communication among parents of children with cancer: the impact of race and ethnicity. Cancer. 2017;123(20):3995–4003. https://doi.org/10.1002/cncr.30960.
89. Bona K, Wolfe J. Disparities in pediatric palliative care: an opportunity to strive for equity. Pediatrics. 2017;140(4):e20171662. https://doi.org/10.1542/peds.2017-1662.
90. Johnston EE, Bogetz J, Saynina O, Chamberlain LJ, Bhatia S, Sanders L. Disparities in inpatient intensity of end-of-life Care for Complex Chronic Conditions. Pediatrics. 2019;143(5):e20182228. https://doi.org/10.1542/peds.2018-2228.
91. Davies B, Larson J, Contro N, Cabrera AP. Perceptions of discrimination among Mexican American families of seriously ill children. J Palliat Med. 2011;14(1):71–6. https://doi.org/10.1089/jpm.2010.0315.
92. Foronda C, Baptiste D-L, Reinholdt MM, Ousman K. Cultural humility: a concept analysis. J Transcult Nurs. 2016;27(3):210–7. https://doi.org/10.1177/1043659615592677.
93. Kraetschmer N, Sharpe N, Urowitz S, Deber RB. How does trust affect patient preferences for participation in decision-making? Health Expect. 2004;7(4):317–26. https://doi.org/10.1111/j.1369-7625.2004.00296.x.
94. Montgomery KE, Sawin KJ, Hendricks-Ferguson V. Communication during palliative care and end of life: perceptions of experienced pediatric oncology nurses. Cancer Nurs. 2017;40(2):E47–57. https://doi.org/10.1097/NCC.0000000000000363.
95. Foster TL, Lafond DA, Reggio C, Hinds PS. Pediatric palliative Care in Childhood Cancer Nursing: from diagnosis to cure or end of life. Semin Oncol Nurs. 2010;26(4):205–21. https://doi.org/10.1016/j.soncn.2010.08.003.
96. Grech A, Depares J, Scerri J. Being on the frontline: nurses' experiences providing end-of-life care to adults with hematologic malignancies. J Hosp Palliat Nurs. 2018;20(3):237–44. https://doi.org/10.1097/NJH.0000000000000433.
97. Mehta A, Chan L. Understanding of the concept of "Total pain": a prerequisite for pain control. J Hosp Palliat Nurs. 2008;10(1):26–32. https://doi.org/10.1097/01.NJH.0000306714.50539.1a.
98. Kaye EC, Kegel A, Weber M, et al. Food is love: partnering with families to provide nourishment at the end of life. J Clin Oncol Off J Am Soc Clin Oncol. 2020;38(16):1864–7. https://doi.org/10.1200/JCO.20.00176.
99. Oxford Textbook of Palliative Nursing. Oxford University Press. https://oxfordmedicine.com/view/10.1093/med/9780199332342.001.0001/med-9780199332342. Accessed 17 Nov 2020
100. Hoell JI, Warfsmann J, Balzer S, Borkhardt A, Janssen G, Kuhlen M. End-of-life care in children with hematologic malignancies. Oncotarget. 2017;8(52):89939–48. https://doi.org/10.18632/oncotarget.21188.
101. Friebert S, Greffe B, Wheeler J. Integrating palliative care with pediatric hematology/oncology. In: Palliative care for infants, children, and adolescents: a practical handbook; 2011. p. 488–520.
102. Puchalski C, Ferrell B, Virani R, et al. Improving the quality of spiritual care as a dimension of palliative care: the report of the consensus conference. J Palliat Med. 2009;12(10):885–904. https://doi.org/10.1089/jpm.2009.0142.
103. Lion AH, Skiles JL, Watson BN, Young JD, Torke AM. Chaplain care in pediatric oncology: insight for interprofessional collaboration. Pediatr Blood Cancer. 2019;66(12):e27971. https://doi.org/10.1002/pbc.27971.
104. Koenig H, King D, Carson VB. Handbook of religion and health. 2nd ed. Oxford University Press; 2012.
105. Purow B, Alisanski S, Putnam G, Ruderman M. Spirituality and pediatric cancer. South Med J. 2011;104(4):299–302. https://doi.org/10.1097/SMJ.0b013e3182083f40.
106. Ennis-Durstine RK, Brown RM. Spiritual Care in Pediatric Oncology. In: Abrams AN, Muriel AC, Wiener L, editors. Pediatric psychosocial oncology: textbook for multidisciplinary care. Springer International Publishing; 2016. p. 327–37. https://doi.org/10.1007/978-3-319-21374-3_18.
107. Fitchett G, Murphy PE, Kim J, Gibbons JL, Cameron JR, Davis JA. Religious struggle: prevalence, correlates and mental health risks in diabetic, congestive heart failure, and oncology patients. Int J Psychiatry Med. 2004;34(2):179–96. https://doi.org/10.2190/UCJ9-DP4M-9C0X-835M.
108. Hui D, Bruera E. Models of integration of oncology and palliative care. Ann Palliat Med. 2015;4(3):898.
109. Wachholtz AB, Pearce MJ. Does spirituality as a coping mechanism help or hinder coping with chronic pain? Curr Pain Headache Rep. 2009;13(2):127–32. https://doi.org/10.1007/s11916-009-0022-0.
110. Ullrich CK, Lehmann L, London WB, et al. End-of-life care patterns associated with pediatric palliative care among children who underwent hematopoietic stem cell transplant. Biol Blood Marrow Transplant. 2016;22(6):1049–55. https://doi.org/10.1016/j.bbmt.2016.02.012.
111. Foster TL, Gilmer MJ, Davies B, et al. Bereaved parents' and siblings' reports of legacies created by children with cancer. J Pediatr Oncol Nurs. 2009;26(6):369–76. https://doi.org/10.1177/1043454209340322.
112. Foster TL, Dietrich MS, Friedman DL, Gordon JE, Gilmer MJ. National survey of children's hospitals on legacy-making activities. J Palliat Med. 2012;15(5):573–8. https://doi.org/10.1089/jpm.2011.0447.
113. Riordan PA, Price M, Robbins-Welty GA, et al. Top ten tips palliative care clinicians should know about bereavement and

grief. J Palliat Med. 2020;23:1098. https://doi.org/10.1089/jpm.2020.0341.
114. Jones BL, Contro N, Koch KD. The duty of the physician to care for the family in pediatric palliative care: context, communication, and caring. Pediatrics. 2014;133(Suppl 1):S8–15. https://doi.org/10.1542/peds.2013-3608C.
115. Jalmsell L, Onelöv E, Steineck G, Henter J-I, Kreicbergs U. Hematopoietic stem cell transplantation in children with cancer and the risk of long-term psychological morbidity in the bereaved parents. Bone Marrow Transplant. 2011;46(8):1063–70. https://doi.org/10.1038/bmt.2010.287.
116. Field MJ, Behrman RE. Institute of Medicine (US) committee on palliative and end-of-life care for children and their families. In: Field MJ, Behrman RE, editors. When children die: improving palliative and end-of-life care for children and their families. National Academies Press (US); 2003; http://www.ncbi.nlm.nih.gov/books/NBK220818/. Accessed 18 Nov 2020.
117. Macdonald ME, Liben S, Carnevale F, et al. Parental perspectives on hospital staff members' acts of kindness and commemoration after a Child's death. Pediatrics. 2005;116:884–90. https://doi.org/10.1542/peds.2004-1980.
118. Rusch R, Greenman J, Scanlon C, Horne K, Jonas DF. Bibliotherapy and bereavement: harnessing the power of Reading to enhance family coping in pediatric palliative care. J Soc Work End--Life Palliat Care. 2020;16(2):85–98. https://doi.org/10.1080/15524256.2020.1745728.
119. Youngblut JM, Brooten D. What children wished they had/had not done and their coping in the first thirteen months after their Sibling's neonatal/pediatric intensive care unit/emergency department death. J Palliat Med. 2021;24(2):226–32. https://doi.org/10.1089/jpm.2019.0538.
120. Gaab EM, Owens GR, MacLeod RD. Siblings caring for and about pediatric palliative care patients. J Palliat Med. 2014;17(1):62–7. https://doi.org/10.1089/jpm.2013.0117.
121. Sanchez-Reilly S, Morrison LJ, Carey E, et al. Caring for oneself to care for others: physicians and their self-care. J Support Oncol. 2013;11(2):75–81.
122. Mills J, Wand T, Fraser JA. Examining self-care, self-compassion and compassion for others: a cross-sectional survey of palliative care nurses and doctors. Int J Palliat Nurs. 2018;24(1):4–11. https://doi.org/10.12968/ijpn.2018.24.1.4.

# Palliative Care for Adolescents and Young Adults (AYAs)

# 21

Natalie Jewitt and Alisha Kassam

## Epidemiology of Hematologic Cancers and Serious Blood Disorders in AYAs

Adolescents and young adults (AYAs) are an important population with age-related challenges that make their illness experience distinct from their younger and older counterparts. Various definitions have been used to define AYAs, although 15–39 years of age is now the standard accepted by the National Cancer Institute [1].

The three most common types of cancers in AYAs are thyroid, breast, and lymphoma [2] (Fig. 21.1). However, the incidence of hematologic cancers varies substantially within AYA cohorts. For example, leukemia and lymphomas account for 36% of cancer diagnoses in younger AYAs (aged 15–19), compared to approximately 11% in older AYAs (aged 30–39) [2]. Importantly, hematologic malignancies are also a major cause of death in AYAs, accounting for over 18% of cancer deaths in males and approximately 11% in females [2] (Fig. 21.2).

For non-malignant, serious blood disorders, exact prevalence in AYAs has not been well defined. Serious blood disorders represent a diverse diagnostic group including bone marrow failure syndromes, aplastic anemias, and sickle cell disease. Bone marrow failure peaks in young childhood due to inherited conditions, and again in early adulthood, typically due to acquired causes [3]. Sickle cell disease is estimated to affect 100,000 Americans across age groups [4] and with improvements in care, most children with sickle cell disease now survive into young adulthood [5]. This heterogenous group therefore represents an increasingly important population of AYAs with distinct needs.

It is well established that AYAs have not benefited from the same improvements in survival over the past few decades compared to children and adults [6]. Over the last 40 years, pediatric mortality rates in sickle cell anemia have declined, while AYA mortality has increased [7]. In hematologic malignancies, despite treatment advances, survival rates for AYAs have not reached the levels achieved by children [8]. These differences are partially related to unique biology, as AYAs are more likely to have unfavorable biologic features than children with the same diagnoses [9]. Additional barriers to achieving optimal outcomes include a delayed presentation [10], difficulties with treatment adherence, and limited or lack of healthcare insurance [8]. Inferior outcomes in AYAs also reflect the historical evolution of separate healthcare sectors devoted to pediatric and adult care [8]. For AYAs with sickle cell disease, the time of transition to adult care in particular is associated with increased mortality [5]. As AYAs exist on the periphery of both pediatric and adult populations, they have not represented the "typical" patient on which research efforts have focused [8]. As a result, they are also less likely to be referred to or participate in clinical trials [11]. Furthermore, AYAs, by definition, live in a period of developmental transition, which leads to countless psychosocial vulnerabilities that can impact treatment success [12].

N. Jewitt
Paediatric Advanced Care Team (PACT), Department of Paediatrics, The Hospital for Sick Children, Toronto, Canada
e-mail: natalie.jewitt@sickkids.ca

A. Kassam (✉)
Department of Pediatric Oncology and Palliative Medicine, Southlake Regional Health Centre, Newmarket, ON, Canada
e-mail: akassam@southlakeregional.org



C. K. Ullrich, E. J. Roeland (eds.), *Palliative Care in Hematologic Malignancies and Serious Blood Disorders*,
https://doi.org/10.1007/978-3-031-38058-7_21

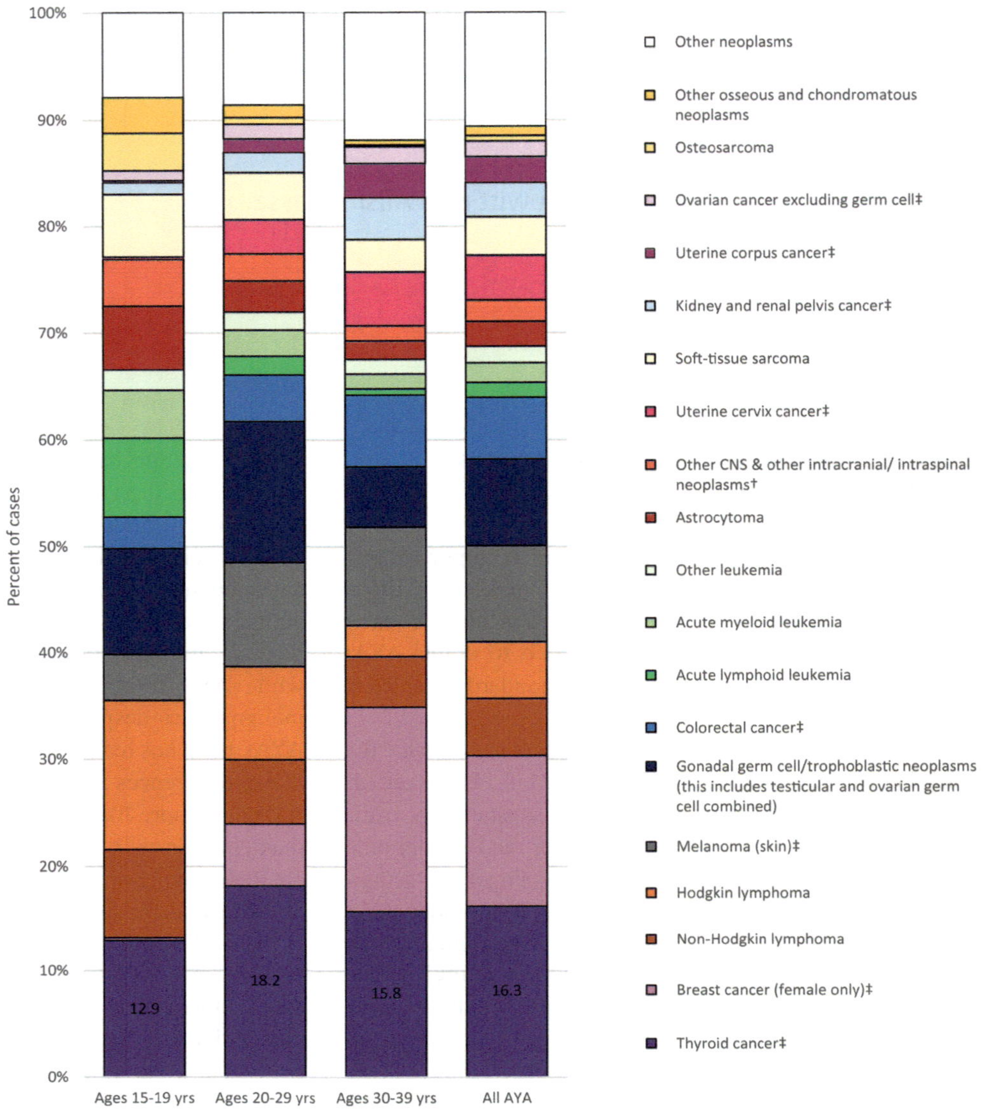


**Fig. 21.1** Case distribution (%) of selected AYA cancer types by age group, 2011 to 2015 [2]. †Excludes benign and borderline brain cancers. ‡Coding for these cancers is based on Surveillance, Epidemiology, and End Results site recode International Classification of Diseases for Oncology, third edition/World Health Organization 2008 definitions. Kidney includes renal pelvis. CNS indicates the central nervous system. Source: Case distribution, North American Association of Central Cancer Registries public use database, 2018, as cited in Close A. Adolescent and young adult oncology—past, present, and future. *CA* cancer journal for clinicians 69 (6):2019

**Fig. 21.2** Percent of AYA cancer deaths (2012–2016) for patients ages 15–39 years [2]. Reproduced with permission of Close et al. (2019). Abbreviations: AAPC, average annual percent change; CNS, central nervous system. [a]AAPCs are based on joinpoint models using 1970 to 2016 mortality data, allowing for up to 5 joinpoints. [b]Percentages are not shown because of sparse data (<10 deaths during 2012–2016). [c]The AAPC is statistically different from zero ($P < 0.05$)

| CANCER TYPE | CANCER DEATHS 2012-2016, % | | AAPC 2007-2016, %[a] | |
|---|---|---|---|---|
| | MALES | FEMALES | MALES | FEMALES |
| Leukemia | | | | |
| Acute lymphocytic | 5.0 | 2.4 | −0.8[b] | −2.0[b] |
| Acute myeloid | 5.1 | 4.2 | −0.7[b] | −1.7[b] |
| Brain and CNS | 13.8 | 8.4 | 0.6 | 1.0 |
| Colorectal | 11.0 | 8.1 | 1.1[b] | 0.6[b] |
| Lymphoma | | | | |
| Non-Hodgkin lymphoma | 6.0 | 3.2 | −4.1[b] | −4.9[b] |
| Hodgkin lymphoma | 2.0 | 1.3 | −5.1[b] | −10.0[b] |
| Soft tissue | 6.1 | 4.1 | −0.3[b] | −0.7[b] |
| Bone and joints | 5.3 | 2.6 | 0.6[b] | 0.5[b] |
| Melanoma of the skin | 4.3 | 2.9 | −3.4[b] | −2.8[b] |
| Thyroid | 0.3 | 0.3 | −0.6 | −1.0[b] |
| Kidney and renal pelvis | 2.4 | —[c] | 2.2 | −1.4[b] |
| Testis | 4.1 | —[c] | 0.2 | |
| Breast | —[c] | 22.2 | | −0.2 |
| Ovary | —[c] | 4.6 | | −1.5[b] |
| Uterine cervix | —[c] | 9.5 | | −0.1 |
| Uterine corpus | —[c] | 2.3 | | 2.8[b] |

## Challenges Facing AYAs with Hematologic Cancer and Serious Blood Disorders

The AYA life stage is one of transition and personal growth; it often includes finishing school, pursuing a career, and starting a family. It is typically a time of increasing independence, where youth progressively form their individual adult identities [13] and personal social networks [14]. AYAs living with chronic serious blood disorders must adapt to the challenges of emerging adulthood while simultaneously navigating the transition from pediatric to adult care. These challenges include shifting parental-AYA healthcare responsibilities, finding a new adult healthcare provider, learning the nuances of emergency care, and understanding medications and symptoms [15]. In contrast, AYAs newly diagnosed with cancer experience an unexpected disruption to their future plans [16]. These implications are far-reaching, impacting many aspects of life, such as peer relations, family dynamics, fertility, and educational plans [16] (Fig. 21.3). Rather than increasing independence, AYAs facing an oncologic diagnosis may find themselves unable to study or work, which can have long-term career implications [17]. AYAs with cancer may find themselves unexpectedly financially and physically reliant on others for their day-to-day necessities. This regressive dependency on parents or loved ones can have a significant impact on one's sense of identity [17] and lead to increased distress and decreased treatment adherence [18].

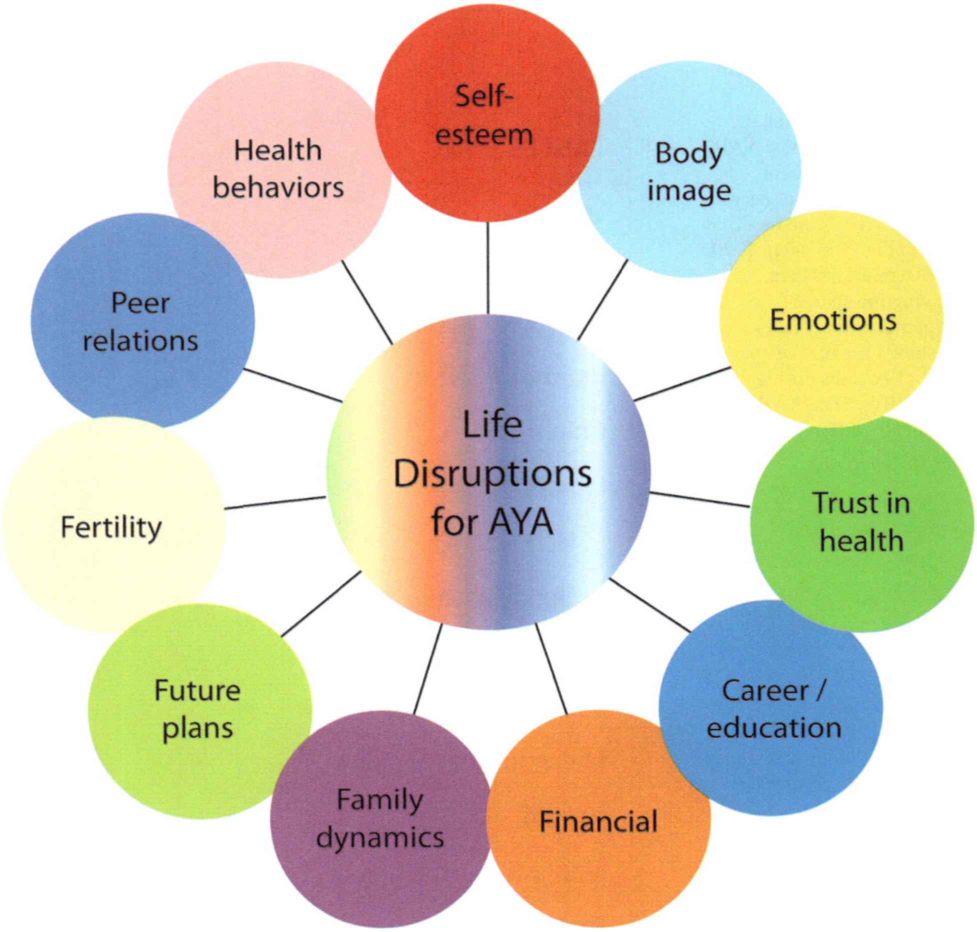


**Fig. 21.3** Possible life disruptions for AYA patients with cancer [54]. Reproduced with permission from Nass et al. (2015)

Late teenage and early adult years often involve developing intimate and romantic relationships. While typical AYAs establish their own sexual identity, AYAs may face disease or treatment-related physical changes that can impact self-esteem [18]. These physical differences may impact AYAs' interest in engaging in sexual relationships and their ability to form romantic connections. Approximately half of AYAs endorse their cancer diagnosis has harmed sexual function [19]. Sexual dysfunction remains an unmet concern for many AYAs up to 2 years after diagnosis [20]. Rather than forming or building on existing relationships, AYAs may feel unable to form new romantic relationships and experience strain on existing relationships [17]. In long-term relationships, youth may question their partners' motivations to stay together and wonder if their partner is experiencing feelings of guilt and obligation [10].

Due to the transitional life stage of AYAs and challenges developing and maintaining romantic relationships, youth may reside with their parents, their spouse, or a combination. This situation can lead to various preferences for individual or shared decision-making when it comes to treatment choices [21]. Decision-making preferences are often a process, and do not abruptly change when an adolescent turns 18. Many AYAs want to make medical decisions after reflection on their parents' opinions, and others prefer shared decision-making with their spouse [21]. Some patients may bring both their spouse and parent to medical appointments with them for support. These preferences may evolve over one's illness journey, and it is important for clinicians to continually check-in with AYAs about their wishes.

The AYA life stage is also a time where healthy youth engage in experimentation and substance use. Preconceptions about substance use and misuse in AYAs can negatively impact care. Specifically, healthcare providers' assumptions about drug-seeking behavior in AYAs with sickle cell disease can lead to inadequate pain management and avoidance of emergency care [15]. There are often concerns that AYAs with cancer are at increased risk for substance abuse due to access to legitimate opioid prescriptions [22]. However,

AYAs with cancer have reported similar substance and illicit drug use as age-matched peers [22]. Furthermore, rates of opioid misuse are similar in AYAs with cancer to adult oncology patients [23].

There are also differences in how AYAs routinely interact with the healthcare system. Compared to pediatric patients, AYAs are more likely to delay seeking medical care following symptom development [10]. This delay may be related to feelings of invincibility, embarrassment, or denial [24]. AYAs also less often identify with a clear primary care clinician, leading to less frequent routine health checks [10]. In the sickle cell population, this leads to increased reliance on emergency room care during the adolescent and young adult years [25]. Furthermore, AYAs face significant challenges complying with treatment recommendations [26, 27]. As many as half of AYAs may not adhere to outpatient therapy plans [26]. Cognitive-emotional factors, lack of peer and family support, and the youth's relationship with their clinician have all been shown to impact treatment adherence [27].

## Symptom Distress in AYAs with Hematologic Cancer and Serious Blood Disorders

Advanced illness in AYAs leads to symptoms of physical, psychological, and existential distress. Many physical symptoms may be similar to those experienced by younger and older populations; however, unique psychosocial factors may influence the symptom burden experienced by AYAs.

In AYAs with cancer referred for palliative care, pain is the most commonly reported physical symptom (endorsed by 91% of patients) [28]. As a result, most adolescents with cancer reportedly use pain medication at the end of life (EOL) [29]. Diminished well-being, fatigue, and anorexia are also frequently experienced (endorsed by 76%, 75%, and 67% of patients, respectively) [28]. Pain, fatigue, and edema are the most common physical symptoms reported in AYAs post-hematopoietic cell transplantation (HCT), documented in over 80% of patients in the last month of life [30] (Fig. 21.4). Compared to patients with central nervous sys-

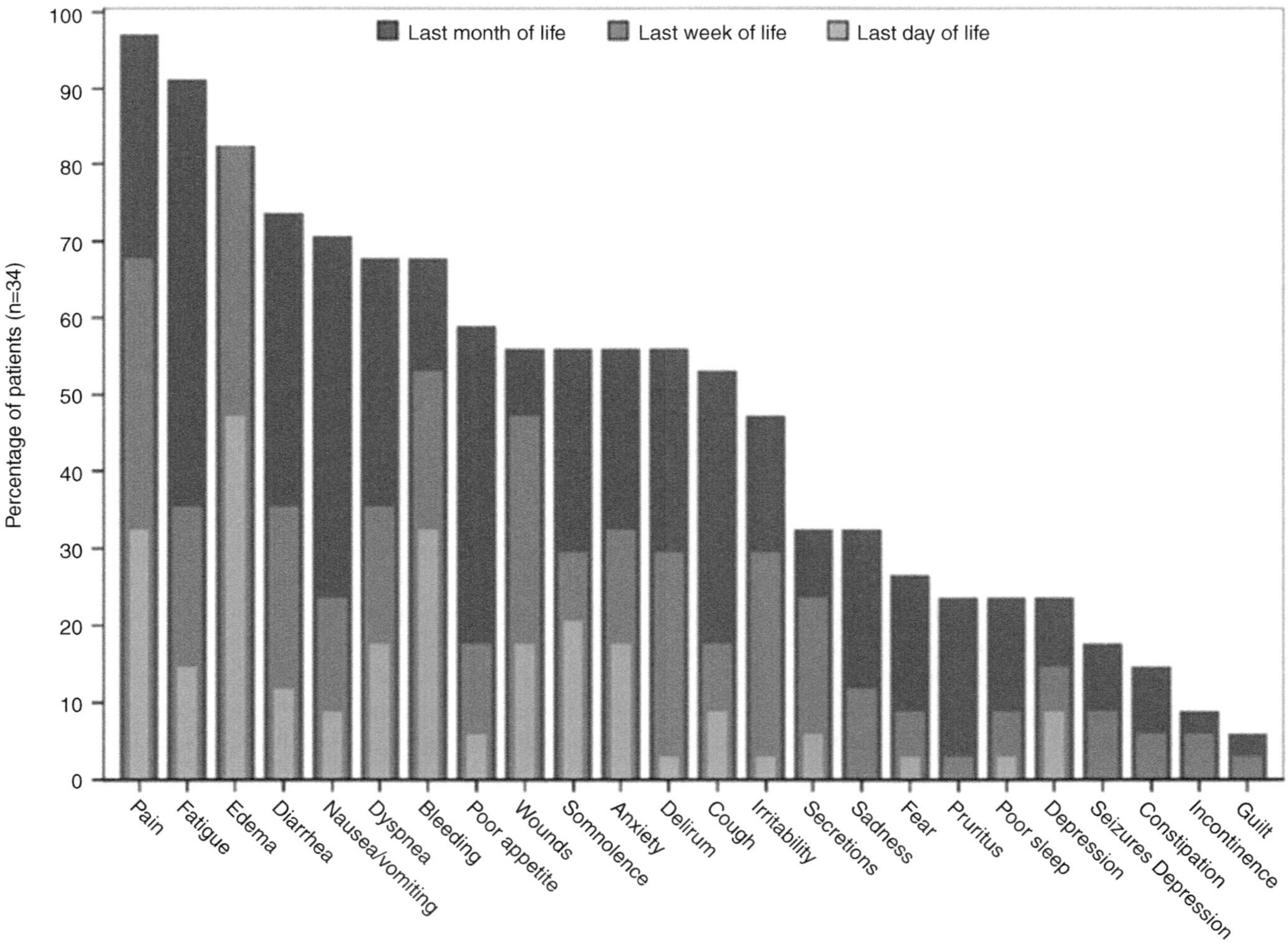


**Fig. 21.4** Symptoms present during the last month, last week, and last day of life for AYA patients who received allogeneic hematopoietic cell transplant and died while inpatient at St Jude ($n = 34$) [30]. Reproduced with permission from Snaman (2017)

tem (CNS) tumors, adolescents diagnosed with leukemia or lymphoma are more likely to use oxygen at EOL [29].

In AYAs with sickle cell disease, death is often due to a sudden deterioration such as an acute pulmonary or cardiovascular event [31]. The experience of physical symptoms is therefore specific to the presenting event, such as dyspnea in acute chest syndrome, or neurological symptoms associated with stroke. Moreover, the real possibility of sudden death can lead to significant fear [32]. Psychological suffering, such as symptoms of depression and anxiety, is common in adolescents with sickle cell disease [33]. AYAs with cancer also report higher mental health concerns than age-matched peers [19]. Although feelings of anxiety, fear, and sadness are common across all ages at the EOL, AYAs experience more anxiety and depression than their younger counterparts [34]. At EOL, the use of anti-anxiety medications has been reported as significantly higher in late adolescents (aged 18–21) compared to early adolescents (aged 10–13) [29]. Anxiety and delirium were the most commonly experienced psychological symptoms in AYAs post-HCT, occurring in over 50% of patients admitted to hospital in the last month of life [30]. This pattern of increased psychological symptoms may reflect higher rates of intensive medical interventions when compared to non-HCT AYA oncology patients. Frequent assessments and prompt management of psychological symptoms in this high-risk population is essential.

Grappling with advanced illness and EOL, many AYAs also face existential distress. Rather than feelings of invincibility enjoyed by their healthy peers, premature awareness of mortality confronts AYAs with life-limiting illnesses [35]. Many adolescents also worry about being a burden to their loved ones [36]. Compared to older adults, what is important to AYAs at EOL is undoubtedly different [37]. Facing death while parenting young children, rather than adult offspring, brings a unique distress level [37]. Young adults facing EOL, who are parents themselves, often worry about being a strain on their children [38]. Processing some of these complex emotions during the experience of illness can lead to inward reflection and a search for purpose. For some AYAs who identify as religious, faith can remain a source of support and meaning, whereas others question their beliefs and faith in God [39]. Regardless of religiosity, most AYAs endorse spiritual concerns such as quests for purpose and legacy creation [39]. At the EOL, having adequate pain control, feeling physically comfortable, and finding spiritual peace, has been reported as most important for adolescents [36].

Given the transitional period of the AYA life stage, the importance of social support is paramount. AYAs with chronic hematologic conditions such as sickle cell disease, often lean on existing peer support to navigate transition [15]. Unfortunately, AYAs facing cancer frequently experience isolation from healthy peers due to their increased medical needs [40]. With advancing disease, AYAs may experience further isolation from those AYAs with cancer still pursuing curative treatment [40]. Interestingly, a study by Geue et al. (2019) found that AYAs with hematologic malignancies reported similar positive social supports to older oncology patients [14]. However, AYAs were more likely to report detrimental social interactions (e.g., people in their lives made suggestions that they found unhelpful or upsetting) than older counterparts [14]. These interactions may be related to larger social networks or less well-established social relationships in AYAs. Alternatively, it may reflect younger peer supports who are less familiar with advanced illness and uncertain about how to support their friend. Recognizing the unique social networks of AYAs and offering to help AYAs navigate those relationships is essential in providing appropriate care. Clinicians with psychosocial expertise (such as social workers) can be an excellent resource.

In terms of the care received, most AYAs are high users of medically intensive care towards EOL [13]. In the sickle cell population, compared to children and older adults, young adults (aged 22–40 years) had the highest rates of emergency room deaths, with 20% dying in the emergency room [32]. In a cross-sectional study using cancer registry data, Mack et al. (2015) explored EOL care in AYA oncology patients [13]. They found that the majority of AYAs received at least one form of high-intensity medical care in the last month of life (22% were admitted to the intensive care unit (ICU); 22% had >1 emergency room visit, and 62% were hospitalized) [13]. In their cohort, AYAs with leukemia were higher users of medically intensive EOL care than patients with soft tissue or gastrointestinal cancers [13]. Snaman et al. (2018) similarly found that nearly 80% of AYA after HCT died in hospital, and many received high-intensity care such as mechanical ventilation and dialysis in the last month of life [30]. Bell et al. (2010) looked at the EOL experience of younger adolescents aged 10–21 years [29]. They found that in adolescents who continued to receive aggressive life-sustaining measures at EOL, most were patients with leukemia or lymphoma [29]. Furthermore, more adolescents with leukemia or lymphoma died in the ICU than patients with solid tumors or CNS cancers [29]. This finding in part may be due to higher rates of treatment related mortality in AYAs with hematologic cancers. Additionally, AYAs with hematologic malignancies or serious blood disorders may have unique disease specific needs that can be challenging to manage as an outpatient. For example, AYAs with refractory leukemia may derive symptomatic benefit from frequent transfusion support that practically may not be feasible in certain community settings.

Although the use of high-intensity care has consistently been demonstrated in AYAs, it remains unclear if continued hospitalization or medical intensive care is aligned with the goals of care of those patients that receive it. These findings emphasize the need to explore further the wishes of AYAs and optimal strategies to ease suffering.

## Easing Suffering in AYAs with Hematologic Malignancies and Serious Blood Disorders

Exploring the goals of care of AYAs with advanced illness is essential to ease suffering and deliver optimal care. Numerous practice guidelines highlight the importance of the early introduction of a palliative care team to an AYA before symptom escalation or the discontinuation of curative treatment [41]. This early introduction allows for exploration of goals of care and rapport building while decreasing time pressure on challenging EOL conversations. Early introduction of palliative care is also essential for AYAs with serious blood disorders who are at risk for premature death [32]. Many patients and clinicians may want to avoid the early introduction of palliative care due to perceptions that palliative care means "giving up" or discontinuing active therapy [40]. Educating patients, families, and caregivers on an expanded definition of palliative care can help increase comfort and normalize palliative care involvement. Clinicians should highlight that palliative care focuses on quality of life, not only for the patient but the entire family [42]. The focus on quality of life is often beneficial independent of prognosis and/or treatment goals. Symptom management and EOL care are important although only partial, parts of delivering optimal palliative care.

For the alleviation of EOL pain and dyspnea in AYAs, similar to children and adults, opioids remain the mainstay of treatment [43]. Studies to date have not demonstrated differences in pharmacodynamics in AYAs compared to older adults [43]. Methadone has also been shown to provide effective analgesia of both nociceptive and neuropathic pain in adolescents with leukemia and lymphoma [44]. Consider gabapentin/pregabalin and duloxetine for neuropathic pain management, such as vincristine-related neuropathy [45, 46]. Of note, gabapentinoids require titration and time to reach therapeutic levels [47], and therefore should be introduced before the last weeks of life. In AYAs with leukemia and lymphoma, other EOL symptoms, such as bleeding, can be treated with similar strategies for younger and older patients.

To address psychological symptoms in AYAs, providing professional support through social workers, music therapists, and psychologists is invaluable [40]. Asking about an AYA's spiritual beliefs can be a helpful starting point to explore hopes and worries and to determine how to best provide support [39] (Fig. 21.5). Flexible scheduling that accommodates late awakenings in AYAs can promote connection and continuity of care [48]. Using virtual care where possible, may also decrease travel time and minimize disruption to an AYA's school or work commitments. Clinicians must also recognize the unique social networks of AYAs and find creative solutions to combat feelings of social isolation. To facilitate connection, hospice facilities should include shared spaces that promote interaction [40]. Furthermore, the innovative use of technology for video conferencing and social networking can provide an alternative medium to

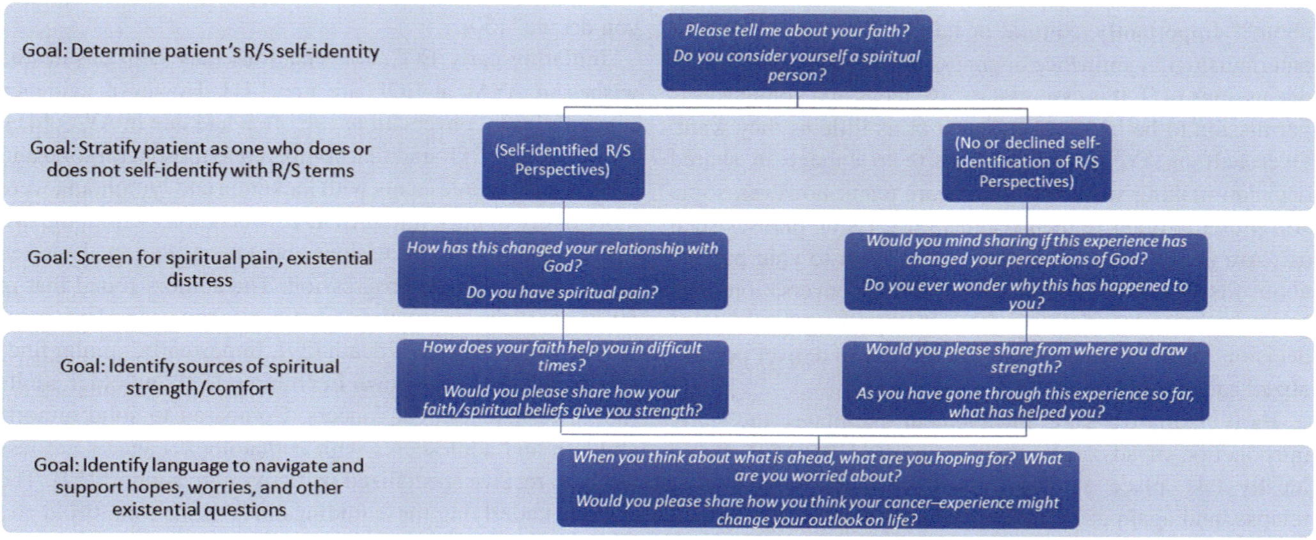


**Fig. 21.5** A conceptual framework for navigating discussions of religion, spirituality, and hope with AYA who do/do not immediately endorse religious/spiritual (R/S) beliefs [39]. Italicized phrases are sample questions to use in conversation. This framework does not necessarily reflect a single discussion; rather, clinicians may use it to navigate ongoing discussions spanning screening, spiritual history taking, and assessments of religious/spiritual supportive needs. Reproduced with permission from Barton (2018)

maintain relationships between AYAs [40]. For AYAs who are parents themselves, supporting AYAs in communication with their own children is essential. Parents want assistance and resources from care providers to help explain their illness to their children [49]. Connecting families with child life and grief support specialists can help parents navigate these difficult conversations.

In addition to addressing physical and psychological symptoms, clear communication and planning around EOL are essential for AYAs. Adolescents report that honesty from their healthcare team is important [36]. However, many clinicians find EOL conversations with AYAs challenging. As experts in communication, palliative care clinicians have unique expertise in navigating difficult discussions. Involving a palliative care team also provides an opportunity for AYAs to share fears or worries that they may not wish to share with their primary treating team. Effective communication with AYAs requires recognition of the complex interaction of their social context and developmental stage [41]. First asking about an AYA's understanding of their illness and specific worries or wishes they have may provide a starting place for more difficult EOL discussions. AYAs may still be developing their cognitive capacities to reflect on EOL issues and may have limited or no experience with death and dying [41]. Recognizing a youth's developmental stage and adjusting language and concepts to their cognitive abilities is essential. Providing examples of questions other patients have asked about death and dying, and acknowledging feelings of distress in others can also normalize the experience and create a space for further discussion [48]. For example, clinicians may ask, "Other patients in a similar situation have asked me what will happen if there is progression on their next scan. Is that something you have been wondering about?" Importantly, cultural or family beliefs in protective paternalism may influence openness to involve AYAs in EOL discussions [41]. It is essential to give teens and young adults permission to be involved as much or as little as they want. Over half of AYAs express a desire to engage in shared decision-making with their healthcare team; however, some still prefer to defer to their parents [21]. Using phrases such as, "Are there things you would rather I talk to your parents about first?" can help introduce difficult conversations and honor individual preferences [50]. Recognizing the range of decision-making preferences is imperative to deliver personalized care for AYAs.

Early palliative care involvement facilitates the early introduction of advance care planning (ACP). ACP should ideally take place at diagnosis, throughout treatment, at relapse, and again at EOL [42]. Transitions in the treatment plan, such as stem cell transplant, can create a natural opportunity to discuss uncertainty and EOL [29]. Gentle but recurring ACP discussions create numerous opportunities to explore AYAs' wishes [50]. To assess AYAs' readiness to engage in ACP, clinicians can utilize the Advance Care Planning Readiness Assessment (2008) developed by Pao and Wiener [51]. The measure asks three questions:

1. "Whether talking about what would happen if treatments were no longer effective would be helpful
2. Whether talking about medical care plans ahead of time would be upsetting
3. Whether they would be comfortable writing down/discussing what would happen if treatments were no longer effective" [51].

An adolescent's answers to these questions can be a practical starting point for conversation. If adolescents report such conversations would be upsetting, allowing space and time before revisiting these topics is important. For some patients, talking in advance is unhelpful, and following the lead of each individual AYA is essential. Additional strategies to introduce and normalize discussions about EOL include the concept of parallel planning. It can help to explain that we continue to hope for the best while simultaneously plan for the rest [29]. This explanation promotes discussion without eliminating hope. This can be particularly important for AYAs who continue to discuss future plans, such as school or career goals. Remaining future oriented does not necessarily indicate a lack of illness understanding or denial. Rather, it may highlight holding hope and worry simultaneously. Again, sharing experiences of other patients can be helpful when exploring goals of care. For instance, when discussing disease progression, consider stating, "Some people say they want to be home with their family and others say it is important to keep trying new medications. There is no wrong answer here, and we will support you no matter what you decide" [50].

Initiating early EOL conversations may help ensure the wishes of AYAs at EOL are met [41]. However, evidence suggests EOL conversations are often had late in AYAs [41]. Bell et al. (2010) found that compared to those with solid and CNS tumors, adolescents with leukemia and lymphoma were more likely to have initial EOL conversations within the last 7 days of life [29]. Discussions about resuscitation also often occur late in disease progression. The authors found that in 50% of their population, donot-resuscitate orders were signed within 7 days of death [29]. Importantly, similar findings have also been shown in children [52] and older adults [53] with hematologic cancers. Compared to solid tumors, children and adolescents with hematologic cancers are less likely to receive specialized palliative care support [52]. The reasons underlying these findings in AYAs are multifold and include provider inexperience with advanced care planning discussions, clinician desire to protect the AYA and pressure from caregivers to focus on anti-cancer treatments when facing the loss of a young person.

**Table 21.1** AYA Advance Care Planning Tools

| Resource | Description | Link |
|---|---|---|
| *Voicing my choices* | An AYA focused advance care planning document | https://store.fivewishes.org/ShopLocal/en/p/VC-MASTER-000/voicing-my-choices [55] |
| *Five wishes* | A legal document that designates a healthcare decision-maker for EOL and medical care | https://www.fivewishes.org/for-myself/ [55] |
| *Living out loud* | An online Canadian resource with significant patient contributions and a comprehensive resource section for discussing EOL and advance care planning with AYAs | https://livingoutloud.life [56] |
| *Together for short lives* | A UK website that contains helpful resources to guide difficult discussions with AYAs | https://www.togetherforshortlives.org.uk/get-support/supporting-you/family-resources/difficult-conversations-young-adults/ [57] |

The majority of AYAs express a wish to discuss EOL care in advance; however, many AYAs had never heard of an advance directive [36]. The use of ACP tools can help facilitate and structure EOL conversations with AYAs and their families [41]. Multiple tools exist and are outlined in Table 21.1.

Location of care is also a critical discussion to initiate with AYAs and their families. In a study conducted by Jacobs et al. (2015), 88% of AYAs did not know that hospice care was available or what it entailed [36]. Individual factors such as having children or elderly parents in the home may influence preferred location of care. Most adolescents discuss a preference for dying at home [36]. However, this preference contrasts findings that many AYAs receive medically intensive care in the ICU or inpatient ward in their final weeks of life [13]. This fact highlights the importance of educating patients and their families on available care options and exploring patients' wishes in advance. Only then can clinicians facilitate the care plan that most closely reflects the AYA and their family's values.

## Summary

AYAs represent an important group of patients facing serious hematologic disease. Their unique position, bridging pediatric and adult populations, is associated with unfavorable outcomes and complex psychosocial challenges. Recognizing the impact of an existing serious blood disorder or a cancer diagnosis during this pivotal time of identity formation and establishing relationships is essential. Early exploration of communication preferences and goals of care can improve the care team's ability to provide personalized EOL care aligned with patient values. Many tools exist to aid the clinician in ACP and EOL discussions. Early involvement of palliative care teams can assist primary teams in navigating these difficult discussions, aid in symptom management and ensure focus on quality of life. AYAs with cancer and serious blood disorders are not simply big children or small adults; they are a distinctive group that requires customized expert care.

## References


1. Henley SJ, Ward EM, Scott S, Ma J, Anderson RN, Firth AU, et al. Annual report to the nation on the status of cancer, part I: national cancer statistics. Cancer. 2020;126(10):2225–49. https://doi.org/10.1002/cncr.32802.
2. Close AG, Dreyzin A, Miller KD, Seynnaeve BKN, Rapkin LB. Adolescent and young adult oncology-past, present, and future. CA Cancer J Clin. 2019;69(6):485–96. https://doi.org/10.3322/caac.21585.
3. Moore C, Krishnan K. Bone marrow failure. Treasure Island, Fl: StatPearls Publishing; 2020. https://www.ncbi.nlm.nih.gov/books/NBK459249/
4. Hassell KL. Population estimates of sickle cell disease in the U.S. Am J Prev Med. 2010;38(4 Suppl):S512–21. https://doi.org/10.1016/j.amepre.2009.12.022.
5. Quinn CT, Rogers ZR, McCavit TL, Buchanan GR. Improved survival of children and adolescents with sickle cell disease. Blood. 2010;115(17):3447–52. https://doi.org/10.1182/blood-2009-07-233700.
6. Veal GJ, Hartford CM, Stewart CF. Clinical pharmacology in the adolescent oncology patient. J Clin Oncol. 2010;28(32):4790–9. https://doi.org/10.1200/jco.2010.28.3473.
7. Kayle M, Docherty SL, Sloane R, Tanabe P, Maslow G, Pan W, et al. Transition to adult care in sickle cell disease: a longitudinal study of clinical characteristics and disease severity. Pediatr Blood Cancer. 2019;66(1):e27463. https://doi.org/10.1002/pbc.27463.
8. Wood WA, Lee SJ. Malignant hematologic diseases in adolescents and young adults. Blood. 2011;117(22):5803–15. https://doi.org/10.1182/blood-2010-12-283093.
9. Tricoli JV, Bleyer A. Adolescent and young adult cancer biology. Cancer J(Sudbury, Mass). 2018;24(6):f–74. https://doi.org/10.1097/ppo.0000000000000343.
10. Albritton K, Bleyer WA. The management of cancer in the older adolescent. Eur J Cancer (Oxford, England: 1990). 2003;39(18):2584–99. https://doi.org/10.1016/j.ejca.2003.09.013.
11. Burke ME, Albritton K, Marina N. Challenges in the recruitment of adolescents and young adults to cancer clinical trials. Cancer. 2007;110(11):2385–93. https://doi.org/10.1002/cncr.23060.
12. Ferrari A, Barr RD. International evolution in AYA oncology: Current status and future expectations. Pediatr Blood Cancer. 2017;64(9):e26528. https://doi.org/10.1002/pbc.26528.
13. Mack JW, Chen LH, Cannavale K, Sattayapiwat O, Cooper RM, Chao CR. End-of-life care intensity among adolescent and young adult patients with cancer in Kaiser Permanente Southern California. JAMA Oncol. 2015;1(5):592–600. https://doi.org/10.1001/jamaoncol.2015.1953.
14. Geue K, Götze H, Friedrich M, Leuteritz K, Mehnert-Theuerkauf A, Sender A, et al. Perceived social support and associations with

health-related quality of life in young versus older adult patients with haematological malignancies. Health Qual Life Outcomes. 2019;17(1):145. 10.1186/s12955-019-1202-1
15. Porter JS, Wesley KM, Zhao MS, Rupff RJ, Hankins JS. Pediatric to adult care transition: perspectives of young adults with sickle cell disease. J Pediatr Psychol. 2017;42(9):1016–27. https://doi.org/10.1093/jpepsy/jsx088.
16. IOM (Institute of Medicine). Identifying and addressing the needs of adolescents and young adults with cancer: workshop summary. Washington, DC: The National Academies Press; 2013.
17. Place AE, Frederick NN, Sallan SE. Therapeutic approaches to haematological malignancies in adolescents and young adults. Br J Haematol. 2014;164(1):3–14. https://doi.org/10.1111/bjh.12556.
18. Shaw PH, Reed DR, Yeager N, Zebrack B, Castellino SM, Bleyer A. Adolescent and young adult (AYA) oncology in the United States: a specialty in its late adolescence. J Pediatr Hematol Oncol. 2015;37(3):161–9. https://doi.org/10.1097/mph.0000000000000318.
19. Smith AW, Keegan T, Hamilton A, Lynch C, Wu XC, Schwartz SM, et al. Understanding care and outcomes in adolescents and young adult with cancer: A review of the AYA HOPE study. Pediatr Blood Cancer. 2019;66(1):e27486. https://doi.org/10.1002/pbc.27486.
20. Wettergren L, Kent EE, Mitchell SA, Zebrack B, Lynch CF, Rubenstein MB, et al. Cancer negatively impacts on sexual function in adolescents and young adults: the AYA hope study. Psycho-Oncology. 2017;26(10):1632–9. https://doi.org/10.1002/pon.4181.
21. Mack JW, Fasciano KM, Block SD. Adolescent and young adult cancer patients' experiences with treatment decision-making. Pediatrics. 2019;143(5):e20182800. https://doi.org/10.1542/peds.2018-2800.
22. Rosenberg AR, Bona K, Ketterl T, Wharton CM, Wolfe J, Baker KS. Intimacy, substance use, and communication needs during cancer therapy: a report from the "resilience in adolescents and young adults" study. J Adolesc Health. 2017;60(1):93–9. https://doi.org/10.1016/j.jadohealth.2016.08.017.
23. Oberoi-Jassal R, Chang YD, Smith J, Rajasekhara S, Desai V, Fenech AL, et al. Illicit substance use and opioid misuse in adolescent and young adult (AYA) patients with cancer. J Clin Oncol. 2017;35(31_suppl):205. https://doi.org/10.1200/JCO.2017.35.31_suppl.205.
24. Barr RD, Ferrari A, Ries L, Whelan J, Bleyer WA. Cancer in adolescents and young adults: a narrative review of the current status and a view of the future. JAMA Pediatr. 2016;170(5):495–501. https://doi.org/10.1001/jamapediatrics.2015.4689.
25. Blinder MA, Duh MS, Sasane M, Trahey A, Paley C, Vekeman F. Age-related emergency department reliance in patients with sickle cell disease. J Emerg Med. 2015;49(4):513–22.e1. https://doi.org/10.1016/j.jemermed.2014.12.080.
26. Festa RS, Tamaroff MH, Chasalow F, Lanzkowsky P. Therapeutic adherence to oral medication regimens by adolescents with cancer. I. Laboratory assessment. J Pediatr. 1992;120(5):807–11. https://doi.org/10.1016/s0022-3476(05)80256-2.
27. KyngAs HA, Kroll T, Duffy ME. Compliance in adolescents with chronic diseases: a review. J Adolesc Health. 2000;26(6):379–88. https://doi.org/10.1016/s1054-139x(99)00042-7.
28. Hughes RE, Holland LR, Zanino D, Link E, Michael N, Thompson KE. Prevalence and intensity of pain and other physical and psychological symptoms in adolescents and young adults diagnosed with cancer on referral to a palliative care service. J Adolesc Young Adult Oncol. 2015;4(2):70–5. https://doi.org/10.1089/jayao.2014.0015.
29. Bell CJ, Skiles J, Pradhan K, Champion VL. End-of-life experiences in adolescents dying with cancer. Support Care Cancer. 2010;18(7):827–35. https://doi.org/10.1007/s00520-009-0716-1.
30. Snaman JM, Talleur AC, Lu J, Levine DR, Kaye EC, Sykes A, et al. Treatment intensity and symptom burden in hospitalized adolescent and young adult hematopoietic cell transplant recipients at the end of life. Bone Marrow Transplant. 2018;53(1):84–90. https://doi.org/10.1038/bmt.2017.187.
31. Payne AB, Mehal JM, Chapman C, Haberling DL, Richardson LC, Bean CJ, et al. Trends in Sickle Cell Disease-Related Mortality in the United States, 1979 to 2017. Ann Emerg Med. 2020;76(3s):S28–s36. https://doi.org/10.1016/j.annemergmed.2020.08.009.
32. Johnston EE, Adesina OO, Alvarez E, Amato H, Paulukonis S, Nichols A, et al. Acute care utilization at end of life in sickle cell disease: highlighting the need for a palliative approach. J Palliat Med. 2020;23(1):24–32. https://doi.org/10.1089/jpm.2018.0649.
33. Jerrell JM, Tripathi A, McIntyre RS. Prevalence and treatment of depression in children and adolescents with sickle cell disease: a retrospective cohort study. Prim Care Companion CNS Disord. 2011;13(2):PCC.10m01063. https://doi.org/10.4088/PCC.10m01063.
34. Rosenberg AR, Wolfe J. Palliative care for adolescents and young adults with cancer. Clin Oncol Adolesc Young Adults. 2013;2013(3):41–8. https://doi.org/10.2147/coaya.S29757.
35. Zebrack BJ. Psychological, social, and behavioral issues for young adults with cancer. Cancer. 2011;117(10 Suppl):2289–94. https://doi.org/10.1002/cncr.26056.
36. Jacobs S, Perez J, Cheng YI, Sill A, Wang J, Lyon ME. Adolescent end of life preferences and congruence with their parents' preferences: results of a survey of adolescents with cancer. Pediatr Blood Cancer. 2015;62(4):710–4. https://doi.org/10.1002/pbc.25358.
37. Bleyer A. The death burden and end-of-life care intensity among adolescent and young adult patients with cancer. JAMA Oncol. 2015;1(5):579–80. https://doi.org/10.1001/jamaoncol.2015.2038.
38. Park EM, Deal AM, Yopp JM, Edwards TP, Wilson DJ, Hanson LC, et al. End-of-life experiences of mothers with advanced cancer: perspectives of widowed fathers. BMJ Support Palliat Care. 2016;6(4):437–44. https://doi.org/10.1136/bmjspcare-2015-000976.
39. Barton KS, Tate T, Lau N, Taliesin KB, Waldman ED, Rosenberg AR. "I'm Not a Spiritual Person." How hope might facilitate conversations about spirituality among teens and young adults with cancer. J Pain Symptom Manag. 2018;55(6):1599–608. https://doi.org/10.1016/j.jpainsymman.2018.02.001.
40. Pritchard S, Cuvelier G, Harlos M, Barr R. Palliative care in adolescents and young adults with cancer. Cancer. 2011;117(10 Suppl):2323–8. https://doi.org/10.1002/cncr.26044.
41. Sansom-Daly UM, Wakefield CE, Patterson P, Cohn RJ, Rosenberg AR, Wiener L, et al. End-of-life communication needs for adolescents and young adults with cancer: recommendations for research and practice. J Adolesc Young Adult Oncol. 2020;9(2):157–65. https://doi.org/10.1089/jayao.2019.0084.
42. National Cancer Policy Forum; Board on Health Care Services. Identifying and addressing the needs of adolescents and young adults with cancer: workshop summary (a Livestrong and Institute of Medicine Workshop). Washington, DC: National Academies Press (US); 2014.
43. Wein S, Pery S, Zer A. Role of palliative care in adolescent and young adult oncology. J Clin Oncol. 2010;28(32):4819–24. https://doi.org/10.1200/jco.2009.22.4543.
44. Anghelescu DL, Faughnan LG, Hankins GM, Ward DA, Oakes LL. Methadone use in children and young adults at a cancer center: a retrospective study. J Opioid Manag. 2011;7(5):353–61. https://doi.org/10.5055/jom.2011.0076.
45. Wood H, Dickman A, Star A, Boland JW. Updates in palliative care - overview and recent advancements in the pharmacological management of cancer pain. Clin Med (London, England). 2018;18(1):17–22. https://doi.org/10.7861/clinmedicine.18-1-17.
46. Loprinzi CL, Lacchetti C, Bleeker J, Cavaletti G, Chauhan C, Hertz DL, et al. Prevention and Management of Chemotherapy-Induced Peripheral Neuropathy in survivors of adult cancers: ASCO guide-

line update. J Clin Oncol. 2020;38(28):3325–48. https://doi.org/10.1200/JCO.20.01399.
47. Hauer J, Duncan J, Scullion BF. Pediatric pain and symptom management guidelines. Boston, MA: Dana Farber Cancer Institute; Boston Children's Hospital; Pediatric Advanced Care Team; 2014.
48. Wiener L, Weaver MS, Bell CJ, Sansom-Daly UM. Threading the cloak: palliative care education for care providers of adolescents and young adults with cancer. Clin Oncol Adolesc Young Adults. 2015;5:1–18. https://doi.org/10.2147/coaya.S49176.
49. Turner J, Clavarino A, Yates P, Hargraves M, Connors V, Hausmann S. Development of a resource for parents with advanced cancer: what do parents want? Palliat Support Care. 2007;5(2):135–45. Epub 2007/06/21. https://doi.org/10.1017/s1478951507070204.
50. Rosenberg AR, Wolfe J, Wiener L, Lyon M, Feudtner C. Ethics, emotions, and the skills of talking about progressing disease with terminally ill adolescents: a review. JAMA Pediatr. 2016;170(12):1216–23. https://doi.org/10.1001/jamapediatrics.2016.2142.
51. Zadeh S, Pao M, Wiener L. Opening end-of-life discussions: how to introduce Voicing My CHOiCES™, an advance care planning guide for adolescents and young adults. Palliat Support care. 2015;13(3):591–9. https://doi.org/10.1017/s1478951514000054.
52. Widger K, Sutradhar R, Rapoport A, Vadeboncoeur C, Zelcer S, Kassam A, et al. Predictors of specialized pediatric palliative care involvement and impact on patterns of end-of-life Care in Children with Cancer. J Clin Oncol. 2018;36(8):801–7. https://doi.org/10.1200/jco.2017.75.6312.
53. Odejide OO, Salas Coronado DY, Watts CD, Wright AA, Abel GA. End-of-life care for blood cancers: a series of focus groups with hematologic oncologists. J Oncol Pract. 2014;10(6):e396–403. https://doi.org/10.1200/jop.2014.001537.
54. Nass SJ, Beaupin LK, Demark-Wahnefried W, Fasciano K, Ganz PA, Hayes-Lattin B, et al. Identifying and addressing the needs of adolescents and young adults with cancer: summary of an Institute of Medicine Workshop. Oncologist. 2015;20(2):186–95. https://doi.org/10.1634/theoncologist.2014-0265.
55. Aging with Dignity. Five wishes. Tallahassee, Florida. 2020; [cited 2020 May 18]. https://www.fivewishes.org/for-myself/.
56. Canadian Virtual Hospice. Living out loud. 2020; [cited 15 May 2020]. https://livingoutloud.life.
57. Together for Short Lives. Difficult conversations for young adults. Bristol, UK: New Bond House; 2020; [cited 04 May 2020]. https://www.togetherforshortlives.org.uk/get-support/supporting-you/family-resources/difficult-conversations-young-adults/.

# Caregivers of Patients with Hematologic Malignancies

# 22

Tara A. Albrecht, Shelby Langer, Marcia A. Winter, J. Nicholas Dionne-Odom, and Laura S. Porter

Individuals with cancer often rely on close family and friends throughout their cancer journey [1]. These close family and friends are commonly identified as caregivers and provide a variety of support that is uncompensated and can include, assistance with personal care, activities of daily living, transportation needs, medical and nursing care, and social, psychological, and spiritual support [1, 2]. (Table 22.1) Caregivers are typically spouses, children, parents, or close friends, who may or may not live in the same house as the person requiring assistance.

Hematologic malignancies are a complex group of cancers that often involve intense treatments, long periods of recovery, and often considerable care both in the hospital and at home [6]. Given the complicated disease trajectory, it is not surprising that the diagnosis of a hematologic malignancy has profound implications not only for the patient but also their caregiver. Those diagnosed with a hematologic malignancy often must rely on a caregiver for physical, emotional, and practical care [7, 8]. This care requires a significant amount of energy and is often physically, emotionally,

T. A. Albrecht (✉)
School of Nursing, Duke University, Durham, NC, USA
e-mail: tara.albrecht@duke.edu

S. Langer
Edson College of Nursing and Health Innovation Arizona State University, Phoenix, AZ, USA
e-mail: shelby.langer@asu.edu

M. A. Winter
Department of Psychology, Virginia Commonwealth University, Richmond, VA, USA
e-mail: mawinter@vcu.edu

J. N. Dionne-Odom
School of Nursing, University of Alabama at Birmingham, Birmingham, AL, USA
e-mail: dionneod@uab.edu

L. S. Porter
Department of Psychiatry and Behavioral Sciences, Duke University Hospital, Durham, NC, USA
e-mail: laura.porter@duke.edu

**Table 22.1** Common responsibilities caregivers assist or assume [3–5]

| |
|---|
| *Medical* |
| Medication management and administration |
| Symptom monitoring and management |
| Ostomy and wound care |
| Tube feedings |
| Catheter care |
| Coordinating medical appointments |
| Decision making |
| *Practical and activities of daily living* |
| House and yard maintenance |
| Shopping |
| Financial management |
| Transportation |
| Meal preparation |
| Laundry |
| Showering |
| Ambulation/transition out of bed and chairs |
| Toileting |
| Child/pet care |
| *Emotional support* |
| Providing hope |
| Discussion of future, possibility of death |
| Managing changes in mood (sadness, anger, irritability) |
| Provide information updates and supporting friends/family |

socially, and/or financially demanding for the caregiver [9, 10]. And, for those who are diagnosed with an acute form of hematologic malignancy there is very little time for the caregiver to adjust to or prepare for their new role. This sudden change can be an overwhelming experience [6]. For example, caregivers have even compared the experience with the health care system to be as challenging as learning a new language [8].

The goal of this chapter is to provide an overview for clinicians of the important role the caregiver has in the care of individuals with hematologic malignancies, detail how the role of caregiver affects the individuals providing care, and how to assess these effects, and to highlight interventions



C. K. Ullrich, E. J. Roeland (eds.), *Palliative Care in Hematologic Malignancies and Serious Blood Disorders*,
https://doi.org/10.1007/978-3-031-38058-7_22

and resources available to support the caregivers through the cancer trajectory. That said, important to note is that compared to solid tumors, the literature focused on caregiving in hematologic malignancies is relatively small. Thus, as critical aspects of caregiving are discussed throughout this chapter, we will introduce current knowledge, but supplement when appropriate, with current evidence from other cancer caregiving areas, such as solid tumors and aggregated samples of multiple cancer types, as appropriate.

## Who Are the Caregivers and What Is their Role?

A survey conducted by the National Alliance on Caregiving [3] reports that the majority of caregivers are women with a mean age of 53.1 years. These caregivers also tend to be white non-Hispanic, without a college degree [3]. Most caregivers are either parents, spouses/partners, or siblings not residing with the care recipient [3]. Importantly, studies that have explored caregivers from more racially diverse populations that include Blacks and Hispanics report that these caregivers tend to be younger (mean age 40.97 years), not a spouse, and also have the responsibility of caring for their own dependents (children and/or parents) [11–13]. Finally, an important consideration for at least minority caregivers in the United States is that there may be additional significant challenges for them related to access to care, health insurance, immigration issues, and challenging work environments and language barriers, that should not be ignored [12].

Caregivers spend on average 32.6 h per week, and approximately 32% of caregivers spend at least 41 h per week, providing care-related services to patients with cancer [3]. However, the time and care delivered is quite fluid, and changes over time, naturally increasing or decreasing depending on the health status of the individual. This is especially true for caregivers caring for individuals with hematologic malignancies, where rapid fluctuations and deterioration of health are quite common [14–16].

Caregivers provide a variety of care, including delivering emotional support, assisting with common everyday household tasks, providing intimate personal care, and coordinating medical care and related transportation, and the delivery of skilled nursing care [3]. Importantly, caregivers of patients with cancer assist with significantly more tasks when compared with non-cancer caregivers [16]. Table 22.1 provides an overview of specific responsibilities that caregivers commonly assist with or assume. Caregivers, also provide a significant input related to treatment decisions [17]. This role may be especially important in hematologic malignancies, when treatment regimens can be quite complicated, a large amount of information regarding the disease and treatment needs to be understood, and prognosis may be uncertain [18–20].

Across the cancer care continuum, caregivers provide the majority of medical care and support in the home setting [3, 4, 21]. There has been a marked shift in settings of care that have impacted the role of caregivers. Inpatient hospital care is costly and hence treatment for cancer is now largely delivered in the outpatient setting [5, 22]. This shift has forced caregivers to assume an extensive amount of responsibility to deliver critical medical care as well as the ongoing support for patients with cancer [9, 23–25]. The reliance on caregivers is anticipated to continue to increase as telehealth grows and health care continues to evolve, allowing more cancer treatment to be delivered in the outpatient settings [22]. For example, even in the case of a hematopoietic cell transplant (HCT), where there are lengthy inpatient stays, portions of the process and recovery has transitioned from the inpatient to the outpatient setting, requiring caregivers to assume a higher burden of delivering complex care in the home [5].

Unfortunately, most caregivers do not feel prepared to assume their role as caregiver. Individuals with hematologic malignancies have complicated treatment regiments and require a large amount of physical and psychological care both in and out of the home. The side effects associated with many hematologic malignancies and their associated treatment can often be sudden life-threatening complications, such as neutropenic fever, hemorrhage, respiratory distress, and anemia which can overwhelm the caregiver and the patient and result in trips to the emergency department and admissions [26]. Thus, caregivers play a significant role in the individual's treatment and recovery and need to be appropriately prepared and recognized for this invaluable role.

## Effect of Delivering Care on the Caregivers

Caregiver burden is defined as a "multidimensional response to physical, psychological, emotional, social, and financial stressors associated with the caregiving experience." [27] This description is most apt in considering demands placed on caregivers of persons with hematologic malignancies. Serving as primary caregiver for a loved one undergoing HCT, for example, involves considerable disruption to multiple life domains. Families often relocate to a transplant center for an extended stay. Employment is either disrupted or managed remotely, necessitating the juggling of multiple roles including parenting for some [28]. Patient isolation for infection control translates to caregiver isolation as well [29]. Financial impacts are great given the high cost of treatment. Aside from role changes and impacts on personal time, the nature of the caregiving itself is quite intense, having to perform medical care tasks, communicate with the medical team, and manage medications. Food preparation must be done in accordance with strict safety guidelines for infection control [30]. Similarly, home environments must be cleaned frequently and thoroughly, again according to strict guidelines [30]. Caregivers report feeling unprepared for the role [29]. As one might expect, this set of demands and the imbalance of demands relative to resources, diminishes quality of life among caregivers [31, 32].

## Psychological Impacts

Psychological distress is perhaps the most frequently cited impact of the caregiving role. The term distress is generally used to refer to depression and anxiety though conceptual confusion exists given reference to theoretically similar constructs such as stress and fear of cancer recurrence [7], a cancer-specific concern. The issue is further exacerbated by administration of different assessments of these myriad constructs [1]. It is not surprising, then, that prevalence rates vary across studies of cancer caregivers, for example, from 12–59% for depression and from 30–50% for anxiety per two systematic reviews that have been conducted since 2013 [33, 34].

Caregivers of patients with hematologic malignancies may be at particular risk for distress given the nature of treatments undergone by their loved ones [35]. HCT, for example, is characterized by intensity, toxicity, and chronicity. Recovery trajectories vary per type of transplant (autologous and allogeneic) but generally involve an acute inpatient period, close monitoring during a post-transplant outpatient period lasting approximately 3 months, and a long-term survivorship period during which late complications may occur, including secondary malignancy and even death [36]. This set of challenges can be likened to a marathon comprised of multiple sprints.

As with the general cancer caregiving literature, prevalence rates of distress among caregivers of patients with hematologic malignancies vary, for example, from 5–67% for depression and from 16–58% for anxiety [35]. As one example, in a study of Australian caregivers of hematologic cancer survivors, 21% were classified as elevated (above norms) with respect to depression and 16% as elevated with respect to anxiety [37]. Prospective, longitudinal investigations have afforded examination of trajectories of distress relative to key clinical points in time. Anxiety levels tend to be elevated relative to norms just after diagnosis and, in the context of HCT, just prior to or at the start of treatment [35, 38, 39]. The pattern of change over time has not yet been fully elucidated. Some research suggests that distress decreases over time [40, 41]; other research suggests that both depression and anxiety remain elevated relative to norms up to 6 months and 1 year post-transplant, respectively [38]. Cross-sectional work, moreover, suggests that depression may be problematic years following the transplant. In a study of 177 survivor-partner dyads ranging from 1.9 to 19.4 years post-transplant (and peer-nominated controls), 20% of partners, and 21.5% of survivors were categorized as depressed (scoring ≥16 on the Center for Epidemiologic Studies Depression), markedly elevated as compared to the value for controls, 7.5% [42]. Importantly, studies have demonstrated that distress levels among caregivers are comparable to those of patients and in some cases higher [38, 40]. This is truly remarkable given the rigors of the transplant experience for patients and underscores the significant emotional toll taken on informal caregivers.

Predictors of distress parallel those identified in the broader general cancer caregiving literature: female caregiver gender [40, 43], younger caregiver age [39], and greater patient symptomatology [35, 40]. These findings offer implications for the design and testing of targeted and perhaps even tailored supportive care interventions.

## Social Impacts

Caregiving for a loved one with a hematologic malignancy confers social risks. The social isolation described above is common [29]. The patient–caregiver relationship is also altered [29, 44], in some cases for the better and in other cases, for the worse [29]. Role shifts are challenging. Other observed social impacts include less social support, more loneliness, and less dyadic satisfaction as compared to both survivors and controls [42].

With respect to dyadic satisfaction, Langer and colleagues [45] examined marital satisfaction among HCT patients and their spousal caregivers repeatedly over time: prior to transplant (baseline), 6 months post-transplant, and 1, 2, 3, and 5-year post-transplant. They also reported on marital status over time. Marital satisfaction was on par with community norms at baseline and stable over time for male and female patients and male spouses, but not for female spouses. Female spouses (also on par with community norms at baseline) reported reductions in marital satisfaction at all follow-up time points relative to baseline. Marital dissolution was uncommon. This suggests that while marriages were stable, female caregivers (not females per se and not caregivers per se) are at risk for long-term relationship dissatisfaction. Additional research is needed to replicate this finding, to identify mechanisms by which relationship satisfaction changes over time, and to develop strategies to support this vulnerable group.

Interpersonal communication may also change. Couples may engage in avoidant behaviors known as holding back and protective buffering. The latter refers to hiding cancer-related thoughts and concerns from one's partner and can be enacted by both patients and caregiving partners though one study found that it was more likely to be enacted by caregivers than patients [46]. This makes sense given that the caregiving role by definition is meant to be protective. However, despite the positive intent, holding back and protective buffering are associated with deleterious outcomes, namely poorer mental health and decreased relationship satisfaction [46]. The importance of adaptive communication is underscored by another study finding that HCT survivors reported less distress when they received more effective support from their partner [47].

## Physical Impacts

Impacts of caregiving extend beyond the psychological and social to the physical. Sleep disruption is common. One study assessed sleep quality among caregivers of allogeneic HCT recipients just prior to or at the start of transplant using the Pittsburgh Sleep Quality Index [48]. Total scores for all 109 participants fell above the cut-off for sleep difficulties based on norms, thus indicating poor sleep quality for the entire sample [39]. Sleep problems have also been observed among caregivers of long-term HCT survivors [42]. In the cross-sectional study of survivor-partner pairs mentioned previously (mean years post-transplant = 6.7), both survivors *and* partners reported more sleep problems as compared to controls [42]. While of course bothersome from an intrapersonal standpoint, caregiver sleep decrements may also adversely impact clinical outcomes in the patient. In an intriguing investigation reported by Sannes and colleagues [49], caregiver sleep quality prior to transplant predicted patient time (days) to neutrophil engraftment, a critical clinical marker of recovery. Specifically, self-reported worse sleep, lower sleep efficiency, and more frequent awakening after sleep onset (measured via actigraphy) were associated with longer time to engraftment, and thus may be a factor in the success of transplant outcomes. The use of an objective measure of sleep quality strengthens this finding and underscores the potential interpersonal detrimental nature of poor physical functioning among caregivers.

Less attention has been paid to other physical effects of caregiving for a family member with hematologic malignancy. One study found elevated levels of fatigue among both survivors and partners relative to controls [42]. Another reported low levels of fatigue [50]. Ross and colleagues [51] assessed self-reported health behaviors and chronic health conditions among 78 transplant caregivers. They also collected weight and height data to determine body mass index. Almost two-thirds of the caregivers (64%) were classified as overweight or obese and 60% reported at least one chronic health condition. Of the health behaviors measured, including nutrition, stress management, and health responsibility (e.g., preventive health care), physical activity was the most infrequent. All of the aforementioned health behaviors, moreover, were inversely related to fatigue (e.g., more physical activity and better nutrition was associated with less fatigue). These findings highlight the need for greater health promotion and self-care among caregivers.

In a study of 24 family members of HCT recipients early in the transplant process, [52] abnormalities in immune markers, including the percentage of circulating T cells, CD4+, CD8+, B cells, and NK cells were greatest prior to the transplant (on the day of hospital admission) and on the day of the transplant, in contrast to days 20 and 34 post-transplant. Similar patterns were observed for negative affect and escape-avoidance coping. These findings suggest that anticipation of transplant and the preparatory phase may be particularly challenging and detrimental to physical health. Interventions to support the psychological needs of caregivers may hold promise in improving the physical health of caregivers as well.

While the state of the science on burdens experienced by caregivers of individuals with hematologic malignancies has expanded significantly in the past decade, limitations in study design limit conclusions that may be drawn. With some exceptions, sample sizes are small, limiting the generalizability of study findings. Comparison across studies is difficult given different measures of burden and distress. Many investigations are cross-sectional in design. While informative, these studies describe functioning and well-being among a wide variety of caregivers. Large cohort studies are needed to follow caregivers prospectively over time and for long periods to capture acute and late effects of caregiving. Bereaved caregivers are also in need of scientific and clinical attention. Very little research has been conducted to examine health behaviors among these caregivers. Given the intensity and chronicity of the role, this is an area of great need. Evidence-based interventions are needed to support caregivers in multiple domains (psychological, physical, and social/ interpersonal) and as well as vulnerable caregivers (e.g., females and younger persons) who may be in particular need of support.

## Benefits of Caregiving for the Caregiver

While the majority of research on caregivers of persons with hematologic malignancies has focused on adverse effects of the role, benefits *do exist*. Qualitative research has been especially useful in identifying these effects and in elucidating the relative preponderance of benefits relative to burdens. A recent qualitative study of spouse caregivers of HCT recipients [28] examined positive and negative psychological themes. Negative psychological impacts far outweighed positive psychological impacts (164 instances versus 34 instances). The latter included optimism, gratitude, relief, hopefulness, and pride. In another study, focus groups with HCT caregivers revealed other benefits, namely personal growth, family cohesion, and a more positive relationship with the patient [53]. Lastly, interviews with HCT survivor-spouse pairs (on average 13 years post-transplant) revealed multiple positive changes since transplant, for example, increased compassion, a different perspective on life (not taking things for granted), and deeper faith [54]. Accordingly, interventions designed to foster positive states, for example, to promote gratitude, are worthy of consideration and could expand the arsenal of supportive care options available to clinicians.

## Unique Impact of Caregiving for Children

Medical advances in the diagnosis and treatment of children with hematologic malignancies and other illnesses have resulted in higher cure rates, such that researchers and clinicians are increasingly concerned with ensuring physical and mental health, and quality of life, over time. As attention to these efforts grows, it has become increasingly clear that the focus must be on the well-being of both children and their families [55]. As heads of families and caregivers of their children, parent-caregivers are both powerful and vulnerable.

Parent caregivers experience high distress. For example, parents of children with cancer, including hematologic malignancies, often experience elevated levels of distress and post-traumatic stress symptoms [56]. This distress can undermine parents' own health as well as their children's health and quality of life. A recent meta-analysis of 28 diverse studies found that parent distress (including overall distress, depression, anxiety, and post-traumatic stress) was consistently associated with overall child distress [57]. Parent-focused interventions, in turn, can improve the adjustment of children as well as parents [58]. Thus, current psychosocial standards of care in pediatric malignancies call for both parent and child distress to be routinely assessed [59].

Even as they cope with their own emotional distress, parents must also tend to the child and the family. Edmond and colleagues [60] identified family financial strain and child pain as especially potent stressors for caregivers of children with oncological and hematologic disorders. Financial stress, child sleep problems, pain, and emotional/behavioral problems were associated with more caregiver distress; financial stress, parent unemployment, and child pain were also correlated with caregiver burden [60]. For example, maintaining employment is challenging for caregivers of children with a hematologic malignancy [60]. While reasons for this have not been explicitly stated, when a child is in the hospital for treatment, the parents often remain at their child's bedside for long periods to both comfort and advocate for their child. If a child is experiencing sleep disruption, chances are the parent's sleep is disrupted as well. Similarly, if a young child is home sick, an adult must be with the child; parents may be loath to leave even older children home alone if they have a life-threatening illness and/or are in distress. Child suffering may also be especially emotionally distressing to parents, who by nature are in the role of protecting their children from hurt and harm.

To understand the experience of parents of children with cancer, it is important for practitioners to appreciate that children are unique in the levels and breadth of their dependence on adult caregivers. Unlike adults, children are largely not self-sufficient in any domain though as they age their capabilities and needs may evolve. Children depend on caregivers to assist with coping and socio-emotional needs in addition to health care needs, and they look to their closest adults as a source of information regarding the meaning their illness has for their well-being [61]. Whereas adult patients may obtain information and support from multiple sources, children—particularly young children—will mainly depend on their parents.

Parents-caregivers, therefore, are responsible for garnering resources, synthesizing information, and communicating to children in child-focused, age-appropriate ways. This can be challenging. For example, Mayer and colleagues found that over half of parents of children undergoing HCT reported needing better access to resources and services [62]. They identified unmet needs pertaining to addressing emotional and social needs of their child, post-transplant and follow-up care, and caring for the family and themselves. Parents specifically reported that they had difficulty finding pediatric-specific HCT information [62]. While some of these needs are applicable to all caregivers, others—for example, addressing the child's socio-emotional and medical follow-up needs—require that parents have access to developmentally appropriate information that is relevant. Intervening to increase parents' understanding of children's medical care has been shown to increase adherence to cancer treatment regimens [63].

Parents also need assistance determining when and how to convey complex information to their children [64]. Although research shows that children—even young children—want to be involved in communication and making decisions, parents can be reluctant to talk to children about the seriousness of their illness [65]. Guidelines of the National Academy of Pediatrics recommend that palliative care be included from diagnosis for children with life-threatening illness [66], which could aid in these communication challenges. Palliative care would also be especially helpful if curative treatments are not effective and families must transition to end-of-life care. Grieving the loss of a child, compared to other losses, is more severe and likely to be unresolved. This may be further complicated by poor end-of-life care, resulting in profound impact on parents such as more unresolved grief, poorer quality of life and mental health, marital problems, and poorer family functioning [67].

Overall, research regarding parent-caregivers highlights the unique needs of parents as well as the importance of information and resources tailored to families. These include, but are not limited to, psychosocial screening, financial counseling, developmentally appropriate information and coaching on how to communicate with children, and supportive referrals.

## Assessing Self-Reported Outcomes in Caregivers

Caregivers commonly experience both positive and negative effects as a result of caring for patients with cancer. Thus, an important consideration for both clinical practice and research is choosing appropriate instruments to measure the impact of the caregiving experience. A wide variety of instruments measuring various important constructs such as burden, strain, satisfaction, quality of life, distress, social isolation, and needs are available. Important to note, many of these instruments were originally developed and tested for use in caregivers of patients with a variety of other chronic conditions and thus may or may not specifically evaluate the unique impact of caring for patients with cancer or other serious blood disorders [68]. A selection of common instruments used in the measurement of important constructs related to caregivers of adults and children with hematologic malignancies are described in Table 22.2.

Understanding the needs of caregivers of individuals with hematologic malignancies and serious blood disorders is important, as this information can be used to guide and tailor interventions support the caregiver and indirectly improve their quality of life [88]. Table 22.2 highlights eight psychometrically tested instruments measuring caregiver needs [88, 89]. Hoenig and Hamilton first conceptualized caregiver burden in the 1960s [90]. Originally, the assessment of caregiver burden focused on necessary patient care tasks and how these tasks impacted the patient on a psychological and emotional level [89]. Since that time, the assessment of caregiver burden has evolved to often include assessments of the caregivers health, finances, well-being, social life, and relationships [89]. A number of instruments provide a multidimensional assessment of burden. The selection of instruments to assess caregiver burden for research purposes should be guided by the subscales/domains needed to answer the research question. For research purposes the Cancer

**Table 22.2** Common instruments used to assess important caregiver constructs

| Instrument | Description | Psychometrics |
|---|---|---|
| *Caregiver needs* | | |
| Health care needs Survey [70] | 90-items; 7-point Likert; domains: Information, household, patient care, personal, spiritual, psychological. | α 0.93, 0.98 |
| Cancer survivors' partners unmet Needs [71] | 40-items; identify need present and Likert for strength of need; domains: Relationships, information, partner issues, comprehensive care, emotional support | α 0.94 |
| The cancer support Person's unmet needs Survey [72] | 78-items; 5-point Likert; domains: Information, relationship, emotional, personal, work and finance, health care access | α 0.99 |
| Supportive care needs of family caregivers-partners and Caregivers [73] | 40-items; 4-point Likert; domains: Healthcare service needs, psychological, emotional, work and social, information | α 0.88–0.94 |
| Comprehensive needs assessment tools for cancer-Caregivers [74] | 41-items; 4-point Likert; domains: Health and psychological problems, family and social support, healthcare staff, information, religious/spiritual support, hospital facilities and services, and practical support | α 0.96 |
| Cancer caregiving tasks consequences and needs Questionnaire [75] | 71-items; 4-point Likert; 9 subscales | α 0.65–0.95 |
| Family inventory of Needs [76] | 20-items; identify need met or unmet and 10-point Likert identifying importance | α 0.83 |
| Distress thermometer [77] | Report distress via numeric rating scale and identify five domains of problems that are contributing to distress (physical, practical, family, emotional or spiritual) | α 0.81 |
| *Caregivers of pediatric patients* | | |
| Family inventory of needs-Pediatrics [78] | 17-items; three Likert like ratings; domains: Importance of care, if needs met, need for information | α 0.83–0.98 |
| *Caregiver burden* | | |
| Appraisal of caregiving Scale [79] | 53-items (and shortened 27-item); 5-point Likert; domains: Harm/loss, threat, challenge, benign | α 0.72–0.91 |
| Caregiver reaction Assessment [80] | 24-items; 5-point Likert; domains: Esteem, family support, finances, schedule, health | α 0.82, 0.90, 0.85, 0.80, 0.81 |
| Caregiver impact Scale [81] | 14-items; 7-point Likert; domains: Health, diet, employment, household responsibilities, recreation | α 0.87 |

**Table 22.2** (continued)

| Instrument | Description | Psychometrics |
|---|---|---|
| Brief assessment scale for the caregivers of the medically Ill [82] | 14-items; 4-point Likert; domains: Personal impact, positive and negative impact, medical issues, concerns | α 0.70, 0.80 |
| *Caregivers of pediatric patients* | | |
| Psychosocial assessment tool 2.0 [83] | 15-items; Total score is 8-point Likert; domains: Family structure and resources, family social support, family problems, parent stress reactions, family beliefs, child problems, sibling problems | α 0.81 |
| *Caregiver quality of life* | | |
| Caregiver quality of life index-cancer [84] | 35-items; 5-point Likert; multidimensional: Burden, financial, disruptiveness, positive adaptation, | α 0.91 |
| Quality of life-family Version [85] | 37-item; 11-point Likert; multidimensional: Social, physical wellbeing, psychological wellbeing, spiritual wellbeing | α 0.89 |
| Quality of life in life-threatening illness- family Carer Version [86] | 16-item; 11-point Likert; multidimensional: Financial, state of carer, patient wellbeing, quality of care, Carer's outlook, environment, relationship | α 0.86 |
| Caregiver quality of life Index [87] | 4-items; visual analog scale (0–100); domains: Physical, psychological, social, financial | α 0.76, 0.88 |
| *Caregivers of pediatric patients* | | |
| Pediatric quality of life inventory family impact Module [88] | 36-items; 5-point Likert; domains: Physical, emotional, social and cognitive functioning, worry, communication, daily activities, family relationships | α 0.90 |

Support Person's Unmet Needs Survey (SPUNS) [71] is a potentially good choice given its test-retest reliability (0.99) and testing in variety of malignancies that support its generalizability across various cancer types and caregiver relationships [88].

For clinical purposes, the Supportive Care Needs Survey-Partners and Caregivers (SNCS-P&C) [71] may be an alternative [88]. However, while the SNCS-P&C is shorter than the SPUNS, there are still 40-items and thus may not be feasible to administer in the clinical setting. The Brief Assessment Scale for the Caregivers of the Medically Ill [81] is a 14-item instrument focusing on both the negative and positive impact of caring for a patient with cancer. Given the concise number of questions, this instrument may be feasible for use in the clinical setting.

An alternative for rapid interpretation in the clinical setting may be the Family Inventory of Needs, which includes 20 items and provides scores for importance of the need on a 0–10 Likert Scale [75]. Additionally, the National Comprehensive Cancer Networks Distress Thermometer is a brief screening instrument designed specifically for its rapid use and interpretation in the clinical setting [76].

Health-related quality of life (QOL) is a multidimensional construct encompassing how a medical circumstance affects an individual's physical, emotional, social, and spiritual well-being as well as their environment [89]. There is an overwhelming selection of instruments designed to measure quality of life for patients and a growing number designed specifically for caregivers. For research purposes, the Quality of Life Index-Cancer [83] has been recommended as it has undergone rigorous development and testing iteratively, in subjects with a variety of cancers [89] and has been successfully used in caregivers of individuals with hematologic malignancies [91]. The simple 4-item Caregiver Quality of Life Index [86] may be useful in the clinical setting for rapid assessment of a caregiver's physical, psychological, social, and financial well-being during the illness trajectory.

## Supporting Caregivers of Patients with Hematologic Malignancies

A small but growing literature describing interventions to assist caregivers of patients with hematologic malignancies exists. A systematic review by Bangerter et al. [92] identified 12 studies, including seven efficacy studies and five feasibility studies of caregivers of HCT recipients. Interventions included problem-solving education, cognitive-behavioral stress management, one-on-one sessions with a palliative care clinician in an inpatient setting, family-based intervention, and massage therapy. Most interventions were conducted with the caregiver alone although some involved patient-caregiver dyads.

These interventions were largely feasible and acceptable, with completion rates of 70–100% and high satisfaction ratings. While findings were inconsistent and difficult to summarize due to the small number of studies and heterogeneity in intervention content and the outcomes assessed, most studies reported a beneficial effect on emotional distress with respect to depression, anxiety, and mood disturbance. Two studies, including a problem-solving intervention and massage therapy, showed reduced fatigue. Only two studies assessed caregiver burden, and neither found a significant effect. Regarding health care utilization and measures of physiological stress, an intervention study led to improvements in mental health use but not medical service use, and some but not all markers of physiological stress. Overall, the review concluded that caregiver interventions were feasible and acceptable, particularly with flexible delivery formats that allowed for a combination of in person and telehealth sessions, and that caregiver interventions show promise in alleviating emotional distress.

Since 2017, there have been two additional randomized clinical trials (RCTs) testing cognitive-behavioral caregiver interventions, shedding additional light on the potential efficacy of this approach. First, Laudenslager and colleagues [93] tested the efficacy of a cognitive behavioral stress management intervention for caregivers of patients receiving allogeneic HCT. Given the potential interaction between caregiver well-being and patient outcomes, the study was designed to test the impact of the intervention on both patient QOL and caregiver distress. The intervention consisted of eight 60-min one-on-one sessions, plus two optional booster sessions, over the 100-day post-transplant period. Content included psychoeducation about the mind-body connection, training in problem solving, cognitive restructuring, and relaxation techniques, along with utilizing social support and setting appropriate goals. Sessions were conducted via video chat when caregivers were unable to attend in-person sessions. Caregivers (n = 155) were randomized to the intervention or to a control group in which they received the intervention workbook but no sessions. Results indicated that at 6 months post-transplant the intervention led to significant improvements in caregiver distress; however, there were no significant effects on patient QOL. The authors speculate that the lack of effect on patient QOL may reflect the choice of instrument (FACT-BMT which focuses on somatic symptoms), or inadequate power to detect this indirect effect. In addition to the assessment of the intervention impact on patient outcomes, study strengths include relatively long follow-up, and a comparison group controlling for the effects of receiving information on stress management.

A second pilot RCT assessed the feasibility, acceptability, and preliminary efficacy of an intervention for caregivers of HCT recipients integrating treatment-related education with self-care and cognitive behavioral skills to promote adaptive coping [94]. The intervention consisted of six 60-min sessions delivered by a psychologist or social worker in person, or via telephone or videoconferencing starting before HCT and continuing until day +60 after HCT. One hundred caregivers were randomized to either the intervention or usual care. At day +60, caregivers assigned to the intervention reported better QOL, lower caregiving burden, less anxiety and depression, and higher self-efficacy and coping skills relative to those in usual care.

Taken together, these studies suggest that a cognitive-behavioral approach may be effective in reducing caregivers' distress and enhancing adaptive coping. These studies can be placed in the broader context of the much larger literature of interventions for cancer caregivers, most of which have focused on caregivers of individuals with solid tumors. A number of systematic reviews and meta-analyses have been published summarizing these studies [95–98]. Overall, these reviews conclude that most interventions have small positive effects on caregiver and patient psychological distress and interpersonal outcomes. However, the heterogeneity of samples and interventions make it difficult to draw firm conclusions about efficacy, and few studies have assessed long-term outcomes.

In designing a caregiver intervention, it is important to consider at least three questions: [1] What need is the intervention addressing? [2] Should the intervention target the caregiver alone, or in combination with the patient? [6] What mode of delivery is best suited for the intervention and population? With regard to the first question, given that caregivers' needs are broad ranging and change over time, it is unlikely that any given intervention will meet every need. Table 22.3 presents a list of caregiver needs, along with relevant intervention strategies and outcomes. To date, the majority of studies conducted with HCT caregivers have focused on the care of the patient and the caregiver's emotional self-care, while few have focused on the caregiver's physical well-being, dyadic or family relationships, or practical concerns.

In addition, most studies have targeted the caregiver alone. This is in contrast to the broader cancer caregiver intervention literature in which approximately 50% of inter-

**Table 22.3** Approaches to caregiver interventions

| Caregiver need | Intervention content | Outcomes |
|---|---|---|
| Care of patient | • Education<br>• Physical care of patient<br>• Symptom management<br>• Advance care planning | • Knowledge<br>• Preparedness<br>• Self-efficacy for caregiving<br>• Caregiver burden |
| Own emotional self-care | • Mindfulness<br>• Relaxation<br>• Cognitive reframing<br>• Behavioral activation<br>• Problem solving | • Psychological distress<br>• Perceived stress<br>• Coping |
| Own physical self-care | • Physical activity<br>• Sleep | • Physical function<br>• Sleep<br>• Health<br>• Health care utilization |
| Relationship/family dynamics | • Communication<br>• Dyadic coping | • Communication quality<br>• Relationship quality<br>• Family functioning |
| Practical (e.g., finances, transportation) | • Financial counseling<br>• Connection to social services | • Financial distress<br>• Caregiver burden |

ventions have focused on patient-caregiver dyads. While there have been a number of descriptive studies documenting the interdependence of HCT patient-caregiver adjustment and the impact of HCT on spousal relationships in particular [99], few intervention studies have targeted patient-caregiver dyads. One example of a promising dyadic approach is a dyadic problem-solving intervention developed by Bevans et al. [100] Findings from this RCT indicated that the intervention, which was delivered jointly to patients and caregivers in three 1-h sessions, led to reductions in patient and caregiver distress, improvements in caregiver self-efficacy, and trends in improvements in caregiver health outcomes [100]. A second approach to dyadic interventions is illustrated by a couple communication intervention designed to improve effective communication and relationship functioning among patients and their spousal caregivers. Results from a pilot feasibility study suggest that the intervention was feasible and acceptable and led to improvements in communication skills [101].

There are a number of factors to consider in deciding whether to target the caregiver alone, or in combination with the patient [21]. Dyadic interventions are, of course, the most appropriate approach for interventions in which the major focus is improving dyadic communication, dyadic coping, or the quality of the patient-caregiver relationship. They may also be preferred for delivery of interventions that focus on patient care, given that patients are usually active agents in their own care, and that caregiving takes place in the context of the interpersonal relationship. When the main focus of the intervention is the caregiver's emotional or physical well-being, conducting the intervention with the caregiver alone may be beneficial in that it gives caregivers a forum to discuss issues and concerns without worrying about upsetting or burdening the patient. However, a dyadic approach should not necessarily be ruled out. As demonstrated by the Bevans et al. dyadic problem-solving intervention [100], patients and caregivers may mutually benefit from learning coping skills together, leading to a "two-for-one" approach. The dyadic approach also provides the opportunity to assist patients and caregivers in working collaboratively to manage illness-related challenges and assisting each other in learning and applying skills. Finally, given that caregivers are often reluctant to seek help for themselves or divert resources away from the patient, they may be more willing to participate in a dyadic intervention that has the potential to benefit the patient as well as themselves.

With regard to mode of delivery, it is clear that flexibility is important, with a combination of in person, video, and/or telephone sessions demonstrating the highest degree of feasibility. There is also growing interest in self-directed, web-based interventions due to their scalability and reach. However, findings from studies evaluating web-based interventions indicate that they are often under-utilized by participants and associated with high attrition, particularly among caregivers with high levels of burden [102]. These findings may speak to the degree to which caregivers are overwhelmed and lack the time and energy to access and use resources without more structured guidance and support. Thus, while web-based delivery may be advantageous for some caregivers, it is clear that feasibility and acceptability should be established among potential participants.

In summary, interventions for caregivers of individuals with hematologic malignancies, including those who have undergone HCT, show promise for improving caregiver outcomes; however, this area of research is still in its infancy. In particular, interventions focused on caregiver physical well-being, dyadic or family relationships, or practical concerns are lacking. Many of the limitations noted in the broader cancer caregiver interventions apply to those conducted in the hematologic malignancy populations: Study quality is often poor to fair, and methodological details are not always fully reported. Samples are often not inclusive of minorities, underserved, and rural populations. Also, among interventions targeted to caregivers alone, few studies have examined patient outcomes, and no studies have examined caregiver improvements as a mediator of longer term patient improvements. Finally, few studies have specifically targeted at-risk caregivers, for instance, those who report high levels of distress, or low self-efficacy for caregiving. In addition to addressing these limitations, researchers should also consider innovative approaches such stepped care designs that provide more intensive interventions to those who need it most, or adaptive just-in-time designs that aim to provide the right type and amount of support at the right time [103]. Finally, organizations such as the American Cancer Society, CancerCare, and the Cancer Support Community (see Table 22.4) have developed excellent resources for cancer caregivers; researchers might partner with such organizations to explore methods for enhancing the use of these resources and evaluating outcomes.

**Table 22.4** Resources for caregivers of persons with hematologic malignancies

| Organization/Resource | Description | Where accessed? |
|---|---|---|
| *General* | | |
| American Cancer Society | Provides educational materials about hematological cancers; offers online support groups and discussion boards and information about in-person support groups through local chapters; road to recovery program offered by some local chapters to assist with transportation; Hope lodges are temporary housing for patients and families traveling long distances for care | www.cancer.org |
| National Cancer Institute Cancer information service | Provides up-to-date information on cancer in easy-to-understand language over the phone, email, or online chat. Trained information specialists provide personalized responses about cancer research and clinical trials, cancer treatment centers, cancer prevention, risk factors, symptoms, and diagnosis and treatment | 1–800-4-CANCER www.cancer.gov/contact |
| Family caregiver Alliance | Comprehensive resource for family caregivers. Provides information and resources for long-term caregiving, including practical skills, how to hold family meetings, decision-making, assistive equipment, online support. Their family care navigator is an online search portal that can identify state-specific resources | www.caregiver.org |
| Cancer support community | Provides support and resources to all individuals impacted by cancer to ensure that they are empowered by knowledge, strengthened by action, and sustained by community | www.cancersupportcommunity.org |
| *Specific to hematologic malignancies* | | |
| Leukemia and Lymphoma society caregiver support | Comprehensive web resource for family caregivers of adults and children with leukemia and lymphoma. Provides information about leukemia and other blood cancers and treatment options; worksheets to help caregivers stay organized (e.g., emergency room plan, daily medication log, communication guides); guidance on communication, including how to talk with children, and relationship changes; financial and legal planning; and links to online leukemia and lymphoma caregiving communities | www.lls.org/support/caregiver-support |
| CML advocates network | For individuals and their families affected by chronic myeloid leukemia, this patient-led international network provides a world-wide directory of CML patient groups, shared best practices on cancer advocacy, and a repository of easy-to-understand, downloadable information | www.cmladvocates.net |
| BMTinfonet.org | Web resource for family caregivers whose relative is undergoing bone marrow or stem cell transplant. Includes treatment information, videos, and what to expect during all phases of the treatment | www.bmtinfonet.org/transplant-article/role-family-caregiver |
| CancerCare—myeloproliferative neoplasms | Resource information for families and patients affected by myeloproliferative cancers. Support resources include information on counseling, support groups, and financial assistance. Information resources include online workshops, podcasts, news articles for lay audiences, and information booklets and fact sheets | www.cancercare.org/diagnosis/myeloproliferative_neoplasms |
| MDS Foundation | The myelodysplastic syndromes foundation was established by an international group of physicians and researchers to provide an ongoing exchange of information relating to MDS. The network and website provide family caregivers and patients with referrals, clinical trial information, new research and treatment options, and a variety of educational support resources | www.mds-foundation.org |

## Conclusions

There has been limited research to date that has examined the caregivers of individuals with hematologic malignancy, with the largest focus on those caregivers of individuals who have undergone HCT. This small body of research indicates that caregivers provide a significant amount of care to individuals with hematologic malignancies and often times to the detriment of their own health. Clinicians may better support caregivers by providing family-centered care and education that is clear, consistent and tailored to patient-specific needs as well as other supportive interventions that will improve their quality of life during these difficult times. Future caregiver research should include specific hematologic malignancies outside of HCT to ensure efficacy of interventions in diverse settings and hematologic diseases.

## References

1. Kent EE, Rowland JH, Northouse L, Litzelman K, Chou WY, Shelburne N, Timura C, O'Mara A, Huss K. Caring for caregivers and patients: research and clinical priorities for informal cancer caregiving. Cancer. 2016;122(13):1987–95. Epub 2016/03/19. https://doi.org/10.1002/cncr.29939.

2. Frambes D, Givens B, Lehto R, Sokorskii A, Wyatt G. Informal caregivers of cancer patients: review of interventions, care activities and outcomes. West J Nurs Res. 2018;40:1069–97.
3. National alliance for caregiving. cancer caregiving in the U.S.: an intense, episodic, and challenging care experience2016. https://www.researchgate.net/profile/Margaret_Longacre/publication/318543389_Cancer_Caregiving_in_the_US_An_Intense_Episodic_and_Challenging_Care_Experience/links/596ff15da6fdccc6c96c161f/Cancer-Caregiving-in-the-US-An-Intense-Episodic-and-Challenging-Care-Experience.pdf. Accessed 24 Apr 2020.
4. Dionne-Odom J, Currie E, Johnston E, Rosenberg A. Supporting family caregivers of adult and pediatric patients with leukemia. Semin Oncol Nurs. 2019;35(6):150954. https://doi.org/10.1016/j.soncn.2019.150954.
5. Cooke L, Grant M, Eldredge DH, Maziarz RT, Nail LM. Informal caregiving in hematopoietic blood and marrow transplant patients. Eur J Oncol Nurs. 2011;15(5):500–7. Epub 2011/02/11. https://doi.org/10.1016/j.ejon.2011.01.007.
6. Hall A, Lynagh M, Carey M, Sanson-Fisher R, Mansfield E. Who are the support persons of haematological cancer survivors and how is their performance perceived? Psychooncology. 2017;26(12):2201–7. Epub 2017/04/30. https://doi.org/10.1002/pon.4449.
7. Gemmill R, Cooke L, Williams AC, Grant M. Informal caregivers of hematopoietic cell transplant patients: a review and recommendations for interventions and research. Cancer Nurs. 2011;34(6):E13–21. Epub 2011/01/19. https://doi.org/10.1097/NCC.0b013e31820a592d.
8. McGrath P. Caregivers insights on the dying trajectory in hematology oncology. Cancer Nurs. 2001;24:413–21.
9. Kent E, Rowland J, Northhouse L, Litzelman K, Chou W, Shelbourne N, Timura C, O'Mara A, Huss K. Caring for caregivers and patients: research and clinical priorities for informal cancer caregiving. Cancer. 2016;122:1987–95.
10. Biegel D, Sales E, Schulz R. Family caregiving in chronic illness: Alzheimer's disease, cancer, heart disease, mental illness, and stroke. Thousand Oaks, CA: SAGE Publications; 1991.
11. Siefert ML, Williams A-L, Dowd MF, Chappel-Aiken L, McCorkle R. The caregiving experience in a racially diverse sample of cancer family caregivers. Cancer Nurs. 2008;31(5):399–407. https://doi.org/10.1097/01.NCC.0000305760.04357.96.
12. Badger TA, Sikorskii A, Segrin C. Contextual and cultural influences on caregivers of Hispanic cancer survivors. Semin Oncol Nurs. 2019;35(4):359–62. Epub 2019/06/24. https://doi.org/10.1016/j.soncn.2019.06.008.
13. Friedemann M-L, Buckwalter KC, Newman FL, Mauro AC. Patterns of caregiving of Cuban, other Hispanic, Caribbean black, and white elders in South Florida. J Cross Cult Gerontol. 2013;28(2):137–52. https://doi.org/10.1007/s10823-013-9193-6.
14. LeBlanc TW, El-Jawahri A. When and why should patients with hematologic malignancies see a palliative care specialist? Hematolog. 2015;2015:471–8.
15. Manitta V, Zordan R, Cole-Sinclair M, Nandurkar H, Philip J. The symptom burden of patients with hematological malignancy: a cross-sectional observational study. J Pain Symptom Manag. 2011;42:432–42. https://doi.org/10.1016/j.jpainsymman.2010.12.008.
16. Button E, Chan R. Palliative care provision for patients with a hematological malignancy: can we do more? Cancer Nurs. 2014;37:239–40.
17. Hobbs GS, Landrum MB, Arora NK, Ganz PA, van Ryn M, Weeks JC, Mack JW, Keating NL. The role of families in decisions regarding cancer treatments. Cancer. 2015;121(7):1079–87. Epub 2015/02/25. https://doi.org/10.1002/cncr.29064.
18. LeBlanc TW, Bloom N, Wolf SP, Lowman SG, Pollak KI, Steinhauser KE, Ariely D, Tulsky JA. Triadic treatment decision-making in advanced cancer: a pilot study of the roles and perceptions of patients, caregivers, and oncologists. Support Care Cancer. 2018;26(4):1197–205. Epub 2017/11/05. https://doi.org/10.1007/s00520-017-3942-y.
19. LeBlanc TW, Fish LJ, Bloom CT, El-Jawahri A, Davis DM, Locke SC, Steinhauser KE, Pollak KI. Patient experiences of acute myeloid leukemia: a qualitative study about diagnosis, illness understanding, and treatment decision-making. Psychooncology. 2017;26(12):2063–8. Epub 2016/11/20. https://doi.org/10.1002/pon.4309.
20. El-Jawahri A, Nelson-Lowe M, VanDusen H, Traeger L, Abel GA, Greer JA, Fathi A, Steensma DP, LeBlanc TW, Li Z, DeAngelo D, Wadleigh M, Hobbs G, Foster J, Brunner A, Amrein P, Stone RM, Temel JS. Patient-clinician discordance in perceptions of treatment risks and benefits in older patients with acute myeloid leukemia. Oncologist. 2019;24(2):247–54. Epub 2018/08/25. https://doi.org/10.1634/theoncologist.2018-0317.
21. National Academy of Medicine. Families caring for an aging America. Washington, DC: The National Academies Press; 2016.
22. Kent EE, Mollica MA, Buckenmaier S, Wilder SA. The characteristics of informal cancer caregivers in the United States. Semin Oncol Nurs. 2019;35(4):328–32. Epub 2019/06/24. https://doi.org/10.1016/j.soncn.2019.06.002.
23. Perreault A, Fothergill-Bourbonnais F, Fiset V. The experience of family members caring for a dying loved one. Int J Palliat Nurs. 2004;10:133–43.
24. Northfield S, Nebauer M. The caregiving journey for family members of relatives with cancer: how do they cope? Clin J Oncol Nurs. 2010;14:567–77.
25. Lambert SD, Ould Brahim L, Morrison M, Girgis A, Yaffe M, Belzile E, Clayberg K, Robinson J, Thorne S, Bottorff JL, Duggleby W, Campbell-Enns H, Kim Y, Loiselle CG. Priorities for caregiver research in cancer care: an international Delphi survey of caregivers, clinicians, managers, and researchers. Support Care Cancer. 2019;27(3):805–17. Epub 2018/08/01. https://doi.org/10.1007/s00520-018-4314-y.
26. Wiese M, Daver N. Unmet clinical needs and economic burden of disease in the treatment landscape of acute myeloid leukemia. Am J Manag Care. 2018;24:347–55.
27. Hiseman JP, Fackrell R. Caregiver burden and the nonmotor symptoms of Parkinson's disease. Int Rev Neurobiol. 2017;133:479–97. Epub 2017/08/15. https://doi.org/10.1016/bs.irn.2017.05.035.
28. Langer S, Yi J, Chi N, Lindhorst T. Psychological impacts and ways of coping reported by spousal caregivers of hematopoietic cell transplant recipients: a qualitative analysis. Biol Blood Marrow Transplant. 2020;26:764–71. https://doi.org/10.1016/j.bbmt.2019.11.023.
29. Jim H, Quinn G, Barata A, Cases M, Cessna J, Gonzalez B, Gonzalez L, Koskan A, Montiel-Ishino F, Pidala J. Caregivers' quality of life after blood and marrow transplantation: a qualitative study. Bone Marrow Transplant. 2014;49(9):1234–6. https://doi.org/10.1038/bmt.2014.118.
30. Yokoe D, Casper C, Dubberke E, Lee G, Munoz P, Palmore T, Sepkowitz K, Young J-A, Donnelly J. Safe living after hematopoietic cell transplantation. Bone Marrow Transplant. 2009;44(8):509–19.
31. Deniz H, Inci F. The burden of care and quality of life of caregivers of leukemia and lymphoma patients following peripheric stem cell transplantation. J Psychosoc Oncol. 2015;33(3):250–62. https://doi.org/10.1080/07347332.2015.1019660.
32. El-Jawahri A, Traeger L, Kuzmuk K, Eusebio J, Vandusen H, Shin J, Keenan T, Gallagher E, Greer J, Pirl W, Jackson V, Ballen K, Spitzer T, Graubert T, McAfee S, Dey B, Chen Y, Temel J. Quality

of life and mood of patients and family caregivers during hospitalization for hematopoietic stem cell transplantation. Cancer. 2015;121:951–9.
33. Applebaum A, Breitbart W. Care for the cancer caregiver: a systematic review. Palliative and Supportive Care. 2013;11(3):231–52. https://doi.org/10.1017/S1478951512000594.
34. Geng H-M, Chuang D-M, Yang F, Yang Y, Liu W-M, Liu L-H, Tian H-M. Prevalence and determinants of depression in caregivers of cancer patients: a systematic review and meta-analysis. Medicine. 2018;97(39):e11863. https://doi.org/10.1097/MD.0000000000011863.
35. Dionne-Odom J, Currie E, Johnston E, Rosenberg A. Supporting family caregivers of adult and pediatric persons with leukemia. Semin Oncol Nurs. 2019;35(6):150954. https://doi.org/10.1016/j.soncn.2019.150954.
36. Inamoto Y, Lee S. Late effects of blood and marrow transplantation. Haematologica. 2017;102(4):614–25.
37. Carey M, Sanson-Fisher R, Paul C, Bradstock K, Williamson A, Campbell H. Psychological morbidity among Australian rural and urban support persons of haematological cancer survivors: results of a national study. Psycho-Oncology. 2017;26:1952–8. https://doi.org/10.1002/pon.4411.
38. Langer S, Abrams J, Syrjala K. Caregiver and patient marital satisfaction and affect following hematopoietic stem cell transplantation: a prospective, longitudinal investigation. Psychooncology. 2003;12(3):239–53.
39. Simoneau T, Mikulich-Gilbertson S, Natvig C, Kilbourn K, Spradley J, Grzywa-Cobb R, Philips S, McSweeney P, Laudenslager M. Elevated peri-transplant distress in caregivers of allogeneic blood or marrow transplant patients. Psychooncology. 2013;22(9):2064–70. https://doi.org/10.1002/pon.3259.
40. Beattie S, Lebel S. The experience of caregivers of hematological cancer patients undergoing a hematopoietic stem cell transplant: a comprehensive literature review. Psychooncology. 2011;20(11):1137–50. Epub 2011/03/23. https://doi.org/10.1002/pon.1962.
41. Fife B, Monahan P, Abonour R, Wood L, Stump T. Adaptation of family caregivers during the acute phase of adult BMT. Bone Marrow Transplant. 2009;43:959–66. https://doi.org/10.1038/bmt.2008.405.
42. Bishop M, Beaumont J, Hahn E, Cella D, Andrykowski M, Brady M, Horowitz M, Sobocinski K, Rizzo J, Wingard J. Late effects of cancer and hematopoietic stem-cell transplantation on spouses or partners compared with survivors and survivor-matched controls. J Clin Psychol. 2007;25(11):1403–11.
43. Langer S. Mood disturbance in the cancer setting: effects of gender and patient/ spouse role. Semin Clin Neuropsychiatry. 2003;8:276–85.
44. Sabo B, McLeod D, Couban S. The experience of caring for a spouse undergoing hematopoietic stem cell transplantation. Cancer Nurs. 2013;36(1):29–40. https://doi.org/10.1097/NCC.0b013e31824fe223.
45. Langer S, Yi J, Storer B, Syrjala K. Marital adjustment, satisfaction and dissolution among hematopoietic stem cell transplant patients and spouses: a prospective, five-year longitudinal investigation. Psycho-Oncol. 2010;19(2):190–200.
46. Langer S, Brown J, Syrjala K. Intrapersonal and interpersonal consequences of protective buffering among cancer patients and caregivers. Cancer. 2009;115(18 Suppl):4311–25. https://doi.org/10.1002/cncr.24586.
47. Rini C, Redd W, Austin J, Mosher C, Meschian Y, Isola L, Scigliano E, Moskowitz C, Papadopoulos E, Labay L, Rowley S, Burkhalter J, Dunkel Schetter C, DuHamel K. Effectiveness of partner social support predicts enduring psychological distress after hematopoietic stem cell transplantation. J Consult Clin Psychol. 2011;79(1):64–74. https://doi.org/10.1037/a0022199.
48. Buysse D, Reynolds C, Monk T, Berman S, Kupfer D. The Pittsburgh sleep quality index: a new instrument for psychiatric practice and research. Psychiatry Res. 1989;28:193–213.
49. Sannes T, Mikulich-Gilbertson S, Natvig C, Brewer B, Simoneau T, Laudenslager M. Caregiver sleep and patient neutrophil engraftment in allogeneic hematopoietic stem cell transplant. Cancer Nurs. 2018;41(1):77–85. https://doi.org/10.1097/NCC.0000000000000447.
50. Gaston-Johansson F, Lachica E, Fall-Dickson J, Kennedy M. Psychological distress, fatigue, burden of care, and quality of life in primary caregivers of patients with breast cancer undergoing autologous bone marrow transplantation. Oncol Nurs Forum. 2004;31(6):1161–9.
51. Ross A, Yang L, Klagholz S, Wehrlen L, Bevans M. The relationship of health behaviors with sleep and fatigue in transplant caregivers. Psychooncology. 2016;25(5):506–12. https://doi.org/10.1002/pon.3860.
52. Futterman A, Wellisch D, Zighelboim J, Luna-Raines M, Weiner H. Psychological and immunological reactions of family members to patients undergoing bone marrow transplantation. Psychosom Med. 1996;58:472–80.
53. Stetz K, McDonald J, Compton K. Needs and experiences of family caregivers during marrow transplantation. Oncol Nurs Forum. 1996;23(9):1422–7.
54. Bishop M, Curbow B, Springer S, Lee J, Wingard J. Comparison of lasting life changes after cancer and BMT: perspectives of long-term survivors and spouses. Psycho-Oncology. 2011;20:926–34.
55. Winter MA, Al Ghriwati N, Devine KA. Pediatric chronic health conditions: Adaptation within the family context. In: MC BHF, Deater-Deckard K, Jouriles EN, Whisman MA, editors. APA handbooks in psychology® APA handbook of contemporary family psychology. Applications and broad impact of family psychology American Psychological Association; 2019. p. 69–84.
56. Pai AL, Drotar D, Zebracki K, Moore M, Youngstrom E. A meta-analysis of the effects of psychological interventions in pediatric oncology on outcomes of psychological distress and adjustment. J Pediatr Psychol. 2006;31(9):978–88. Epub 2006/03/04. https://doi.org/10.1093/jpepsy/jsj109.
57. Bakula DM, Sharkey CM, Perez MN, Espeleta HC, Gamwell KL, Baudino M, Delozier AM, Chaney JM, Matt Alderson R, Mullins LL. Featured article: the relationship between parent and child distress in pediatric cancer: a meta-analysis. J Pediatr Psychol. 2019;44(10):1121–36. Epub 2019/07/02. https://doi.org/10.1093/jpepsy/jsz051.
58. Fedele DA, Hullmann SE, Chaffin M, Kenner C, Fisher MJ, Kirk K, Eddington AR, Phipps S, McNall-Knapp RY, Mullins LL. Impact of a parent-based interdisciplinary intervention for mothers on adjustment in children newly diagnosed with cancer. J Pediatr Psychol. 2013;38(5):531–40. Epub 2013/03/09. https://doi.org/10.1093/jpepsy/jst010.
59. Wiener L, Kazak AE, Noll RB, Patenaude AF, Kupst MJ. Standards for the psychosocial Care of Children with Cancer and Their Families: an introduction to the special issue. Pediatr Blood Cancer. 2015;62(Suppl 5):S419–24. Epub 2015/09/24. https://doi.org/10.1002/pbc.25675.
60. Edmond S, Graves P, Whiting A, Karlson C. Emotional distress and burden among caregivers of children with oncological/hematological disorders. Families, Systems and Health. 2016;34(2):166–71.
61. Winter MA, Fiese BH, Spagnola M, Anbar RD. Asthma severity, child security, and child internalizing: using story stem techniques to assess the meaning children give to family and disease-specific events. J Fam Psychol. 2011;25(6):857–67. Epub 2011/11/09. https://doi.org/10.1037/a0026191.
62. Mayer DK, Tighiouart H, Terrin N, Stewart S, Peterson E, Jeruss S, Parsons SK. A brief report of caregiver needs and resource utilization during pediatric hematopoietic stem cell transplantation. J

Pediatr Oncol Nurs. 2009;26(4):223–9. Epub 2009/09/04. https://doi.org/10.1177/1043454209340409.
63. Rapoff MA, McGrath AM, Smith SD. Adherence to treatment demands. In: Brown RT, editor. Comprehensive handbook of childhood cancer and sickle cell disease: a biopsychosocial approach. New York: Oxford University Press; 2006. p. 138–69.
64. Vannatta K, Salley CG. Pediatric cancer. In: Steele MCRRG, editor. Handbook of pediatric psychology. Fifth ed. New York: The Guilford Press; 2017. p. 284–97.
65. Ellis R, Leventhal B. Information needs and decision-making preferences of children with cancer. Psychooncology. 1993;2(4):277–84. https://doi.org/10.1002/pon.2960020407.
66. National Consensus Project for Quality Palliative Care. Clinical practice guidelines for quality palliative care. 3rd ed. PA: Pittsburgh; 2013. https://www.nationalconsensusproject.org
67. Gerhart CA, Baughcum AE, Fortney C, Lichtenthal WG. Palliative care, end of life, and bereavement. In: Steele MCRRG, editor. Handbook of pediatric psychology. 5th ed. New York: The Guilford Press; 2017. p. 191–200.
68. Shilling V, Matthews L, Jenkins V, Fallowfield L. Patient-reported outcome measures for cancer caregivers: a systematic review. Qual Life Res. 2016;25(8):1859–76. Epub 2016/02/14. https://doi.org/10.1007/s11136-016-1239-0.
69. Hileman JW, Lackey NR, Hassanein RS. Identifying the needs of home caregivers of patients with cancer. Oncol Nurs Forum. 1992;19(5):771–7.
70. Hodgkinson K, Butow P, Hobbs KM, Hunt GE, Lo SK, Wain G. Assessing unmet supportive care needs in partners of cancer survivors: the development and evaluation of the cancer Survivors' Partners unmet needs measure (CaSPUN). Psychooncology. 2007;16(9):805–13. https://doi.org/10.1002/pon.1138.
71. Campbell HS, Sanson-Fisher R, Taylor-Brown J, Hayward L, Wang XS, Turner D. The cancer support Person's unmet needs survey. Cancer. 2009;115(14):3351–9. https://doi.org/10.1002/cncr.24386.
72. Girgis A, Lambert S, Lecathelinais C. The supportive care needs survey for partners and caregivers of cancer survivors: development and psychometric evaluation. Psychooncology. 2011;20(4):387–93. Epub 2010/09/30. https://doi.org/10.1002/pon.1740.
73. Shin DW, Park JH, Shim EJ, Park JH, Choi JY, Kim SG, Park EC. The development of a comprehensive needs assessment tool for cancer-caregivers in patient-caregiver dyads. Psychooncology. 2011;20(12):1342–52. Epub 2011/11/22. https://doi.org/10.1002/pon.1857.
74. Lund L, Ross L, Petersen MA, Groenvold M. The validity and reliability of the 'Cancer caregiving tasks, consequences and needs Questionnaire' (CaTCoN). Acta Oncol. 2014;53(7):966–74. Epub 2014/03/19. https://doi.org/10.3109/0284186x.2014.888496.
75. Kristjanson LJ, Atwood J, Degner LF. Validity and reliability of the family inventory of needs (FIN): measuring the care needs of families of advanced cancer patients. J Nurs Meas. 1995;3:109–26.
76. Zwahlen D, Hagenbuch N, Carley M, Recklitis C, Buchi S. Screening cancer patients' families with the distress thermometer (DT): a validation study. Psychooncology. 2009;17:959–66. https://doi.org/10.1002/pon.
77. Monterosso L, Kristjanson LJ, Dadd G. Content validity and reliability testing of the FIN-PED II: a tool to measure care needs of parents of children with cancer. J Nurs Meas. 2006;14(1):31–44. Epub 2006/06/13. https://doi.org/10.1891/jnum.14.1.31.
78. Oberst MT, Thomas SE, Gass KA, Ward SE. Caregiving demands and appraisal of stress among family caregivers. Cancer Nurs. 1989;12(4):209–15. Epub 1989/08/01
79. Given CW, Given B, Stommel M, Collins C, King S, Franklin S. The caregiver reaction assessment (CRA) for caregivers to persons with chronic physical and mental impairments. Res Nurs Health. 1992;15(4):271–83. Epub 1992/08/01. https://doi.org/10.1002/nur.4770150406.
80. Cameron JI, Franche RL, Cheung AM, Stewart DE. Lifestyle interference and emotional distress in family caregivers of advanced cancer patients. Cancer. 2002;94(2):521–7. Epub 2002/03/20. https://doi.org/10.1002/cncr.10212.
81. Glajchen M, Kornblith A, Homel P, Fraidin L, Mauskop A, Portenoy RK. Development of a brief assessment scale for caregivers of the medically ill. J Pain Symptom Manag. 2005;29(3):245–54. Epub 2005/03/23. https://doi.org/10.1016/j.jpainsymman.2004.06.017.
82. Pai AL, Patino-Fernandez AM, McSherry M, Beele D, Alderfer MA, Reilly AT, Hwang WT, Kazak AE. The psychosocial assessment tool (PAT2.0): psychometric properties of a screener for psychosocial distress in families of children newly diagnosed with cancer. J Pediatr Psychol. 2008;33(1):50–62. Epub 2007/07/05. https://doi.org/10.1093/jpepsy/jsm053.
83. Weitzner MA, Jacobsen PB, Wagner H Jr, Friedland J, Cox C. The caregiver quality of life index-cancer (CQOLC) scale: development and validation of an instrument to measure quality of life of the family caregiver of patients with cancer. Qual Life Res. 1999;8(1–2):55–63. Epub 1999/08/24. https://doi.org/10.1023/a:1026407010614.
84. Ferrell B, Grant M, Borneman T, Juarez G, ter Veer A. Family caregiving in cancer pain management. J Palliat Med. 1999;2:185–95.
85. Cohen R, Leis AM, Kuhl D, Charbonneau C, Ritvo P, Ashbury FD. QOLLTI-F: measuring family carer quality of life. Palliat Med. 2006;20(8):755–67. Epub 2006/12/07. https://doi.org/10.1177/0269216306072764.
86. McMillan SC, Mahon M. The impact of hospice services on the quality of life of primary caregivers. Oncol Nurs Forum. 1994;21(7):1189–95. Epub 1994/08/01
87. Varni JW, Sherman SA, Burwinkle TM, Dickinson PE, Dixon P. The PedsQL™ family impact module: preliminary reliability and validity. Health Qual Life Outcomes. 2004;2(1):55. https://doi.org/10.1186/1477-7525-2-55.
88. Prue G, Santin O, Porter S. Assessing the needs of informal caregivers to cancer survivors: a review of the instruments. Psychooncology. 2015;24(2):121–9. Epub 2014/06/17. https://doi.org/10.1002/pon.3609.
89. Deeken JF, Taylor KL, Mangan P, Yabroff KR, Ingham JM. Care for the caregivers: a review of self-report instruments developed to measure the burden, needs, and quality of life of informal caregivers. J Pain Symptom Manag. 2003;26(4):922–53. https://doi.org/10.1016/s0885-3924(03)00327-0.
90. Hoenig J, Hamilton MW. The schizophrenic patient in the community and his effect on the household. Int J Soc Psychiatry. 1966;12(3):165–76. Epub 1966/01/01. https://doi.org/10.1177/002076406601200301.
91. Mishra VS, Chandrakala S, Saranath D. Assessing the quality of life among caregivers of patients with Haematological cancer. Journal of Global Oncology. 2018;4(Supplement 2):104s. https://doi.org/10.1200/jgo.18.76100.
92. Bangerter LR, Griffin JM, Langer S, Hasan B, Kim WS, Murad MH, Khera N. The effect of psychosocial interventions on outcomes for caregivers of hematopoietic cell transplant patients. Curr Hematol Malig Rep. 2018;13(3):155–63. Epub 2018/05/01. https://doi.org/10.1007/s11899-018-0445-y.
93. Laudenslager ML, Simoneau TL, Kilbourn K, Natvig C, Philips S, Spradley J, Benitez P, McSweeney P, Mikulich-Gilbertson SK. A randomized control trial of a psychosocial intervention for caregivers of allogeneic hematopoietic stem cell transplant patients: effects on distress. Bone Marrow Transplant. 2015;50(8):1110–8. Epub 2015/05/12. https://doi.org/10.1038/bmt.2015.104.
94. El-Jawahri A, Jacobs JM, Nelson AM, Traeger L, Greer JA, Nicholson S, Waldman LP, Fenech AL, Jagielo AD, D'Alotto J. Multimodal psychosocial intervention for family caregivers of

patients undergoing hematopoietic stem cell transplantation: a randomized clinical trial. Cancer. 2020;126:1758.
95. Candy B, Jones L, Drake R, Leurent B, King M. Interventions for supporting informal caregivers of patients in the terminal phase of a disease. Cochrane Database Syst Rev. 2011;6:CD007617.
96. O'Toole MS, Zachariae R, Renna ME, Mennin DS, Applebaum A. Cognitive behavioral therapies for informal caregivers of patients with cancer and cancer survivors: a systematic review and meta-analysis. Psycho-Oncology. 2017;26(4):428–37.
97. Griffin JM, Meis LA, MacDonald R, Greer N, Jensen A, Rutks I, Wilt TJ. Effectiveness of family and caregiver interventions on patient outcomes in adults with cancer: a systematic review. J Gen Intern Med. 2014;29(9):1274–82.
98. Hu Y, Liu T, Li F. Association between dyadic interventions and outcomes in cancer patients: a meta-analysis. Support Care Cancer. 2019;27(3):745–61.
99. Langer S, Lehane C, Yi J. Patient and caregiver adjustment to hematopoietic stem cell transplantation: a systematic review of dyad-based studies. Curr Hematol Malig Rep. 2017;12:324–34. https://doi.org/10.1007/s11899-017-0391-0.
100. Bevans M, Wehrlen L, Castro K, Prince P, Shelburne N, Soeken K, Zabora J, Wallen GR. A problem-solving education intervention in caregivers and patients during allogeneic hematopoietic stem cell transplantation. J Health Psychol. 2014;19(5):602–17. Epub 2013/03/09. https://doi.org/10.1177/1359105313475902.
101. Langer SL, Porter LS, Romano JM, Todd MW, Lee SJ. A couple-based communication intervention for hematopoietic cell transplantation survivors and their caregiving partners: feasibility, acceptability, and change in process measures. Biol Blood Marrow Transplant. 2018;24(9):1888–95.
102. Heynsbergh N, Heckel L, Botti M, Livingston PM. Feasibility, useability and acceptability of technology-based interventions for informal cancer carers: a systematic review. BMC Cancer. 2018;18(1):244.
103. Nahum-Shani I, Qian M, Almirall D, Pelham WE, Gnagy B, Fabiano GA, Waxmonsky JG, Yu J, Murphy SA. Experimental design and primary data analysis methods for comparing adaptive interventions. Psychol Methods. 2012;17:457–77. https://doi.org/10.1037/a0029372.

# Part V

# The Intersection of Palliative Care and Hematologic Malignancies and Serious Blood Disorders: Caring for Patients at End of Life

# End-of-Life Considerations

# 23

Robert Macauley, Jessica Bordley,
Lindsay Wooster-Halberg, and Paul Galchutt

## Introduction

Life for patients with hematologic malignancies is often extremely challenging, having spent on average 28.3% of their post-diagnosis lives in hospital and an additional 13.8% in clinic [1]. End of life (EOL) can be even more burdensome, as these patients tend to receive more medically intensive treatment than those with solid tumors and are twice as likely to die in the hospital [2]. According to one study, in the last month of life, 24% of patients with hematologic cancer receive chemotherapy and 48% a blood transfusion, while 12% are intubated and 18% eventually die in the ICU [3].

In addition to being potentially burdensome, these interventions also highlight other areas of concern. Did the patient have the opportunity to identify their hopes and their fears in crafting a consistent treatment plan with their medical team? Did they get the chance to "say goodbye" and achieve closure with the people they love, and in the process have a sense of continuing to care for those people even after they're gone? And were the patient and their family supported in all ways—not just physical, but also emotional and spiritual—through and after the dying process?

## Goals of Care and Treatment Plans

### Case

*Mr. K is a 64-year-old man who was diagnosed with acute myeloid leukemia 4 years ago. He underwent intensive chemotherapy, during which time he had two ICU admissions for sepsis, one requiring intubation. However, he ultimately achieved remission and had a good quality of life until 3 months ago when routine surveillance revealed that the leukemia had recurred.*

*He is not considered a good bone marrow transplant candidate by virtue of his age and comorbidities. He believes, though, that he is "too young to die" and thus consents to further chemotherapy in the hope of being able to watch his grandchildren grow up. He is subsequently re-admitted to the ICU and intubated, although unlike previous such admissions, his condition continues to deteriorate. No longer able to participate in decision-making, his wife of 32 years is tasked with making decisions on his behalf.*

## Prognostication

As noted in Chap. 10, "Advance Care Planning in Hematologic Malignancies," early advance care planning helps clarify expectations, establish an appropriate treatment plan, and prepare the patient and family for what lies ahead. While every patient will hope for a cure—or, at least, prolonging life—there will come a time when EOL is approaching. Both of those magnify the previously identified needs while also presenting additional ones.

Prognostication is particularly challenging in hematologic malignancies, often characterized by a fluctuating trajectory with intense medical interventions close to death [4–6]. One of the reasons for this unpredictable course is that intensive life-prolonging treatment can often achieve its goal, with half of patients with hematologic cancer surviving ICU admission (as Mr. K did twice) [7]. Most patients with hematologic malignancies die from acute deterioration and critical illness [8], making prognostication more complex that is more comparable to non-oncological conditions such as heart failure than to solid tumors [9, 10].

R. Macauley (✉) · J. Bordley · L. Wooster-Halberg
Department of Pediatrics, Oregon Health and Science University, Portland, OR, USA
e-mail: macauler@ohsu.edu

P. Galchutt
University of Minnesota Medical Center, Minneapolis, MN, USA


C. K. Ullrich, E. J. Roeland (eds.), *Palliative Care in Hematologic Malignancies and Serious Blood Disorders*,
https://doi.org/10.1007/978-3-031-38058-7_23

**Table 23.1** Barriers to optimal EOL care for patients with hematologic malignancies

| | |
|---|---|
| **Illness-specific barriers** | • Variable trajectory and precipitous decline at EOL<br>• Challenges in prognostication at EOL<br>• Transfusion-dependence at EOL |
| **Cultural barriers** | • Unrealistic expectations in terms of outcomes<br>• Worry that EOL discussions could undermine patients' trust in their physician<br>• Oncologists' approach toward prescribing disease-directed therapy at EOL |
| **System-based barriers** | • Inadequate EOL supports<br>• Barriers to providing blood product support at EOL, especially for hospice patients |

The result is these conversations happen quite late in the disease course [11, 12]. In a recent study, for instance, 42% of hematologic oncologists reported the first conversation about resuscitation status at less than optimal times (i.e., acute hospitalization or imminent death), and many waited until death was clearly imminent to discuss hospice (23%) or preferred site of death (39%) [12]. Not surprisingly, studies have shown that advance directives and resuscitation status are rarely addressed and documented for these patients [13].

In addition to more medically intensive treatment at EOL, another result of these delayed conversations is decreased likelihood of enrolling in hospice [14], which only 47% of Medicare beneficiaries with hematologic malignancies utilize [15]. While that likelihood has increased somewhat in recent years, median hospice enrolment for this population remains only 6–9 days [16, 17].

There may also be structural barriers to hospice enrollment for patients with blood diseases. For instance, while the Medicare Hospice Benefit does not specifically preclude blood transfusions, the cost of these may exceed per diem allotment [18]. Not surprisingly, transfusion dependence has been associated with a lower rate of hospice enrolment in myelodysplastic syndrome [19]. Recognizing this barrier, surveyed hematologists harbor concerns about hospice services' adequacy and report that they would be more likely to refer patients to hospice if transfusions could be continued [20]. (Table 23.1).

## Planning for EOL

Many aspects of EOL care apply to all patients, irrespective of their particular condition (i.e., the importance of advance care planning and optimal symptom management). Patients with hematologic malignancies are unique in some respects, though, especially recognizing the increased risk of burdensome procedures at EOL. In identifying the patient's primary hopes and fears [21], it is also crucial to explore what constitutes a "good death" in their mind. For one patient, death may be the worst imaginable outcome, whereas, for another, a life of dependence or neurologic devastation could be even worse. These preferences also impact EOL care, as some patients—if forced to choose—would opt for lucidity over optimal analgesia, even as physicians tend to prioritize the latter [22].

**Table 23.2** NURSE model of expressing empathy [26]

| | Example | Notes |
|---|---|---|
| **Naming** | "It sounds like you are angry." | Naming allows the clinician to empathize with and deescalate the intensity of feeling |
| **Understanding** | "This helps me better understand where you're coming from." | Important not to claim complete understanding, which could make the patient feel more alone |
| **Respecting** | "I can see you have really been trying to adhere to the treatment plan." | Praise is also applicable here (e.g., "I admire how hard you've worked toward reaching your goals") |
| **Supporting** | "I will do everything I can to make sure you have what you need." | Supporting is a profound statement of commitment and solidarity |
| **Exploring** | "Could you say more about what you mean when you say that …" | Usually best to specify what you're inquiring about, or else the patient may not understand the query |

These can be very challenging conversations to hold, often eliciting strong emotion. Physicians are often tempted to shy away from these topics for that very reason, but such emotion reflects the importance of these conversations. Rather than ignoring and moving past the patient's expressed feelings, it is more effective to address them directly. Emotional processes generally occur more quickly than rational thought and thus influence decisions that are made [23]. Attending to those emotions can decrease patient anxiety and improve patient satisfaction [24]. The Vital Talk method of responding to emotion summarizes appropriate responses with the NURSE acronym (Table 23.2) [25].

After the patient's values have been elicited and emotional response honored, the medical team should make a clinical recommendation based on those values. While perhaps initially appearing to be paternalistic by telling the patient what to do, a recommendation based on the patient's values reflects respect for autonomy [24, 26]. Most patients value physician recommendations [27], recognizing them as an integral part of shared decision-making [28]. The recommendation should be framed in terms of the patient's expressed values and explicitly leave room for the patient to disagree or clarify, if the physician has misunderstood the patient's goals.

It may be necessary, in the course of making a recommendation, to clarify common misperceptions. For instance, many patients associate the limitation of treatment with "giving up," or are worried that they will not continue to receive attentive care if they consent to a DNR order. Those letters, however, stand for Do Not Resuscitate, not Do Not *Respond*. The mere fact that a patient has a DNR order is relevant only to situations of cardiopulmonary arrest, not impacting interventions such as antibiotics, supplemental oxygen, or intravenous fluids. Here it should be noted that some physicians may also misunderstand—and inappropriately extend—DNR orders [29], underscoring the need to be clear on what they refer to and what they do not [30].

Many patients express a simultaneous hope for receiving treatment that will prolong their life (which CPR can, in some cases) while also dying comfortably, ideally at home. Given the uncertain trajectory of hematologic malignancies and the likelihood of acute decompensation, it may not be possible to achieve both of these goals. In the case of such seemingly conflicting goals, medical teams should discuss the patient's goals, likelihood of each option, anticipated outcomes, and measures that can be taken to ensure comfort in either scenario. With such information patients are better prepared to identify their greatest priority.

It is also important to recognize that hospitalized patients—especially those receiving intensive care, which patients with hematologic malignancies do more frequently than other patients with cancer—often have compromised decision-making capacity, as befell Mr. K. In that event, a surrogate must make decisions on the patient's behalf. Ideally, the patient will have documented their goals in an advance directive, as well as named a durable power of attorney for health care. But often, neither of these has occurred. In such situations, the surrogate must determine what the patient would have wanted (i.e., provide "substituted judgment").

*Recognizing that it is improbable that Mr. K will survive this hospitalization and thus not achieve his goal of watching his grandchildren grow up, the medical team engages Mrs. K in a conversation about his goals and values. This conversation is understandably extremely emotional, and they spend significant time honoring her love and dedication to her spouse and acknowledging what a challenging position she is in.*

Acting as a loved one's surrogate decision-maker is challenging both emotionally and cognitively in identifying the appropriate treatment course based on the patient's goals. It is difficult to know for sure what another person would choose in a situation that may not have been precisely anticipated, explaining studies showing that surrogates accurately estimate a patient's treatment preferences only two-thirds of the time [31]. It can be helpful to reframe the more precise question of "What would the patient decide if he were still able?" to a more manageable one that emphasizes that it is, indeed, the patient's values driving the decision (e.g., "What would the patient want you to do, in this role of surrogate decision-maker?").

Providing thoughtful guidance and an informed recommendation based on the patient's values may also help spare the surrogate distress by lifting some of the decision-making burden from them. Over one-third of these surrogates who decided to limit treatment report serious symptoms—including stress, doubt, and guilt over the decisions they've made—which in some cases can last for years [32]. In one study, 82% of family members who took part in EOL decision-making had subsequent post-traumatic stress disorder symptoms [33], findings which cross racial and ethnic boundaries [34]. Agreeing to a DNR order specifically—thereby expanding beyond the question of "whether I should" to concretizing the memory "that I *did*" sign a document that prevented my loved one from receiving treatment that had a chance of extending their life—has been found to "raise many negative emotions including guilt, ambivalence, and conflict." [35]

There may be times when a patient or their surrogate decision-maker, such as Mrs. K, cannot explicitly decide to limit treatment, even though that treatment is unlikely to help them achieve their espoused goals (and may cause undue suffering). In those cases where the likelihood of successful CPR, for instance, is negligible [36], the medical team might utilize a technique known as "informed assent." [37] Acknowledging that the patient is unable to bring himself to authorize limitation of treatment explicitly, the team could inform the patient that he is free to accept their recommendation not to pursue CPR. While this may seem like a semantic distinction, accepting a professional recommendation may be more palatable to some patients—especially those who view themselves as "fighters"—than authorizing a DNR order. Taken further (in what might be termed "informed non-dissent"), the team could even inform the patient that the clinical team will enact a DNR order unless the patient objects.

If this is not acceptable to the patient, another option is a time-limited trial (TLT), which some have referred to as "provisional intensive care." [38] Agreeing to either continue or initiate a requested treatment shows respect for the patient's or family's priorities while establishing a clear point of review and reconsideration. By establishing clear markers of either success or failure—as the team did in this section's case—the intervening time may provide greater clarity as to the possibility of success of the intervention, as well as provide the patient or family the opportunity to recognize the low likelihood of meaningful benefit [39]. A TLT also permits framing the expectant treatment approach in terms of "following the patient's lead," with the ensuing course of action determined by the patient's response to therapy, rather than a decision imposed by the surrogate. Obviously, such an agreement on a TLT is not binding, and additional TLTs—perhaps with modified waypoints to guide future care—may be necessary.

*Mrs. K notes that her husband is a "fighter" who did survive two previous ICU admissions. Even when the doctors inform her that this situation is different, she can't bring herself to authorize any limitation of treatment. Therefore, the physi-*

*cians suggest a time-limited trial of continued mechanical ventilation and antibiotics, which will be revisited in 72 h to determine if his counts improved or ventilator settings diminished.*

Another potential response to patients who seemingly "want everything" is a Do Not Escalate Treatment (DNET) order [40]. Rather than withholding a specific treatment a DNET order generally indicates that current life-sustaining medical treatment (LSMT) will not be escalated, and no new forms of LSMT will be initiated. A common application of this occurs after a patient is discharged from the ICU and wishes not to return, where current antimicrobials, blood products, and oxygen support are maintained at current levels.

Potential advantages of a DNET order include providing the patient or family additional time to accept the patient's impending death [41]—thus increasing the likelihood of withdrawal of treatment already in use [42]—as well as "absolving" the decision-maker of ultimate responsibility for the patient's death (which clearly follows a clinical decompensation) [43]. Drawbacks include lack of clinical clarity—for while initiation of vasopressors is clearly an escalation, temporary increase in $FiO_2$ may not be—and the risk of using an acronym as a replacement for a goal-directed plan of care [44].

*When the time-limited trial does not yield the hoped-for improvement, Mrs. K expresses concern that her husband—who she says never wanted to die this way—might be suffering. She still can't bear to stop life-sustaining treatment, so the team recommends that current treatment not be escalated (including instituting a DNR order). She agrees to this.*

Given the intensive nature of EOL care for patients with hematologic malignancies, much of that care necessarily occurs in hospitals. But for those patients who opt for less medically intensive treatment, planning for EOL is no less complicated and just as important. Description of goals in an advance directive and, as applicable, documentation of a treatment plan on a Portable Order for Life-Sustaining Treatment (POLST) form is crucial. POLST forms have been shown to decrease the probability of a patient who cannot communicate from receiving unwanted treatment [45] and increase the probability of patients who want only comfort measures dying at home [46]. (Chap. 24).

## Conclusion of the Case

*The following day when Mr. K's condition has worsened further, the team utilizes an "informed assent" approach by recommending a shift to comfort measures only, which Mrs. K is free to accept. She is grateful for the additional time with her husband and the reassurance that the team has done everything possible for him. He dies comfortably after the withdrawal of life-sustaining treatment.*

## Location for EOL Care

Organizations that set standards for best practice in cancer care, such as the American Society of Clinical Oncology and the National Quality Forum, recognize quality metrics spanning the full spectrum of cancer disease course, including EOL. These quality metrics include: no CPR, intubation, or ICU in the last 30 days of life; hospice enrolment of greater than 7 days; and death outside of an acute care facility [47, 48]. A broad survey of 349 hematologic oncologists in the United States found that clinicians who care for patients with blood cancers believe these broader cancer metrics apply to and appropriately represent quality EOL care for the hematologic malignancy patient population (Table 23.3) [49].

Yet, while the rate of in-hospital deaths among patients with hematologic malignancies has decreased by 30% over the past 17 years, patients with hematologic cancers are still 65% more likely to die in the hospital—and if in the hospital, in the ICU—compared to patients with solid tumors, and 25% less likely to die at home [50]. How can we explain this gap between best practice for high-quality EOL care and the care actually received?

From the Odejide et al. survey, hematologic oncologists' perceive the greatest barrier to high-quality EOL care to be "unrealistic patient expectations" around their disease [49]. Importantly, this patient-focused factor may be an understandable extension of the other recognized clinician-centered barriers, namely clinicians' desire to preserve patient hope combined with clinicians' optimism and the uncertainty of prognostication as addressed above. Solutions, as suggested by this group of clinicians, include increased access to palliative care, early integration of palliative care services at the time of diagnosis, increased availability of inpatient hospice facilities, and the ability to provide concur-

**Table 23.3** Percent of hematologic oncologists who believe a specific quality measure appropriately represents quality EOL care [49]

| Time frame | Quality measure | Reported acceptability |
|---|---|---|
| Within 30 days of death | No CPR | 85.1% |
| | No intubation | 80.5% |
| | No ICU admission | 63.9% |
| | Fewer than 2 hospitalizations | 54.2% |
| | Fewer than 2 ED visits | 53.6% |
| Within 14 days of death | No chemotherapy | 79.9% |
| Within 7 days of death | No platelet transfusions | 59.9% |
| | No red cell transfusions | 58.7% |

rent hospice and disease-directed care, as is available for pediatric hospice patients.

As the quality metrics demonstrate, death at home has come to be thought of as the gold standard for a "good death." Conversely, death in a hospital has been characterized negatively as "proceduralizing" death by turning it into a medical "problem" and offering an environment that fails to promote comfort and peace for patients and their loved ones. The Macmillan Cancer Support non-for-profit in the UK—to improve care and conversations around dying—queried cancer patients and found that only 1% of this population expressed a preference for in-hospital death, while 64% hoped to die at home [51]. Yet, a Belgian survey of family physicians, nurses, and caregivers highlights that this is not quite such a universal perspective. For some patients and families—especially those who have dealt with prolonged and complex illness, such as the hematologic malignancy population—the hospital represents a "safe haven." [52]

Illustrative of this, hematologic malignancy patients continue to prefer death in the hospital at higher rates than the overall cancer population. Howell et al. found that 28% of patients with blood cancer preferred to die in hospital, 18% in a hospice or other facility, and only 46% preferred a home death. As has been discussed elsewhere, the long-standing relationship and trust in the expertise of the hematologic malignancy care team is an important factor in the preference to spend EOL in a hospital. From this study, an important takeaway is not so much that there is one "right" location for death but that there is power in providing the opportunity for patients to express a preference. Of the 74% of hematologic malignancy patients that did die in hospital, there was an 84% in-hospital death rate among patients for whom no preference was documented, while those who had documented EOL conversations had a 62% in-hospital death rate. Relatedly, the highest rates of in-hospital death were in the population who lived less than 1 month from the time of diagnosis to death, thus often missing a window in their disease course that allowed for advance care planning [53, 54].

## Post-Mortem Options

Patients who are able to engage in discussions regarding memorial planning may provide an incredible gift to loved ones. Being newly bereaved and in a position to make decisions regarding post-mortem care, memorial services and disposition can be emotionally and financially burdensome [55]. An important part of legacy building, identifying one's wishes for post-mortem care and disposition can help finalize an individual's sense of "having affairs in order" before death.

For some patients and families, post-mortem rituals and choices about interment are clearly defined by their cultural or spiritual context. For many others, the opportunity to explore how their body could provide benefit after death—to science, education, or other persons—may be an important piece of their legacy work. Many hematologic malignancy patients will have been the recipients and beneficiaries of treatments such as bone marrow donation and chemotherapy clinical trials. They may, therefore, may already have strong feelings and first-hand knowledge around the value of organ donation and contributions to scientific advancement.

Broadly, the potential opportunities that are available to patients include organ donation, body donation, and autopsy. Organ donation is the surgical removal of a healthy organ from a donor for transplantation into an individual's body for whom that organ has stopped working. The ability of cancer patients to participate in organ donation varies by cancer type and treatment status. Having blood cancer at the time of death makes being the donor of an internal organ, such as liver or kidney, unlikely. Still, there may be the important option of donating corneas and other tissues.

The post-mortem decision about whether an individual is a candidate for organ donation lies with the regional organ procurement organization (OPO). OPOs are a collective of non-profit organizations overseen by the United Network for Organ Sharing (UNOS) at the federal level. Organ donation can be an emotionally charged topic, both due to sensitivity around the treatment of a loved one's body and intense feelings of disappointment that can arise upon learning that it is not possible to honor a patient's wishes around donation. The third-party OPO serves the important role of protecting the anonymity of donors and recipients should donation proceed and protecting the relationship between families and care teams if organ donation is not an option.

In the case of body donation, the intent is a gift toward scientific learning. Many medical education and research institutions support whole-body donation for anatomy education or specific research. Loved ones need to know that they will not receive reports or results related to the donation and that the choice of whole-body donation will likely delay their receipt of the patient's remains for burial or other rituals. The desire for organ donation or autopsy may preclude body donation, and factors such as age younger than 18 and extremes of body mass index might be barriers to body donation.

Finally, an autopsy may be requested at the time of death. Autopsy allows a patient's medical team and loved ones to learn more specifically about the medical conditions contributing to the individual's death. An autopsy report will be available to the patient's next of kin and, typically, a medical clinician will be able to review the results with the family if desired. An autopsy may be of particular importance should questions remain around the status of the patient's cancer at the time of death or about the immediate circumstances leading to death.

We know that a family's awareness of their loved one's wishes prior to the time of death is a significant factor influencing participation in and acceptance of EOL choices such as organ donation [56, 57]. This awareness offers another example of the importance of advance care planning and demonstrates how the impact of such planning can extend even beyond the time of death. Whatever the wishes, the most important thing a patient can do is to share them—to ensure they are honored by their loved ones but also that they might offer the best chance at peace for those left behind.

## Beyond the Medical Treatment Plan: Addressing Emotional Distress at EOL

*Brenda, an African American married woman in her 40s with two children, aged 15 and 17, was diagnosed 5 years ago prior with multiple myeloma. Throughout her treatment, her oncology team noted her distress and frustration when treatment regimens interfered with her ability to attend the school functions, drama performances, and track meets of her teenage sons. She often met with the clinic social worker about how to best support her sons but was hesitant to engage around issues of her own coping, voicing a preference to journal about her feelings instead.*

*As her illness progressed, conversations continued with Brenda about her goals. The team learned that the pain related to her myeloma was increasingly making it difficult to spend time with her family. She wanted to use her limited energy to be with her sons instead of coming to the clinic for treatment. Brenda spoke openly about her awareness that she was dying, and tearfully shared her grief and sadness around dying before seeing her sons as adults. She expressed her fear about the caregiving burden her husband already managed, and shared a wish that she could somehow make this easier on him.*

*The decision was made between Brenda and her team to reprioritize her care, focusing on comfort and enjoying time with her family at home, as opposed to treating her multiple myeloma. She was admitted into home hospice care.*

*Brenda met multiple times with the hospice social worker, who invited her to engage in life review. By sharing memories that she had not given thought to for some years, Brenda remembered some of the more poignant parenting moments wherein she felt that she could instill her values toward her sons. In exploring her grief about not seeing them grow to adults, she was urged by the social worker to use her journaling skills to write letters that could be shared with them during milestones throughout the remainder of their teenage years and into adulthood.*

*As Brenda confronted her emotional distress, she and her husband were increasingly able to communicate their concurrent worries. Brenda learned that her husband shared many of the same fears about caring for her and being the sole support for their children after she died. In his sadness, he also voiced feeling overwhelmed about knowing "what to do" when she died, allowing Brenda the opportunity to identify and share her wishes about a memorial service. With support from her hospice social worker, she even called the funeral home to make her own arrangements—one final way she could try to make this easier on her family.*

In addition to eliciting patient preferences and wishes regarding medical care, practitioners and professional staff who serve patients at EOL also have the unique opportunity to alleviate emotional distress in conjunction with advance care planning.

Advance care planning, which promotes emotional health through education and enhancement of autonomy, can act as both a conduit to and a reciprocal intervention alongside evidenced-based psychotherapeutic modalities that address emotional well-being and distress at EOL. Emotional health and well-being must be prioritized throughout a patient's illness, particularly as practitioners appropriately anticipate both cognitive and emotional reactions as a normalized response to illness progression. Individuals with cancer may especially describe a renewed sense of reflection at EOL compared to prior life stages due to their illness trajectory, prognosis fears, and time already spent in processing and adjustment since the time of diagnosis. Multiple psychotherapeutic interventions, such as meaning-centered psychotherapy, dignity therapy, therapeutic life review, and family therapy, draw upon the lived experience of a patient and may be appropriate to support this population.

## Meaning-Centered Psychotherapy

Developed by palliative psychiatrist William Breitbart, meaning-centered psychotherapy is an evidence-based therapeutic approach that focuses on helping patients find meaning and purpose as they "confront terminal illness and death." [58] Heavily influenced by psychiatrist Viktor Frankl, who in his memoir, *Man's Search for Meaning*, draws from his experience as a Holocaust survivor in observing that "despair is suffering without meaning" [59] and that life can hold meaning even while suffering. Meaning-centered psychotherapy, which recognizes humans as inherently holistic, emphasizes humans' capacity to identify meaning amid suffering and illness. Proven effective in individual and group settings, meaning-centered psychotherapy can reduce emotionally distressing depression and anxiety symptoms [60].

## Dignity Therapy

Dignity therapy, developed and introduced by palliative researcher Harvey Max Chochinov in 2002, is a brief, time-limited psychotherapy designed to reduce feelings of emotional distress commonly identified at EOL [61]. Dignity therapy interventions invite participants to reflect on a series of nine questions targeted toward personal reflection and the exploration of hopes that one most wants to share with their loved ones. Following a narrative interview guided by these questions, which is recorded, edited, and transcribed by a dignity therapy trained healthcare professional, a transcription of the interview is then provided to the patient to share with their family as a generativity document. A 2005 study [62] found that dignity therapy decreased suffering and self-reports of depressed mood and confirmed that dignity therapy is beneficial for patients reporting higher initial psychosocial distress levels. These results were validated by a multi-site randomized controlled trial considering dignity therapy in relation to standard palliative care and client-centered care in 2011 [63].

## Therapeutic Life Review

Therapeutic life review is an intervention focused intentionally on helping patients tell and find peace with, their story. Often utilizing prompts or items from a person's past to elicit memories and experiences to facilitate memories, life review focuses on identifying accomplishments or memories that give "new significance to an individual's life." [64] Less structured than either meaning-centered psychotherapy or dignity therapy, life review techniques are easily accessible and adaptable for patients experiencing cognitive decline.

## Family Therapy

For many families, family therapy may effectively promote adaptive functioning and maintain healthy attachments within a family system facing a crisis resulting from a patient's illness. Research demonstrates that family functioning factors (such as cohesiveness, support, conflict-management, and communication) decrease throughout the progression of a cancer illness [65] and that maintaining strong family relationships can help support a patient's sense of purpose [66]. Family therapy provides an underlining opportunity for a skilled practitioner to emphasize, enhance, and validate a patient's continued role within an active system, along with providing opportunities for families to find reconciliation with past or current conflict.

All conversations surrounding meaning, legacy, and dignity deserve absolute authenticity and presence. Thus, it may be prudent for those working with EOL care teams to consider their feelings related to death and dying before helping others. Self-assessment of one's experiences with illness and dying—inclusive of a familial, cultural, spiritual, and personal lens—requires continuous consideration throughout a career [67]. If such feelings inhibit an ability to engage with patients around EOL issues, practitioners must have access to professional and institutional mental health and bereavement support.

## Legacy Work

The creation of a legacy is profoundly personal. As patients approaching EOL identify worries and anxieties related to being forgotten, legacy conversations and projects can be initiated in tandem with the interventions discussed above while providing comforting reassurance to a patient that they will be remembered.

Widely utilized in hospitals and hospice programs for patients who are near EOL, legacy projects are an important modality "to process the emotions associated with anticipatory grief." [68] Tangible legacy projects can include handprints or molds, photo collages, artwork, pieces of writing, or videos/songs. These are best initiated amongst a multidisciplinary team including art therapists, child-life therapists, chaplains, and social workers.

In addition to creating space to process feelings and identify meaningful priorities, legacy work also creates palpable memories for loved one's post-death. Research shows that such keepsakes are incredibly meaningful [69]. For bereaved family members navigating the realms of sadness and grief, finding meanings in memories can provide indisputable comfort but can be an incredibly heavy and daunting task.

## Addressing Emotional Distress at EOL with Children

Children are remarkably perceptive about mortality and loss. However, often due to adult anxiety and a desire to protect the child, many practitioners report discomfort in sharing news about diagnosis and prognosis with pediatric patients. Thus, children are more likely to be isolated in their distress, which becomes problematic as they also likely have less developed coping skills than adult patients. When information regarding prognosis is withheld from children, "it not only gives them less time to process it and adapt, but also denies them the opportunity to observe adults modeling how to cope" as well as robbing "them of the opportunity to share fears and seek comfort." [70] By including children in discussions about their illness, prognosis, and care goals, practitioners and families have the opportunity to reduce emotionally distressing feelings such as worry, loneliness, alienation, and isolation [67]. Families will appropriately look to practitioners for guidance on sharing information about an illness or prognosis with a child, and all members of the healthcare team have a role in guiding, coaching, and modeling these conversations.

Both the American Academy of Pediatrics and World Health Organization advise that youth should be involved in care decisions as they are developmentally and emotionally ready, and research overwhelmingly supports that conversations about a child's diagnosis, hopes, and fears can be incredibly meaningful for both the pediatric patient and their family [71]. As such, discussions about illness, coping, and planning need to be especially patient-centered and individually tailored for pediatric patients and their families. When considering how to engage pediatric patients and their parents best, a practitioner needs to work alongside the healthcare team for an interdisciplinary assessment of how the family understands the child's illness and prognosis. As part of this assessment, the team should pay special attention to exploring already-established communication patterns within the child's family system, understanding that these patterns are likely influenced by the family's cultural and spiritual framework.

Additionally, communication with the child will be guided by assessing a child's developmental functioning, which will serve as a stronger factor than age when considering a child's questions, wonderings, and thoughts about illness and potential mortality. Assessment of developmental functioning includes a child's intellectual skills, social/language skills, and adaptive functioning and is also influenced by exposures to adverse childhood and social experiences.

Armed with an understanding of family functioning and a developmental assessment, clinicians can provide targeted education to empower parents in their ability to initiate and maintain an open dialogue about the illness with their children. A multi-conceptual understanding of death includes universality, personal mortality, irreversibility, nonfunctionality, and causality [71]. There is empirical support that children can likely grasp these concepts around age 10 as they typically start to transcend from the concrete operational stage to a more abstract level of thinking [72]. Often, children with cancer—especially if they have been in treatment for many months or years—might display even an advanced grasp. Alternatively, children who have had treatment that impacts cognitive functioning may be developmentally behind their peers and struggle with these concepts.

## Spiritual Considerations in EOL Care

*David (pseudonym) was in his mid-60s and 8 years out from his allogeneic hematopoietic cell transplantation (HCT). Approximately 1 year following his HCT, he began to develop graft rejection and associated complications. As a result, David's need for outpatient care within the HCT clinic increased. David's affable nature and penchant for gentle jocularity endeared him to the HCT clinic's interprofessional staff, especially the nurses. He would often describe them as his "second family," given the frequency of his clinic visits over the years and the whole person and the compassionate, skillful care he consistently received.*

*David identified his spirituality to be central to his positive coping. Religious aspects of his spirituality were evident in his devotion to his Christian (Episcopal) faith and his active involvement with Alcoholics Anonymous (AA). Both his Bible and his AA's "Big Book" were sacred texts helping him cope with his serious illness's distressing complications. Chaplaincy care also became a fixture of his care team within both the outpatient and inpatient settings. As he slowly experienced a functional decline with worsening comorbidities and progressed toward his death, he unsurprisingly requested more opportunities to discuss the religious aspects of life that he held sacred* [73] *through his faith and the sense of meaning, connection, and purpose evident in his spirituality embraced through this AA identity and community* [74].

*David's sobriety was critical to his sense of personhood and his behavioral disavowal to pain medications. During one of his final inpatient admissions, he shared a story about how one of his HCT physicians who knew him well resolved a physical pain crisis through her spiritual care. David described being in immersive pain as his physician rounded with him during that hospitalization. He recalled defending against her resolute persuasion to receive the pain medications until she stated that he needed to "get off his cross because we needed the wood." David reported being initially stunned before transitioning to uproarious laughter. He took the medications he needed receiving much-improved pain management because of his physician's skillful spiritual care.*

## Desire for Spiritual Care

As a patient with advanced cancer, David was not alone in his desire to receive spiritual care from his HCT interprofessional medical team members [75]. A focus group study was used within the HCT outpatient clinic environment to understand the importance and efficacy of addressing spiritual matters from both the patient and the interprofessional team. The research team discovered that both patients and the team agreed that providing spiritual care was the team's responsibility, that it was not being addressed as desired, and that a chaplain (spiritual care professional) was needed as a specialist within that clinic environment. Although this research team recognized the transferability limits of their data to other settings (based in the Alberta province, Canada), other quantitative, more broadly-based advanced cancer research projects based in the United States confirm their results. In one study, patients (78%) wanted spiritual care from their team members [76], and in another, patients (72%) indicated that the entire care team minimally met their spiritual needs [77].

The desire for patients with advanced cancer to have the religious and spiritual aspects of their lives attended to was also shown in a randomized controlled trial through the patients' wishes for the end of their lives. The need for the religious and spiritual aspects of their lives to be attended to was prioritized to be higher than several other wishes among 35 total. Participants either used the Go-Wish™ card game or the same 35 wishes placed on a sequential list to be ranked. The investigators discovered that whether using the card game or the list, patients ranked their top two wishes as (1) to be at peace with God; (2) to pray. Notably, the wish to be free from physical pain appeared as the fourth most important wish [78]. While this study asked patients with advanced cancer to consider their EOL wishes, a separate project using a national, cross-sectional survey asked seriously ill patients, bereaved family members, physicians, and interprofessional team members to rank, among 26 factors, those they believed to be most important. Among their patients' findings, peace with God was similarly ranked high as the second most important factor. In this study, however, freedom from physical pain ranked as the most important factor. Unsurprisingly, among patients who received an HCT, the experience of physical pain, as well as other high comorbidities, and the decision to pursue more intensive medical interventions such as an ICU admission are common [22].

Data show that the ICU can be a familiar environment for patients who received an HCT. In a retrospective data analysis from California, nearly half (49%) of these patients (pediatric and adult populations) who experienced death within 1 year of their transplantation were transferred at some point to the ICU [79]. Sometimes admission to the ICU cannot be avoided. Sometimes, however, other less medically intensive care options could be a viable alternative for care, especially within the context of poor performance status, high morbidity, and increased mortality. The opportunity to invite additional advance care planning from either the primary team or through an extra layer of support with the palliative consult service can ideally lead to goals-of-care conversations within a family care conference. These goals-of-care conversations often surface narrative aspects of the patient and family, what is most important to them, and what they value most at this time. Among these values, patients and their loved ones often want their religious and spiritual needs to be addressed.

Family care conferences in the ICU are an opportunity for providing multidimensional support from contributing medical team members. The importance of providing this care cannot be understated as evidence suggests most patients and family members amid serious illness and EOL circumstances desire spiritual care from their medical team. In an extended study involving 13 ICUs and 249 goals-of-care conferences, the research team pursued how frequently surrogate decision-makers and interprofessional ICU care team members discussed religious or spiritual considerations. They found that 78% of the surrogate decision-makers endorsed religion or spirituality to be fairly or very important in their life. This endorsement contrasts with how often (16%) religious or spiritual considerations occurred during these care conferences. Including a chaplain as the specialist to help address these religious and spiritual needs could help the medical team. This inclusion can be logistically challenging as chaplains were present in only 2 of the 249 family care conferences. Providing spiritual care during episodes of treatment such as in ICUs makes a difference and provides more desirable evidence-based outcomes [80]. This provision of spiritual care comes from all members on the healthcare team and not from chaplains alone.

## Outcomes from Spiritual Care

A generalist-specialist model of spiritual care proposes that each interprofessional member of the medical team provides spiritual care. While each member of the team is a generalist, the chaplain is the spiritual specialist [81]. The white paper on spirituality within palliative care details this model focusing on the type of care, including the functions of screening, history, and assessment. A screen is most often conducted by spiritual generalists, noting when a person is in a crisis, such as feeling punished by God or severely disconnected from loved ones. The outcome of this screen can then prompt a timely referral to a chaplain. A spiritual history, also addressed by a generalist, is a brief, interview-based intervention designed to invite basic information. In the acute care setting, this history is often conducted by a bedside nurse at admission. An example of this history is the FICA tool. This tool is designed to provide brief information about a patient's faith/beliefs, whether important, whether there is a supportive community, and whether needs can be addressed [82]. A spiritual assessment is a more involved, detailed, time-intensive process conducted by a chaplain [83].

Evidence suggests this spiritual generalist-specialist model offered by the entire medical team produces desirable outcomes concerning decision-making and quality of life. Among this evidence base, Balboni and colleagues have conducted many studies with advanced cancer populations investigating relationships with spiritual care provision. Some of the variables explored have been to what degree spiritual care from the medical team impacts decision-making toward medically intensive treatment and other outcomes such as quality of life. They discovered that when

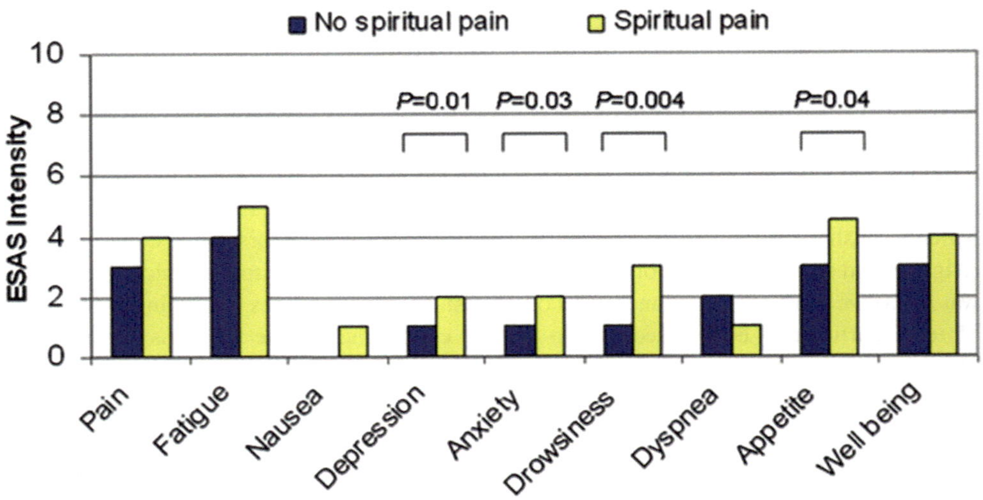


**Fig. 23.1** Association of spiritual pain with physical/emotional symptoms. Delgado-Guay MO, Hui D, Parsons HA, Govan K, De la Cruz M, Thorney S, Bruera E. Spirituality, religiosity, and spiritual pain in advanced cancer patients. J Pain Symptom Manage. 2011;41(6):986–994. With permission from Elsevier

spiritual care is provided by the medical team (especially the hospital chaplains), terminally ill patients are more likely to enroll in hospice. They also found that with spiritual care provision from the medical team among high religious copers, medically intensive interventions at the EOL were pursued less. Consistent with these findings, spiritual care was also associated with patients experiencing a better patient quality of life as death drew near [84]. In a separate but related investigation, "spiritual care and EOL discussions by the medical team may reduce medically intensive treatment, highlighting spiritual care as a key component of EOL medical care guidelines." ([85], p. 1110) There is clarity with these generalized outcomes showing that less intensive measures are pursued when the medical team provides spiritual care at EOL with patients and their loved ones. However, what is less clear is when more medically intensive measures are pursued by patients and family members based on their faith that a miracle is possible when the clinical picture is an irreversible illness and non-beneficial treatment.

This treatment preference for medically intensive measures hoping that a miracle will occur is fairly prevalent among the public. In a study regarding trauma death with the public and trauma professionals, 57% of the public and 20% of trauma professionals believe that divine intervention could save a patient even if the treatment course was determined to be non-beneficial by a physician [86]. Additionally, in a US-based survey with over 1000 clergy (98% Christian) of varying denominations, 86% affirmed the possibility of God performing a miracle [87]. Amid complicated clinical circumstances, there is no standardized, evidence-based intervention to guide clinicians on how to navigate these emotionally charged, religiously guided, and ethically weighted situations. There is some help from expert opinion with a published model, the AMEN (affirm, meet, educate, no matter what) protocol. The authors designed this protocol to be a tool for medical team members to facilitate challenging conversations involving a patient with a poor prognosis and religious beliefs involving the possibility of a miracle [88].

Beyond decision-making, other components of spirituality within the advanced cancer population are associated with physical symptoms or psychosocial distress such as depression or anxiety. In an MD Anderson Cancer study involving interviews ($n$ = 100) of patients with advanced cancer, 44% of them experienced spiritual pain. Notably, "the patients with spiritual pain reported that it contributed adversely to their physical/emotional symptoms. There was a trend toward increased depression, anxiety, anorexia, and drowsiness, as measured by the Edmonton Symptom Assessment Scale [89], among patients with spiritual pain." ([90], p. 986) (Fig. 23.1).

This evidence suggests the need for consistent screening for spiritual distress and/or religious struggle by nurses and physicians. Adding to this evidence, with a population of those who had undergone an HCT, ranging from 6 months to 40 years, King and team identified that 27% experienced religious struggle. This finding is of concern as religious struggle was associated with depression and poorer quality of life [91]. Screening for spiritual distress or religious struggle also needs to be recognized as an essential aspect and practice of HCT team spiritual care [92].

## Barriers to Providing Spiritual Care

There are barriers, however, for nurses and physicians in providing spiritual care at EOL. In a research project conducted by Balboni and colleagues within four Boston hospitals, they investigated why spiritual care provided by nurses and doctors is infrequent at EOL. Among their results, participants identified lack of time as a barrier, but it was not identified as a predictor concerning spiritual care provision. Instead, the strongest predictor for providing spiritual care was training [93]. Another study also identified that physicians and nurses name offending the patients as a possible barrier [94]. As discussed above, instead of offending patients with the exploration of the religious and/or spiritual aspects of their lives, especially amid serious illness, patients desire it. This cultivation of religious and spiritual components also surpasses a theoretical argument for being a part of an ideal patient-centered care model.

It simply yields better evidence-based outcomes with decision-making as well as physical and psychosocial outcomes. As the HCT field continues to move forward identifying evidence-based EOL spiritual care training practices for all team members, some shared spiritual practices already exist, especially for those patients who experience a transplant. Within many care settings, a ritual for an HCT is often available. With the existential stakes being heightened, a ritual creatively and memorably holds a moment in time for what is sacred for a patient to be shared with loved ones and staff [95].

## Necessity of Ritual within Spiritual Care

At the most fundamental level of spiritual care, when all HCT team members of the HOT team engage in meaningful conversation [96] and hear the stories of their patients, like David, something like a "secular healing ritual" ([97], p. 293) can occur. Ritual marks and orders time by the creation and expression of meaning. Ritual supports the heightened narration of the story of someone's existence, especially during an uncertain and unpredictable time where the outcome is unknown as is the case with HCT [98].

Where medical centers offer HCTs, many chaplains provide HCT blessing rituals commensurate with the representative faith, spirituality, or worldviews of the patients and/or their family members. In other words, many chaplains use a framework of a blessing service that is adapted and personally customized in partnership with the patient to reflect the person, their culture, and their beloved community of family and loved ones. This framework contains a basic past, present, and future structure that honors the past with the gravity of the serious illness journey leading to transplant that speaks to the present hope of healing and life being continued with the cells received, and that imagines cure venturing forward in time. Whether through a theistic faith or humanist perspective, these personalized, co-created blessing services become representative artifacts or keepsakes [70] in time as they are also printed like a program for patients and family members.

The significance of these blessing services is that they become thickened moments when recognizing and holding the palpable significance of the unknown outcome with the high mortality and morbidity of the patients who come to an HCT as their best, arguably only, chance of survival. Patients have frequently identified their transplant day as a "second birthday," or they attach a religious meaning of new life through the desired healing of the HCT. Often patients and families, when tearfully remarking on the significance of the transplant during the blessing service, comment on the irony of the hanging of the cells as it visually appears as just another intravenous fluid bag.

The occasion of these ritual/blessing services has also become opportunities for shared spiritual care with the chaplain and interprofessional team members. One of my most memorable HCT co-created blessing services occurred when a Jewish patient and his Christian spouse designed a ritual weaving in words of scripture and meaning, respectively, relevant to the healing desired. On the morning of this patient's HCT, we had also arranged for it to be attended by one of the patient's physicians, who happened to be Jewish, and one of the patient's advanced practice nurses, who happened to be Christian. These interprofessional team members attended and participated by reading words of scripture as part of the service. For a suspended moment in time, they were indistinguishably a physician and an advanced practice nurse, and brothers and sisters in faith and humanity with the shared hope of healing and a longing for life to continue.

## References


1. El-Jawahri AR, Abel GA, Steensma DP, LeBlanc TW, Fathi AT, Graubert TA, DeAngelo DJ, Wadleigh M, Ballen KK, Foster JE, Attar EC, Amrein PC, Bruner AM, Stone RM, Temel JS. Health care utilization and end-of-life care for older patients with acute myeloid leukemia. Cancer. 2015;121(16):2840–8.
2. Howell DA, Roman E, Cox H, Smith AG, Patmore R, Garry AC, Howard MR. Destined to die in hospital? Systematic review and meta-analysis of place of death in haematological malignancy. BMC Palliat Care. 2010;9:9.
3. Beaussant Y, Daguindau E, Chauchet A, Rochigneux P, Tournigand C, Aubry R, Morin L. Hospital end-of-life care in haematological malignancies. BMJ Support Palliat Care. 2018;8(3):314–24.
4. Manitta VL, Philip JAM, Cole-Sinclair MF. Palliative care and the hemato-oncological patient: can we live together? A review of the literature. J Palliat Med. 2010;13(8):1021–5.
5. Cheng BHW, Sham MMK, Chan KY, Li CW, Au HY. Intensive palliative care for patients with hematological cancer dying in hospice: analysis of the level of medical care in the final week of life. Am J Hosp Palliat Care. 2015;32(2):221–5.
6. Brück P, Pierzchlewska M, Kaluzna-Oleksy M, Ramos Lopez ME, Rummer M, Hoelzer D, Böhme A. Dying of hematologic patients—treatment characteristics in a German University hospital. Support Care Cancer. 2012;20(11):2895–902.
7. Azoulay E, Mokart D, Pène F, Lambert J, Kouatchet A, Mayaux J, Vincent F, Nyunga M, Bruneel F, Laisne LM, Rabbat A, Lebert C, Perez P, Chaize M, Renault A, Meert AP, Benoit D, Hamidfar

R, Jourdain M, Darmon M, Schlemmer B, Chevret S, Lemaile V. Outcomes of critically ill patients with hematologic malignancies: prospective multicenter data from France and Belgium—a groupe de recherche respiratoire en reanimation onco-hematologique study. J Clin Oncol. 2013;31(22):2810–8.
8. Habib AR, Cronin AM, Earle CC, Tulsky JA, Mack JW, Abel GA, Odejide OO. How do blood cancer doctors discuss prognosis? Findings from a national survey of hematologic oncologists. J Palliat Med. 2019;22(6):677–84.
9. Lunney JR, Lynn J, Foley DJ, Lipson S, Guralnik JM. Patterns of functional decline at the end of life. JAMA. 2003;289(18):2387–92.
10. Murray SA, Kendall M, Boyd K, Sheikh A. Illness trajectories and palliative care. BMJ. 2005;330(7498):1007–11.
11. McCaughan D, Roman E, Smith AG, Garry AG, Johnson MJ, Patmore RD, Howard MR, Howell DA. Palliative care specialists' perceptions concerning referral of haematology patients to their services: findings from a qualitative study. BMC Palliat Care. 2018;17(1):33.
12. Odejide OO, Cronin AM, Condron N, Earle CC, Wolfe J, Abel GA. Timeliness of end-of-life discussions for blood cancers: a national survey of hematologic oncologists. JAMA Intern Med. 2016;176(2):263–5.
13. LeBlanc TW. Advance care planning and palliative care specialists in malignant hematology and stem-cell transplantation: on why it takes a village. J Oncol Pract. 2018;14(1):3–5.
14. Earle CC, Landrum MB, Souza JM, Neville BA, Weeks JC, Ayanian JZ. Aggressiveness of cancer care near the end of life: is it a quality-of-care issue? J Clin Oncol. 2008;26(23):3860–6.
15. Egan P, LeBlanc T, Olszewski A. End-of-life care quality care outcomes among Medicare beneficiaries with hematologic malignancies. Presented at: 60th American Society of Hematology Annual Meeting & Exposition; 2018 Dec 3; San Diego, CA. Abstract 829.
16. LeBlanc TW, Egan PC, Olszewski AJ. Transfusion dependence, use of hospice services, and quality of end-of-life care in leukemia. Blood. 2018;132(7):717–26.
17. Odejide OO, Li L, Cronin AM, Murillo A, Richardson PG, Anderson KC, Abel GA. Meaningful changes in end-of-life care among patients with myeloma. Haematologica. 2018;103(8):1380–9.
18. Odejide OO. A policy prescription for hospice care. JAMA. 2016;315(3):257–8.
19. Fletcher SA, Cronin AM, Zeidan AM, et al. Intensity of end-of-life care for patients with myelodysplastic syndromes: findings from a large national database. Cancer. 2016;122:1209–15.
20. Odejide OO, Cronin AM, Earle CC, et al. Why are patients with blood cancers more likely to die without hospice? Cancer. 2017;123:3377–84.
21. Bernacki RE, Block SD. American College of Physicians High Value Care Task Force. Communication about serious illness care goals: a review and synthesis of best practices. JAMA Intern Med. 2014;174(12):1994–2003.
22. Steinhauser KE, Christakis NA, Clipp EC, McNeilly M, McIntyre L, Tulsky JA. Factors considered important at the end of life by patients, family, physicians, and other care providers. JAMA. 2000;284(19):2476–82.
23. Pollak KI, Alexander SC, Tulsky JA, Lyna P, Coffman CJ, Dolor RJ, Gulbrandsen P, Ostbye T. Physician empathy and listening: associations with patient satisfaction and autonomy. J Am Board Fam Med. 2011;24(6):665–72.
24. Scheunemann LP, Arnold RM, White DB. The facilitated values history: helping surrogates make authentic decisions for incapacitated patients with advanced illness. Am J Respir Crit Care Med. 2012;186(6):480–6.
25. Rose BL, Leung S, Gustin J, Childers J. Initiating advance care planning in primary care: a model for success. J Palliat Med. 2019;22(4):427–31.
26. Childers JW, Back AL, Tulsky JA, Arnold RM. REMAP: a framework for goals of care conversations. J Oncol Pract. 2017;13(10):e844–e50.
27. Curtis JR, Wenrich MD, Carline JD, Shannon SE, Ambrozy DM, Ramsey PG. Understanding physicians' skills at providing end-of-life care perspectives of patients, families, and health care workers. J Gen Intern Med. 2001;16(1):41–9.
28. Murray E, Pollack L, White M, Lo B. Clinical decision-making: patients' preferences and experiences. Patient Educ Couns. 2007;65(2):189–96.
29. Beach MC, Morrison RS. The effect of do-not-resuscitate orders on physician decision-making. J Am Geriatr Soc. 2002;50(12):2057–61.
30. Macauley R. You keep using that term. J Palliat Med. 2014;17(7):747–8.
31. Shalowitz DI, Garrett-Mayer E, Wendler D. The accuracy of surrogate decision makers: a systematic review. Arch Intern Med. 2006;166(5):493–7.
32. Wendler D, Rid A. Systematic review: the effect on surrogates of making treatment decisions for others. Ann Intern Med. 2011;154(5):336–46.
33. Azoulay E, Pochard F, Kentish-Barnes N, et al. Risk of post-traumatic stress symptoms in family members of intensive care unit patients. Am J Respir Crit Care Med. 2005;171(9):987–94.
34. Braun UK, Beyth RJ, Ford ME, McCullough LB. Voices of African American, Caucasian, and Hispanic surrogates on the burdens of end-of-life decision making. J Gen Intern Med. 2008;23:267–74.
35. Handy CM, Sulmasy DP, Merkel CK, Ury WA. The surrogate's experience in authorizing a do not resuscitate order. Palliat Support Care. 2008;6(1):13–9.
36. Stapleton RD, Ehlenbach WJ, Deyo RA, Curtis JR. Long-term outcomes after in-hospital CPR in older adults with chronic illness. Chest. 2014;146(5):1214–25.
37. Curtis JR. Point: the ethics of unilateral "do not resuscitate" orders: the role of "informed assent". Chest. 2007;132(3):748–56.
38. Giannini A, Messeri A, Aprile A, Casalone C, Jankovic M, Scarani R, Viafora C, SARNePI Bioethics Study Group. End-of-life decisions in pediatric intensive care. Recommendations of the Italian Society of Neonatal and Pediatric Anesthesia and Intensive Care (SARNePI). Paediatr Anaesth. 2008;18(11):1089–95.
39. Quill TE, Holloway R. Time-limited trials near the end of life. JAMA. 2011;306(13):1483–4.
40. Jacobsen J, Billings A. Easing the burden of surrogate decision making: the role of a do-not-escalate-treatment order. J Palliat Med. 2015;18(3):306–9.
41. Vig EK, Starks H, Taylor JS, Hopley EK, Fryer-Edwards K. Surviving surrogate decision making: what helps and hampers the experience of making medical decisions for others. J Gen Intern Med. 2007;22(9):1274–9.
42. Morgan CK, Varas GM, Pedroza C, Almoosa KF. Defining the practice of "no escalation of care" in the ICU. Crit Care Med. 2014;42(2):357–61.
43. Seymour JE. Negotiating natural death in intensive care. Soc Sci Med. 2000;51(8):1241–52.
44. Curtis JR, White DB. Practical guidance for evidence-based ICU family conferences. Chest. 2008;134(4):835–43.
45. Turnbull AE, Ning X, Rao A, Tao JJ, Needham DM. Demonstrating the impact of POLST forms on hospital care requires information not contained in state registries. PloS One. 2019;14(6):e0217113.
46. Fromme EK, Zive D, Schmidt TA, Cook JN, Tolle SW. Association between physician orders for life-sustaining treatment for scope of treatment and in-hospital death in Oregon. J Am Geriatr Soc. 2014;62(7):1246–51.
47. American Society of Clinical Oncology: Measures Overview. http://www.instituteforquality.org/qopi/measures. Accessed 10 Sep 2020.

48. National Quality Forum: National Voluntary Consensus Standards: Palliative Care and End-of-Life Care: A Consensus Report. https://www.qualityforum.org/Publications/2012/04/Palliative_Care_and_End-of-Life_Care%E2%80%94A_Consensus_Report.aspx. Accessed 10 Sep 2020.
49. Odejide OO, Cronin AM, Condron NB, Fletcher SA, Earle CC, Tulsky JA, Abel GA. Barriers to quality end-of-life care for patients with blood cancers. J Clin Oncol. 2016;34(26):3126–32.
50. Chino F, Kamal AH, Chino J, LeBlanc TW. Disparities in place of death for patients with hematological malignancies, 1999 to 2015. Blood Adv. 2019;3(3):333–8.
51. Macmillan Cancer Support, No Regrets: How talking more openly about death could help people die well. http://www.macmillan.org.uk/_images/no-regrets-talking-about-death-report_tcm9-311059.pdf. Accessed 10 Sep 2020.
52. Reyniers T, Houttekier D, Cohen J, Pasman HR, Deliens L. The acute hospital setting as a place of death and final care: a qualitative study on perspectives of family physicians, nurses and family carers. Health Place. 2014;27:77–83.
53. Howell DA, Wang HI, Roman E, Smith AG, Patmore R, Johnson MJ, Garry A, Howard M. Preferred and actual place of death in haematological malignancy. BMJ Support Palliat Care. 2015;7(2):150–7.
54. McCaughan D, Roman E, Smith AG, Johnson MJ, Patmore RD, Howard MR, Howell DA. Palliative care specialists' perceptions concerning referral of haematology patients to their services: findings from a qualitative study. BMJ Support Palliat Care. 2018;17(1):33.
55. Kelly CM, Masters JL, DeViney S. End-of-life planning activities: an integrated process. Death Stud. 2013;37(6):529–51.
56. Ralph A, Chapman JR, Gillis J, Craig JC, Butow P, Howard K, Irving M, Sutanto B, Tong A. Family perspectives on deceased organ donation: thematic synthesis of qualitative studies. Am J Transplant. 2014;14(4):923–35.
57. Miller C, Breakwell R. What factors influence a family's decision to agree to organ donation? A critical literature review. London J Prim Care. 2018;10(4):103–7.
58. Rosenfeld B, Cham H, Pessin H, Breitbart W. Why is Meaning-Centered Group Psychotherapy (MCGP) effective? Enhanced sense of meaning as the mechanism of change for advanced cancer patients. Psychooncology. 2018;27(2):654–60.
59. Frankl VE. The unconscious god. New York: Washington Square Press; 1985. p. 137.
60. Breitbart W, Pessin H, Rosenfeld B, Applebaum AJ, Lichtenthal WG, Li Y, Saracino RM, Marziliano AM, Masterson M, Tobias K, Fenn N. Individual meaning-centered psychotherapy for the treatment of psychological and existential distress: a randomized controlled trial in patients with advanced cancer. Cancer. 2018;124(15):3231–9.
61. Martínez M, Arantzamendi M, Belar A, Carrasco JM, Carvajal A, Rullán M, Centeno C. 'Dignity therapy', a promising intervention in palliative care: a comprehensive systematic literature review. Palliat Med. 2017;31(6):492–509.
62. Chochinov HM, Hack T, Hassard T, Kristjanson LJ, McClement S, Harlos M. Dignity therapy: a novel psychotherapeutic intervention for patients near the end of life. J Clin Oncol. 2005;23(24):5520–5.
63. Chochinov HM, Kristjanson LJ, Breitbart W, McClement S, Hack TF, Hassard T, Harlos M. Effect of dignity therapy on distress and end-of-life experience in terminally ill patients: a randomised controlled trial. Lancet Oncol. 2011;12(8):753–62.
64. Wang CW, Chan CAY, CL. The effects of life review interventions on spiritual well-being, psychological distress, and quality of life in patients with terminal or advanced cancer: a systematic review and meta-analysis of randomized controlled trials. Palliat Med. 2017;31(10):883–94.
65. Persson C, Ostlund U, Wennman-Larsen A, Wengström Y, Gustavsson P. Health-related quality of life in significant others of patients dying from lung cancer. Palliat Med. 2008;22(3):239–47.
66. Zaider T, Kissane D. The assessment and management of family distress during palliative care. Curr Opin Support Palliat Care. 2009;3(1):67–71.
67. Pao M, Mahoney MR. "Will You Remember Me?": talking with adolescents about death and dying. Child Adolesc Psychiatr Clin N Am. 2018;27(4):511–26.
68. Neville TH, Clarke F, Takaoka A, Sadik M, Vanstone M, Phung P, Hjelmhaug K, Hainje J, Smith OM, LeBlanc A, Hoad N, Tam B, Reeve B, Cook DJ. Keepsakes at the end of life. J Pain Symptom Manage. 2020;60(5):941–7.
69. Neville TH, Clarke F, Takaoka A, Sadik M, Vanstone M, Phung P, Hjelmhaug K, Hainje J, Smith OM, LeBlanc A, Hoad N, Tam B, Reeve B, Cook DJ. Keepsakes at the end of life. J Pain Symptom Manage. 2020, S0885-3924(20)30525-X. Advance online publication.
70. Bates AT, Kearney JA. Understanding death with limited experience in life: dying children's and adolescents' understanding of their own terminal illness and death. Curr Opin Support Palliat Care. 2015;9(1):40–5.
71. Stein A, Dalton L, Rapa E, Bluebond-Langner M, Hanington L, Stein KF, Ziebland S, Rochat T, Harrop E, Kelly B, Bland R, Communication Expert Group. Communication with children and adolescents about the diagnosis of their own life-threatening condition. Lancet. 2019;393(10176):1150–63.
72. Panagiotaki G, Hopkins M, Nobes G, Ward E, Griffiths D. Children's and adults' understanding of death: cognitive, parental, and experiential influences. J Exp Child Psychol. 2018;166:96–115.
73. Pargament KI. The psychology of religion and coping: theory, research, practice. Guilford press; 2001.
74. Puchalski C, Ferrell B, Virani R, Otis-Green S, Baird P, Bull J, Chochinov H, Handzo G, Nelson-Becker H, Prince-Paul M, Pugliese K, Sulmasy D. Improving the quality of spiritual care as a dimension of palliative care: the report of the Consensus Conference. J Palliat Med. 2009;12(10):885–904.
75. Sinclair S, McConnell S, Raffin Bouchal S, Ager N, Booker R, Enns B, Fung T. Patient and healthcare perspectives on the importance and efficacy of addressing spiritual issues within an interdisciplinary bone marrow transplant clinic: a qualitative study. BMJ Open. 2015;5(11):e009392.
76. Alcorn SR, Balboni MJ, Prigerson HG, Reynolds A, Phelps AC, Wright AA, Block SD, Peteet JR, Kachnic LA, Balboni TA. "If God wanted me yesterday, I wouldn't be here today": religious and spiritual themes in patients' experiences of advanced cancer. J Palliat Med. 2010;13(5):581–8.
77. Balboni TA, Vanderwerker LC, Block SD, Paulk ME, Lathan CS, Peteet JR, Prigerson HG. Religiousness and spiritual support among advanced cancer patients and associations with end-of-life treatment preferences and quality of life. J Clin Oncol. 2007;25(5):555–60.
78. Delgado-Guay MO, Rodriguez-Nunez A, De la Cruz V, Frisbee-Hume S, Williams J, Wu J, Liu D, Fisch MJ, Bruera E. Advanced cancer patients' reported wishes at the end of life: a randomized controlled trial. Support Care Cancer. 2016;24(10):4273–81.
79. Johnston EE, Muffly L, Alvarez E, Saynina O, Sanders LM, Bhatia S, Chamberlain LJ. End-of-life care intensity in patients undergoing allogeneic hematopoietic cell transplantation: a population-level analysis. J Clin Oncol. 2018;36(30):3023–30.
80. Ernecoff NC, Curlin FA, Buddadhumaruk P, White DB. Health care professionals' responses to religious or spiritual statements by surrogate decision makers during goals-of-care discussions. JAMA Intern Med. 2015;175(10):1662–9.
81. Robinson MR, Thiel MM, Meyer EC. On being a spiritual care generalist. Am J Bioeth. 2007;7(7):24–6.

82. Puchalski CM. The FICA spiritual history tool #274. J Palliat Med. 2014;17(1):105–6.
83. Puchalski C, Ferrell B, Virani R, et al. Improving the quality of spiritual care as a dimension of palliative care: the report of the Consensus Conference. J Palliat Med. 2009;12(10):885–904.
84. Balboni TA, Paulk ME, Balboni MJ, Phelps AC, Loggers ET, Wright AA, Block SD, Lewis EF, Peteet JR, Prigerson HG. Provision of spiritual care to patients with advanced cancer: associations with medical care and quality of life near death. J Clin Oncol. 2010;28(3):445–52.
85. Balboni TA, Balboni M, Enzinger AC, Gallivan K, Paulk ME, Wright A, Steinhauser K, VanderWeele TJ, Prigerson HG. Provision of spiritual support to patients with advanced cancer by religious communities and associations with medical care at the end of life. JAMA Intern Med. 2013;173(12):1109–17.
86. Jacobs LM, Burns K, Bennett JB. Trauma death: views of the public and trauma professionals on death and dying from injuries. Arch Surg. 2008;143(8):730–5.
87. Balboni MJ, Sullivan A, Enzinger AC, et al. U.S. clergy religious values and relationships to end-of-life discussions and care. J Pain Symptom Manage. 2017;53(6):999–1009.
88. Cooper RS, Ferguson A, Bodurtha JN, Smith TJ. AMEN in challenging conversations: bridging the gaps between faith, hope, and medicine. J Oncol Pract. 2014;10(4):e191–5.
89. Bruera E, Kuehn N, Miller MJ, Selmser P, Macmillan K. The Edmonton Symptom Assessment System (ESAS): a simple method for the assessment of palliative care patients. J Palliat Care. 1991;7(2):6–9.
90. Delgado-Guay MO, Hui D, Parsons HA, Govan K, De la Cruz M, Thorney S, Bruera E. Spirituality, religiosity, and spiritual pain in advanced cancer patients. J Pain Symptom Manage. 2011;41(6):986–94.
91. King SD, Fitchett G, Murphy PE, Pargament KI, Martin PJ, Johnson RH, Harrison DA, Loggers ET. Spiritual or religious struggle in hematopoietic cell transplant survivors. Psychooncology. 2017;26(2):270–7.
92. King SD, Fitchett G, Murphy PE, Pargament KI, Harrison DA, Loggers ET. Determining best methods to screen for religious/spiritual distress. Support Care Cancer. 2017;25(2):471–9.
93. Balboni MJ, Sullivan A, Amobi A, Phelps AC, Gorman DP, Zollfrank A, Peteet JR, Prigerson HG, Vanderweele TJ, Balboni TA. Why is spiritual care infrequent at the end of life? Spiritual care perceptions among patients, nurses, and physicians and the role of training. J Clin Oncol. 2013;31(4):461–7.
94. Sinclair S, Booker R, Fung T, Raffin-Bouchal S, Enns B, Beamer K, Ager N. Factors associated with post-traumatic growth, quality of life, and spiritual well-being in outpatients undergoing bone marrow transplantation: a pilot study. Oncol Nurs Forum. 2016;43(6):772–80.
95. Remen RN. Kitchen table wisdom: stories that heal. New York: Riverhead Books; 1996.
96. Gadamer HG. Truth and method. 2nd rev ed. [Weinsheimer J, Marshall DG, trans]. New York: Continuum; 2004.
97. Couser GT. Recovering bodies: Illness, disability, and life writing. Univ of Wisconsin Press; 1997.
98. Anderson H. How rituals heal. Word World. 2010;30(1):41–50.

# Care of the Imminently Dying Patient with a Hematologic Malignancy or Serious Blood Disorder

# 24

Kevin Madden and Eduardo Bruera

## Introduction

Over 56,000 Americans will die this year of a hematological malignancy such as leukemia, lymphoma, or multiple myeloma. This is more than those with breast cancer, colon cancer, or pancreatic cancer. (1) There is a gap in quality end-of-life care for patients with hematological malignancies (2) and so before one can consider the end-of-life care in patients with hematological malignancies, it is important to examine how these patients differ than other patients with solid tumors. The differences mainly stem from a more unpredictable course of illness that ultimately shapes how patients with hematological malignancies integrate (or don't) with palliative care and enroll (or don't) in hospice. The choices hematologic oncologists and their patients make directly influence where and what care they receive at the end of life. Only after understanding the unique characteristics of this patient population one can approach the end-of-life care with the mindfulness, empathy, and compassion that are the hallmarks of high-level palliative care.

## Early Integration with Palliative Care

Patients with hematological malignancies are less likely to be referred to palliative care compared to patients with solid tumors (3, 4). There are many reasons for this, including prognostic uncertainty (5), the attitudes and beliefs of hematologic oncologists, and the perceived attitudes and beliefs of patients. The chronicity of hematologic malignancies and serious blood disorders forges an intimate and enduring relationship between the patient and their physician. Not surprisingly, hematologic oncologists possess a strong sense of obligation and professional duty to be the "whole doctor" for their patients, able to manage all aspects of the care delivered, from chemotherapy to quality of life. Consequently, hematologic oncologists are often uncertain about what palliative care specialists can provide to their patients that they do not already receive (6, 7) and thus hesitant to refer their patients (8). For some, there is a misperception that palliative care is only end-of-life care (6) and a referral may "send the wrong message" (9), resulting in depression, despair, and a loss of hope (10). Additionally, both physicians and nurses report that their patients may have unrealistic hopes of a cure which precludes them from being amenable to a referral to palliative care (5, 11–13). Patients, on the other hand, report that they prefer to talk about one particular set of issues with their palliative care provider and other distinct issues with their oncologist (14). There is room for both in the care of patients.

There is progress, however. Recent studies have demonstrated that the use of the "Surprise Question" ("Would you be surprised if this patient died within the next *x* months?" as a suggested trigger for referrals to a palliative care specialist (15, 16)) enabled hematological oncologists to consider more patient-centered goals, identify unmet needs of their patients, and to identify patients with a poor quality of life and depression (17, 18). This is encouraging as palliative care provided early in treatment and concurrently with disease-directed therapy is associated with increased prognostic awareness, improved quality of life, and a decreased frequency of depression (19). Patients with hematologic malignancies or serious blood disorders who underwent hematopoietic cell transplantation with concurrent palliative care are reported to have lower frequencies of depression and posttraumatic stress symptoms (20) while their caregivers coped better with administrative and financial stressors (20). The benefits of palliative care clearly extend beyond the patient and encompass family members and friends.

K. Madden (✉) · E. Bruera
Department of Palliative, Rehabilitation, & Integrative Medicine, Division of Cancer Medicine, The University of Texas, MD Anderson Cancer Center, Houston, TX, USA
e-mail: kmadden@mdanderson.org; ebruera@mdanderson.org



C. K. Ullrich, E. J. Roeland (eds.), *Palliative Care in Hematologic Malignancies and Serious Blood Disorders*,
https://doi.org/10.1007/978-3-031-38058-7_24

## Advance Care Planning

Goals of care conversations are a crucial intervention that can shape the end-of-life care for patients with any type of cancer. These discussions are indispensable and associated with accepted outcomes measures of high-quality end-of-life such as increased use of hospice, fewer intensive interventions near death, and care that is aligned with what patients desire (21–23). Early goals of care conversations are recommended and part of established guidelines for patients with a life-threatening illness (24, 25). Despite recommendations that these conversations occur early and in the outpatient setting, (25, 26) a majority of hematologic oncologists believe end-of-life discussions occur too late (27) and most initial goals of care conversations occurred less than 30 days before death (28).

The lack of clarity in distinguishing a potentially curable hematologic malignancy from the beginning of the end-of-life phase of the illness is what makes prognostication difficult (5), and this may be a factor in delayed advance care planning conversations (29). In one study, documented advance care planning was only present for 1 out of 4 patients with a hematological malignancy and minority patients are at risk for even lower rates of advance directives (30, 31). Yet even with high levels of uncertainty, the value of timely goals of care conversations cannot be underscored (32). Unfortunately, the long-standing, close relationships that hematologic oncologists have with their patients may paradoxically lead them to delay or even avoid goals of care conversations (33). This may be driven by an existential distress that they feel, as many hematologic oncologists feel a sense of "failure" more frequently compared to solid tumor oncologists when their patients are dying (34, 35). Hematologic oncologists at tertiary care centers were more likely to report the belief that end-of-life discussions happen too late than those at community hospitals (27).

Prognostic uncertainty combined with difficulty in initiating advance care planning conversations leads to an unspoken agreement to avoid talking about a patient's goals should their hopes of cure not be possible. This lack of open and transparent communication ostensibly leads to many common features of patients with hematologic malignancies and the care they receive in the last month of life. When compared to patients with advanced solid tumors, they are more likely to:

- Receive chemotherapy in the last month of life (36–39).
- Less likely to be referred to a palliative care specialist (40).
- Less likely to enroll in hospice (41–43).
- Visit the emergency department in the last month of life (36–38).
- Be admitted to the hospital in the last month of life (36, 38).
- Be admitted to the intensive care unit in the last month of life (36–38, 44).
- Die in an acute care setting (2).
- Die in the hospital (36, 38, 45).
- Die in the intensive care unit in the last month of life (36).

Many of these outcomes are associated with poor quality-of-life and end-of-life care, and so a timely referral to Palliative Care can help patients and families be clear in their choices in the context of the prognosis.

## End-of-Life Care

### Intensive Care Unit (ICU)

The intensive care unit can provide medical interventions to sustain and prolong life that other areas of a hospital cannot. This includes noninvasive ventilation such as bilevel positive airway pressure (BiPAP), mechanical ventilation through an endotracheal tube, peritoneal dialysis (PD) or continuous renal replacement therapy (CRRT), and extracorporeal membrane oxygenation (ECMO). There are sequelae to receiving care in the intensive care unit, however, as it can add significant physical and psychological suffering to both patients and their families (46–48). The paradox and conundrum of specific interventions the ICU can provide, such as mechanical ventilation and dialysis, is that they often prove to be more challenging to discontinue than not start in the first place. It is often helpful to suggest "time-limited" trials and mutually agreed upon dates to reassess the benefit and burden of each intervention. Additionally, the unpredictability of critical illnesses is compounded by the aforementioned unpredictability of how hematologic malignancies respond to second, third, or even fourth lines of chemotherapy. The resultant difficulties in making reliable predictions directly affect the choices and decisions that families face; the future is unclear and the burden of making life and death decisions acute with intensely real consequences (49–51).

### Home Hospice

Patients with hematological malignancies are less likely to use hospice compared with those patients with advanced solid tumors (2, 41–43) and are the most likely patients to enroll in hospice within the last 3 days of their life (2, 43). A hematologic malignancy is also an independent predictor of patients' not using hospice at all (2, 42, 43). These phenomena are not limited to the United States, and similar patterns are observed in Australia and Europe (3, 52, 53). While there is an increasing trend towards utilizing hospice (39), the continued late enrollment of patients with hematological malignancies translates to sub-optimal symptom management and being deprived of added layers of psychosocial support that hospice services can provide to both the patient and the family (23).

The question of why these patients use hospice less frequently again ties back to the often rapid and unpredictable progression of most hematologic malignancies, which makes prognostication difficult. Many hematologic oncologists report they wait until death is clearly imminent before initiating conversations about hospice (27). Patients with solid tumors typically follow a trajectory of slow decline with a clear, rapid decline that represents the natural end of their life. Their rather predictable decline translates into a better ability to prognosticate and provide the patient and family with the option of hospice while quality time remains. Patients with hematological malignancies, however, often have an undulating disease trajectory similar to patients with chronic organ failure, such as heart or lung failure (54, 55) This trajectory is characterized by a gradual decline, with intermittent episodes of acute deterioration and with some recovery, but never returning to their previous baseline condition. Near the end of the life, there are more sudden, precipitous declines that can lead to a seemingly unexpected death (56). This inability to accurately prognosticate is certainly a factor in both not utilizing hospice and in patients that do, typically do so in the last few days of life.

While hematologic oncologists perceive the benefits of hospice, many simultaneously felt that the services provided by hospice would not meet the unique needs of their patients (7). The access—or namely, the lack of access—to blood transfusions is a major barrier to patients enrolling in hospice services (7, 29, 39, 44, 57, 58). From the perspectives of hospice agencies, transfusions are cost-prohibitive given the relatively small amount the US Medicare Hospice Benefit allots to cover costs. And yet, this is a patient population that due to their underlying disease, have been transfusion dependent for large swaths of time. This creates a normalcy around transfusions that becomes very difficult for them to abandon when faced with the choice of enrollment in hospice (59). Furthermore, although generally counseled that continued transfusions at best do no harm, and at worst can worsen volume overload leading to worsening symptoms, there are prospective studies that report improvement in symptoms of fatigue and dyspnea with transfusions (60, 61). Reflecting the difficulty of decision to continue transfusion or enroll in hospice of forego this intervention, almost half of all patients with hematological malignancies receive a blood transfusion within the last month of their life (62).

Patients with hematologic malignancies have many sources of physical and psychological suffering (63–66) and late enrollment in hospice may mean that their quality of life and quality of symptom control at the end of life may be compromised. Enrollment in hospice is associated with an improved quality of life when compared to those patients who died in a hospital (23).

Patients with advanced cancer that enrolled in hospice had fewer number of hospital admissions, fewer number of intensive care unit admissions, and fewer invasive procedures during the last 12 months of their life, (67) all accepted outcome measures of high-quality end-of-life care. As with caregivers of patients that receive early palliative care, the caregivers of patients with advanced cancer who were enrolled in hospice had a reduced frequency of depression and perceived that their loved one received excellent end-of-life care compared to those caregivers whose loved one died in a hospital (68, 69).

## Symptom Management

The most common symptoms in patients with advanced cancer that are dying are uncontrolled pain, delirium, dyspnea, and xerostomia (70, 71) and the same holds true for patients with hematologic malignancies. Caregivers and families simultaneously report a high prevalence of psychological and physical symptoms during the end-of-life phase (72) and even though earlier involvement of palliative care is preferred, these "late" referrals can help alleviate suffering as evidenced by a higher completion rate of advance directives and less use of non-beneficial life-sustaining therapies or interventions (46, 70). Palliative care can also assist in the management of the common symptoms at the end of life. For patients with capacity for medical decision-making and can self-report, the Edmonton Symptom Assessment Scale (ESAS) is a validated tool to measure physical, psychology, financial, and spiritual suffering (73). The ESAS has been validated in many settings (71, 74) and has a high retest reliability.

### Pain

The definition of pain is "an unpleasant sensory and emotional experience associated with, or resembling that associated with, actual or potential tissue damage" (75) and is one of the most common physical symptoms in patients with any type of cancer. It is important to both characterize the type of pain syndrome (nociceptive somatic, nociceptive visceral, neuropathic, or mixed; acute, chronic, or acute-on-chronic) as well as the etiology of pain syndrome to formulate the appropriate plan of care. While non-opioid analgesics such as acetaminophen, ibuprofen, ketorolac, gabapentin, and pregabalin can be helpful, and are always the starting point for the treatment of pain, patients at the end of life likely have more intense pain that will require the use of opioids. Table 24.1 summarizes the most commonly used medications for the treatment of pain.

Many patients at the end of life are not opioid-naïve and rather require aggressive titration to control pain, usually

**Table 24.1** Brief overview of commonly used opioids

| Opioid | Route | Onset (min) | Peak effect (hours) | Duration (hours) | Initially scheduled dosing in an opioid naïve patient | Available oral dose formulations | Comments |
|---|---|---|---|---|---|---|---|
| Codeine | PO | 30–60 | 1–1.5 | 4–8 | Short-acting: 30–60 mg every 6 h Long-acting: N/A | Short-acting: 15, 30, 60 mg tablets Long-acting: N/A | Available alone or in combination with 300 mg acetaminophen. Ceiling effect around 400 mg. |
| Tramadol | PO | 30–60 | 1.5 | 3–7 | Short-acting: 25 mg PO every 6 h Long-acting: 100 mg ER daily | Short-acting: IR from 50 mg tablets Long-acting: ER from 100, 200, 300 mg tablets | Additional SNRI effect. Some formulations contain acetaminophen Caution: risk of hypoglycemia, seizure, serotonin syndrome. |
| Tapentadol | PO | <60 | 1.25–1.5 | 4–6 | Short-acting: PO every 4–6 h Long-acting: N/A | Short-acting: 50, 75, 100 mg tablets | A dual opioid agonist and norepinephrine reuptake inhibitor. Avoid MAOIs, SSRIs, and SNRIs due to the potential for serotonin syndrome. |
| Hydrocodone | PO | 10–20 | 1–3 | 4–8 | Short-acting: 5–10 mg PO every 4–6 h Long acting: Every 12 or 24 h preparations | Short-acting: 5, 7.5, 10 mg tablets; 2.5 mg/5 mL liquid, in combination with acetaminophen Long-acting: 10, 15, 20, 30, 40, 50, 60, 80, 100, 120 mg. | All short-acting analgesic formulations contain either acetaminophen or ibuprofen |
| Morphine | PO<br>IV/SC | 30<br>5–10 | 0.5–1 | 3–6 | Short-acting: PO: 5–10 mg every 4 h; IV: 2–4 mg every 4 h. Long-acting: 15 mg every 12 h, or 20 or 30 mg once daily. | Short-acting: 15, 30 mg tablets; 10 mg/5 mL, 20 mg/mL liquid Long-acting: 15, 30, 60, 100 mg as every 12-h preparations | Available tablet or liquid preparation. Short-acting preparations can be given via PEG tube. Rectal preparations (5, 10, 20 mg) available. |
| Oxycodone | PO | 10–15 | 0.5–1 | 3–6 | Short-acting: 5 mg PO every 4 h Long-acting: 10 mg PO every 12 h | Short-acting: 5, 15, 30 mg tablets; 5 mg/5 mL, 20 mg/mL liquid<br>Long-acting: 10, 20, 30, 40, 80 mg tablets as 12-h preparations. | Available alone or in combination with acetaminophen. Not available for parenteral or rectal administration. |
| Oxymorphone | PO<br>IV/SC | 5–10 | 0.5–1 | 3-6 | Short-acting: 5 mg PO every 4 h Long-acting: 5 mg PO every 12 h | Short-acting: 5,10 mg tablets Long-acting: 5, 10, 20, 40 mg as 12-h preparation | Poor bioavailability, must be taken on empty stomach. |
| Hydromorphone | PO<br>IV/SC | 15–30<br>15–20 | 0.5–1 | 3–5<br>4–5 | Short-acting: PO 2 mg every 4 h<br>IV/SC: 0.5–1 mg every 4 h | Short-acting: 2, 4, 8 mg tablets; 1 mg/mL liquid Long acting: 8, 12, 16, 32 mg as 24 h preparations | Available as tablet or liquid preparation. Short-acting can be given via PEG tube. Rectal preparations (3 mg) available. |

*Source:* The MD Anderson Supportive and Palliative Care Handbook, Sixth edition-2018
Permission obtained from Dr. Eduardo Bruera, MD

through the intravenous route. The type and dose of the opioid is both practitioner dependent, but largely stems from the patient's own history of pain. Many patients have been exposed to opioids and generally are reliable reporters of which opioid has been helpful and what has not. The goal with opioid therapy is to titrate to effect, but to minimize the significant and serious side effects of hallucinations, myoclonus, and excessive somnolence (opioid-induced neurotoxicity). Upward titration of opioids is common due to developing tolerance over time, as well as opioid rotation when escalating doses of opioids fail to control pain, or who develop opioid-induced neurotoxicity (76).

## Dyspnea

Dyspnea is one of the most common and distressing symptoms in patients with advanced cancer (77). It is defined as "a subjective experience of breathing discomfort that consists of qualitatively distinct sensations that vary in intensity" by the American Thoracic Society (78) and can be classified into different subtypes. The incidence and intensity of dyspnea significantly increases in cancer patients 10 days prior to death and appears to peak again three days prior to death (79). Unfortunately, even with a heightened awareness of how physically and psychologically debilitating dyspnea can be, only 3% of caregivers report that their family member was breathing comfortably at the end of their life (80). The etiology of dyspnea in advanced cancer patients is often multifactorial, and so the interventions demand a multifaceted approach that includes pharmacological and non-pharmacological treatments.

### Pharmacological Treatments

Opioids are the most reliable and effective intervention for dyspnea; no one opioid is superior to others in providing relief. Randomized controlled studies have demonstrated that opioids can relive dyspnea without diminishing the underlying respiratory drive (81). Opioids primarily exert their effect by acting on the right posterior cingulate gyrus, which decreases the underlying neuromechanical dissociation (81–83) and the anxiety that comes with it. The first step in management is the administration of short acting intravenous or oral opioids on an as needed basis (84), but it is not uncommon for a continuous infusion or oral long acting opioids to be added. Historically, benzodiazepines have been used for the management of dyspnea, yet a recent Cochrane review showed no benefit and their use was associated with adverse side effects including excessive somnolence (85). In patients with a hematologic malignancy, specific comorbidities that might cause swelling, inflammation, and edema anywhere from the oropharynx to distal bronchioles may benefit from a pulse of corticosteroids (86). Additionally, the judicious use of diuretic medications may be beneficial for those with underlying congestive heart failure or renal insufficiency (87). The evidence supporting the efficacy of nebulized opioids and diuretics to treat dyspnea is equivocal at best, and not generally recommended (88).

### Non-pharmacological Treatments

The use of noninvasive ventilation strategies including BiPAP and high flow nasal cannula (HFNC) is gaining ground. Both modalities have been shown to reduce the work of breathing and improve oxygenation (89). Other non-pharmacological interventions include a fan aimed at the face where the trigeminal nerve distribution is located, frequent repositioning, and chest physiotherapy can be used to relieve symptoms (87, 90). Integrative therapies such as acupuncture and guided imagery are useful interventions in the treatment of dyspnea and can be considered in patients who can participate in these techniques (91, 92).

## Delirium

At the most basic level, delirium is "decompensation of cerebral function in response to one or more pathophysiological stressors," (93) and it is the most common neuropsychiatric condition in patients with cancer. It is estimated to occur in 50%–85% of patients at the end of life (94–96). Technically, the Diagnostic and Statistical Manual of Mental Disorders (DSM-5) defines delirium as "a disturbance in attention and awareness" that "develops over a short period of time," is a change from baseline, fluctuates during the course of the day with an "additional disturbance in cognition not explained by another neurocognitive disorder that is caused by a direct physiological consequence of another medical condition, substance intoxication or withdrawal (i.e., due to a drug of abuse or to a medication), or exposure to a toxin, or is due to multiple etiologies" (93).

There are three types of delirium: hyperactive, hypoactive, and mixed (97). Hypoactive delirium is the most common clinical manifestation of delirium, but it is almost certainly underdiagnosed as it is often mistaken for somnolence or sleeping. Hyperactive delirium is the form most commonly recognized and diagnosed, as it is often readily apparent with confusion, agitation, and restlessness (98). Patients with mixed delirium have features of both that can fluctuate quickly between these states, at times making the diagnosis challenging. The diagnosis of delirium was missed by the primary referring team in almost two-thirds of patients referred to a palliative care specialist (99). One of the sentinel signs of emerging delirium is disinhibition, which is often misinterpreted as worsening pain (99).

There are many different validated assessment tools, but the most commonly used are the Memorial Delirium Assessment Scale (MDAS) (100) and Delirium Rating Scale (DRS) (101, 102). The MDAS is widely used and is appropriate for patients with hematologic malignancies; it is composed of 10 items, each rated 0–3 points for a maximum total score of 30 points. Scores $\geq$13 indicate the presence of delirium (100). Given that symptoms can fluctuate rapidly it is imperative to maintain vigilance. Caregivers who remain at the bedside and nursing staff are invaluable sources and often notice subtle changes in the patient, especially at night when delirium is often worse.

### Pharmacological Treatments

The use of antipsychotics to control the hyperactive features of delirium including confusion, agitation, and restlessness is well substantiated and documented, and should be considered the drugs of choice (103). Table 24.2 summarizes the most commonly used medications for the treatment of delirium. The most commonly used antipsychotic is haloperidol. Other antipsychotics including chlorpromazine, olanzapine, and quetiapine are considered appropriate therapy for patients with delirium. It is important to counsel families that the purpose of using medications is to protect the patient from harming themselves through actions they would otherwise not do, such as pulling out central venous catheters, attempting to get out of bed and risking a catastrophic fall, or removing Foley catheters and supplemental oxygen—the intent is never to deliberately sedate their loved one.

**Table 24.2** Overview of treatment of delirium

| Medication | Class | Dose, route | Adverse effects | Additional comments |
|---|---|---|---|---|
| Haloperidol | Typical Antipsychotic | 0.5–2 mg every 2–12 h<br>PO, IV, IM, SC | Extrapyramidal syndrome, prolonged QTc | First line<br>Oral bioavailability is approximately 60–70%<br>May add Lorazepam for agitated patients. |
| Chlorpromazine | Typical Antipsychotic | 12.5–50 mg every 4–6 h<br>PO, IV, IM, SC, PR | Sedation, Hypotension | More sedating and anticholinergic when compared to haloperidol |
| Olanzapine | Atypical Antipsychotic | 2.5–5 mg every 12–24 h<br>PO | Extrapyramidal syndrome, prolonged QTc, Hyperglycemia, Weight gain, Hyperlipidemia | |
| Risperidone | Atypical Antipsychotic | 0.25–1 mg every 12–24 h<br>PO | Extrapyramidal syndrome, prolonged QTc, Weight gain | |
| Quetiapine | Atypical Antipsychotic | 12.5–100 mg every 12–24 h<br>PO | Extrapyramidal syndrome, prolonged QTc, Weight gain | |
| Lorazepam | Benzodiazepine | 0.5–3 mg every 2–12 h<br>PO, IV | Sedative, Respiratory depression | Can have paradoxical effect causing worsening delirium |

*Abbreviation: PO* Per Oral, *IV* Intravenous, *IM* Intramuscular, *SC* Subcutaneous, *PR* Per Rectum
*Source:* The MD Anderson Supportive and Palliative Care Handbook, Sixth edition-2018
Permission obtained from Dr. Eduardo Bruera, MD

The use of benzodiazepines has been debated; on the one hand, their sedative qualities may calm a patient while on the other hand their use can lead to further disinhibition and worsening of delirium. There is emerging evidence that the addition of lorazepam to haloperidol in patients with delirium and persistent agitation was beneficial in controlling the symptoms (104) and the alpha-2 agonist dexmedetomidine may be useful as well (105).

### Non-pharmacological Treatments

There are many non-pharmacological treatments that may be helpful as adjunctive therapies in the prevention of delirium. It is important for the healthcare staff to be aware if a patient has visual and hearing aids that have been forgotten about in the emotional turmoil that is present when someone approaches the end of life. Minimizing extraneous noise, adherence to a "lights on during daytime" and "lights off during nighttime" routine, and placement of familiar keepsakes all may be useful as well (106–108).

## Palliative Sedation

Palliative sedation refers to the deliberate attempt to reduce or minimize consciousness in order to alleviate suffering from refractory symptoms at the end of life (109–112). Pain, dyspnea, and delirium are the most common indications for the use of palliative sedation. It is an important and necessary intervention that should be approached cautiously, and deliberately. In the context of palliative sedation, the term "refractory" has a very specific definition (113):

1. Intensive efforts short of sedation fail to provide relief.
2. Additional invasive or noninvasive treatments are incapable of providing relief.
3. Additional therapies are associated with excessive or unacceptable morbidity or are unlikely to provide relief within a reasonable time frame.

Building on this definition, other conditions should be met before starting palliative sedation including a full spiritual and psychological assessment, a do-not-resuscitate order is placed in the medical record, informed consent is provided by the patient or medical power of attorney, and a conversation occurs and is documented regarding the use or limits of artificial nutrition and hydration (114). Lastly, it is imperative that before palliative sedation starts all parties involved including the patient, the caregiver, bedside nursing, pharmacy, physicians, respiratory therapists, and any other party that will provide care to the patient understand clearly that the intent is to provide relief but not to hasten death (115).

There are numerous medications that can be used to reduce consciousness and alleviate suffering. The most commonly used medications are benzodiazepines, and midazolam is the drug of choice due to its rapid onset and short half-life (116). These pharmacological qualities make initiation and titration easier, safer, and more predictable than longer acting benzodiazepines such as lorazepam (117). Propofol is another agent that can be used, and interestingly enough appears in the pediatric medical literature (118–120) more so than in the adult literature (121). The use of propofol is largely limited due to hospital policies regarding who can administer and where propofol can be used, as it is usually restricted to ICU physicians and anesthesiologists in the operating room, ICU, or for procedural sedation. The rapidly acting intravenous alpha-2 agonist dexmedetomidine may be a consideration as its application for intractable pain and delirium is gaining wider acceptance (105). There is no consensus (122, 123) on the objective assessment of a patient's level of consciousness and the optimal level of sedation needed for the relief of suffering, but the use of bispectral index (BIS) monitoring holds promise for future areas of research in palliative sedation (124).

## Spiritual Care

Spirituality is defined as "the aspect of humanity that refers to the way individuals seek and express meaning and purpose, and the way they experience their connectedness to the moment, to self, to others, to nature, and the significant or sacred" (125) and religion is the formalized structure through which spiritual beliefs can be expressed individually or collectively in a larger community. Providing spiritual care to advanced cancer patients and their caregivers is associated with increased hospice utilization, improved quality of life, fewer aggressive medical or surgical interventions near the end of life, and a decreased risk that they will die in an intensive care unit (126–128). The best palliative care is always delivered in an interdisciplinary fashion, and so all healthcare providers should systemically screen patients and their families for spiritual distress and have a low threshold for referring patients to qualified, trained spiritual care providers such a chaplains (129).

## Communication

The cornerstone of quality palliative care at the end of life is communication. It is essential to understand the structure and functioning components of the family as a whole (130). It is only through this knowledge can comprehensive psychosocial, emotional, and spiritual support for the entire family—while maintaining focus on the well-being of the patient—be provided (131). The primary intervention of communication is the family meeting, whose main purpose is to assist with transparent and open communication, ensure understanding of the plan of care, minimize distress among healthcare providers, and mitigate complicated and pathological grief in the bereaved (131–133).

## Discontinuation of Medical Technology

Many patients and families choose life-sustaining therapies with the hope that they will recover and return to the previous baseline performance status, and not an insignificant number choose these interventions under the rubric of "not giving up." There is, however, an enormous burden on healthcare providers, patients, and families around the notion of discontinuing any intervention that is sustaining life. The discontinuation of medical interventions is often viewed through the lens of morals and ethics; however, this is complicated as it can be difficult to distinguish the boundary between ethics and morals in real-world clinical practice (134–136). It is wise to consider the expertise of a consultation to the Ethics Service, and reliance on professional guidelines when there is not agreement in the decision-making process.

## Discontinuation of Artificial Hydration and Nutrition

Often when patients are starting to approach the end of their life, eating and drinking can technically become a risk factor for aspiration into the tracheobronchial tree and further into the lungs, precipitating edema and possibly infection. There is great distress, however, among caregivers about not providing food or drink to their loved one. After all, the importance of providing nutrition and hydration appears to be a basic socioanthropological expression of caring, and withholding food and drink can be intensely felt as "not caring" or not fulfilling one of the core human characteristics—the desire to care for those who are ill. It is best to not "throw the baby out with the bathwater," and discuss the risks and benefits of "feeding to comfort" as many patients and caregivers will feel relief staking out and claiming this middle ground. As time draws closer, and the difficulty of safe handling of oral secretions becomes more evident, a gentle suggestion to dip a green oral care brush into the patient's favorite beverage (or even small amounts of food) sustains the pleasure of taste while minimizing the distress that can come with choking on larger volumes of food or drink.

A common request near the end of life is to provide artificial nutrition and hydration (ANH) through the intravenous route or through a gastric or intestinal feeding tube. This can be seen as one sees any other medical intervention. Risks and benefits need to be discussed, and it is important that the request is not benign and can actually increase suffering. Volume overload leading to pulmonary edema and resultant dyspnea are real possibilities (137). Conversely, as ANH is a medical invention it is legally indistinguishable from other medical interventions and has been affirmed by the Supreme Court of the United States (138, 139). Furthermore, the American Medical Association (140) and the Hastings Center (141) have agreed that providing ANH is not always necessary.

## Impending Death and Anticipatory Guidance

"Anticipatory guidance" is proactive counseling to both patients and caregivers that addresses the physical, emotional, and psychological changes that occur as death nears. A structured approach to the changes one may see in the physical condition, for example, can help to alleviate the stress associated with the intense scrutiny that caregivers give as they search for clues as to "how much time" their loved one has. Days to months of absorbing subtle cues as to the relative health or sickness based on vital signs, laboratory values, and interpretations of diagnostic imaging can leave caregivers disoriented when the end-of-life approaching. It is important to counsel that research shows that vital signs at the end of life are a poor predictor (142) of how much time a patient has to life. While monitors in the room displaying vital signs have in the past provided reassurance, at the end-of-life they can serve as distractors and so gently recommending turning the monitors off can allow caregivers to be fully present with their loved one. Additionally, it is important to describe—if the family would like—what changes they can expect to see as time gets shorter. The first change observed as one enters the active phase of dying is "sleeping" more, and almost for a majority of the day. "Sleeping," in reality, is most likely hypoactive delirium. Next, the hands and feet will begin to cool as the body shifts blood towards the vital organs and away from peripheral vasculature beds. For those with a Foley catheter, it is expected that urine output will start to diminish. A change from the normal rhythmic ebb and flow of breathing towards an erratic pattern rhythmic breathing interspersed with rapid shallow breaths, deep long breaths, and increasing periods of apnea. These signs, combined with mandibular respirations and flattening of the nasolabial fold are more predictive of death with 72 h (143, 144). Even with this guidance, the most commonly asked question will remain: "How long do they have?" In general, the accuracy of clinician prediction of survival is quite low (145) and it may be helpful to reframe the question as, "What would you like to do with the time you have left?" as it provides a small modicum of control over what is essentially an uncontrollable situation. Conscious decisions about how to spend time with a loved one who is dying is likely to be more beneficial than being fixated on a specific amount time that is certain to be inaccurate.

Many families believe that discontinuation of medical technology such as mechanical ventilation, BiPAP, CPAP, PD, and CRRT will result in a rapid death. This may occur under specific clinical conditions, such as the discontinuation of ECMO, but generally is not true. Therefore, it is incumbent that to prepare the family that death will likely not be immediate, but rather a process that advances over minutes to hours to days.

## Bereavement

Studies have shown that family members and caregivers report poorer end-of-life care when a loved one dies in the hospital, requires admission to the ICU in the last month of life, or if hospice enrollment occurred late or not at all (146). Furthermore, surviving family members and caregivers can experience remorse, a decreased quality of life, and have an increased risk of developing psychological disorders including anxiety and depression when there is not goal-concordant care at the end of life (23). The dilemma that follows is that almost a third of patients with a hematologic malignancy or blood disorder prefer to die in the hospital (147).

Given that surviving caregivers suffer after the death of their loved one, the provision of psychological counseling to surviving family members should be considered a standard of care but is not routine even at large tertiary cancer centers. Prior to death, caregivers provided early counseling (less than 60 days of diagnosis of advanced cancer) had lower rates of depression compared to those caregivers given delayed counseling (greater than 12 weeks of diagnosis of advanced cancer) 3 months after the counseling sessions (148), but there was no difference between the groups in rates of complicated grief or depression 2–3 months after death (149). More research is necessary to better understand how to support family and caregivers, and how to integrate this care into a financially feasible model of healthcare delivery.

## References

1. Siegel RL, Miller KD, Jemal A. Cancer statistics, 2019. CA Cancer J Clin. 2019;69(1):7–34.
2. Earle CC, Landrum MB, Souza JM, Neville BA, Weeks JC, Ayanian JZ. Aggressiveness of cancer care near the end of life: is it a quality-of-care issue? J Clin Oncol. 2008;26(23):3860–6.
3. Howell DA, Shellens R, Roman E, Garry AC, Patmore R, Howard MR. Haematological malignancy: are patients appropriately referred for specialist palliative and hospice care? A systematic review and meta-analysis of published data. Palliat Med. 2011;25(6):630–41.
4. El-Jawahri AR, Abel GA, Steensma DP, LeBlanc TW, Fathi AT, Graubert TA, et al. Health care utilization and end-of-life care for older patients with acute myeloid leukemia. Cancer. 2015;121(16):2840–8.
5. Odejide OO, Cronin AM, Condron NB, Fletcher SA, Earle CC, Tulsky JA, et al. Barriers to quality end-of-life care for patients with blood cancers. J Clin Oncol. 2016;34(26):3126–32.
6. LeBlanc TW, O'Donnell JD, Crowley-Matoka M, Rabow MW, Smith CB, White DB, et al. Perceptions of palliative care among hematologic malignancy specialists: a mixed-methods study. J Oncol Pract. 2015;11(2):e230–8.
7. Odejide OO, Cronin AM, Earle CC, Tulsky JA, Abel GA. Why are patients with blood cancers more likely to die without hospice? Cancer. 2017;123(17):3377–84.

8. Epstein AS, Goldberg GR, Meier DE. Palliative care and hematologic oncology: the promise of collaboration. Blood Rev. 2012;26(6):233–9.
9. Tricou C, Munier S, Phan-Hoang N, Albarracin D, Perceau-Chambard É, Filbet M. Haematologists and palliative care: a multicentric qualitative study. BMJ Support Palliat Care. 2019;
10. Mack JW, Smith TJ. Reasons why physicians do not have discussions about poor prognosis, why it matters, and what can be improved. J Clin Oncol. 2012;30(22):2715–7.
11. Lin RJ, Elko TA, Perales MA, Alexander K, Jakubowski AA, Devlin SM, et al. End-of-life care for older AML patients relapsing after allogeneic stem cell transplant at a dedicated cancer center. Bone Marrow Transplant. 2019;54(5):700–6.
12. McCaughan D, Roman E, Smith AG, Garry AC, Johnson MJ, Patmore RD, et al. Haematology nurses' perspectives of their patients' places of care and death: a UK qualitative interview study. Eur J Oncol Nurs. 2019;39:70–80.
13. McCaughan D, Roman E, Smith AG, Garry A, Johnson M, Patmore R, et al. Determinants of hospital death in haematological cancers: findings from a qualitative study. BMJ Support Palliat Care. 2018;8(1):78–86.
14. Back AL, Park ER, Greer JA, Jackson VA, Jacobsen JC, Gallagher ER, et al. Clinician roles in early integrated palliative care for patients with advanced cancer: a qualitative study. J Palliat Med. 2014;17(11):1244–8.
15. White N, Kupeli N, Vickerstaff V, Stone P. How accurate is the 'Surprise Question' at identifying patients at the end of life? A systematic review and meta-analysis. BMC Med. 2017;15(1):139.
16. Weissman DE, Meier DE. Identifying patients in need of a palliative care assessment in the hospital setting: a consensus report from the Center to Advance Palliative Care. J Palliat Med. 2011;14(1):17–23.
17. Gerlach C, Goebel S, Weber S, Weber M, Sleeman KE. Space for intuition—the 'Surprise'-question in haemato-oncology: qualitative analysis of experiences and perceptions of haemato-oncologists. Palliat Med. 2019;33(5):531–40.
18. Hudson KE, Wolf SP, Samsa GP, Kamal AH, Abernethy AP, LeBlanc TW. The surprise question and identification of palliative care needs among hospitalized patients with advanced hematologic or solid malignancies. J Palliat Med. 2018;21(6):789–95.
19. Temel JS, Greer JA, Muzikansky A, Gallagher ER, Admane S, Jackson VA, et al. Early palliative care for patients with metastatic non-small-cell lung cancer. N Engl J Med. 2010;363(8):733–42.
20. El-Jawahri A, Traeger L, Greer JA, VanDusen H, Fishman SR, LeBlanc TW, et al. Effect of inpatient palliative care during hematopoietic stem-cell transplant on psychological distress 6 months after transplant: results of a randomized clinical trial. J Clin Oncol. 2017;35(32):3714–21.
21. Mack JW, Cronin A, Keating NL, Taback N, Huskamp HA, Malin JL, et al. Associations between end-of-life discussion characteristics and care received near death: a prospective cohort study. J Clin Oncol. 2012;30(35):4387.
22. Mack JW, Cronin A, Taback N, Huskamp HA, Keating NL, Malin JL, et al. End-of-life care discussions among patients with advanced cancer: a cohort study. Ann Intern Med. 2012;156(3):204–10.
23. Wright AA, Zhang B, Ray A, Mack JW, Trice E, Balboni T, et al. Associations between end-of-life discussions, patient mental health, medical care near death, and caregiver bereavement adjustment. JAMA. 2008;300(14):1665–73.
24. Levy MH, Smith T, Alvarez-Perez A, Back A, Baker JN, Block S, et al. Palliative care, version 1.2014. J Natl Compr Canc Netw. 2014;12(10):1379–88.
25. Gilligan T, Coyle N, Frankel RM, Berry DL, Bohlke K, Epstein RM, et al. Patient-clinician communication: American Society of Clinical Oncology consensus guideline. Obstet Gynecol Surv. 2018;73(2):96–7.
26. Dans M, Smith T, Back A, Baker JN, Bauman JR, Beck AC, et al. NCCN guidelines insights: palliative care, version 2.2017. J Natl Compr Canc Netw. 2017;15(8):989–97.
27. Odejide OO, Cronin AM, Condron N, Earle CC, Wolfe J, Abel GA. Timeliness of end-of-life discussions for blood cancers: a national survey of hematologic oncologists. JAMA Intern Med. 2016;176(2):263–5.
28. Odejide OO, Uno H, Murillo A, Tulsky JA, Abel GA. Goals of care discussions for patients with blood cancers: association of person, place, and time with end-of-life care utilization. Cancer. 2020;126(3):515–22.
29. Odejide OO, Salas Coronado DY, Watts CD, Wright AA, Abel GA. End-of-life care for blood cancers: a series of focus groups with hematologic oncologists. J Oncol Pract. 2014;10(6):e396–403.
30. Freeman AT, Wood WA, Fox A, Hanson LC. Access to palliative care consultation and advance care planning for adults with high-risk leukemia. J Palliat Med. 2018;21(2):225–8.
31. Kirtane K, Downey L, Lee SJ, Curtis JR, Engelberg RA. Intensity of end-of-life Care for Patients with hematologic malignancies and the role of race/ethnicity. J Palliat Med. 2018;21(10):1466–71.
32. Temel JS, Shaw AT, Greer JA. Challenge of prognostic uncertainty in the modern era of cancer therapeutics. J Clin Oncol. 2016;34(30):3605–8.
33. Christakis NA, Smith JL, Parkes CM, Lamont EB. Extent and determinants of error in doctors' prognoses in terminally ill patients: prospective cohort study Commentary: why do doctors overestimate? Commentary: prognoses should be based on proved indices not intuition. BMJ. 2000;320(7233):469–73.
34. Hui D, Bansal S, Park M, Reddy A, Cortes J, Fossella F, et al. Differences in attitudes and beliefs toward end-of-life care between hematologic and solid tumor oncology specialists. Ann Oncol. 2015;26(7):1440–6.
35. Granek L, Mazzotta P, Tozer R, Krzyzanowska MK. Oncologists' protocol and coping strategies in dealing with patient loss. Death Stud. 2013;37(10):937–52.
36. Hui D, Didwaniya N, Vidal M, Shin SH, Chisholm G, Roquemore J, et al. Quality of end-of-life care in patients with hematologic malignancies: a retrospective cohort study. Cancer. 2014;120(10):1572–8.
37. Ho TH, Barbera L, Saskin R, Lu H, Neville BA, Earle CC. Trends in the aggressiveness of end-of-life cancer care in the universal health care system of Ontario. Canada J Clin Oncol. 2011;29(12):1587–91.
38. Tang ST, Wu S-C, Hung Y-N, Chen J-S, Huang E-W, Liu T-W. Determinants of aggressive end-of-life care for Taiwanese cancer decedents, 2001 to 2006. J Clin Oncol. 2009;27(27):4613–8.
39. Wang R, Zeidan AM, Halene S, Xu X, Davidoff AJ, Huntington SF, et al. Health care use by older adults with acute myeloid leukemia at the end of life. J Clin Oncol. 2017;35(30):3417–24.
40. LeBlanc TW. Palliative care and hematologic malignancies: old dog, new tricks? J Oncol Pract. 2014;10(6):e404–7.
41. Sexauer A, Cheng MJ, Knight L, Riley AW, King L, Smith TJ. Patterns of hospice use in patients dying from hematologic malignancies. J Palliat Med. 2014;17(2):195–9.
42. Odejide OO, Cronin AM, Earle CC, LaCasce AS, Abel GA. Hospice use among patients with lymphoma: impact of disease aggressiveness and curability. JNCI: Journal of the National Cancer Institute. 2016;108(1).
43. O'Connor NR, Hu R, Harris PS, Ache K, Casarett DJ. Hospice admissions for cancer in the final days of life: independent predictors and implications for quality measures. J Clin Oncol. 2014;32(28):3184.
44. Fletcher SA, Cronin AM, Zeidan AM, Odejide OO, Gore SD, Davidoff AJ, et al. Intensity of end-of-life care for patients with myelodysplastic syndromes: findings from a large national database. Cancer. 2016;122(8):1209–15.

45. Howell DA, Wang H-I, Smith AG, Howard MR, Patmore RD, Roman E. Place of death in haematological malignancy: variations by disease sub-type and time from diagnosis to death. BMC Palliat Care. 2013;12(1):42.
46. Mercadante S, Gregoretti C, Cortegiani A. Palliative care in intensive care units: why, where, what, who, when, how. BMC Anesthesiol. 2018;18(1):1–6.
47. Davidson JE, Aslakson RA, Long AC, Puntillo KA, Kross EK, Hart J, et al. Guidelines for family-centered care in the neonatal, pediatric, and adult ICU. Crit Care Med. 2017;45(1):103–28.
48. Davidson JE, Jones C, Bienvenu OJ. Family response to critical illness: Postintensive care syndrome–family. Crit Care Med. 2012;40(2):618–24.
49. Myburgh J, Abillama F, Chiumello D, Dobb G, Jacobe S, Kleinpell R, et al. End-of-life care in the intensive care unit: report from the task force of world Federation of Societies of intensive and critical care medicine. J Crit Care. 2016;34:125–30.
50. Downar J, Delaney JW, Hawryluck L, Kenny L. Guidelines for the withdrawal of life-sustaining measures. Intensive Care Med. 2016;42(6):1003–17.
51. Edwards JD, Voigt LP, Nelson JE. Ten key points about ICU palliative care. Intensive Care Med. 2017;43(1):83–5.
52. Hunt R, McCaul K. Coverage of cancer patients by hospice services, South Australia, 1990 to 1993. Aust N Z J Public Health. 1998;22(1):45–8.
53. Davison D, Johnston G, Reilly P, Stevenson M. Where do patients with cancer die in Belfast? Ir J Med Sci. 2001;170(1):18.
54. Lunney JR, Lynn J, Foley DJ, Lipson S, Guralnik JM. Patterns of functional decline at the end of life. JAMA. 2003;289(18):2387–92.
55. Lehman R. How long can I go on like this? Dying from cardiorespiratory disease. Br J Gen Pract. 2004;54(509):892–3.
56. Murray SA, Kendall M, Boyd K, Sheikh A. Illness trajectories and palliative care. BMJ. 2005;330(7498):1007–11.
57. LeBlanc TW, Egan PC, Olszewski AJ. Transfusion dependence, use of hospice services, and quality of end-of-life care in leukemia. Blood. 2018;132(7):717–26.
58. Odejide OO, Li L, Cronin AM, Murillo A, Richardson PG, Anderson KC, et al. Meaningful changes in end-of-life care among patients with myeloma. Haematologica. 2018;103(8):1380–9.
59. McCaughan D, Roman E, Smith AG, Garry AC, Johnson MJ, Patmore RD, et al. Perspectives of bereaved relatives of patients with haematological malignancies concerning preferred place of care and death: a qualitative study. Palliat Med. 2019;33(5):518–30.
60. Martinsson U, Lundström S. The use of blood transfusions and erythropoietin-stimulating agents in Swedish palliative care. Support Care Cancer. 2009;17(2):199–203.
61. To TH, LeBlanc TW, Eastman P, Neoh K, Agar MR, To LB, et al. The prospective evaluation of the net effect of red blood cell transfusions in routine provision of palliative care. J Palliat Med. 2017;20(10):1152–7.
62. Beaussant Y, Daguindau E, Chauchet A, Rochigneux P, Tournigand C, Aubry R, et al. Hospital end-of-life care in haematological malignancies. BMJ Support Palliat Care. 2018;8(3):314–24.
63. Hochman MJ, Yu Y, Wolf SP, Samsa GP, Kamal AH, LeBlanc TW. Comparing the Palliative Care Needs of Patients With Hematologic and Solid Malignancies. J Pain Symptom Manage. 2018;55(1):82–8.e1.
64. Zimmermann C, Yuen D, Mischitelle A, Minden MD, Brandwein JM, Schimmer A, et al. Symptom burden and supportive care in patients with acute leukemia. Leuk Res. 2013;37(7):731–6.
65. Manitta V, Zordan R, Cole-Sinclair M, Nandurkar H, Philip J. The symptom burden of patients with hematological malignancy: a cross-sectional observational study. J Pain Symptom Manage. 2011;42(3):432–42.
66. Kiely F, Cran A, Finnerty D, O'Brien T. Self-reported quality of life and symptom burden in ambulatory patients with multiple myeloma on disease-modifying treatment. Am J Hosp Palliat Care. 2017;34(7):671–6.
67. Obermeyer Z, Makar M, Abujaber S, Dominici F, Block S, Cutler DM. Association between the Medicare hospice benefit and health care utilization and costs for patients with poor-prognosis cancer. JAMA. 2014;312(18):1888–96.
68. Wright AA, Keating NL, Balboni TA, Matulonis UA, Block SD, Prigerson HG. Place of death: correlations with quality of life of patients with cancer and predictors of bereaved caregivers' mental health. J Clin Oncol. 2010;28(29):4457–64.
69. Kumar P, Wright AA, Hatfield LA, Temel JS, Keating NL. Family perspectives on hospice care experiences of patients with cancer. J Clin Oncol. 2017;35(4):432–9.
70. Delgado-Guay MO, Parsons HA, Li Z, Palmer LJ, Bruera E. Symptom distress, interventions, and outcomes of intensive care unit cancer patients referred to a palliative care consult team. Cancer. 2009;115(2):437–45.
71. Nelson JE, Meier DE, Oei EJ, Nierman DM, Senzel RS, Manfredi PL, et al. Self-reported symptom experience of critically ill cancer patients receiving intensive care. Crit Care Med. 2001;29(2):277–82.
72. McAdam JL, Dracup KA, White DB, Fontaine DK, Puntillo KA. Symptom experiences of family members of intensive care unit patients at high risk for dying. Crit Care Med. 2010;38(4):1078–85.
73. Bruera E, Kuehn N, Miller MJ, Selmser P, Macmillan K. The Edmonton Symptom Assessment System (ESAS): a simple method for the assessment of palliative care patients. J Palliat Care. 1991;7(2):6–9.
74. Richardson LA, Jones GW. A review of the reliability and validity of the Edmonton Symptom Assessment System. Curr Oncol. 2009;16(1):55.
75. Raja SN, Carr DB, Cohen M, Finnerup NB, Flor H, Gibson S, et al. The revised International Association for the Study of Pain definition of pain: concepts, challenges, and compromises. Pain. 2020;161(9):1976–82.
76. Dalal S, Tanco KC, Bruera E. State of art of managing pain in patients with cancer. Cancer J. 2013;19(5):379–89.
77. Barnes H, McDonald J, Smallwood N, Manser R. Opioids for the palliation of refractory breathlessness in adults with advanced disease and terminal illness. Cochrane Database Syst Rev. 2016;3
78. Society AT. Dyspnea: mechanisms, assessment, and management: a consensus statement. Am J Respir Crit Care Med. 1999;159:321–40.
79. Currow DC, Smith J, Davidson PM, Newton PJ, Agar MR, Abernethy AP. Do the trajectories of dyspnea differ in prevalence and intensity by diagnosis at the end of life? A consecutive cohort study. J Pain Symptom Manage. 2010;39(4):680–90.
80. Mularski RA, Heine CE, Osborne ML, Ganzini L, Curtis JR. Quality of dying in the ICU: ratings by family members. Chest. 2005;128(1):280–7.
81. Mahler DA, Mahler, Parshall, et al. Opioids for refractory dyspnea. Expert Rev Respir Med. 2013;7(2):123–35.
82. Jennings A, Davies A, Higgins J, Gibbs J, Broadley K. A systematic review of the use of opioids in the management of dyspnoea. Thorax. 2002;57(11):939–44.
83. Currow DC, McDonald C, Oaten S, Kenny B, Allcroft P, Frith P, et al. Once-daily opioids for chronic dyspnea: a dose increment and pharmacovigilance study. J Pain Symptom Manage. 2011;42(3):388–99.
84. Puntillo K, Nelson JE, Weissman D, Curtis R, Weiss S, Frontera J, et al. Palliative care in the ICU: relief of pain, dyspnea, and thirst—a report from the IPAL-ICU Advisory Board. Intensive Care Med. 2014;40(2):235–48.

85. Simon ST, Higginson IJ, Booth S, Harding R, Bausewein C. Benzodiazepines for the relief of breathlessness in advanced malignant and non-malignant diseases in adults. Cochrane Database Syst Rev. 2010;1
86. Lossignol D. A little help from steroids in oncology. J Transl Intern Med. 2016;4(1):52–4.
87. Pisani L, Hill NS, Pacilli AMG, Polastri M, Nava S. Management of dyspnea in the terminally ill. Chest. 2018;154(4):925–34.
88. Wilcock A, Walton A, Manderson C, Feathers L, El Khoury B, Lewis M, et al. Randomised, placebo controlled trial of nebulised furosemide for breathlessness in patients with cancer. Thorax. 2008;63(10):872–5.
89. Hui D, Morgado M, Chisholm G, Withers L, Nguyen Q, Finch C, et al. High-flow oxygen and bilevel positive airway pressure for persistent dyspnea in patients with advanced cancer: a phase II randomized trial. J Pain Symptom Manage. 2013;46(4):463–73.
90. Schwartzstein RM, Lahive K, Pope A, Weinberger SE, Weiss JW. Cold facial stimulation reduces breathlessness induced in normal subjects. Am Rev Respir Dis. 2012;136(1):58–61.
91. Lai W-S, Chao C-SC, Yang W-P, Chen C-H. Efficacy of guided imagery with theta music for advanced cancer patients with dyspnea: a pilot study. Biol Res Nurs. 2010;12(2):188–97.
92. Huang ET-Y, Di PhD YM. Acupuncture therapies for chronic obstructive pulmonary disease: a systematic review of randomized, controlled trials. Altern Ther Health Med. 2014;20(6):10.
93. Association ED. The DSM-5 criteria, level of arousal and delirium diagnosis: inclusiveness is safer. BMC Med. 2014;12(1):141.
94. de la Cruz M, Noguera A, San Miguel-Arregui MT, Williams J, Chisholm G, Bruera E. Delirium, agitation, and symptom distress within the final seven days of life among cancer patients receiving hospice care. Palliat Support Care. 2015;13(2):211–6.
95. Casarett DJ, Inouye SK. Diagnosis and management of delirium near the end of life. Ann Intern Med. 2001;135(1):32–40.
96. Alici-Evcimen Y, Breitbart W. An update on the use of antipsychotics in the treatment of delirium. Palliat Support Care. 2008;6(2):177.
97. Meagher DJ, O'Hanlon D, O'Mahony E, Casey PR, Trzepacz PT. Relationship between symptoms and motoric subtype of delirium. J Neuropsychiatry Clin Neurosci. 2000;12(1):51–6.
98. Meagher D. Motor subtypes of delirium: past, present and future. Int Rev Psychiatry. 2009;21(1):59–73.
99. de la Cruz M, Fan J, Yennu S, Tanco K, Shin S, Wu J, et al. The frequency of missed delirium in patients referred to palliative care in a comprehensive cancer center. Support Care Cancer. 2015;23(8):2427–33.
100. Breitbart W, Rosenfeld B, Roth A, Smith MJ, Cohen K, Passik S. The memorial delirium assessment scale. J Pain Symptom Manage. 1997;13(3):128–37.
101. Adamis D, Slor CJ, Leonard M, Witlox J, de Jonghe JF, Macdonald AJ, et al. Reliability of delirium rating scale (DRS) and delirium rating scale-revised-98 (DRS-R98) using variance-based multivariate modelling. J Psychiatr Res. 2013;47(7):966–71.
102. Trzepacz PT, Baker RW, Greenhouse J. A symptom rating scale for delirium. Psychiatry Res. 1988;23(1):89–97.
103. Slooter A, Van De Leur R, Zaal I. Delirium in critically ill patients. Handbook of clinical neurology. 141. Elsevier; 2017. p. 449–66.
104. Hui D, Frisbee-Hume S, Wilson A, Dibaj SS, Nguyen T, De La Cruz M, et al. Effect of lorazepam with haloperidol vs haloperidol alone on agitated delirium in patients with advanced cancer receiving palliative care: a randomized clinical trial. JAMA. 2017;318(11):1047–56.
105. Hofherr ML, Abrahm JL, Rickerson E. Dexmedetomidine: a novel strategy for patients with intractable pain, opioid-induced hyperalgesia, or delirium at the end of life. J Palliat Med. 2020;23(11):1515–7.
106. Siddiqi N, Harrison JK, Clegg A, Teale EA, Young J, Taylor J, et al. Interventions for preventing delirium in hospitalised non-ICU patients. Cochrane Database Syst Rev. 2016;3
107. Bannon L, McGaughey J, Clarke M, McAuley DF, Blackwood B. Impact of non-pharmacological interventions on prevention and treatment of delirium in critically ill patients: protocol for a systematic review of quantitative and qualitative research. Syst Rev. 2016;5(1):1–9.
108. Hshieh TT, Yue J, Oh E, Puelle M, Dowal S, Travison T, et al. Effectiveness of multicomponent nonpharmacological delirium interventions: a meta-analysis. JAMA Intern Med. 2015;175(4):512–20.
109. Cherny N. The use of sedation to relieve cancer patients' suffering at the end of life: addressing critical issues. Oxford University Press; 2009.
110. Cherny NI, Radbruch L. Care BotEAfP. European Association for Palliative Care (EAPC) recommended framework for the use of sedation in palliative care. Palliat Med. 2009;23(7):581–93.
111. Quill TE, Byock IR. Responding to intractable terminal suffering: the role of terminal sedation and voluntary refusal of food and fluids. Ann Intern Med. 2000;132(5):408–14.
112. Quill TE, Lo B, Brock DW, Meisel A. Last-resort options for palliative sedation. American College of Physicians; 2009.
113. Cherny NI, Portenoy RK. Sedation in the management of refractory symptoms: guidelines for evaluation and treatment. J Palliat Care. 1994;10(2):31–8.
114. Rousseau P. Palliative sedation in the management of refractory symptoms. J Support Oncol. 2004;2(2):181.
115. Lo B, Rubenfeld G. Palliative sedation in dying patients: "we turn to it when everything else hasn't worked". JAMA. 2005;294(14):1810–6.
116. Gamblin V, Berry V, Tresch-Bruneel E, Reich M, Da Silva A, Villet S, et al. Midazolam sedation in palliative medicine: retrospective study in a French center for cancer control. BMC Palliat Care. 2020;19(1):1–10.
117. Bruera E. Palliative sedation: when and how? American Society of Clinical Oncology; 2012.
118. Anghelescu DL, Hamilton H, Faughnan LG, Johnson L-M, Baker JN. Pediatric palliative sedation therapy with propofol: recommendations based on experience in children with terminal cancer. J Palliat Med. 2012;15(10):1082–90.
119. Johnson L-M, Frader J, Wolfe J, Baker JN, Anghelescu DL, Lantos JD. Palliative sedation with propofol for an adolescent with a DNR order. Pediatrics. 2017;140(2)
120. Miele E, Angela M, Cefalo MG, Del Bufalo F, De Pasquale MD, Annalisa S, et al. Propofol-based palliative sedation in terminally ill children with solid tumors: a case series. Medicine. 2019;98(21)
121. Fredheim OM, Skulberg IM, Magelssen M, Steine S. Clinical and ethical aspects of palliative sedation with propofol—a retrospective quantitative and qualitative study. Acta Anaesthesiol Scand. 2020;64(9):1319–26.
122. Gurschick L, Mayer DK, Hanson LC. Palliative sedation: an analysis of international guidelines and position statements. Am J Hosp Palliat Med. 2015;32(6):660–71.
123. Maltoni M, Scarpi E, Rosati M, Derni S, Fabbri L, Martini F, et al. Palliative sedation in end-of-life care and survival: a systematic review. J Clin Oncol. 2012;30(12):1378–83.
124. Monreal-Carrillo E, Allende-Pérez S, Hui D, García-Salamanca M-F, Bruera E, Verástegui E. Bispectral index monitoring in cancer patients undergoing palliative sedation: a preliminary report. Support Care Cancer. 2017;25(10):3143–9.
125. Puchalski C, Ferrell B, Virani R, Otis-Green S, Baird P, Bull J, et al. Improving the quality of spiritual care as a dimension of palliative care: the report of the Consensus Conference. J Palliat Med. 2009;12(10):885–904.

126. Silvestri GA, Knittig S, Zoller JS, Nietert PJ. Importance of faith on medical decisions regarding cancer care. J Clin Oncol. 2003;21(7):1379–82.
127. Thune-Boyle IC, Stygall JA, Keshtgar MR, Newman SP. Do religious/spiritual coping strategies affect illness adjustment in patients with cancer? A systematic review of the literature. Soc Sci Med. 2006;63(1):151–64.
128. Balboni T, Balboni M, Paulk ME, Phelps A, Wright A, Peteet J, et al. Support of cancer patients' spiritual needs and associations with medical care costs at the end of life. Cancer. 2011;117(23):5383–91.
129. Puchalski CM. Spirituality in the cancer trajectory. Ann Oncol. 2012;23(suppl_3):49–55.
130. Azhar A, Bruera E. Outcome measurement and complex physical, psychosocial and spiritual experiences of death and dying. Ann Palliat Med. 2018;7(Suppl 3):S231–S43.
131. Dev R, Coulson L, Del Fabbro E, Palla SL, Yennurajalingam S, Rhondali W, et al. A prospective study of family conferences: effects of patient presence on emotional expression and end-of-life discussions. J Pain Symptom Manage. 2013;46(4):536–45.
132. Shear MK. Complicated grief. N Engl J Med. 2015;372(2):153–60.
133. Shear MK, Ghesquiere A, Glickman K. Bereavement and complicated grief. Curr Psychiatry Rep. 2013;15(11):406.
134. Glick S. Withholding versus withdrawal of life support: is there an ethical difference? BMJ. 2011;342:d728.
135. Dickenson DL. Are medical ethicists out of touch? Practitioner attitudes in the US and UK towards decisions at the end of life. J Med Ethics. 2000;26(4):254–60.
136. Rebagliato M, Cuttini M, Broggin L, Berbik I, de Vonderweid U, Hansen G, et al. Neonatal end-of-life decision making: Physicians' attitudes and relationship with self-reported practices in 10 European countries. JAMA. 2000;284(19):2451–9.
137. Winter SM. Terminal nutrition: framing the debate for the withdrawal of nutritional support in terminally ill patients. Am J Med. 2000;109(9):723–6.
138. Bouvia v. Superior Court. Cal App 3d: Cal: Court of Appeal, 2nd Appellate Dist., 2nd Div.; 1986. p. 1127.
139. Cruzan v. Director, Mo. Dept. of Health. US: Supreme Court; 1990. p. 261.
140. American Medical Association. Decisions near the end of life. Council on Ethical and Judicial Affairs. JAMA. 1992;267(16):2229–33.
141. Turnbull J. The Hastings center guidelines for decisions on life-sustaining treatment and care near the end of life. Crit Care Med. 2014;42(1):e87.
142. Bruera S, Chisholm G, Dos Santos R, Crovador C, Bruera E, Hui D. Variations in vital signs in the last days of life in patients with advanced cancer. J Pain Symptom Manage. 2014;48(4):510–7.
143. Hui D, dos Santos R, Chisholm G, Bansal S, Silva TB, Kilgore K, et al. Clinical signs of impending death in cancer patients. Oncologist. 2014;19(6):681–7. https://doi.org/10.1634/theoncologist.2013-0457. Epub 2014 Apr 23.
144. Hui D, dos Santos R, Chisholm G, Bansal S, Souza Crovador C, Bruera E. Bedside clinical signs associated with impending death in patients with advanced cancer: preliminary findings of a prospective, longitudinal cohort study. Cancer. 2015;121(6):960–7.
145. Farinholt P, Park M, Guo Y, Bruera E, Hui D. A comparison of the accuracy of clinician prediction of survival versus the palliative prognostic index. J Pain Symptom Manage. 2018;55(3):792–7.
146. Wright AA, Keating NL, Ayanian JZ, Chrischilles EA, Kahn KL, Ritchie CS, et al. Family perspectives on aggressive cancer care near the end of life. JAMA. 2016;315(3):284–92.
147. Howell DA, Wang HI, Roman E, Smith AG, Patmore R, Johnson MJ, et al. Preferred and actual place of death in haematological malignancy. BMJ Support Palliat Care. 2017;7(2):150–7.
148. Dionne-Odom JN, Azuero A, Lyons KD, Hull JG, Tosteson T, Li Z, et al. Benefits of early versus delayed palliative care to informal family caregivers of patients with advanced cancer: outcomes from the ENABLE III randomized controlled trial. J Clin Oncol. 2015;33(13):1446.
149. Dionne-Odom JN, Azuero A, Lyons KD, Hull JG, Prescott AT, Tosteson T, et al. Family caregiver depressive symptom and grief outcomes from the ENABLE III randomized controlled trial. J Pain Symptom Manage. 2016;52(3):378–85.

# Bereavement in Hematologic Malignancies and Serious Blood Disorders

# 25

Sue E. Morris, Holly E. Barron, Kathleen A. Lee, Jennifer M. Snaman, and Sarah J. Tarquini

## Introduction

Bereavement, defined as the "objective situation of having lost someone significant" through death [1], is a complex, multidimensional process that involves the physical, psychological, sociological, and spiritual domains of the human experience [2]. Individual differences, both within and between cultures, highlight the importance of interventions tailored to meet the individual needs of the bereaved. Within a preventive model of care, identifying those individuals at risk of poor bereavement outcomes is an essential task for health professionals [3]. Interdisciplinary palliative care clinicians are well positioned to provide support and guidance to caregivers prior to and after a patient's death. How an individual copes following a significant death is influenced by a range of factors, including their personality style, the relationship they shared with the patient, the course of the illness, the nature of the death, and the cultural and social context in which bereavement is experienced [4, 5].

Within hematological malignancies and serious blood disorders, the duration of a patient's illness and often intensive treatment course, coupled with ongoing prognostic uncertainty and witnessing tremendous suffering, can greatly impact a caregiver's bereavement. Integrating interdisciplinary palliative care early in the disease trajectory is recommended to support patients and their families during treatment and improve bereavement outcomes. In this chapter, drawing upon the palliative care and bereavement literature, we provide an overview of the grief experience, focusing predominantly on the bereavement of caregivers of both adult and pediatric patients with hematological malignancies. The same principles, however, apply to supporting bereaved caregivers of patients with other serious blood disorders, such as sickle cell anemia and hemophilia. We provide guidelines on how clinicians can best support caregivers before a patient's death, in addition to psychological strategies that can be used either with bereaved individuals or as part of bereavement support group programs. Two case studies are included that highlight some of the themes identified throughout.

## Background

The death of a loved one, especially the death of a child, is believed to be the most powerful stressor in everyday life [6, 7]. While most individuals adapt to their loss over time without requiring professional intervention [8], bereaved individuals are at heightened risk of serious physical and mental health problems, including sleep disturbance, increased sub-

S. E. Morris (✉)
Division of Adult Psychosocial Oncology, Department of Psychosocial Oncology and Palliative Care, Dana-Farber Cancer Institute, Boston, MA, USA
e-mail: sue_morris@dfci.harvard.edu

H. E. Barron
Division of Social Work, Department of Psychosocial Oncology and Palliative Care, Dana-Farber Cancer Institute, Boston, MA, USA
e-mail: hollye_barron@dfci.harvard.edu

K. A. Lee
Section of Palliative Care, Division of General Medicine, Beth Israel Deaconess Medical Center, Boston, MA, USA
e-mail: klee17@bidmc.harvard.edu

J. M. Snaman
Pediatric Advanced Care Team, Department of Pediatric Oncology, Department of Psychosocial Oncology and Palliative Care, Dana-Farber Cancer Institute, Boston, MA, USA
e-mail: jennifer_snaman@dfci.harvard.edu

S. J. Tarquini
Division of Pediatric Psychosocial Oncology, Department of Psychosocial Oncology and Palliative Care, Dana-Farber Cancer Institute, Boston, MA, USA
e-mail: sarah_tarquini@dfci.harvard.edu



C. K. Ullrich, E. J. Roeland (eds.), *Palliative Care in Hematologic Malignancies and Serious Blood Disorders*,
https://doi.org/10.1007/978-3-031-38058-7_25

stance use, depression, and increased risk of suicide [5]. A recent meta-analysis reported that 2–3% of the general population and approximately 10% of bereaved individuals suffer from prolonged grief disorder (PGD) [9], with bereaved parents at even higher rates [10–12].

Distinguishing normal bereavement from complicated bereavement reactions has been the focus of considerable research over the past two decades [13–15]. Cultural norms of mourning can be hard to distinguish from individual responses, and different grief responses may be considered "normal" based on the type of loss. Current integrative models view grief as a process of constructing a meaning to life following a significant death, an event that changes one's life forever [4].

Given that approximately 2.8 million people die each year in the United States [16], and an estimated average of five people are impacted by each death [17], a significant number of individuals are likely to experience difficulty coping, requiring mental health intervention. From a public health perspective, these numbers have important implications regarding how our society cares for the bereaved and the types of support we provide both before and after a death.

## Palliative Care Model

Bereavement care is considered a core component of high-quality end-of-life (EOL) care by the hospice and palliative care movement [18, 19]. In the United States, the importance of providing specialized bereavement services to bereaved families as a preventive model of care is endorsed by the National Consensus Project for Quality Palliative Care [18] and the National Hospice and Palliative Care Organization [19]. In the pediatric setting, best practice guidelines for hospital-based bereavement care [20] and evidence-based psychological standards of care for children with cancer, including two standards about bereavement [21], have been published.

## Integration of Palliative Care Principles Throughout the Disease Course

The disease trajectory and disease-directed therapy, including its duration, the nature of the interventions, the symptoms experienced by the patient and witnessed by family members, all impact the bereavement experience of bereaved caregivers. Recent expert consensus practice guidelines from the American Society of Clinical Oncology recommend palliative care concurrent with oncological care for individuals with advanced cancer and/or high symptom burden [22]. Early interdisciplinary palliative care improves quality of life (QOL) and symptoms for patients with cancer, including from the time of diagnosis [23, 24]. Research also shows that the provision of palliative care and hospice services is associated with improved family reported quality end-of-life care [25] and better bereavement outcomes in both the adult [26–28] and pediatric populations [29].

Supporting the family is an integral part of the care model of palliative care, in which the treatment of the patient and the family's physical, psychological, social, and spiritual needs are integrated with treatments aimed at addressing the underlying disease. The establishment and maintenance of a trusting, therapeutic relationship between the clinician, the patient, and their caregiver is paramount to the delivery of high-quality care. Showing compassion, being receptive to the needs and concerns of the patient and their caregiver, and communicating in a way that conveys empathy, all positively impact the bereavement experience, as does receiving "honest facts" and "accurate information" about the end-of-life period and the dying process [29, 30].

Figure 25.1 outlines the palliative care model and shows how as a serious illness progresses, care that is focused on comfort, pain management, and decreasing other burdensome symptoms plays an increasingly larger role. Throughout the disease course, hope plays an important role. However, the specific hopes of the patient and family may shift over time from hopes for cure, life extension or a miracle, perhaps toward hope for comfort and meaning at the EOL and into bereavement. (Fig. 25.1).

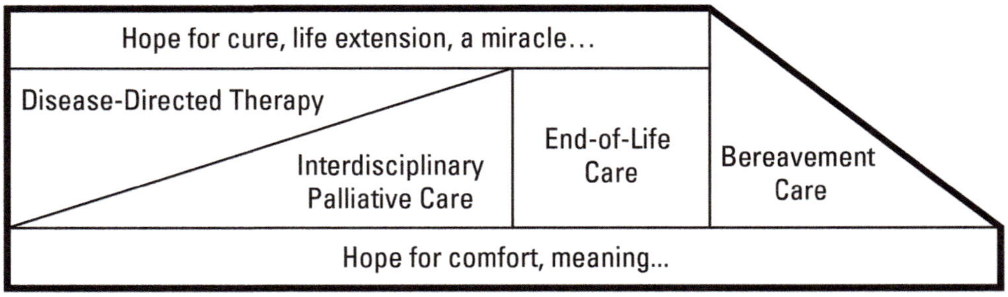


**Fig. 25.1** Palliative Care Model of Treatment. Liben, S., Papadatou, D., Wolfe, J. Paediatric palliative care: challenges and emerging ideas. Lancet 2008;371:852–64

## Disease Trajectory and Treatment

High stakes and tremendous uncertainty, balancing the risk of toxicity and death with a chance of cure, characterize the disease trajectory and treatment course for patients with hematological malignancies. For other serious blood disorders, such as sickle cell anemia and hemophilia, the disease trajectory typically involves ongoing treatments and planning for emergency situations, throughout the often-shortened lifespan [31, 32]. There has been increasing recognition of the chronic stress experienced by family caregivers associated with the burden of caregiving for patients with serious illness, particularly those with hematological malignancies [33–35]. (see Chap. 22) Caregiving tasks often involve assisting the individual in all aspects of their daily life, including administering medications, providing transportation, preparing meals, managing finances, advocating for health care, and providing ongoing emotional support [36]. Caring for children with serious illness brings its own set of challenges for parents depending on the age and developmental stage of the child and whether or not there are siblings whose lives are also greatly impacted by the diagnosis and course of treatment.

### Adult-Specific Treatment Considerations

Unlike the treatment of many solid cancers, the treatment of hematological malignancies often consists of intensive therapies, prolonged hospitalizations, and times of high infection risk and prognostic uncertainty [37]. Individuals with hematological malignancy often need to immediately start treatment shortly after diagnosis. Despite great advancements in the treatment of adult hematological malignancies and improved survival rates, the clinical course can vary significantly. For some, their condition responds to curative treatment attempts with long-term remission, and after a period of time, are considered cured. For others, their condition initially responds to therapy but later relapses at an unpredictable time. Additional treatment may result in remission for far fewer. Yet still, for other patients, their cancer is so advanced at the time of diagnosis that they experience a rapid clinical decline and death. In addition to the unpredictability of their disease response, intense hematological malignancy treatment modalities, such as hematopoietic cell transplantation (HCT) and chimeric antigen receptor T-cell therapy, may also cause toxicity, worsening a patient's existing symptom burden [38, 39] and neuropsychiatric outcomes [40].

Even though patients living with hematological malignancies have palliative care needs, especially high symptom burden [41], they are less likely to receive palliative care referrals compared to those with solid tumors [42, 43]. (see Chaps. 19 and 23) Unique barriers to palliative care involvement in hematological malignancy care exist, including in the pediatric setting [44]. Given the prognostic uncertainty related to the diagnosis of many hematological malignancies and the benefit of blood transfusions, patients are more likely to receive intensive measures (e.g., chemotherapy, hospital admissions, intensive care unit admissions, intubation and/or mechanical ventilation, and/or cardiopulmonary resuscitation) in the last 2–4 weeks of life [45] and are less likely to enroll in hospice at EOL or die at home [46–48]. Furthermore, many hematologic oncologists still view palliative care as EOL care [49].

Although caregivers of individuals with hematological malignancies experience significant stressors during their loved one's illness [33–36], which increases the risk of developing complicated grief reactions, there is currently a lack of studies focusing on the bereavement of family members of adult patients who die of hematological malignancies [50] and from other serious blood disorders.

### Adult-Specific Psychological Considerations

Within the adult population, family members and loved ones are tasked with taking on the role of caregiver for the individual, in addition to their existing roles of spouse, parent, employee, and so on. The caregiver responsibilities are dependent upon the patient's diagnosis and treatment plan. If transplant is part of the treatment plan, the caregiver may have to take a leave of absence from work, make alternative plans for childcare, and forego their own self-care practices to be able to care for the patient. Financial stress is also likely to compound existing stress within the family, especially if the caregiver needs to take unpaid leave or the patient is the primary provider.

While caregivers are usually encouraged to continue taking care of themselves during this period, many report that they can no longer prioritize themselves when caregiving. Even with significant planning, they often cite the unforeseen stressors and challenges that come with this role, including sleep deprivation, social isolation, depression, uncertainty, and guilt when doing something for themselves [51]. Caregivers can also experience anger and frustration about aspects of the patient's transplant recovery process that are beyond their control, often feeling as though there is something more they should be able to do. They might take ownership over the patient's recovery, assigning undue blame to themselves for what they see as short-comings in their ability to provide care if the patient's health declines. While the patient's well-being is assessed regularly throughout the transplant recovery process by their medical team, there is currently no standard approach to address emotional concerns of the caregiver [52].

Given the high level of caregiver distress throughout the disease trajectory, and while acknowledging the potential barriers to palliative care in hematological malignancy care, we recommend that interdisciplinary palliative care be introduced early to support both patients and their caregivers during treatment as well as improve bereavement outcomes. Anne B's story of her husband's diagnosis with lymphoma and his death 20 months later highlights the emotional roller coaster that caregivers endure during treatment. She describes how guidance from clinicians both during her husband's treatment and her bereavement, social support and having realistic expectations of progress, positively impacted her bereavement.

**Case Study: Anne B**

My husband was diagnosed with diffuse large b-cell lymphoma at age 54 and died 20 months later. When we got the diagnosis, we were very optimistic because it had a 90% cure rate. He underwent many treatments, each of which worked initially but then stopped before the treatment was complete. Eventually, he had an allogeneic stem cell transplant, which we thought would be the cure. When that failed, about 5 months before his death, we finally realized he might die from the cancer. During those final 5 months, he had treatments to jump-start the stem cell transplant and entered a clinical trial for CAR-T therapy.

The hardest things about the treatment course were (1) the emotional ups and downs, (2) the shifts between periods of being able to maintain a semblance of our previous life and periods when my husband was incapacitated or hospitalized unexpectedly, and (3) taking our kids along on the journey of the success and failure of each treatment. The cycle of success and failure takes an emotional toll. You'd think after a few such cycles we would have been more guarded in our optimism, but the mind does what it wants. We were two smart, realistic, analytic, data-driven people. Yet, we truly and wholeheartedly believed each treatment would be the one that cured him. When the statistical prognosis was on our side, we relied on that. When it wasn't, we relied on the fact that my husband was always in the minority statistical group, so wouldn't he be one of the few who were cured?

We were able to maintain life, as it was pre-cancer, during many of the treatments. But cancer is fickle. A treatment would fail and we would have to immediately shift into a different mode. On one occasion, my husband had an unexpected bad reaction to a treatment, and a routine visit to the hospital ended up in a Code Blue with a chaplain running into the room. Conversely, he had one course of treatment that required 3 days in the hospital every 2 weeks, but during those days he was allowed to leave to go to our son's basketball games or have dinner at home. The unexpectedness takes a toll.

It was extraordinarily hard to strike the balance between being open with our children about what was going on and causing unnecessary anxiety. Our boys were 15 and 18 when my husband was diagnosed. At those ages, they deserved to know the truth but not to bear the burden of the entire truth. We struggled with how much to sanitize each conversation. We didn't want to be unrealistically optimistic but also didn't want to cause undue alarm. As the 20 months progressed and each treatment failed, we also struggled with when to tell them about new developments. The most difficult conversations were the final 2, about 10 weeks apart. First, we had to tell them that the stem cell transplant—which we all viewed as the "cure"—had failed. Then, when it was apparent that our last hope, the CAR-T Therapy trial, did not work, we struggled with how to guide them through the final months of my husband's life: Should our college freshman come home? Should the boys spend as much time as possible with their dad, or try to retain a sense of normalcy by living their regular lives? How could we help them make choices they wouldn't regret or resent later?

We talked with a family therapist at the hospital as we prepared to tell our boys that he would die. She gave us advice that was infinitely helpful. When we asked what we should tell the boys about how to interact with their father in the final months, for example, whether they should stay at school or come home, she told us there was nothing they could do to avoid regrets. Whatever path they chose, they would have second thoughts. That was a freeing concept and we shared it with the boys: there's no "right" way to do this, so the best guide is what your gut tells you to do. That helped even as my husband lay unconscious in his final days. I told the boys they could sit with him and talk to him as much as they wanted, but if they didn't want to go into the room, that was okay too. And I truly believe both my sons feel comfortable about how they handled those final days, even though one talked to his dad at great length and the other decided not to see him.

The only "glitch" that happened near the end of my husband's life was with the timing of hospice. We couldn't have his "intake" until he was no longer receiving treatment. Although he was clearly dying, his doctors scheduled injections that could potentially minimally extend his life. I was unwilling to stop the injections solely to have the hospice intake. As a result, my husband was scheduled for intake 2–3 weeks in the future. In his final days, I spent way too much time on the phone to the hospice trying to move up the appointment, and crying to the Palliative Care doctor that I needed help speeding up the process. My greatest fear was that my husband would end up in the ER and die in a hospital against his wishes. Ultimately, after many days of pleading, his intake was moved up. In the end, his intake was 4 days before he died. We could have used help earlier.

In bereavement, by far the most helpful thing has been the Dana-Farber Bereavement Program. I'm not a "therapy" person, especially not group therapy. Nevertheless, I can't overestimate how helpful it was to be with a cohort of people who also lost partners to cancer, and to be guided through the process by an experienced professional. Before my husband died, I committed to myself that after he passed, I would "say yes to everything." I was terrified of turning inward and grieving in solitude. I accepted every invitation and every offer of help. Even now, almost 2 years later, I still say "yes" to a lot more than I really want to do. It keeps me busy and in contact with people who want to support me. I have a tendency to not ask for help. If I were sitting home alone, I'd probably never get it.

Sue Morris from the Bereavement Program gave me two pieces of advice that were extremely helpful. First, in the initial weeks, as I despaired about the future, Sue said, "Don't think about the long-term future. Take it day by day." That sounds simple, but at the time it was profound. My natural instinct is to look ahead; I'm a planner. I had to let go of that to get through the first year or so. Second, when I told Sue, many months in, that I still cried every day, she said, "Yes, but maybe you cry for a minute less." That made me realize my progress would be incremental and maybe even invisible day to day, but it was there.

Many of the "exercises" in the support group helped, but one stood out. The exercise asked us to articulate something about our greatest fears going forward. Then we were to consider those fears from other perspectives: If your friend told you she had those fears, what advice would you give? What would your partner say? That last question resonated with me. I could easily imagine what my husband would have told me. That helped and motivated me in ways nothing else had during my bereavement.

## Pediatric-Specific Treatment Considerations

Grief that results from the death of a child is intense and prolonged; bereaved parents noting that their grief may change over time but is never-ending [11, 53]. Many factors related to the child and their EOL experience affect parental grief and bereavement, including location of death, type, and severity of symptoms and associated distress at EOL [54]. Given the unique disease and treatment characteristics, and that pediatric patients with hematological malignancies are more likely to receive intensive end-of-life care [55], parents of children who die from hematological malignancies may require additional or targeted support in their bereavement. The same is true for parents whose children die from serious blood disorders considering the chronic nature of the disease and their long association with the team.

Acute lymphoblastic leukemia (ALL), the most common childhood cancer, has survival rates of greater than 90%; however, curative treatment may require years of intensive medical care and certain subtypes or other hematological malignancies continue to have high mortality [56]. Similar to adult patients with hematological malignancy, pediatric patients with high-risk or relapsed hematologic malignancies may be offered HCT as a curative option [57]. Despite significant advances in supportive care and transplant techniques, HCT remains an intensive and high-risk therapy, with an associated high level of suffering and risk of mortality [58]. Pediatric patients who undergo HCT are more likely to suffer greatly from their last therapy and die in the ICU, with less opportunity for end-of-life care planning, and hospice enrollment [58, 59].

Further, parents of children who received HCT report higher levels of depression, anxiety, and stress compared to parents of children who did not receive HCT, most likely because of the treatment intensity and high symptom burden. Similarly, parents whose children died in the hospital after receipt of HCT had a greater likelihood of meeting the criteria for PGD [60].

## Pediatric-Specific Psychological Considerations

Regarding pediatric best practices, strong recommendations have been made for early, integrated access to family-centered palliative care for children and adolescents diagnosed with hematological malignancies [24], and in other serious blood disorders, such as sickle cell anemia [31]. These recommendations specify that such services should be made available to the entire family system, however defined by the patient. The primary goals of these services are similar when provided in adult oncology settings, namely, to reduce symptom burden, ease suffering, and provide preventive bereavement care. However, when applied in pediatric settings, the following should be considered:

1. It is common for multiple individuals to be involved in and responsible for caregiving, including more than one guardian who shares medical decision-making rights. Having several individuals sharing the immense burden of medical care can be very helpful, and it can also add significant complexities. Navigating the delicate territory of end-of-life decision-making can be complex given that each individual brings their own coping style, strengths and vulnerabilities, communication preferences, and quality of relationship to the patient and to one another.
2. Adding to that complexity is the fact that communications must also be individualized to meet the dynamic

developmental needs and preferences of the pediatric patient, given that patients with hematological malignancies and other serious blood disorders may be in treatment for many years. Psychosocial and palliative care clinicians can assist families in providing developmentally appropriate information, continually assessing patient goals and preferences, and facilitating age-appropriate adjustment and coping.

3. Siblings of children with cancer have been identified as a high-risk group for psychosocial distress. It is strongly recommended that teams provide guidance, support, and resources to families so that they can appropriately meet the needs of siblings throughout the patient's disease trajectory [61]. In particular, siblings who have served as bone marrow donors may experience unique psychosocial vulnerabilities in the event of the recipient sibling's death, as they may worry that they somehow contributed to or are at "fault" in some way [62, 63]. With this in mind, a donor advocate should be identified by the medical team and made available to all minor sibling donors and their families, to provide an added layer of support throughout the treatment trajectory. A donor advocate can assist donor siblings and their caregivers in understanding both the significant contributions they make, as well as the limits of their role in medical treatment, with the goal of optimizing adjustment in the event of their sibling's death.

These considerations are highlighted in Jack S's case study. Here Jack describes his young daughter's diagnosis with acute myelogenous leukemia and treatment course, which included HCT with his son serving as the donor. In Jack's case, the way in which the grueling nature of treatment impacts coping is evident, and how continuing to speak about his daughter, finding ways to honor her memory, and being with other bereaved parents, helps him as he grieves.

**Case Study: Jack S**

My daughter Kaylee was diagnosed with Acute Myeloid Leukemia (AML) 2 weeks after her seventh birthday. Her treatment lasted 5 months. The standard treatment at the time was three rounds of chemotherapy. The doctors said that if her brother was a bone marrow match they would give her a bone marrow transplant. She went through her first round of chemotherapy and went into remission. During this time, her brother Liam was tested to see if he was a bone marrow match and he was. The plan was for her to receive another round of chemotherapy before the bone marrow transplant. She received her second round of chemotherapy and went into remission. Next was to prepare her for the transplant. She was transferred to the bone marrow unit and when the attending physician was checking her, he noticed that her liver felt enlarged so he held off on the preparation for bone marrow. A few days later, he noticed a little mole on her arm that wasn't there before and when it was biopsied, she had relapsed. Kaylee was transferred back to the oncology unit and received another round of chemotherapy and chemotherapy shots in her skin. She went into remission again and was transferred back to the bone marrow unit. Her preparation for bone marrow was 4 days of chemotherapy followed by 4 days of full body radiation. Her brother was prepared to be her bone marrow donor and we brought him in for surgery and the doctors took about 24 ounces of bone marrow from him and later that day he pushed the button and Kaylee received his bone marrow. About 22 days later, Kaylee engrafted and was targeted to go home in 2 weeks. During the following 2 weeks, she got sicker and sicker; her white blood cell count was up to 15,000. She was in a lot of pain and 1 day when the doctors where rounding on her, she said her arm hurt. The doctor noticed a swollen lymphoid in her right armpit. They biopsied it and the AML came back. She had absolutely no immune system. The doctors said they had never seen a patient relapse this soon. On April 23, 2011, we were told that she would not make it through the night and she passed away in our arms on April 24, 2011, and it was Easter Sunday.

Looking back, the hardest things about her treatment for me was constantly seeing her in pain—she was vomiting a lot. She had surgeries all the time, bone marrow aspirations and lumbar punctures. The worst morning was during her second round of chemotherapy. She woke up crying and I asked her what was wrong and she said that she didn't want to die. I consoled her with her primary nurse and we told her that she was not going to die. No child should ever have to think that.

Kaylee's team was the best—they always where upfront and straightforward with us. They covered everything from the best-case scenario to the worst-case scenario. They were very thorough. I have never seen a group of doctors and nurses so dedicated to their patients and families. After her funeral one of the biggest things that helped was a friend would come over every day for about 2 weeks to bring us coffee and get us out of bed. Once I got up, I found that I could go about my day. We have a golf tournament in her honor and donate the money to two great organizations that help children and families going through treatment. I am in therapy and that has help immensely. I have found that when I talk about her and her journey to doctors, nurses, or anybody, I feel better. Hopefully, I can help them understand what patients and families go though. There is also a bereavement cruise I go on every year and we have all lost children to cancer. It is a day of healing.

**Table 25.1** Considerations for family members before the patient's death [18, 21, 24, 30, 66, 68]

1. Provide and facilitate honest, developmentally appropriate communications with the patient and family members at the time of diagnosis and throughout the disease trajectory.
2. Following a patient's diagnosis, acknowledge and respond to the patient and caregiver's emotions, e.g., *I know this news is hard to hear.* Ongoing normalization and validation of emotions and experiences can be helpful. Acknowledge that emotional reactions and coping strategies are expected to vary for all family members.
3. Conduct an initial psychosocial assessment at the time of diagnosis, as well as distress screenings for the patient, caregivers, and siblings (especially sibling donors), at significant time points across the treatment trajectory. Provide or refer to supportive services, as indicated.
4. Provide the patient and family members with accurate, developmentally appropriate information about the disease trajectory and what to expect, especially at different time points, including at diagnosis, beginning treatment, following a recurrence and during the end-of-life period.
5. Recommend that caregivers and family members monitor and attend to their own physical and mental health needs. Encourage engagement in indicated medical services. Provide indicated emotional support via hospital-based services and/or provide indicated community-based referrals.
6. Involve palliative care early in the disease trajectory as part of usual care to offer an additional layer of support to both the patient and family system.
7. Offer patient, sibling, and caregiver support groups that create safe places for family members to share their experiences with others.
8. Offer hospital or clinic based supportive counseling with psychosocial clinicians with an expertise in psycho-oncology. Individual, couples, and/or family based sessions can be tailored to support the family in navigating all forms of distress associated with end-of-life care.
9. Facilitate conversations between the patient and family members as appropriate, involving psychosocial clinicians.
10. For family members with risk factors for difficult bereavement outcomes, refer them to a community mental health clinician for additional support prior to the patient's death. If indicated, coordinate a safety assessment at the time of the patient's death.
11. Continually assess the patient and family's hopes, goals, and medical care preferences. If discrepancies emerge, facilitate individual and family discussions, as needed. For families who wish to discharge from the hospital, make an early referral to hospice if possible, to maximize support for both the patient and the family.
12. Introduce the concept of memory making. For pediatric patients, if consistent with family values and culture, refer to a Child Life Specialist who can facilitate individual and/or family-centered memory making activities.
13. If discharged to home or hospice, continue to assess patient and family coping by phone and provide indicated emotional support, if possible.

## Consideration for Family Members before the patient's Death

As we have described, in hematological malignancies and serious blood disorders, there is often considerable caregiver distress throughout the disease trajectory associated with treatment and caregiving demands. Together, this distress can likely impact the bereavement outcomes of caregivers. Adopting a preventive model of care, Table 25.1 lists recommendations to support caregivers and family members before the death of an adult or child that can be adapted to the social and cultural context of the family as indicated. (Table 25.1).

## End-of-Life Care

When it has been determined that survival will not be possible, helping to prepare the family emotionally and physically for their loved one's death, is an essential role of the palliative care team. Psychosocial clinicians can play an integral part in preparing a family for what they might experience as the death of their loved one approaches [64]. While the phenomenon of family anticipatory grief is well accepted within serious illness and palliative care, it currently is not clearly defined in the literature [65, 66].

### Helping the Family Prepare for an Adult patient's Death

Given the prognostic uncertainty associated with hematologic malignancies, the transition toward a patient's end-of-life process can be sudden. In a national survey of hematologic oncologists, the majority of respondents reported discussing prognosis with most of their patients (>95%), preferring the use of general or qualitative terms [67]. Further, even though prognosis evolves during the hematological malignancy trajectory, nearly one in five hematologic specialists reported never readdressing prognosis or only doing so near death, which potentially increases the risk for the development of difficult grief reactions for caregivers. These findings suggest the need for structured interventions to improve prognostic communication for those with hematological malignancy [68], which also likely benefits the bereavement experience of family members [30].

Finding the balance of maintaining hope and holding uncertainty is a significant psychological stressor faced by both the patient and their caregiver throughout the patient's treatment. When the patient's disease relapses and there are no longer treatment options available, or treatment-related toxicity proves insurmountable, goals of care may shift. As part of the interdisciplinary team, the palliative care social worker (or other psychosocial clinician) typically works with the patient and their loved ones to help prepare for EOL, addressing whether or not final arrangements are in place, as well as identifying goals and what is most important to them [69]. Through empathic and reflective listening, emotional support, and counseling, the social worker can help the patient and caregiver explore the existential challenges they face. For the caregiver, many of whom have devoted what can feel like every part of themselves to caring for their loved one, they now might experience a range of emotions, including anger, sadness, fear, and loss of control. In our experience, caregivers frequently struggle to find meaning in what is happening to their loved one and are sometimes left with unanswerable questions. It can be helpful to have the social worker or palliative care chaplain engage with the caregiver around these existential issues and facilitate a conversation between the patient and caregiver, creating an environment that feels safe to do so. This important role helps to normalize and validate both the patient and caregiver experience and helps to bridge the feelings of isolation that anticipatory grief can foster.

In anticipating the patient's death, the social worker can also explore together with the patient and caregiver the types of memory-making activities that might be meaningful to them, for example, writing letters, creating art, recording videos, sharing meals, or visiting favorite places. Such activities can help create space for the patient and caregiver to discuss their hopes for now and for the future, acknowledging that hope might in fact be a good day spent sharing quality time together. These conversations often include painful yet important explorations around hopes and wishes the individual might have for their loved ones, permitting the caregiver to envision the possibility of what life might look like after the patient's death. When the patient is a parent of dependent children, the social worker often plays an integral role in helping them (and the caregiver) find appropriate language to talk with their children about anticipating their death, and ways in which they can remain connected to their parent after they have died. The social worker can also help the family access community bereavement resources, such as support group programs for bereaved spouses and children, including bereavement camps.

In situations where a person dies unexpectedly or in the ICU, both of which are risk factors for complicated bereavement outcomes (see Table 25.2), much of this work around meaning-making and legacy must be done during bereavement. While some conversations might have occurred before their loved one's death, bereaved individuals are encouraged to engage in activities to facilitate maintaining a connection with the deceased, such as journaling, creating memory photo albums, and reminiscing with others. Within a prevention model, it is essential for families to be given opportunities to speak with the team soon after an unexpected death to help them understand to the extent possible, the reasons that lead to their loved one's death. Some might benefit from individual professional support to help reframe or restructure their experience.

**Table 25.2** Risks factors for poor bereavement outcomes [2, 5, 11, 80–84]

| |
|---|
| **Bereaved Individual risk factors** |
| History of psychiatric disorders, e.g., depression, substance use |
| Female gender/mother |
| Poor social support |
| Concurrent stressors, including financial burden |
| Close or dependent relationship with the deceased |
| Previous losses |
| **Risks factors associated with the death** |
| Death of a child |
| Death of a spouse |
| Unexpected diagnosis |
| High initial distress |
| Sudden/traumatic death |
| Hospital-based death |
| Death in an intensive care unit (ICU) |
| Unable to find meaning in the death |

## Helping the Family Prepare for a Pediatric Patient's Death

The death of a child is commonly referred to as the "worst loss" a person can endure [70], describing something of the deep suffering parents experience after the death of a child. For parents or caregivers of seriously ill children, letting go of the goal for cure, and moving toward hope for a comfortable death, is an extremely challenging transition [64]. Helping parents and families, including siblings, prepare for a child's death is therefore a very important role of the palliative care team.

Conversations that address challenging decisions about different aspects of end-of-life care ideally should be held when it is understood that cure is no longer a possibility. Such decisions include resuscitation status, memory-making or legacy activities, desired location of death and funeral arrangements. Depending on the age of the child, they should be included in these discussions to the extent possible or desired, acknowledging that each family will have different preferences. Allowing children and adolescents to participate in these conversations and decision-making helps maintain their autonomy at a time when they have little control over their situation [71].

Memory-making activities prior to a child's death or immediately afterwards, can help families maintain a connection to the child. Typically provided by certified child life specialists, social workers, and chaplains, these activities include making hand tracings or prints of the child with different family members, taking individual and family photos, and recording videos. However, the decision by some children and parents to decline participating in such activities should be respected.

## The Psychological Impact of Treatment on Bereavement

There is no doubt that family caregivers experience great distress throughout the course of their loved one's illness that impacts their subsequent bereavement. Bereaved individuals often describe this experience as being on an emotional roller coaster, referring to the psychological toll that they have endured, characterized by distress, uncertainty, hope, feelings of helplessness, and bearing witness to great suffering. By the time the individual dies, caregivers are often exhausted both physically and emotionally, which makes the challenge of coping with significant loss even more difficult. In the next section, we discuss the nature of grief from a psychological perspective, including the risk factors for poor bereavement outcomes, and outline strategies that psychosocial clinicians can use to help the bereaved cope with the death of their loved one.

## The Nature of Grief

Grief is defined as the "anguish experienced after significant loss, usually the death of a significant loved one" [72], where attachment is central [73]. Grief is characterized not only by profound sadness but also by yearning or longing to be with that person again. Loss and change are two major components of grief that are important in understanding an individual's bereavement experience [74]. Following the death of a loved one, the bereaved individual loses many things in addition to the person themselves. These losses can include practical roles, such as the person who managed the finances or who organized the social calendar, to their hopes and dreams for the future. The grief associated with lost hopes and dreams is particularly relevant when a young child or adolescent dies and are important issues to explore in bereavement counseling. How much a person's life changes following a significant death tends to reflect how much their lives overlapped, such as an elderly couple who married at a young age or a parent of a young, dependent child. As such, the difficulty in adjusting to a death tends to reflect the amount of change an individual has to navigate, not the length of the relationship per se.

Given grieving involves adaptation to change and integrating the loss, the role of the psychosocial clinician is to help facilitate this adjustment so that the bereaved individual can continue to live their life with a sense of purpose, acknowledging that it may not be the life they originally planned. In addition to loss and change, the concept of control is also central, especially in bereavement following prolonged illness and arduous treatment regimens, where the bereaved typically have little control over the course of the illness and the circumstances surrounding the death. Part of bereavement care is therefore to help individuals regain a sense of control and restore balance in their lives.

## A Cognitive Perspective

A person's worldview, including how they think about life and death, also impacts their bereavement experience [4, 74]. Most people expect that parents will die before their children and that adults will live well into their later years. The death of a child at any age is a devastating life event that occurs "off-time" [75], challenging one's beliefs about the world and its natural order. Similarly, when someone dies suddenly or unexpectedly, even within the context of a cancer diagnosis, many of these basic assumptions about life are challenged, often resulting in a discrepancy between what they expected to happen in their life and what actually happened in reality [74]. Exploring these assumptions early in bereavement counseling can help individuals begin to make sense of their loss.

Expectations about the trajectory or outcome of treatment are also important to explore. It is not uncommon for bereaved individuals to express that their loved one's death was unexpected even though the patient was very sick. This is often because the caregiver thought the chances of cure were high or the patient had always "rallied" before. In these cases, it is helpful to conceptualize and name the bereavement experience as a "sudden or unexpected death within the context of a serious illness," creating space for the bereaved to grapple with what they expected and what actually happened. It also underscores the important role of palliative care clinicians in helping families balance hope and realism during treatment and to prepare psychologically for death, when all treatment options have been exhausted and the goals of care shift to end-of-life care.

Similarly, in the early months of bereavement, individual and societal expectations about progress also play a role [74]. Bereaved individuals often express comments such as "It's been three months and I thought I'd be better by now" or "It's been six months and it seems as though it is getting harder, not easier." These beliefs reflect western society's "fix-it" mentality and view that grief should be something an individual can "get over quickly" and return to "normal" in the much the same way that they would recover from a common cold. This view of grief is inaccurate—grief is not an illness with a prescribed cure, nor does it follow a linear pattern. Rather it is a highly individualized process, typically following a wave-like pattern that involves accommodation or adaptation to change following significant loss [74]. For many, especially bereaved parents, this adaptation to loss can take years [7].

## Acute Grief

In the initial weeks following a loved one's death, many bereaved caregivers describe a feeling of being on "automatic pilot," where they are just "going through the motions," preparing for services, attending to financial and administrative tasks as well as visiting with family and friends. Sleep and appetite disturbance and concentration difficulties are common, as are feelings of numbness, shock, and disbelief. In addition to profound sadness, the predominant emotion is that of intense yearning or pining for the deceased [74, 76].

Although there is no set timetable, many bereaved people often report feeling as though they are getting worse in the weeks after the death. This feeling tends to coincide with the lives of those around them returning to their normal routines coupled with society's expectation that the bereaved "should" be getting over the death. During this time, intense feelings of sadness, yearning, and anxiety about the future are common as the reality starts to take hold. Replaying the events of the deceased's last days, in an attempt to make sense of what happened, is also common. Unanswered questions, especially about treatment decisions, "what ifs?" and regret may arise, making this a particularly challenging time [74, 76]. Addressing these questions and regrets in bereavement counseling can help bereaved individuals reconcile in some way, their experience.

## The Wave-Like Pattern of Grief

Grief was popularly conceptualized as a stage model based on psychiatrist Elisabeth Kubler-Ross's work with dying patients [77]. Now grief is considered to be a highly individualized process without distinct stages where waves of intensified emotion or "pangs" of grief characterized by yearning are considered central [78]. Conceptualizing grief as coming in waves provides a useful cognitive framework to help the bereaved understand their experience [74]. Most people report that the intensity and frequency of the waves decrease over time even though there will always be "trigger waves" that result in an intensification of emotion and yearning (see Fig. 25.2). Triggers that set off these larger waves or "pangs" can include significant dates that can be anticipated, such as the deceased's birthday or a couple's wedding anniversary, to triggers that "come out of the blue," such as hearing a song on the radio or seeing an ad on television related to leukemia. Understanding that grief follows a wave-like pattern helps illustrate why people grieve in different ways. It is especially relevant in helping bereaved parents understand why their experiences might differ, even though they are grieving the same child. Anticipating potential difficult days and making a plan to deal with them helps the bereaved increase their sense of control. Discussing these plans in counseling, particularly for major "firsts," can be very beneficial [74, 76].

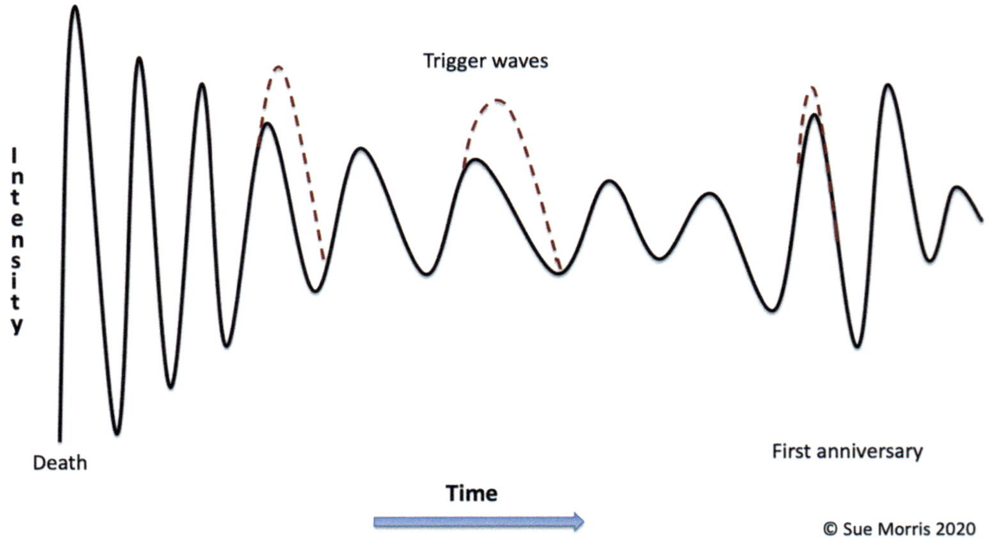


**Fig. 25.2** Wave-like pattern of grief. Courtesy of Sue E. Morris

## Dual Process Model

One current model developed to understand how bereaved individuals adjust to the death of a loved one is the Dual Process Model of coping with bereavement [79]. This model views normal grief as an oscillation between confronting the loss (loss orientation stressors) and avoiding or compartmentalizing it to allow the bereaved time to focus on changes in their life as a result of their loss (restoration orientation stressors). According to Stroebe and Schut [79], the key theoretical mechanism in healthy grieving is the confrontation-avoidance mechanism, in which a balance between the two needs to be achieved after a significant death. Yearning for the deceased or sorting through belongings are examples of loss orientation stressors and mastering new skills, such as paying the bills, is an example of a restoration orientation stressor.

Because caregivers often play a significant role in caring for a patient diagnosed with a hematological malignancy or other serious blood disorder, one important focus of bereavement support is helping the caregiver build a new or different life for themselves given their social connections have often dwindled over the course of treatment as the demands of caregiving increased. For parents of pediatric-aged children, their lives have typically been put on hold, especially if children are hospitalized for long periods of time. The same is true for spouses who have often been housebound as they care for partners with compromised immune systems. Bereavement support therefore needs to target helping the individual gradually reinvest in social activities, while also carving out time to grieve for their loved one, potentially including processing difficult memories of what they witnessed during the course of their loved one's illness.

## Risk Factors for Poor Bereavement Outcomes

A number of risk factors for poor bereavement outcomes, including PGD, have been identified in the literature and are listed in Table 25.2. Some risk factors are individual factors and others are death-related factors, with the implication being that some death-related risk factors are potentially modifiable [28, 53, 83]. An essential task of the palliative care team is to identify those factors that are potentially modifiable and intervene as possible. For those family members believed to be at risk of a poor bereavement outcome, it is recommended that psychosocial support be implemented prior to the death of the patient to help mitigate the risk. Given the high toll that caregivers of hematological patients experience, we recommend that psychosocial support be offered regularly to caregivers throughout the course of treatment, especially at times of increased stress.

## Diagnostic Formulations

Historically, there has been a lack of agreement in the literature about the diagnostic criteria describing the debilitating set of symptoms experienced by individuals who suffer from intense bereavement reactions. Complicated grief and PGD have often been used interchangeably, and Persistent Complex Bereavement Disorder, up until recently, was a condition of further study in DSM-5 (ICD.who.int, [78, 85–87]).

## Prolonged Grief Disorder

Currently, PGD is listed in ICD-11 as a disorder associated with stress (ICD.who.int) and was added as a new diagnostic category to the revised version of DSM-5 [78]. Both of these diagnostic categories describe a state of intense yearning for the deceased, considered to be an attachment figure. Persistent thoughts or memories, rumination, and an inability to accept the reality of the loss are common as is avoidance of situations that remind them of the loss, including withdrawing from family and friends [87]. The diagnosis of PGD should not be made until at least 6 months post-loss (ICD.who.int) and 12 months post-loss in DSM-5 [78]. Symptoms for each must cause significant impairment in social, occupational, or other important areas of functioning. Of note, for bereaved parents, the literature indicates that their grief experiences are more intense, lasting much longer than other types of loss and as such, clinicians should be cautious not to pathologize their grief reactions [7, 10–12, 88, 89].

## Bereavement Versus Depression

The diagnosis of major depression in a bereaved individual represents a clinical challenge [76]. While only a small percentage of recently bereaved individuals develop significant depression, prolonged morbidity is likely to occur [90]. Clinical indications of major depression following a significant death include generalized feelings of hopelessness, helplessness, worthlessness, guilt, lack of enjoyment and active suicidal thoughts, in addition to the symptoms of acute grief. Referral to a medical provider is recommended where treatment with antidepressants and psychotherapy specifically addressing the loss, represents a reasonable therapeutic approach [76].

## Caring for Bereaved Family Members

The literature describing the experience of family members caring for patients with hematological malignancies and other blood disorders offers clinicians important insights into avenues for improving care of family members both during the treatment phase and after a patient's death.

### Preventive Model of Care

Bereavement care is best conceptualized as a preventive model of care, where different types of support, including formal and informal support, are offered to individuals based on level of risk [3, 18, 91]. Even though the development of bereavement services has fallen behind that of other elements of palliative care, bereavement is considered a core element of hospice care where support is offered to families for 13 months following the patient's death [19]. Given that bereaved individuals are at heightened risk of physical and psychological problems [5], structured bereavement programs have the potential to benefit bereaved individuals by identifying those possibly at risk of a difficult bereavement, intervening early and providing bereavement outreach soon after their loved one's death [3, 92].

### Cultural Considerations

Bereavement is a universal experience that is heavily steeped in culture and traditions [76]. When caring for bereaved families, clinicians need to be aware not only of the role that culture plays in the bereavement experience of family caregivers, but also how culture influences their own responses to the grief of others. Being aware of one's biases and adopting a stance of curiosity is a helpful starting point for clinicians. Some general questions when caring for bereaved individuals from other countries or cultures include the following [76]:

- What is the cultural background of the bereaved?
- How is death and dying viewed in their particular culture?
- What terms are used to refer to death?
- How is grief expressed? Are there specific mourning rituals?
- Are their differences between men and women? How are children included in the grieving process?
- What is the role of the wider community?
- What support does the family want from the clinician or team?

### Team Condolences and Bereavement Outreach

Following a hospital death of a patient, the physician should immediately contact the family members not present at the death to notify them, express condolences, answer any initial questions and offer them the opportunity to view the body [76]. Bereavement care at this stage is primarily focused on attending to the family's basic needs, offering emotional support, and helping with arrangements. Child life specialists also play an important role in supporting bereaved siblings. For family caregivers who present with safety concerns, a safety assessment should be coordinated.

In the first weeks following the death, clinicians and teams ideally should send a letter of condolence, considered an important component of quality end-of-life care, found to positively impact a caregiver's bereavement experience [3, 30]. Incorporating writing condolence letters or sympathy cards into a clinician's routine practice not only benefits the family but can also help clinicians process their feelings about the patient's death. Table 25.3 lists guidelines for writing condolence letters or sympathy cards that can easily be adapted for condolence telephone calls. Making calls also provide an opportunity for the clinician to offer condolences, check in with the family to assess coping, and make recom-

**Table 25.3** Guidelines for offering condolences [74, 76]

| |
|---|
| 1. Use simple language and refer to the deceased and bereaved caregiver by name as you knew them. |
| 2. If you call, expect emotion and set aside adequate time so as not to feel rushed. |
| 3. Avoid euphemisms, such as 'passed away', unless indicated by the culture of the bereaved. |
| 4. Articulate how you have been affected or what you will miss about the patient. *For example, 'I was so sorry/saddened to hear of ___'s death last week'.* |
| 5. Mention something that reflects the patient's personality or the history you shared. If possible, include a personal memory of the deceased or share a story about how the patient touched your life. This is especially important following the death of a pediatric patient. *For example, 'I will always remember the way he lit up the room with his smile'.* |
| 6. Remember that for many bereaved family members, learning more about how their loved one touched other's lives, helps them as they grieve. |
| 7. If possible, emphasize the good job the family did in caring and supporting the patient. This can be especially helpful if they begin to doubt the care they provided their loved one. |
| 8. It's always better to send a card or make a condolence call late than not at all. If some time has elapsed since the patient's death, acknowledge the delay. *For example, 'I am sorry this card arrives late. I wanted to write to express my deepest sympathy', or 'I only learned last week of ____'s death—please accept my condolences'.* |
| 9. If possible, send a card from the medical team and encourage each clinician to include a personal reflection or memory. |

mendations for support as needed. If there are unanswered questions, many families benefit from the opportunity to meet with the team at a later date.

## Psychological Strategies to Help the Bereaved

Bereavement support following the death of a patient varies greatly by institution and service, depending on funding and available resources, as well as the clinician's discipline and experience [3]. Typically, bereavement support comes in different forms, including individual counseling, peer-led and clinician-led group support, and family bereavement programs and camps. A range of organizations and professionals offer bereavement support, including hospital-based palliative care programs, hospices, nonprofit community organizations, and faith-based groups, in addition to the informal care provided by funeral directors, primary care physicians, and other clinicians.

At our cancer center, we adopted an education, guidance, and support model for our bereavement program [3]. We provide psychoeducational information about the grieving process and the option for bereaved family members to return to the cancer center to attend individual counseling or group and seminar programs, free of charge. Within hematological malignancies and serious blood disorders, even if the patient was enrolled in hospice, it is not uncommon for bereaved family members to contact the team who cared for their loved one for bereavement support, especially in the initial months given their history and connection. Sometimes, families might want to visit to express their appreciation for the care their loved one received or meet with the oncologist and team to ask questions. This is especially true in the case of children. These visits can be very beneficial, particularly if bereaved caregivers are second-guessing their actions or have questions about their loved one's end-of-life period. Answering their questions, while acknowledging the extent of the caregiving role, can provide both reassurance and validation, which in turn, can positively impact their bereavement experience. These visits also provide an opportunity for the family to say "goodbye" to the institution as a whole and/or to acknowledge their changed relationship with the clinical team.

### Major Approaches

Within a public health model, Aoun et al. [91] propose a model of bereavement risk and support, which predicts that 30% of bereaved individuals have a "moderate risk" of developing complex grief issues and might benefit from group support, and a further 10% are at "high risk," possibly requiring mental health intervention. To date, research findings about the effectiveness of psychological interventions for normal and complicated grief responses are mixed varying according to the study design, sample composition, types of death and interventions targeted. Cognitive-behavior therapy (CBT) treatment approaches for complicated grief are encouraging [4, 87, 93], including internet-based therapist assisted interventions to prevent prolonged grief disorder [94] and manualized interventions targeting family dysfunction [95]. Meaning-centered grief therapy (MCGT), for example, is a therapeutic model for addressing challenges in finding meaning that shows promise, especially with bereaved parents [96]. It is a manualized, one-on-one cognitive-behavioral-existential intervention that uses psychoeducation and experiential exercises to explore themes related to meaning, identity, purpose, and legacy.

### Individual and Group Support

In general, the aims of bereavement support for recently bereaved individuals are:

1. To help the bereaved individual integrate the loss and adapt to life without the deceased
2. To help them maintain a connection with their loved one that is now based on memory and legacy [74, 76].

#### Bereavement Assessment

Depending on the service, the psychosocial clinician who provides bereavement support may or may not have previously met the bereaved caregiver during the patient's treatment. If meeting a bereaved caregiver for the first time, whether it is for individual counseling or screening for participation in a group program, routine issues to be addressed are described in Box 25.1.

**Box 25.1 Routine Issues in Bereavement Assessment [74, 76]**

1. The bereaved's story, including a brief description of the patient's illness from diagnosis to death, paying attention to the burden of caregiving, possible regrets and what they have witnessed
2. What they have lost with the death of their loved one, for example, hopes and dreams for the future, the roles the deceased played in their life, and their "job" as a caregiver
3. Family situation, including other family members who might be in need of support, such as children

4. Social, cultural, and religious/spiritual background
5. Support system, including friends, family, and mental health clinicians
6. Concurrent stressors, for example, financial concerns, unemployment, attending to administrative tasks
7. Previous losses and coping skills
8. Things left unsaid or unresolved with the deceased
9. Mental health history, including depression and substance use
10. Suicidal ideation
11. Goals for seeking support—individual counseling or group support

If the clinician is already known to the bereaved, acknowledging the transition in the therapeutic role is important. Similarly, if the clinician is handing over bereavement care to another clinician, a joint session can help facilitate this given that starting new with someone can be challenging. This can be especially beneficial in pediatrics given that parents often prefer to obtain bereavement support from members of the care team who knew their child [20].

### Support Groups

Shortly after the death of a loved one, many bereaved individuals express a desire to join a support group in an attempt to alleviate their emotional pain. While we don't hold to strict rules about group participation, some organizations suggest waiting 3 months. The reasoning behind this is that not only do participants have to share their own story, but also they have to listen to the stories of the other participants. If not managed appropriately by the group facilitator, this sharing may be overwhelming for others, especially if the participant recounts details of their loved one's final days. Often timing, however, for groups is determined by logistics, including scheduling and having enough participants. Our recommendation is to be flexible about timing given how isolating grief can be, and screen potential members for their readiness to attend a group either in person or by telephone.

We recommend that where possible, participants join groups that are facilitated by trained clinicians with other participants who have shared the same type of loss, in a similar time frame. For example, the groups we offer for adults at our cancer center are typically 6-session closed groups, based on CBT strategies [74]. Our two most common groups are for bereaved spouses or partners, and for adult children whose parents have died. For parents of pediatric aged children who have died at our center, we offer an 8-session closed group facilitated by palliative care social workers over the course of 16 weeks, in addition to drop-in groups and educational seminars [97, 98].

### Strategies

Strategies to help the bereaved based on CBT and self-help principles [74, 76, 99] can be grouped into the following eight categories as shown in Table 25.4 and adapted for individual or group work. When meeting with a bereaved family member for the first time, it is important to pay attention to the "rollercoaster" of the illness trajectory and how this experience impacted them. Individuals typically benefit from being able to tell the story of their loved one's illness and treatment course, including what they witnessed. In an initial meeting, hearing their story can take up the majority of the visit. Painful emotions, such as anger, regret, or guilt, can subsequently be addressed and lend themselves to CBT interventions, including challenging unhelpful thoughts that persist. Family members also benefit from meeting with the clinical team to answer lingering questions and to say "goodbye." Responding to emotion, normalizing their experience and emphasizing the good job they did in caring for their loved one, can also help them as they begin to reconcile their loss.

## Community-Based Bereavement Programs for Children and Adolescents

Specialized, age-appropriate support for bereaved children, adolescents and young adults bereaved by cancer is essential to help them adapt to their loss. When siblings or parents of young children die, children benefit from participating in grief support programs ideally within their own community where they can meet other children who have experienced similar losses and participate in legacy and memory-making activities. Usually, a parent or caregiver attends a group at the same time as the child, where they also have the opportunity to meet others in a similar situation.

For bereaved adolescents and young adults, research indicates that they experience significant distress often associated with witnessing the deteriorating health of a parent or sibling and have unmet psychological needs [100, 101]. Grief support groups offered through school or university counseling centers and other community-based organizations are one way to support bereaved adolescents and young adults with others their own age.

Bereavement family camp programs also provide developmentally appropriate opportunities for families to process the death of a child, sibling, or parent. Such camps provide creative and artistic activities for legacy and memory-making activities as well as model how to talk about the deceased and integrate their loss into their lives. Often children, ado-

**Table 25.4** Psychological strategies to help the bereaved based on cognitive behavior therapy and self-help principles [74, 76, 99]

| Category | Strategies |
|---|---|
| 1. Education and guidance about the nature of grief and expectations about progress | • Grief follows a wave-like pattern that usually eases over time<br>• Grief is a normal response to loss and involves adaptation to change<br>• Grief is unique—no two individuals will experience grief in the same way |
| 2. Opportunities to share the story of their loved one's illness and death, and their subsequent grief | • Counseling<br>• Attending a support group with other caregivers whose loved ones died from cancer<br>• Meeting with the clinical team to review certain aspects of care; express appreciation and/or say 'goodbye'<br>• Writing a journal<br>• Attending a memorial service at the hospital or hospice where their loved one died |
| 3. Regaining control | • Establishing a routine for weekdays and weekends, especially given weekends can be more difficult<br>• Writing a daily 'to-do' list, prioritizing what needs to be done and checking off one or two items each day<br>• Carving out 'grief time' |
| 4. Self-care | • Making an appointment with their primary care physician<br>• Scheduling overdue medical appointments<br>• Daily physical activity or exercise<br>• Re-engaging in hobbies or activities that were not possible during their loved one's illness |
| 5. Reinvesting in social connections | • Identifying friends or family who are empathic and who can provide the best support<br>• Accepting invitations even if they don't feel like it<br>• Being proactive about contacting others, especially given that contact with others has likely lessened because of high caregiving demands and long periods of isolation due to compromised immunity |
| 6. Navigating new or difficult situations and tackling barriers | • Graded exposure to situations that are difficult, avoided or new; developing a hierarchy beginning with the easiest first<br>• Decision-making framework<br>• Making a plan for dealing with 'firsts' e.g., birthdays and anniversaries |
| 7. Coping with painful memories, difficult emotions, and unhelpful thoughts | • Sharing or re-visiting painful memories in a contained way in counseling<br>• Journaling or letter writing, especially about things left unsaid<br>• Meeting with the clinical team to discuss lingering issues or unanswered questions<br>• Exploring difficult emotions in counseling e.g., regret, remorse, guilt, anger<br>• Challenging unhelpful thoughts, especially those leading to feelings of guilt or anger based on CBT: *What would your loved one say if they were here now? How would you advise a friend in the same situation?* |
| 8. Maintaining a connection with the deceased | • Creating new traditions related to special events such as birthdays, anniversaries and the Holidays, finding opportunities to reminisce<br>• Using online applications to make a photo book of their loved one and life together, which can facilitate remembering happier times before their loved one's diagnosis<br>• Legacy exercises—answering questions such as: *What did they learn from them? What values did they impart? What would their loved one want for them now? How would their loved one want to be remembered?*<br>• Supporting a cause in their loved one's memory that has meaning<br>• Opportunities for legacy and memory-making activities for young children |
| 9. Moving forward | • Creating a support system<br>• Seeking opportunities to try new things<br>• Setting goals for the next 6, 12 months<br>• Challenging unhelpful thoughts about moving forward |

lescents, and adults alike, form lasting friendships that exist beyond the camp setting, which helps to lessen the sense of isolation that bereaved individuals often experience.

## Conclusion

Family caregivers of patients with hematological malignancies and serious blood disorders typically endure high levels of prolonged stress associated with the length of their loved one's illness and the demanding course of treatment. Ongoing prognostic uncertainty and witnessing great suffering can both negatively impact their bereavement experience and are best addressed throughout the illness course and early in bereavement. Given that bereavement care is best conceptualized as a preventive model of care and that the provision of hospice and palliative care is associated with better bereavement outcomes, integrating interdisciplinary palliative care at the time of diagnosis is strongly recommended. Psychological services tailored to support caregivers during both the individual's illness and in bereavement are greatly needed. Structured hospital-wide bereavement programs, hospice bereavement programs and community-based family bereavement programs improve access to bereavement support and have the potential to identify those family members possibly at risk of a difficult bereavement, facilitating early intervention with a mental health clinician. Such programs also provide opportunities for bereaved caregivers and families to connect with others who have experienced a similar loss helping to lessen their sense of isolation.

**Acknowledgments** We would like to thank the many bereaved caregivers who have shared their experiences of loss with us over the years. We'd particularly like to thank Jack S. and Anne B. who kindly offered to share their stories for this chapter.

*Financial Disclosures:* Ms. Barron, Dr. Lee, Dr. Snaman, and Dr. Tarquini have no financial disclosures. Dr. Morris receives royalties for her self-help books, *Overcoming grief*, and *An Introduction to Coping with Grief*.

## References

1. Stroebe MS, Stroebe W, Hansson RO. Bereavement research and theory: an introduction to the handbook. In: Stroebe MS, Stroebe W, Hansson RO, editors. Handbook of bereavement: theory, research, and intervention. Cambridge: Cambridge University Press; 1999. p. 3–19.
2. Sanders CM. Risk factors in bereavement outcome. In: Stroebe MS, Stroebe W, Hansson RO, editors. Handbook of bereavement: theory, research, and intervention. Cambridge: Cambridge University Press; 1999. p. 255–67.
3. Morris SE, Block SD. Adding value to palliative care services: the development of an institutional bereavement program. J Palliat Med. 2015;18(11):915–22.
4. Malkinson R. Cognitive grief therapy: constructing a rational meaning to life following loss. New York: Norton; 2007.
5. Stroebe M, Schut H, Stroebe W. Health outcomes of bereavement. Lancet. 2007;370:1960–73.
6. Holmes TH, Rahe RH. The social readjustment rating scale. J Psychosom Res. 1967;1:213–8.
7. Rando TA. Parental loss of a child. Illinois: Research Press; 1986.
8. Prigerson H. Complicated grief: when the path of adjustment leads to a dead-end. Bereave Care. 2004;23:38–40.
9. Lundorff M, Holmgren H, Zachariae R, et al. Prevalence of prolonged grief disorder in adult bereavement: a systematic review and meta-analysis. J Affect Disord. 2017;212:138–49.
10. Goldstein RD, Lederman RI, Lichtenthal WG, et al. The grief of mothers after the sudden unexpected death of their infants. Pediatrics. 2018;141(5):e20173651.
11. Morris S, Fletcher K, Goldstein R. The grief of parents after the death of a young child. J Clin Psychol Med Settings. 2019;26(3):321–38.
12. Pohlkamp L, Kreicbergs U, Sveen J. Bereaved mothers' and fathers' prolonged grief and psychological health 1 to 5 years after loss—a nationwide study. Psycho-Oncology. 2019;28(7):1530–6.
13. Lichtenthal WG, Cruess DG, Prigerson HG. A case for establishing complicated grief as a distinct mental disorder in DSM-V. Clin Psychol Rev. 2004;24(6):637–62.
14. Maciejewski PK, Zhang B, Block SD, Prigerson HG. An empirical examination of the stage theory of grief. JAMA. 2007;297(7):716–23.
15. Prigerson HG, Horowitz MJ, Jacobs SC, et al. Prolonged grief disorder: psychometric validation of criteria proposed for DSM-5 and ICD-11. PLoS Med. 2009;6(8):e10000121.
16. Murphy SL, Xu JQ, Kochanek KD, Arias E. Mortality in the United States, 2017. NCHS Data Brief, no 328. Hyattsville, MD: National Center for Health Statistics. p. 2018.
17. Shear K, Frank E, Houck PR, Reynolds CF III. Treatment of complicated grief: A randomized controlled trial. JAMA. 2005;293:2601–8.
18. National Consensus Project for Quality Palliative Care. Clinical practice guidelines for quality palliative care. 4th ed. Richmond: National Coalition for Hospice and Palliative Care; 2018. https://www.nationalcoalitionhpc.org/ncp.
19. National Hospice and Palliative Care Organization. Guidelines for bereavement care in hospice. Alexandria: NHPCO; 2018.
20. Donovan LA, Wakefield CE, Russell V, Cohn RJ. Hospital-based bereavement services following the death of a child: a mixed study review. Palliat Med. 2015;29(3):193–210.
21. Wiener L, Kazak AE, Noll RB, et al. Standards for psychosocial care for children with cancer and their families: An introduction to this special issue. Pediatr Blood Cancer. 2015;62:S419–24.
22. Ferrell BR, Temel JS, Temin S, et al. Integration of palliative care into standard oncology care: American Society of Clinical Oncology clinical practice guideline update. J Clin Oncol. 2017;35:96–112.
23. Temel JS, Greer JA, Muzikansky A, et al. Early palliative care for patients with metastatic non-small-lung cancer. N Engl J Med. 2010;363(8):733–42.
24. Weaver MS, Heinze KE, Kelly KP, et al. Palliative care as a standard of care in pediatric oncology. Pediatr Blood Cancer. 2015;62(Suppl 5):S829–33.
25. Wachterman MW, Pilver C, Smith D, et al. Quality of end-of-life care provided to patients with different serious illnesses. JAMA Intern Med. 2016;176(8):1095–102.
26. Bradley EH, Prigerson H, Carlson MDA, et al. Depression among surviving caregivers: does length of hospice enrollment matter? Am J Psychiatry. 2004;161(12):2257–62.
27. Christakis NA, Iwashyna TJ. The health impact of health care on families: a matched cohort study of hospice use by decedents and morality outcomes in surviving, widowed spouses. Soc Sci Med. 2003;57:465–75.
28. Higgins PC, Garrido MM, Prigerson HG. Factors predicting bereaved caregiver perception of quality of care in the final week of life: implications for health care providers. J Palliat Med. 2015;18(10):849–57.
29. van der Geest IM, Darlington AS, Streng IC, et al. Parents' experiences of pediatric palliative care and the impact of long-term parent grief. J Pain Symptom Manag. 2014;47(6):1043–53.
30. Morris SE, Nayak MM, Block SD. Insights from bereaved family members about end-of-life care and bereavement. J Palliat Med. 2020; https://doi.org/10.1089/jpm.2019.0467.
31. Wilkie DJ, Johnson B, Mack AK, Labotka R, Molokie RE. Sickle cell disease: an opportunity for palliative care across the life span. Nurs Clin North Am. 2010;45(3):375–97.
32. Wiley RE, Khoury CP, Snihur AWK, et al. From the voices of people with haemophilia A and their caregivers: Challenges with current treatment, their impact on quality of life and desired improvements in future therapies. Haemophilia. 2019;25(3):433–40.
33. Beattie S, Lebel S. The experience of caregivers of hematological cancer patients undergoing a hematopoietic stem cell transplant: a comprehensive literature review. Psychooncology. 2011;20:1137–50.
34. Kumari R, Kohli A, Malhotra P, Grover S, Khadwal A. Burden of caregiving and its impact in the patients of acute lymphoblastic leukemia. Ind Psychiatry J. 2018;27(2):249–58.
35. Wulff-Burchfield EM, Jagasia M, Savani BN. Long-term follow-up of informal caregivers after Allo-SCT: a systematic review. Bone Marrow Transplant. 2013;48:469–73.
36. Bevans M, Sternberg EM. Caregiving burden, stress, and health effects among family caregivers of adult cancer patients. JAMA. 2012;307(4):398–403.

37. Fann JR, Levy M. Hematopoietic dyscrasias and stem cell transplantation. In: Holland JC, Breitbart WS, editors. Psychooncology. New York: Oxford University Press; 2017. p. 144–59.
38. Albrecht TA, Rosenzweig M. Management of cancer related distress in patients with a hematological malignancy. J Hosp Palliat Nurs. 2012;14:462–8.
39. Manitta V, Zordan R, Cole-Sinclair M, Nandurkar H, Philip J. The symptom burden of patients with hematological malignancy: a cross-sectional observational study. J Pain Symptom Manag. 2011;42:432–42.
40. Ruark J, Mullane E, Cleary N, et al. Patient-reported neuropsychiatric outcomes of long-term survivors after chimeric antigen receptor T cell therapy. Biol Blood Marrow Transplant. 2020;26(1):34–43.
41. Shaulov A, Rodin G, Popovic G, et al. Pain in patients with newly diagnosed or relapsed acute leukemia. Support Care Cancer. 2019;27(8):2757–97.
42. LeBlanc TW. In the sandbox: palliative care and hematologic malignancies. J Community Support Oncol. 2014;12:44–5.
43. Rao V. Billing palliative care services and end of life care in patients with hematologic malignancies. Abstract Presentation, Supportive Care in Oncology Symposium 2019.
44. Szymczak JE, Schall T, Hill DL, et al. Pediatric oncology providers' perceptions of a palliative care service: the influence of emotional esteem and emotional labor. J Pain Symptom Manag. 2018;55(5):1260–8.
45. Hui D, Didwaniya N, Vidal M, et al. Quality of end-of-life care in patients with hematologic malignancies: a retrospective cohort study. Cancer. 2014;120(10):1572–8.
46. Howell DA, Shellens R, Roman E, et al. Haematological malignancy: are patients appropriately referred for specialist palliative and hospice care? A systematic review and meta-analysis of published data. Palliat Med. 2011;25:630–41.
47. Odejide OO, Cronin AM, Earl CC, et al. Hospice use among patients with lymphoma: Impact of disease aggressiveness and curability. J Natl Cancer Inst. 2015;108(1):djv280.
48. McCaughan D, Roman E, Smith AG, et al. Palliative care specialists' perceptions concerning referral of haematology patients to their services: findings from a qualitative study. BMC Palliat Care. 2018;17(1):33.
49. El-Jawahri LBTW, Burns LJ, et al. What do transplant physicians think about palliative care? A national survey study. Cancer. 2018;124(23):4556–66.
50. Hoffmann R, Große J, Nagl M, et al. Internet-based grief therapy for bereaved individuals after loss due to Haematological cancer: study protocol of a randomized controlled trial. BMC Psychiatry. 2018;18(1):52.
51. Cooke L, Gemmill R, Kravits K, Grant M. Psychological consequences of hematopoietic stem cell transplant. Semin Oncol Nurs. 2009;25(2):139–50.
52. Bevans M, Wehrlen L, Prachenko O, et al. Distress screening in allogeneic hematopoietic stem cell (HSCT) caregivers and patients. Psychooncology. 2011;20(6):615–22.
53. Snaman JM, Kaye EC, Torres C, et al. Parental grief following the death of a child from cancer: the ongoing odyssey. Pediatr Blood Cancer. 2016;63(9):1594–602.
54. Aschenbrenner AP, Winters JM, Belknap RA. Integrative review: parent perspectives on care of their child at the end of life. J Pediatr Nurs. 2012;27:514–22.
55. Yotani N, Shinjo D, Kato M, Matsumoto K, Fushimi K, Kizawa Y. Current status of intensive end-of-life care in children with hematologic malignancy: a population-based study. BMC Palliat Care. 2021;20(1):82.
56. Pui CH. Childhood acute lymphoblastic leukemia: progress through collaboration. J Clin Oncol. 2015;33(27):2938–48.
57. Majhail NS, Farnia SH, Carpenter PA, et al. Indications for autologous and allogeneic hematopoietic cell transplantation: guidelines from the American Society for Blood and Marrow Transplantation. Biol Blood Marrow Transplant. 2015;21:11863–9.
58. Ullrich CK, Lehmann L, London WB, et al. End-of-life care patterns associated with pediatric palliative care among children who underwent hematopoietic stem cell transplant. Biol Blood Marrow Transplant. 2016;22:1049–55.
59. Brock KE, Steineck A, Twist CJ. Trends in end-of-life care in pediatric hematology, oncology, and stem cell transplant patients. Pediatr Blood Cancer. 2016;63:516–22.
60. Drew D, Goodenough B, Maurice L, Foreman T, Willis L. Parental grieving after a child dies from cancer: is stress from stem cell transplant a factor? Int J Palliat Nurs. 2005;11:266–73.
61. Gerhardt CA, Fairclough DL, Grossenbacher JC, et al. Peer relationships of bereaved siblings and comparison classmates after a child's death from cancer. J Pediatr Psychol. 2012;37(2):209–19.
62. Weaver MS, Diekema DS, Carr A, Triplett B. Matched marrow, sibling shadow: The epidemiology, experience, and ethics of sibling donors of stem cells. J Adolesc Young Adult Oncol. 2015;4(3):100–4.
63. American Academy of Pediatrics. Policy statement—children as hematopoietic stem cell donors. Pediatrics. 2010;125:392–404.
64. Lockwood B, Humphrey L. Supporting children and families at a child's end of life: Pediatric palliative care pearls of anticipatory guidance for families. Child Adolesc Psychiatr Clin N Am. 2018;27(4):527–37.
65. Coelho A, Barbosa A. Family anticipatory grief: An integrative literature review. Am J Hosp Palliat Care. 2017;Se34(8):774–85.
66. Coelho A, de Brito M, Barbosa A. Caregiver anticipatory grief: phenomenology, assessment and clinical interventions. Current Opin Support Palliat Care. 2018;12(1):52–7.
67. Habib AR, Cronin AM, Earle CC, et al. How do blood cancer doctors discuss prognosis? Findings from a national survey of hematologic oncologists. J Palliat Med. 2019;22(6):677–84.
68. Childers JW, Back AL, Tulsky JA, et al. REMAP: a framework for goals of care conversations. J Oncol Pract. 2017;13:e844–50.
69. Levine D, Baker J, Wolfe J, et al. Strange bedfellows no more: how integrated stem-cell transplantation and palliative care programs can together improve end-of-life care. J Oncol Pract. 2017;13(9):569–77.
70. Rosof BD. The worst loss. New York: Henry Holt; 1994.
71. Wicks L, Mitchell A. The adolescent cancer experience: loss of control and benefit finding. Eur J Cancer Care. 2010;19(6):778–85.
72. VandenBos GR. APA dictionary of psychology. Washington, D.C.: American Psychological Association; 2007.
73. Bowlby J. Attachment and loss. New York: Basic Books; 1980.
74. Morris SE. Overcoming grief: a self-help guide using cognitive behavioural techniques. London: Robinson; 2018.
75. Neugarten BL. Time, age and the life cycle. Am J Psychiatry. 1979;136(7):887–94.
76. Morris SE, Block SD. Grief and bereavement. In: Grassi L, Riba M, editors. Clinical psycho-oncology: An international perspective. Oxford: Wiley-Blackwell; 2012. p. 271–80.
77. Kübler-Ross E. On death and dying. New York: Macmillan; 1969.
78. American Psychiatric Association. Diagnostic and statistical manual of mental disorders. 5th ed. Arlington: American Psychiatric Publishing; 2013.
79. Stroebe M, Schut H. The dual process model of coping with bereavement: rationale and description. Death Stud. 1999;23(3):197–224.
80. Lobb EA, Kristjanson LJ, Aoun SM, et al. Predictors of complicated grief: a systematic review of empirical studies. Death Stud. 2010;34:673–98.

81. Kentish-Barnes N, Chaize M, Seegers V, et al. Complicated grief after death of a relative in the intensive care unit. Eur Respir J. 2015;45:1341–52.
82. Wright AA, Keating NL, Balboni TA, et al. Place of death: correlations with quality of life of patients with cancer and predictors of bereaved caregivers' mental health. J Clin Oncol. 2010;28:4457–64.
83. Goldstein RD, Petty CR, Morris SE, Human M, Odendaal H, Elliott A, Tobacco D, Angal J, Brink L, Kinney HC, Prigerson HG. PASS Network. Pre-loss personal factors and prolonged grief disorder in bereaved mothers. Psychol Med. 2019;49(14):2370–8. https://doi.org/10.1017/S0033291718003264.
84. Bogensperger J, Lueger-Schuster B. Losing a child: finding meaning in bereavement. Eur J Psychotraumatol. 2014;5:1. https://doi.org/10.3402/ejpt.v5.22910.
85. Boelen PA, Prigerson HG. The influence of symptoms of prolonged grief disorder, depression, and anxiety on quality of life among bereaved adults: a prospective study. Eur Arch Psy Clin N. 2007;257(8):444–52.
86. Maciejewski PK, Maercker A, Boelen PA, Prigerson HG. "Prolonged grief disorder" and "persistent complex bereavement disorder", but not "complicated grief", are one and the same diagnostic entity: an analysis of data from the Yale Bereavement Study. World Psychiatry. 2016;15(3):266–75.
87. Shear MK. Complicated grief. N Engl J Med. 2015;372(2):153–60.
88. Goodenough B, Drew D, Higgins S, Trethewie S. Bereavement outcomes for parents who lose a child to cancer: Are place of death and sex of parent associated with differences in psychological functioning? Psycho-Oncology. 2004;13(11):779–91.
89. Kreicbergs UC, Lannen P, Onelov E, Wolfe J. Parental grief after losing a child to cancer: Impact of professional and social support on long-term outcomes. J Clin Oncol. 2007;25(22):3307–12.
90. Zisook S, Shuchter SR. Uncomplicated bereavement. J Clin Psychiatry. 1993;54:365–72.
91. Aoun SM, Breen LJ, Howting DA, et al. Who needs bereavement support? A population based survey of bereavement risk and support need. PLoS One. 2015;10(3):e0121101.
92. Morris SE, Anderson CM, Tarquini SJ, et al. A standardized approach to bereavement risk-screening: a quality improvement project. J Psychosoc Oncol. 2019:1–12.
93. Shear MK, Reynolds CF, Simon NM, et al. Optimizing treatment of complicated grief: a randomized clinical trial. JAMA Psychiatry. 2016;73(7):685–94.
94. Litz BT, Schorr Y, Delaney E, et al. A randomized controlled trial of an internet-based therapist-assisted indicated preventive intervention for prolonged grief disorder. Behav Res Ther. 2014;61:23–34.
95. Kissane DW, Zaider TI, Li Y, et al. Randomized controlled trial of family therapy in advanced cancer continued into bereavement. J Clin Oncol. 2016;34(16):1921–7.
96. Lichtenthal WG, Catarozoli C, Masterson M, et al. An open trial of meaning-centered grief therapy: rationale and preliminary evaluation. Palliat Support Care. 2019;17(1):2–12.
97. Jonas D, Scanlon C, Rusch R, et al. Bereavement after a child's death. Child Adolesc Psychiatr Clin N Am. 2018;27(4):579–90.
98. Morris SE, Dole OR, Joselow M, et al. The development of a hospital-wide bereavement program: ensuring bereavement care for all families of pediatric patients. J Pediatr Health Care. 2017;31(1):88–95.
99. Kavanagh DJ. Towards a cognitive-behavioural intervention for adult grief reactions. Br J Psychiatry. 1990;157:373–83.
100. Patterson P, Rangganadhan A. Losing a parent to cancer: a preliminary investigation into the needs of adolescents and young adults. Palliat Support Care. 2010;8:255–65.
101. Patterson P, McDonald FEJ, Costa DSJ, et al. Initial validation of a needs instrument for young people bereaved by familial cancer. Support Care Cancer. 2020;28(8):3637–48.

# Index




C. K. Ullrich, E. J. Roeland (eds.), *Palliative Care in Hematologic Malignancies and Serious Blood Disorders*,
https://doi.org/10.1007/978-3-031-38058-7

**D**

**I**



**K**



**L**

GPSR Compliance

*The European Union's (EU) General Product Safety Regulation (GPSR) is a set of rules that requires consumer products to be safe and our obligations to ensure this.*

*If you have any concerns about our products, you can contact us on ProductSafety@springernature.com*

In case Publisher is established outside the EU, the EU authorized representative is:

Springer Nature Customer Service Center GmbH
Europaplatz 3
69115 Heidelberg, Germany

**Batch number: 10731667**

Printed by Printforce, the Netherlands